Learning to Consult

Edited by
Rodger Charlton
Associate Clinical Professor
The Medical School
University of Warwick

Forewords by

Professor Dame Carol Black

and

Roger Neighbour

Radcliffe Publishing
Oxford • Seattle

Radcliffe Publishing Ltd
18 Marcham Road
Abingdon
Oxon OX14 1AA
United Kingdom

www.radcliffe-oxford.com
Electronic catalogue and worldwide online ordering facility.

British Library Cataloguing in Publication Data

A catalogue record for this book is available from the British Library.

ISBN-10 1 85775 852 8
ISBN-13 978 185775 852 8

Typeset by Aarontype Ltd, Easton, Bristol
Printed and bound by TJI Digital, Padstow, Cornwall

Contents

Foreword

This is a captivating book. That, perhaps, is an unexpected remark from a doctor who trained rather long ago. It is captivating because it rings wonderfully true. It captures the very heart of what it means to be a doctor. There is no single feeling that adequately describes the limitless range of experiences contained in clinical consultation, the encounters that contain and reveal the very essence of medicine.

Without science there would be little understanding of the mechanisms of disease; there would be no modern medicine. Medical science and its translation into daily practice is a marvellously humane achievement: *Cum Scientia Caritas*. Yet, to many people, the dominant place of science seems to have displaced caring, kindness and compassion. I believe that may be true of some doctors, but not of most, in my experience, and certainly untrue of those teaching medicine today.

This book is about the humanity of medicine, not just the management of disease. Illness and loss of well-being may follow in the wake of disease. It is a challenge for medicine to help minimise those consequences. It is done through the partnerships that increasingly characterise medicine today. Partnership makes the traditional formal steps of history taking, investigation and diagnosis, and decisions about treatment and care, a shared enterprise. Done well they enhance the self-esteem, confidence, and dignity which minimise the loss of well-being, the loss that comes with illness.

That is why, for example, a chapter on treatment, even of common disorders, does not detract from the chief and, in my view, most valuable purpose of the book. The way the authors, teachers and mentors all, deal with the subject aligns it nicely with the central themes of communication, partnership and understanding.

This book reflects well the changed and changing environment in which we work today. It is one in which, increasingly we are required to account for what we do. The high public trust in our profession is tested daily; each clinical encounter may be the subject of scrutiny. This book is stuffed with good sense and sound tips – but more, it offers wise guidance for those setting out on their careers and gentle reminders for doctors in decline. Reflecting on its spirit and precepts, as individuals or as a profession, will help us warrant the high trust we are still given.

Professor Carol Black
Chairman of the Academy of Medical Royal Colleges
November 2006

Foreword

Not so many years ago, an orthopaedic surgeon friend of mine told me how he had mentioned to one of his colleagues that he was just on his way to meet me at the Royal College of General Practitioners. 'Oh,' said the colleague, sniffily raising an eyebrow, 'you're off to the college of cardigan-wearers, are you?'

I think – I hope – that the era of such intra-professional disdain is drawing to a close. If not, without condoning it, we might at least understand a point of view that thought GPs were specialists in not much more than niceness, lack of which never killed anybody. But if it is, and GPs are gradually coming to be appreciated for their ability to combine clinical competence with an expertise in complexity, uncertainty, communication and the doctor-patient relationship, it is in large measure thanks to the rigorous eclecticism of which this book is a fine example.

Its title, *Learning to Consult*, perhaps belies its comprehensiveness. There has in the past, perhaps, been a tendency to separate the process of the consultation from the clinical agenda in which it occurs and to whose success it is crucial. But what the reader will find in these pages is a compendium of diverse authors' views of how the principles of effective consulting impact on, and are affected by, all the many facets of clinical thinking. Its relevance is by no means confined to the aspiring general practitioner: even the most stereotypical hospital doctors consult, and both they and their patients will fare better if they can do it well!

If evidence were needed of how the best medical teams underpin the strengths of individuals with a culture of cooperation, this book from a network centred on Warwick Medical School would be Exhibit A. The contributors represent a wide range of disciplines, experience and career stages. Between them, they come at things from a variety of different angles, each shedding light on the other. From this approach (which we now have to call 'triangulation'), a clearer and broader view emerges of how the consultation process fits into the bigger picture of how good doctors 'do their medicine'.

So the reader will find not only a comprehensive account of the theory and practice of effective communication, but also how it supports such basic medical activities as history taking, examination, diagnosis, problem solving, referring, prescribing and so on. Moreover, these possibly mundane-sounding fundamentals are linked through the common denominator of the consultation to some of medicine's more arcane considerations, such as narrative, ethics and spirituality.

Yesterday's man that perhaps I am, it is rare that I find a new book on the consultation to be a genuine page-turner. But this one is and I thank Rodger Charlton and his colleagues enormously for it.

Roger Neighbour MA DSc FRCP FRACGP FRCGP
Past President, Royal College of General Practitioners
November 2006

Preface

This book has been written for trainees in medicine whether undergraduates or postgraduates. *Learning to Consult* is what it says it is. In order to be an effective doctor good consulting skills including good communication skills are required. This book comprises 15 chapters written by myself and a team of colleagues at Warwick Medical School and also colleagues in Birmingham, and finally edited by myself. The following areas are covered in relation to consulting:

- forming a working relationship and rapport with a patient
- taking a history
- undertaking a physical examination
- making a diagnosis as part of problem solving
- treating a patient as part of the management of their illness.

We are not the first to write in this area and I am sure we will not be the last. This is a subject which is pivotal in the training of doctors that is gaining increasing emphasis and so is an ongoing area of medical education research.

The book covers many other important areas in medical consulting including preventive medicine, keeping good medical records and how to write a prescription. Each chapter is accompanied by a bibliography should the reader wish to read more widely about a particular aspect of consulting. Practical summary points appear regularly and common terms used in consulting are defined.

Learning to consult and gaining the skills to become a 'good' doctor is a privilege and this is summarised by the medical educator and orthopaedic surgeon, Professor Lorin Stephens, who died in 1974:

To be a physician – to be permitted, to be invited by another human being into his life in the circumstances of that crucible which is illness – to be a trusted participant in the highest of dramas – for these privileges I am grateful beyond my ability to express ...[1]

I hope that this book will be a useful resource during undergraduate and postgraduate training.

Rodger Charlton
November 2006

Reference

1 Werner ER and Korsch BM. The vulnerability of the medical student: posthumous presentation of LL Stephens' ideas. *Pediatrics*. 1976; **57**: 321–8.

About the editor

Rodger Charlton qualified from Birmingham in 1983. During vocational training in Nottingham he completed an MPhil thesis in Medical Ethics. Shortly afterwards he became a GP principal in Derby in a five-doctor partnership and part-time Lecturer in General Practice at Nottingham University. In 1991–2, he was a visiting fellow at the Department of General Practice, University of Otago Medical School, New Zealand, researching into the perceived needs of undergraduates in palliative medicine education. This formed the basis of his MD thesis. He also worked as a GP in New Zealand gaining his MRNZCGP in 1992.

In 1994 he was appointed as a Senior Lecturer in primary healthcare at the Postgraduate School of Medicine, Keele University, and in 1995 he took over a single-handed general practice in Hampton-in-Arden, close to the Warwickshire border. In 1997 he became a GP trainer and in 1998 he became editor of the Royal College of General Practitioners' (RCGP) Members' Reference Book (MRB) for two years. He is now the editor of RCGP publications excluding the College Journal and *The New Generalist*.

His research interests and published papers are in palliative care and bereavement with a strong focus on research in education and professional development in primary care. In September 2000 he was appointed as Senior Lecturer in continuing professional development at Warwick University and in January 2003 he became the Director of GP Undergraduate Medical Education at Warwick Medical School and is now working as the Co-Director and an Associate Clinical Professor. He received the John Fry Award of the RCGP in April 2001 for being a GP who has 'promoted the discipline of general practice through research and publishing as a practising GP'.

In November 2003 he was awarded a fellowship of the Society of Medical Writers (SOMW) of which he became the chairman in April 2004 for a year. He maintains an interest in postgraduate education by being a GP tutor and a vocational training scheme course organiser and helping GPs move through the recent changes in relation to the Postgraduate Education Allowance (PGEA), personal development plans (PDPs) and appraisal. He has now become a GP Appraiser.

Rodger has been a GP principal for 18 years and during this time has acquired knowledge in the day-to-day running of a general practice. He has worked in a large group practice in Derby before spending five years as a solo practitioner until he went into partnership in September 2000 with Dr Ryan Prince. As well as being an academic GP he remains a practical 'hands-on' GP both in patient care and the running of a practice with his GP partner. Much of his time is spent helping undergraduates and postgraduates in training how to *Learn to Consult* and the aim of this book is to further this process.

About the contributors

Dr Abhijit Bhattacharyya MBBS (Calcutta, India 1986) MRCOG DFFP MRCGP is a full-time GP in North Solihull and a part-time lecturer at Warwick Medical School, Warwick University.

Dr Madhu Garala JP MBChB DRCOG MRCGP has been a single-handed GP principal in Coventry for 19 years. Madhu is a GP trainer and GP appraiser and was a previous GP tutor for Coventry. Madhu is a part-time lecturer at Warwick Medical School.

Dr Emma Hopgood MBChB MSc DRCOG MRCGP graduated from Birmingham University in 1997. She completed her GP training in Hereford before moving to South Warwickshire in order to pursue her interests in continuing medical education and portfolio learning. She helps to deliver the DISC and Clinical Methods course.

Martyn Hull MRCGP DCH DRCOG is a GP in Birmingham and a Lecturer Emeritus at Warwick Medical School, with an interest in communication skills and assessment. He also works as a GP with a specialist interest in substance misuse, and is Honorary Secretary of the Midland Faculty of the Royal College of General Practitioners.

Sqn Ldr Peter Lavallee MBBS is a lecturer in General Practice, Department of Primary Care and General Practice, Royal Centre for Defence Medicine, ICT Centre, Birmingham. Peter has many years' experience of developing and teaching general practice and the processes underpinning the consultation in particular.

Colonel Jonathan Leach MSc FRCGP is Director of General Practice Education at the Defence Postgraduate Deanery, ICT Centre, Birmingham. Jonathan has considerable experience of assessing and examining doctors and other health professionals both at national and international levels, some of which is in core general practice but also in his other main interest, which is pre-hospital care

Dr Catti Moss MBBS LRAM MA FRCGP is a GP in rural Northamptonshire. She became involved in general practice education, becoming a GP trainer in 1989, and local GP tutor from 1994 to 1996. She has been involved with the Royal College of General Practitioners since 1984, when she became the Northampton representative, and has worked for her local Faculty as treasurer, and education division member. From 1994 she has been a member of the Council of the RCGP, with a brief break: first as representative of the Thames Valley Faculty, and now as an independently elected member. She was a member of the Maternity Services and Sexual Health groups, and has been a member of the Rural Standing

Group of the RCGP since 1999. She was Medical Vice-Chair of the Patients' Liaison Group from 1995 until 1999. She was a part-time lecturer in general practice medical education at Warwick Medical School from 2000 to 2005 and is now an honorary clinical senior lecturer.

Dr William Murdoch MRCGP has spent two years receiving academic training at the University of Birmingham and is now a full-time GP in Handsworth, Birmingham. He was awarded a distinction in the MRCGP examination in 2003. He also works as a Primary Care Medical Educator for the West Midlands Postgraduate Medical Education Deanery.

Dr Teresa RB Pawlikowska BSc MBBS MRCP is a part-time general practitioner and a senior lecturer in primary care at Warwick Medical School and director of undergraduate GP medical education. She has been teaching consultation and communication skills to undergraduates and postgraduates in the UK and abroad for over a decade. Her research interests include the assessment of communication and patient enablement.

Dr Joanna Piercy MBChB MSc MRCP MRCGP is a part-time GP lecturer at Warwick Medical School with a responsibility for quality assurance of the clinical methods course and is a salaried GP in a rural practice in Shipston-on-Stour and also a GP non-principal appraiser. Prior to her appointment at Warwick, Jo was a clinical lecturer in communication skills at the University of Birmingham in the Department of Primary Care and General Practice.

Dr Ryan Prince MBChB MRCGP was born in Wales and studied medicine at Birmingham, qualifying in 1995. He became a GP principal in Hampton-in-Arden, Solihull, in 2000 and shortly afterwards was appointed as a lecturer in general practice at the Medical School, University of Warwick. He is also involved in postgraduate medical education as a GP tutor in Solihull and a vocational training scheme course organiser. He was awarded a merit in the MRCGP examination in 2003.

Dr Iram Sattar MBChB BSc (Hons) MRCGP qualified from Leicester University Medical School in the year 2000 during which time she gained an intercalated BSc. She went on to complete vocational training to become a general practitioner and in 2004 she gained her MRCGP. She has a keen interest in medical education and hopes to pursue this further.

Dr Sarah Shannon BSc (Hons) MBChB DCH DRCOG MRCGP DCP is a GP Principal in General Practice in Coleshill, Warwickshire, and a part-time lecturer at Warwick Medical School with responsibilities for the delivery of undergraduate teaching of communication skills and Clinical Methods course.

Dr Jag Sihota MBChB (Birmingham) MRCGP MEd is a full-time GP in Coventry north and part-time lecturer at Warwick Medical School, with an interest in assessment and evaluation. He also has a special interest in diabetes and post-graduate medical education.

Dr Gary Smith MB ChB BMedSci qualified in 2006. He has a BSc in genetics and was the first author on a peer-reviewed paper in a medical journal before he became a medical student.

Dr Ian Ward MBChB DRCOG MMed Ed graduated from Leeds University in 1980 and has completed a Master's in Medical Education at Warwick University. He went in to vocational training in Coventry where he became a principal in his present practice (Phoenix Family Care) in August 1985.

Miss Liz Winborn BA (Hons) Business Studies is an Administrative Officer at Warwick Medical School responsible for organising general practice placements during both Phase I and Phase II of the MBChB degree. She is involved in course development and working with students on the feedback and evaluation process.

List of abbreviations

ABC	Airway, Breathing and Circulation
ALSG	Advanced Life Support Group
ASCOT	Anglo-Scandinavian Cardiac Outcomes Trial
BASIC	British Association for Immediate Care
bd or bid	twice daily (*bis die*)
BLS	basic life support
BMA	British Medical Association
BMI	body mass index
BMJ	*British Medical Journal*
BNF	*British National Formulary*
BOCHS	Basic life support, Observation, remain Calm, History taking, Secondary survey
BP	blood pressure
BTS	British Thoracic Society
CBT	cognitive behavioural therapy
CD	controlled drug
CFS	chronic fatigue syndrome
CHD	coronary heart disease
CME	continuing medical education
COPD	chronic obstructive pulmonary disease
CPD	continuing professional development
CPR	cardiopulmonary resuscitation
DCH	Diploma in Child Health
DENs	Doctors' Educational Needs
DFFP	Diploma in Family Planning
DGM	Diploma in Geriatric Medicine
Dip Derm	Diploma in Dermatology
Dip IMC	Diploma in Immediate Care
Dip OccMed	Diploma in Occupational Medicine
DMD	Drug Misuse Database
DoH	Department of Health
DPA	Data Protection Act
DRCOG	Diploma of the Royal College of Obstetricians and Gynaecologists
DRCOphth	Diploma in Ophthalmology
DVT	deep vein thrombosis
EBM	evidence-based medicine
ECG	electrocardiogram
EURACT	European Academy of Teachers in General Practice
FOI	Freedom of Information (Act)
FOM	Faculty of Occupational Medicine
GMC	General Medical Council

GORD	gastro-oesophageal reflux disease
GP	general practitioner
GTN	glyceryl trinitrate
H	histamine
HbA1c	glycosylated haemoglobin
HBM	Health Belief Model
HIV	human immunodeficiency virus
IBS	irritable bowel syndrome
ICD	International Classification of Diseases
ICE	ideas, concerns and expectations
ICEE	ideas, concerns, effects and expectations
IM	intramuscular
IT	information technology
IV	intravenously
LAB	long-acting bronchodilator
LAP	Leicester Assessment Package
LFTs	liver function tests
LLL	lifelong learning
MCQ	multiple-choice question
MEQ	modified essay question
NAD	no abnormality detected
NCRS	National Care Record Service
NHS	National Health Service
NICE	National Institute for Health and Clinical Excellence
NLP	neuro-linguistic programming
NPfIT	National Programme for IT
NSF	National Service Framework
od	once daily (*omni die*)
OSCE	objective structured clinical examination
OTC	over the counter
PBL	problem-based learning
PCT	primary care trust
PDP	personal development plan
PEI	Patient Enablement Instrument
PLP	personal learning plan
po	orally, by mouth (*per os*)
PPAR-gamma	peroxisome proliferator-activated receptor gamma
PPDP	practice professional development plan
PPI	proton pump inhibitor
pr	rectally (*per rectum*)
prn	as required (*pro re nata*)
PSA	prostate specific antigen
PUNs	Patients' Unmet Needs
pv	vaginally (*per vaginum*)
qid or qds	four times daily (*quater in die*)
RAPRIOP	Reassurance, Advice, Prescription, Referral, Investigation, Observation, Prevention
RCGP	Royal College of General Practitioners
RCT	randomised controlled trial

RTA	road traffic accident
sc	subcutaneously
SDL	self-directed learning
SLS	selected list scheme
sos	if necessary (*si opus sif*)
SQITAS	Site, Quality, Intensity, Timing, Arrows, Symptoms
SSRI	serotonin specific reuptake inhibitor
stat	straight away (*statim*)
tid or tds	three times daily (*ter in die*)
VLE	virtual learning environment
WBL	work-based learning
WHO	World Health Organization

To all medical students and doctors in training that this text may be an aid to them as they care for patients during their career

Chapter 1

Communication skills

Dr Catti Moss

Catti Moss traditionally delivered the contents of this chapter as a lecture to the first-year medical students at Warwick Medical School in their induction week and so introduced them right at the start on the basics of the doctor–patient encounter, which we refer to as the consultation. The chapter also provides a useful revision for doctors at any stage in the training or career.

The desire to communicate with each other is a basic human drive and a social instinct in all human societies. We start to develop our communication skills at the age of four weeks, when the average human baby starts smiling. For most of us the development never stops, and we continue to become more sophisticated communicators throughout our lives.

This chapter is divided into the following sections.

- Essential communication skills.
- Good communication.
- The communication tasks.
- Practice and feedback.

Practical point
Throughout the book will be sections entitled **Practical point**, which will emphasise consultation issues and so alert readers to areas which can enhance communication and so performance and patient satisfaction.

Essential communication skills

So why do we want to talk about communication skills? Why include it in a book about consulting? Surely our instincts can be allowed to sort out any problems.

The sad fact is that not all of us are brilliant at communicating. We will see countless examples of poor communication every day. This is common even in a profession such as medicine, where talking and listening are fundamental to our art. However, the heartening fact is that communication skills can be learned.

Unfortunately, it will not be sufficient to read this book to become an instant successful communicator; you will need practice as well. However, this book will help you to get started, and show you ways to improve your performance.

Good communication

For doctors, the rewards of good communication can be immediate, and the costs of poor communication are potentially devastating.

We can sum them up as in Table 1.1.

Poor communication inevitably results in complaints for doctors.

Practical point

The last point is a very important one for practising doctors because a large proportion of successful complaints against doctors are caused by communication problems.

Complaints against doctors are a major cause of distress, and burnout. They cost the health service millions of pounds, and they cost many doctors their careers, and their emotional and psychological health.

So what is good communication?

It has three basic components.

Non-verbal communication:
- posture
- gestures
- expression.

Table 1.1 Outcomes of good and poor communication

Good communication – rewards	Poor communication – punishments
You know why the patient has come	You miss the real reasons for seeing the doctor
You can make a diagnosis	You miss important diagnoses
The patient understands your explanation	The patient fails to understand
The patient takes the treatment advised	Patients don't do what you advise
The patient likes you	The doctor receives complaints

Paralinguistic communication:
- voice quality
- tone
- pitch changes
- volume
- the noises we make, e.g. the hmms and ers.

Verbal communication:
- the words we use
- how words are used
- when words are used.

The effect that these components can have is quite remarkable. Ex Prime Minister, Lady Margaret Thatcher, was a very ambitious young politician, but her progress was hampered by an unfortunately shrill voice. When she went to a voice coach, and learned how to lower the pitch, and speak in a clear way, her career path was made much easier.

Doctors are fortunate that they don't in general have to make long speeches, and influence large numbers of people at once. Nevertheless, the wrong body language can have a large effect on the single person being interviewed during a consultation. Seeing an expert doctor talking to a patient, the skills seem so easy.

Practical point

When doctors get it right, the patients enjoy talking to them, and tell doctors about their problems in a way that can easily be understood. When any of the ingredients is wrong, the interview may go completely adrift.

Non-verbal communication

If you watch a good doctor talking to a patient, he or she will be demonstrating with their body that they are interested in what the patient is saying. They do this by positioning themselves the correct distance away from the patient:

- not too close (feels threatening)
- not too distant (feels uninterested)
- sitting slightly forward (shows interest)
- looking at the patient directly.

Their gaze will be directed at the face when the patient is talking, and their hands will be still while they are listening. When they start to talk they will transfer their gaze to the patient's shoulder, and they will emphasise their points by using gestures.

On videotape we can speed up a consultation and cut out the sound, and the complexity of the rules that we follow with our bodies can be shown very effectively.

Paralinguistic communication

The good listener will use lots of little almost meaningless noises, e.g. um, ah, etc., to punctuate what the other person is saying. This encourages the contribution of the speaker: in effect saying 'I'm listening'.

When talking to someone who is upset, the good communicator will lower the volume and pitch of their voice, with a calming and non-threatening effect.

Verbal communication

The words used by doctors in the consultation are extremely important. Just by saying one question in several different ways, we can discover how differently a patient will respond.

The communication tasks

Another way of looking at communication skills is to look at what doctors are trying to do, and then look at the best ways of doing it. In practice, this approach is easier to use in order to practise and improve. Rather than thinking about the exact position of one's head, and the way one's hands are moving, it is easier to think about the whole task, and the ways of achieving it.

The basic tasks that doctors set out to do in the consultation are:

- listening
- questioning
- reflection
- summarising
- empathising
- responding
- explaining.

Let us consider each of these in turn.

Listening

You will often hear people say of someone: 'He's a good listener'. This is always a positive comment. Being able to listen is a very valuable skill.

The first component is about **looking interested**. When we are really listening, we often sit slightly forward. We always look at the face of the person we are listening to, and may adopt their posture.

The next component is about **giving the person space to talk**. One of the most common things that inexperienced people do is to talk too much. Only one person can talk at a time, and you can't listen when you are talking. Allowing the patient to say what they want to without interrupting, and giving them time to think about what they say, is essential.

> A wise old owl sat in an oak,
> The more he heard, the less he spoke;
> The less he spoke, the more he heard;
> Why aren't we all like that wise old bird? (Anon)

Next comes the delicate business of **encouraging the patient to go on talking and so elaborate**. If you watch someone listening, you will notice that they make all sorts of little encouraging noises and movements. Nods, hmms and yesses are encouraging. The intonation is best if rising, and the interjections should be very brief. Very often experienced doctors use reflective techniques like just repeating one word that the patient has just said with a rising inflexion. In general, though, the golden rule is that the less you say, the more the patient will say.

Sometimes there are barriers that make it very difficult for the patient to talk about the things you want to know. Being able to break these barriers down often requires a great deal of skill. The first skill is in recognising when barriers exist. A feeling of discomfort in the interviewer often means that there is discomfort for the person being interviewed. Knowing how to empathise, and to share that discomfort, can help to break down barriers. Simply saying something like 'It's very difficult, isn't it?' can work well. **Sometimes just having the courage to stay silent and wait** is the best thing to do.

If you are going to be any good at listening, you must be really interested in what the patient is saying and so be sympathetic. This entails valuing the patient's contribution as equal to your own.

Practical point

It also means that you have to make the effort to cross over to the patient's world and try to see it from his or her point of view and so demonstrate **empathy**.

Questioning

A medical interview can sometimes degenerate into a spoken questionnaire. The doctor wants to know specific items, and if asked in the wrong way, the consultation can be no more productive than a series of computer generated yes/no answers. In contrast, the really skilled doctor seems to ask very few questions, and the patient tells him or her all the important pieces of information very quickly.

Questions can be divided into two categories: closed and open.

A **closed question** is one that can be answered by yes or no. It usually starts with a verb. Examples are:

'Have you had your bowels open today?'
'Are you married?'
'Is the pain sharp and burning?'

An **open question** cannot be answered by yes or no. It usually starts with a questioning word such as what, who, why, where, when or how. Examples are:

'When did you last have your bowels open?'
'Who lives at home with you?'
'What is the pain like?'

The main problem with closed questions is that if they are answered by yes or no, they give no new information other than that supplied by the question. Looking at the two sets of examples, you can see how much more information comes with the second version than the first.

Unfortunately for those in training, open questions may not come naturally at first, but rather come in the guise of ideas that they would like to confirm or deny. It is therefore quite difficult to stop oneself from using closed questions at first.

Experienced doctors often don't ask direct questions at all. They will use phrases like 'Tell me about ...'. Consider the 'tell me' versions below:

'Tell me about your bowels.'
'Tell me about your home.'
'Tell me about the pain.'

These will get even more information than the open questions, mainly because the words 'tell me' encourage the patient to give you a **narrative** of what has been happening to them, and reinforce the idea that you are listening.

Reflection

Repeating the last statement a patient makes will often encourage them to take the story up again and continue it from that point, if you say it with a rising inflection in your voice. For example:

'... I was woken last night by this awful pain in my back. It was sort of burning.'
' Burning ?' [Doctor]
'Yes, it shot through my back like an electric shock, sort of.'

Summarising

If you give a summary back to the patient with all the important points you have picked up, they will very often come back with the important detail that they had left out, and that you didn't know existed. Even if there is no missing information, this process helps both the doctor and the patient to formulate the problem, and start to understand it. For example:

'So you woke up at 4 am with a shooting pain that went from your lower back down the back of your leg, that lasted for about four seconds.' [Doctor]
'Well, it went right down into the top of my foot actually.'

Empathising

Picking up on the feeling that the patient has expressed will very often allow them to express things that they couldn't have otherwise said. Something very simple, like 'That must be very worrying', can release all sorts of important information. If you detect any powerful emotion in a patient, it is a useful practice to mention it, and find out more about it. For example:

'You seem very concerned . . .' [Doctor]
'Well, my neighbour's son had a headache like this yesterday, and he's in hospital with suspected meningitis.'

Responding

One of the big fears of inexperienced consulters is that they will 'waste time' on irrelevant details, and fail to achieve the important tasks of the consultation.

Experienced consulters are listening out for these details that do not seem to fit in with the main story. We call these details '**cues**'.

Practical point
Anything that the patient says that you don't understand, or that makes you unsure why they mentioned it, is a **cue**.

If you hear a cue, you will probably be unable to proceed effectively until you respond to it. You can either respond straight away, or come back to it later. Nearly always a cue is hiding important and relevant information that would be difficult to get hold of by asking routine questions.

The way to respond to a cue is to refer back to the word that you didn't understand, and ask about it. For example:

'I've got this sore throat that everyone's been having recently, and what with the assessment and everything I thought I'd better get it checked out.'
'You talked about an assessment . . . ?' [Doctor]
'Well, you see I've got an important assessment where I have to give a presentation with slides and everything, and there isn't a microphone . . . '

Explaining

This is probably the most difficult of the basic communication tasks. In order to explain something we must translate our own medical understanding of something into words and concepts that the patient will understand. In effect we want to take the patient's existing understanding, and move it towards our understanding to achieve a '**shared understanding**'.

Stating things clearly in simple language is obviously essential for this. We don't stand a chance of explaining something if the patient doesn't understand our explanation. We need to use words that he or she knows the meaning of, and express ideas that he or she can grasp.

However, a good explanation needs more than just clear language. It needs to start from the patient's existing understanding, and to take account of the patient's beliefs, e.g. asking the patient what they understand by the diagnosis you have given or the treatment you have recommended. This is why explaining comes last in our list. We cannot start on an explanation without having first completed the other communication tasks, and found out quite a bit about the patient and his or her world.

Practice and feedback

So how can we start becoming aware of our strengths and weaknesses, and improving our communication skills?

Practical point
Any skill has to be practised in order to improve it.

We could read all about playing the piano for years and years, and we still wouldn't be able to play. The way we improve our skills is by developing awareness of what we are doing, and how it is working. We can then choose to repeat things that have worked well, and try different solutions when things haven't worked well.

The difficult bit is to become aware of what we are doing. For most of us, we don't think about what we are saying, or the way we are saying it, or the position we adopt while talking. We do things so automatically that we are totally unaware of what we are doing. We need some help to become aware of ourselves.

The most effective way of improving self-awareness is to get feedback from someone else. Most communication skills work is done on a one-to-one basis or in small groups with a skilled teacher. If the feedback is positive, this reinforces our strengths. Similarly, suggestions of alternatives can be made where we have demonstrated weaknesses to help us improve.

Practical point
The most effective way of improving is to do something well, and work out why it went well, and then to practise.

This is because it is always easier to repeat something you have already done than something you have never done.

When things don't go well, it is important to translate the feeling that something is wrong into a positive suggestion that can then be tried out in the future. Instead of saying 'that was awful', try to work out what different thing you could have done or said that might have worked better. The more specifically you can formulate your suggestion, the easier it will be to try it out, and change for the better.

It is important that all doctors in training and those who are qualified become aware of their communication strengths and weaknesses, and aim to get better and adopt changes as appropriate. The use of video recording of consultations as a method to do this is discussed in Chapter 13.

Bibliography

This is a personal account of an experienced practitioner. However, there are many different **consultation models** that those in training can adopt and these are described in Chapter 12 with an extensive list of references at the end of the chapter for further reading.

At the end of most chapters is a reference list. These are general references and sources of further reading and, where appropriate, relevant websites. Where an author is quoted, any relevant publications will be cited in the text and will appear in the Bibliography at the end but not numbered in the text, with the exception of Chapters 7 and 12. In addition, details of some references are given in the text, e.g. well-known quotations.

Chapter 2

History taking

Dr Jag Sihota, Dr Sarah Shannon and Dr Abhijit Bhattacharyya

Jag Sihota has looked in depth at the taking of a medical history and breaking it down into its component parts. This is taken further in Chapter 5 in relation to problem solving and making a diagnosis. Sarah Shannon has looked at the vital area of ICE (or ideas, concerns and expectations) in history taking and Abhijit Bhattacharyya at the importance of the patient's story or illness narrative.

It has been said that the majority of diagnoses can be made from the history alone. History taking is therefore a vital part of the consultation if a doctor is to be successful in their objective of making a correct diagnosis.

This chapter is divided into the following sections.

- Taking a history.
- Different methods.
- Familiarisation.
- Rapport.
- Information gathering.
- Exploring health beliefs and ideas, concerns and expectations (ICE).
- The illness narrative.
- Conclusion.

During this chapter and Chapter 5 on problem solving, some quotations are made from the writings of Sherlock Holmes by the author Sir Arthur Conan Doyle. Why? Although Sir Arthur Conan Doyle was a writer of fiction, he was also a medical doctor and qualified from Edinburgh University Medical School in 1881. In relation to 'history taking', further enquiry and problem solving, some of the comments of the famous detective, Sherlock Holmes, help to illustrate the text in these two chapters.

Taking a history

The history part of the consultation is centred around discovering why the patient has come to see the doctor. Doctors essentially listen to patients' stories and read the notes or patient records of these stories to create patient biographies. Information is not only gathered but it is actively interpreted by paying close attention to the patient's language and its context. Cognitive processes both generate possible diagnoses and evaluate them through specific questions and clinical reasoning.

Good and effective history taking is an important part of the consultation process.

Practical point
A vital aim of a consultation is to arrive at a diagnosis.

As the majority of diagnoses can be determined on the basis of history alone, this makes communication and so the history the most effective tool for a successful consultation. History taking is therefore optimum when it is discriminating and each question being asked has a purpose.

Like all other arts, the science of deduction and analysis is one which can only be acquired by long and patient study, nor is life long enough to allow any mortal to attain the highest possible perfection in it. Let the inquirer begin by mastering more elementary problems. (From *A Study in Scarlet* by Sir Arthur Conan Doyle)

Different methods

Diagnosing illness is a process and this process takes place within a physician's mind using the raw ingredients of the patient's:

- history
- examination findings
- social and psychological influences
- investigations.

The internalisation of this process, together with the resultant output of a logical diagnosis by the clinician, is often seen as daunting to students. (The problem-solving process is discussed further in Chapter 5.) They often blame their inexperience or lack of medical knowledge as a reason for 'failure' to make a diagnosis. It is actually more a failure to understand the formulas or methods involved that is at fault.

This is rather like the analogy of a mathematics exam, where more points are awarded for demonstration of the workings than the actual numerical result (the answer) or, in this situation, the diagnosis. By having the skills to follow a logical stepwise process of data interpretation, the correct diagnosis or an appropriate working diagnosis should be a natural outcome.

There are three commonly used methods or 'formulas' of reaching a diagnosis:

- inductive
- hypothetico-deductive
- pattern recognition.

Each clinician selects which method is most appropriate depending upon the clinical problem presented or the external constraints put upon them, e.g. time within the working environment.

The inductive method

The easiest way to describe this method is to imagine a fisherman. The fisherman knows that the fish he seeks lie somewhere in the ocean before him. There is no way of him knowing exactly what will turn up in his nets, so he casts them as wide as possible. He then reviews the contents and selects those of use and throws back that which is of no use.

Translating this into a medical model, we know the diagnosis we seek is out there somewhere in the 'sea' of symptoms. By asking many questions on all the systems of the body we 'cast our nets wide' in the hope of catching something of use.

This is the 'traditional' method employed by medical students when first embarking on making diagnoses. Perhaps due to a lack of knowledge of some specific diseases, a wide-reaching, non-focused line of questioning is taken, searching for any positive responses.

In this traditional or **inductive** method of history taking, students are encouraged to take a comprehensive history irrespective of the **presenting complaint(s)**. Take the example of a patient presenting with a headache. An inductive history could be a history about the headache, but would also be a systemic review of questions, e.g. relating to the cardiovascular and other systems. However, this inductive process is only useful for difficult cases, where there is no obvious presenting complaint or a patient is just unwell and no obvious possible cause is apparent and so a general rather than a focused **deductive** enquiry is more appropriate.

Practical point
This method of multi-systems enquiry is very time consuming as many questions need to be asked.

It is therefore more often used as a fall-back technique by experienced doctors, when they really have no clue as to the diagnosis facing them. Usually they opt for the two more focused methods which shall now be discussed.

The hypothetico-deductive model

This method of producing a diagnosis is the one most commonly used by GPs and hospital doctors alike. It involves the proposal of the most likely diagnoses from information that has been given in the initial history and any prior knowledge. Specific lines of focused questioning are then used in order to make each diagnosis more or less likely.

Using an analogy as before, this is similar to the process used by a police detective when solving a crime. Using information from the scene and prior knowledge of crimes and criminals within the area, the detective draws up a list of suspects. Then using interviews and specific information such as fingerprints, he or she is able to make a judgement that certain individuals are more or less likely of being guilty of the offence. After all the specific information has been reviewed, it may be that all suspects are cleared and have alibis. The detective must then start again and return to the original crime scene and information in order to elicit more suspects, i.e. the entire process can become a loop.

> We balance probabilities and choose the most likely. (From *The Hound of the Baskervilles* by Sir Arthur Conan Doyle)

Translating this again back into medicine, the loop is an important part of this process as often our initial differential diagnoses are subsequently ruled out by further questioning or investigations. Thus we must return to our original information in order to create further **diagnostic hypotheses** that can again be tested.

Using a **hypothetico-deductive** method, relevant and discriminating questions based on the present complaint(s) are asked in an attempt to confirm or refute a possible diagnosis or hypothesis rather than an inductive systemic enquiry. Using either method of history taking, patients are allowed to narrate their stories. The narrative-based approach to history taking is discussed later in this chapter.

Problem solving and so making a diagnosis is usually hypothetico-deductive. So, when a doctor is faced with a patient who is unwell and has symptoms and signs of being unwell, there is in scientific terms a 'problem' which needs to be solved.

Practical point

The ideal approach is therefore to think of possible solutions and test these hypotheses.

This leads to what is frequently termed differential diagnoses where doctors tend to rank what appear to be the most likely diagnoses or solutions first, but not dismissing lesser possibilities until they have been tested with further enquiry. This way of thinking, 'The Diagnosing Mind', arose at McMaster University in Canada and others in the 1970s onwards and has become an important component of the Leicester Assessment Package as detailed in Robin Fraser's *Clinical Method* (2000).

The pattern-recognition process

This is the final method of reaching a diagnosis.

> 'Name a black-and-white animal that "moos".'

The question is not aimed at being patronising; it is merely used as a simplistic example of pattern recognition. We would all respond with the answer of a cow as we recognise both the colour and noise and tie them together. If I ask a slightly briefer question, the response is slightly more varied:

> 'Name a black-and-white animal.'

Now the response may still be a cow but could also be a zebra, dog or cat.
It has to be appreciated that there are simple and complex stories.

In diagnosing illness, clinicians are able to recognise key symptoms and link them together quickly as they have seen them before in specific illnesses. The symptoms must be uncommon and relatively pathopneumonic of a condition for this pattern recognition process to work, e.g. in making a diagnosis of type I diabetes.

A simple pattern recognition of the symptoms polydipsia, polyuria and weight loss may lead to a swift diagnosis of diabetes.

> I never guess. It is a shocking habit – destructive to the logical faculty. (From *The Sign of Four* by Sir Arthur Conan Doyle)

Practical point

Pattern recognition is a method used by experienced doctors who have often seen many patients presenting with similar 'patterns' of symptoms, enabling them to spot diagnoses very quickly.

However, one should issue a cautionary note about pattern recognition. This is a form of the **heuristic diagnosic process** where a diagnosis is based on knowledge accumulated from the experience of human experts. In a paper on the subject Professor Klein, who is an associate professor of marketing in Singapore, points out:

> Doctors often have to make rapid decisions, either because of medical emergency or because they need to see many patients in a limited time. Psychologists have shown that rapid decision making is aided by heuristics – strategies that provide shortcuts to quick decisions – but they have also noted that these heuristics frequently mislead us. Good decision making is further impeded by the fact that we often fall prey to various cognitive biases.

Professor Klein goes on to say:

> Doctors may believe that, as highly trained professionals, they are immune to these pitfalls. Unfortunately, they are just as prone to errors in decision making as anyone else. Even worse, it is common for people who are particularly prone to cognitive biases to believe that they are good decision makers. (Klein 2005)

As Shakespeare put it:

> The fool doth think he is wise, but the wise man knows himself to be a fool. (From William Shakespeare's play, *As You Like It*)

The ability to utilise these three different techniques provides doctors with a toolkit from which the correct instrument for the task of 'making a diagnosis' can be selected. Each has its own qualities and limitations and the professional must learn not only how each 'tool' is used, but also when its use is appropriate.

Familiarisation

Before seeing a patient it is necessary to know some basic information and this hopefully may be readily available prior to the consultation. Name, age and gender of the patient are obvious details but a lot more information is available without too much effort, e.g. family history and medications. This is a distinct advantage of the registered populations and the medical notes 'following' the patient in primary care under the umbrella of the National Health Service. Computer records can reveal active problems, past medical history, health-promotion data, current medication, occupation and details of other members of the household such as family history. Manual records have a summary sheet which may detail active problems and repeat medication. The consultation frequency and details of the last consultation are particularly useful. This process should not be exhaustive and last no more than 2–3 minutes.

Practical point
A universal NHS electronic patient record is being worked towards to help clinicians in this familiarisation process whether working in primary or secondary care.

There is a school of thought that this process may 'colour' your thinking and bias the thought process. However, it would be stupid not to use this information as it augments continuity of care, clinical and time efficiency and does not overburden a patient with questions which they are likely to assume the doctor should already know.

Rapport

Practitioners need to have the ability to communicate and these skills are first assessed during student selection interviews. These attributes are essential for the consultation process and are developed and refined at both undergraduate and postgraduate levels. It is important and advisable that doctors dress in a conservative style and present a professional image. The patient should be greeted in a formal way, using Mr, Miss or Mrs accordingly, despite the general relaxation of attitudes by the public. The formal approach, in turn, may be reciprocated by the patient. If you are seeing the patient for the first time, you must introduce yourself too, despite having a name plate on the consulting room door or a name badge on your clothing. This is to avoid confusion and set the tone for the rest of the consultation. Above all, minimise the potential to start off on the 'wrong foot'. Generally, rapport and respect may be enhanced by personally calling the patient from the waiting area.

Practical point
Establishing a good working relationship and so rapport with a patient will facilitate communication and so problem solving.

It needs to be stated that the observation part of the physical examination/ assessment starts as soon as you see the patient. The appearance, behaviour, body language and other features of the patient are all important in making your assessment and determining the initial approach. For instance, patients may:

- be angry and flustered
- be overtly depressed and withdrawn
- be unkempt and smell of body odour
- smell of alcohol or urine
- have obvious injuries
- limp in due to back pain/sciatica or inflamed joints
- be pale, jaundiced or cyanosed
- have breathing difficulty or other physical distress.

The reality is that doctors work under intense pressures and may run late. Given that patients can be very tense and frustrated due to their own time pressures and circumstances, it is worth acknowledging and accounting for such delays and apologising as appropriate.

Opening question – starting the history

This should be a gentle enquiry with an open question:

- How may I help you?
- What brings you in today?
- What can I do for you?
- Your reason for coming today was . . . [pause, invitingly]?

Information gathering

The patient is then encouraged to give details, in their own words, of the presenting complaint without interference or leading questions. That is to say, those initial 2–3 questions must be open questions with lots of encouraging noises and phrases:

- um . . . go on
- yes, I see . . .
- tell me more.

The **body language** needs to be open and receptive in order to convey the doctor's interest in the patient. The eye contact is also important, but each practitioner will need to develop their own style and vary their responses according to circumstances. At a sensitive point in the consultation, perhaps it would be inappropriate to be looking straight into their eyes. This sort of social skills training is best done through **video analysis** of the consultation. Practitioners learn to adjust their behaviours through constructive critical analysis and feedback from colleagues and tutors.

The consultation is a dynamic process and practitioners need to have heightened perception in order to pick up on **verbal and non-verbal** cues. While all of these may need to be explored, the response may be immediate or delayed. In the initial phase, it may be more productive to allow the patient to talk without interruption. There may be a lot of emotional energy within consultations which also requires appropriate handling and processing.

It is normal, and one hopes, for patients to have a single complaint, e.g. 'I have a chest pain', 'I have a pain in the right knee', 'I have an earache'. This is referred to as the '**presenting complaint**'. Chest pain is used as the example for further analysis.

The prior knowledge of the patient can be 'married' to the presenting complaint, formulating a pre-diagnostic interpretation (Fraser 2000). This is a broad-brush assessment to identify affected systems and gives a strategic aim for the history taking. (Further details on diagnostics can be found in Chapter 5.)

Practical point
Pre-diagnostic interpretation is the marrying up of the prior knowledge about the patient to the presenting complaint.

The doctor needs to allow the patient to **expand on the presenting complaint** by opening up the discussion, e.g. 'Tell me more'. The use of positive and open body language should be augmented by eye contact and encouraging noises. If patients are allowed to talk, they usually give lots of information by themselves, leaving the doctor to make mental notes. This may need further development using the same or similar tactics and then follow it up with systematic and structured enquiry of the presenting complaint (say, chest pain) using an acronym such as SQITAS which is used at the Leicester–Warwick Medical Schools. This can be adapted for analysis of any presenting complaint including rashes. The acronym SQITAS is detailed below:

- S – Site
- Q – Quality
- I – Intensity
- T – Timing
- A – Arrows refers to what makes the pain better or worse
- S – associated Symptoms.

Similar mnemonics can be seen at the following website:
www.medicalmnemonics.com.

Like all other arts, the science of deduction and analysis is one which can only be acquired by long and patient study, nor is life long enough to allow any mortal to attain the highest possible perfection in it. Before turning to those moral and mental aspects of the matter which present the greatest difficulties, let the inquirer begin by mastering more elementary problems. Let him, on meeting a fellow-mortal, learn at a glance to distinguish the history of man, and the trade or profession to which he belongs. Puerile as such an exercise may seem, it sharpens the faculties of observation, and teaches one where to look and what to look for. (From *A Study in Scarlet* by Sir Arthur Conan Doyle)

Exploring health beliefs and ideas, concerns and expectations (ICE)

This can greatly enhance the diagnostic process and reveal more of the history and its impact on the presenting complaint as patients come in to the consultation with their own ideas, concerns and expectations.

During this initial phase, one should attempt to get as much information about the individual patient so that you can replace the 'passport'-like picture of the patient in front of you with a family portrait or perhaps even an album. This information is discretionary and non-essential in terms of diagnostics, but may prove to be very useful for the management phase of the consultation. Practitioners may spend more time on this information if they can see its relevance in difficult, complex and serious cases.

This section explores why a patient's thoughts – traditionally described as their ideas, concerns and expectations (ICE) – should always carefully be considered during the consultation. It also explores when and how this is best done.

The **purpose of the consultation** is to find out what is wrong with the patient and to do something about it.

Practical point

A patient's ideas, concerns and expectations can provide vital clues in the problem-solving process regarding their illness and so making a diagnosis.

The patient's thoughts, worries and hopes yield clues to the social and psychological aspects of their problems.

This section is subdivided as follows.

- Why explore ICE?
- Reassurance and ICE.
- Preventing complaints.
- When to elicit ICE.
- How to elicit ICE.

Why explore ideas, concerns and expectations?

1 Improves communication.
2 Helps problem solving and so making a diagnosis.
3 Aids management of a patient.
4 Reduces medical errors.
5 It's in the job description!

The patient's ideas, concerns and expectations are formulated when he or she first notices symptoms that suggest illness. They arise from his or her innate health beliefs and many external influences. A **health belief model** can be used to decipher the process through which a patient decides to consult a doctor. This is a psychological model illustrating the determinants of health behaviour; it is outlined in Figure 2.1 using the 'decision to consult' as the health behaviour.

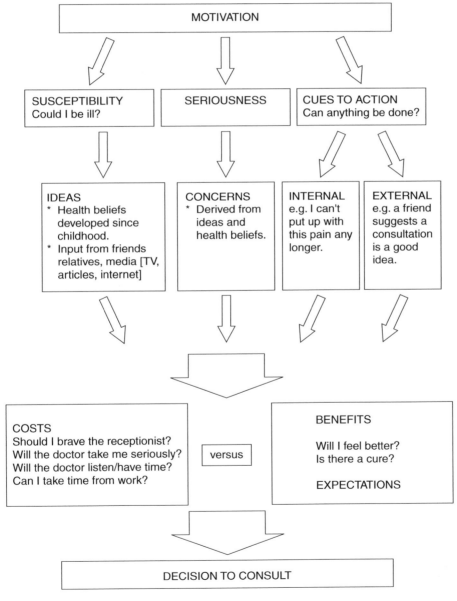

Figure 2.1 A health belief model.

(The **Health Belief Model (HBM)** was first developed in the USA in the 1950s by social psychologists to explain and predict health behaviours.)

Reassurance and ICE

The management of the patient's problem always requires reassurance by the doctor. This may be reassurance that the problem has a solution or, more often, that there is some help available. The reassurance can only be complete if the patient's concerns are addressed.

Practical point
A key to successful doctor–patient partnerships is to recogise that patients are experts too.

The doctor has the knowledge of the causes of the illness and the ways in which it can be treated; the patient knows about his or her personal experience of the illness and will come to the consultation with some expectations of the outcome.

These expectations need to be known and so discussed during the negotiation of the management plan if it is to be successful and the patient is to adhere to it. One of the factors in communication difficulties is a lack of patient involvement in the discussion. This should not arise if expectations are elicited and discussed. For example, patients' unvoiced agendas can lead to inappropriate prescribing by the doctor. A full understanding of the patient's ideas and concerns can minimise such medical error. **Avoid assuming that you think that you know what a patient's expectations are!** Ask them instead.

Preventing complaints

Practical point
Most patient complaints about doctors are due to problems of communication rather than clinical competency.

The commonest complaint is that doctors do not **listen** to their patients. One way to prevent this from happening is to summarise back to the patient the information you have gleaned including their thoughts, worries and hopes. This allows a check of accuracy while demonstrating careful and empathic listening.

> A wise old owl sat in an oak,
> The more he heard, the less he spoke;
> The less he spoke, the more he heard;
> Why aren't we all like that wise old bird? (Anon)

The General Medical Council (GMC) in their recommendations on undergraduate medical education state that graduates must know about and understand how to take account of patients' own views and beliefs when suggesting treatment options. Many reasons have been put forward for eliciting ideas, concerns and expectations; and it should be part of an ideal description.

When to elicit ideas, concerns and expectations

- Not at the start of the consultation.
- Not at the end of the consultation.
- Preferably in response to cues.

Eliciting ideas, concerns and expectations is not always straightforward. Timing can be important if it is to be successful. Rapport is developed as the consultation proceeds if communication is good. Asking questions about the patient's feelings too early may be inappropriate and can hinder disclosure until sufficient trust has been established. However, waiting until the end of the consultation will probably be too late for meaningful answers. The patient may perceive that the doctor does not attach sufficient importance to his or her viewpoint. The ideal time to pose those questions is in response to cues. For example:

> Patient: 'It was when the rash developed I really started to worry.'
> Doctor: 'What in particular worried you about the rash?'
> Patient: 'Well, you hear so much about meningitis . . .'

How to explore ideas, concerns and expectations

- Emphasise 'you'.
- Don't ask for information if it has already been given.
- Explain why you want to know.
- Experiment with words and phrases.

The way in which a question is asked about ideas, concerns and expectations can affect the reply. If the interview is conducted well then some further information regarding ideas, concerns and expectations will emerge. This is illustrated by the following possible consultation questions by the doctor and the responses they might generate by a patient:

> Doctor: '*What* do you think is wrong with you?'
> Patient: 'I don't know; you are the doctor' or 'If I knew that, I wouldn't be here!'

Similarly:

> Doctor: 'Are *you* worried by this?'
> Patient: 'Of course I am! Wouldn't you be?'

Such information therefore needs to be carefully extracted. One needs to use neutral language and tone so that negative responses are avoided.

The question by the doctor, 'What do you think is wrong with you?', might be more appropriately rephrased: ''Have *you* any ideas of your own as to what is wrong with you?'

The patient might then respond, 'Well . . .'.

Similarly, when the doctor asked, 'Are you worried by this?', it may work better if the doctor said, 'Are there any particular worries you may have regarding your symptoms?'

Emphasis matters, for example:

Doctor: 'What do you *think* is wrong with you?'
Patient: 'I'm not a hypochondriac.'

It can be seen therefore that **emphasis** matters!

When asking about a patient's expectations:

Doctor: 'What did you *expect* me to do for you?'
Patient: 'To make me better.'

This might be better phrased by the doctor as: 'What were you hoping I could do for you?'

When asking about ideas, concerns and expectations the question is likely to be successful if it emphasises the patient's viewpoint ('you') and it is asked with empathy and interest.

This is further enhanced if the doctor explains why he or she wants the answer, for example:

Doctor: 'I can see you are worried. Perhaps if you could tell me what is worrying you I may be able to help.'

The question is less likely to succeed if the patient has already voiced a concern and it has not been recognised, for example:

Patient: 'When I coughed up blood I was scared it could be lung cancer.'

If the doctor later in the same consultation asks, 'What are your concerns?', there is a failure of communication. A rigid line of questioning has displaced **active listening**.

It is possible to develop one's own preferred techniques for eliciting ideas, concerns and expectations in communication skills work with simulated patients (actors) and by observing tutors or colleagues in consultations. It is important to try to find out what works best for you.

The illness narrative

The illness process can be seen as an enactment of a narrative in the patient's life. This is often witnessed by health professionals in their continued care, a core value of clinical practice. This gives a unique and privileged access to people's lives allowing deeper understanding and generation of empathic attitudes.

Practical point
Attentive listening to patients' stories is intrinsically therapeutic and serves to set patient-centred agendas and goals in their management.

A narrative is a **story** used by a patient (the narrator) to communicate their experiences and thoughts to a doctor (the listener). The choice of what to tell and what to omit lies with the patient and can be modified at their discretion or by the doctor's questions. The story should engage the listener and invite an interpretation. Narrative-based medicine views doctor–patient encounters (consultations) as agreeing on a narrative or story that satisfies both the patient and the doctor's understanding of the problem or problems being presented. This process is facilitated by the doctor.

Considering symptoms as a narrative is a new conceptual framework that brings medicine into alignment with social sciences and the humanities. Patients bring stories to doctors about their lives which are often complex and one role of a doctor is to provide an opportunity for patients to **find a meaning to their illness experiences**. Most important, perhaps, is the formulation of a therapeutic narrative of an action plan of what to do based on shared understanding and decision making.

This is encouraged with open questions and an expression of both interest and concern. But, nevertheless, doctors may be perceived as steering patients towards 'therapeutic plots'.

The **narrative-based** medicine approach is in its embryonic stages of development. It is interesting to read in a paper by Professor Trisha Greenhalgh of University College London:

> Science is concerned with the formulation and attempted falsification of hypotheses using reproducible methods that allow the construction of generalisable statements about how the universe behaves. Conventional medical training teaches students to view medicine as a science and the doctor as an impartial investigator who builds differential diagnoses as if they were scientific theories and who excludes competing possibilities in a manner akin to the falsification of hypotheses. This approach is based on the somewhat tenuous assumption that diagnostic decision making follows an identical protocol to scientific inquiry – in other words, that the discovery of 'facts' about a patient's illness is equivalent to the discovery of new scientific truths about the universe. The evidence based approach to clinical decision making is often incorrectly held to rest on the assumption that clinical observation is totally objective and should, like all scientific measurements, be reproducible.

Such an argument strongly supports the view held by some doctors that medicine is both a science and an art and that the 'good doctor' is one who has developed **the art of applying the science**. In some clinical scenarios, the evidence of a scientific theory may be overwhelming. Take the example of a patient presenting with tiredness and a blood glucose which is found to be 30 mmol. A diagnosis of diabetes is made. It is likely that their symptom of tiredness will resolve with appropriate treatment and control of their diabetes. But what if it does not? There may be many other factors to be found in the patient's narrative that may explain their tiredness.

It is interesting to read that the *New Zealand Family Physician* has a section entitled 'Swamp rat'. This is a column written from the swamp. The term is taken from Donald Schon where he talks about the crisis of confidence in professional knowledge:

In the varied topography of professional practice, there is a high, hard ground overlooking a swamp. On the high ground, manageable problems lend themselves to solution through the application of research-based theory and technique. In the swampy lowland, messy, confusing problems defy technical solutions. (Schon 1990)

History taking can be **patient-centred** or doctor-centred.

Practical point

Narrative illness enquiry is an example of a patient-centred approach to the consultation.

In a doctor-centred consultation, more closed questions are asked regarding the cardinal symptoms of different systems and so may not consistently focus on the patient's illness narrative. Figure 2.2 illustrates the use of open and closed questions in focused history taking.

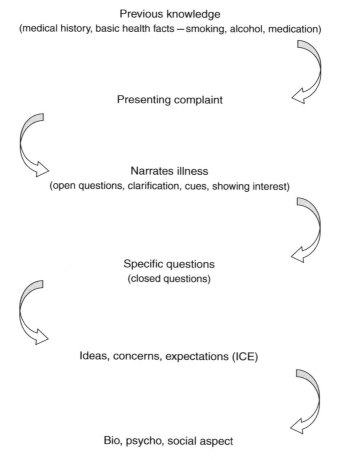

Previous knowledge
(medical history, basic health facts — smoking, alcohol, medication)

Presenting complaint

Narrates illness
(open questions, clarification, cues, showing interest)

Specific questions
(closed questions)

Ideas, concerns, expectations (ICE)

Bio, psycho, social aspect

Figure 2.2   Principles of focused history taking.

Narrative illness

During a consultation, practitioners listen to stories from patients about their illnesses, health beliefs and what have they done to help themselves. Each story frequently starts at the beginning of their illness and how the illness unfolded which prompted them to come to a doctor to seek alleviation of their symptoms.

Practical point
It is hoped by patients that, through the making of a diagnosis, treatment may provide a cure and so an end to the story.

This is not always the case and the **breaking of bad news** to a patient that they have a malignancy is the start of a cancer journey and so a story that continues until they die. A patient's illness narrative may span more than one consultation and so be a **continuing story**.

Some patients find it difficult to make a correlation of their story with the experience of other people. They look to health professionals for the following answers.

- What is wrong with me?
- How long will it last?
- What is the cause?
- Where will the story go from here – how will it affect my work and family?
- Can the illness be cured or controlled?

These questions relating to the illness are evident as the story or narrative unfolds. With modern-day emphasis on patient-centred consultations and a holistic approach, narrative style to medical history taking and therapy is becoming an increasing focus of attention.

Doctors practise this approach every day, often without realising it. Each consultation with a patient is a further part of their health life story and so illness narrative. One doctor recently coined the phrase, 'Life is a consultation', and maybe they have a point. Take the following example of an illness narrative. A patient starts their story: 'Ten days ago when I came back from work ... backache ... I tried some pain killers ... it is not shifting ...'

Practical point
The aim of a successful consultation is not a prescription, but helping the patient to complete his or her illness narrative. This can be cathartic and so therapeutic. Where possible agree the end to the story through mutual understanding and negotiated decision making.

In fact, a new construct addressing the issues, explaining the process and description of the possible outcome of the illness with its effect on patient's family and work, may end in a new narrative. **So no story really ends, but evolves.**

Take another example:

A 25-year-old girl on anticonvulsant treatment comes to see you for a repeat prescription and contraception. She had her last fit five years ago. Her story goes on – epilepsy since childhood, but she could not enjoy life like other children, not being allowed to go swimming or camping with the family. However, her brothers and sisters could participate in any activity. For the first time she is now free of convulsions, but she is not willing to take the risk of stopping anticonvulsant drugs even on an experimental basis. She does not want to go back to her old life and she does not want to lose her driving licence. She has seen her friend, who also has epilepsy and has lost her driving licence.

She narrates her story with emphasis of this illness on her social life. The doctor agrees and narrates the illness of another patient who had a similar problem. The patient feels better after sharing her feelings and being reassured by the doctor's story.

Although the doctor remains objective in his or her efforts to explain an illness, they also wrap it in a narrative: 'I saw a patient a few days ago with similar problems ... and he got better following ...'

Practical point
A prescription may be a helpful option, but is not necessarily the end of a story.

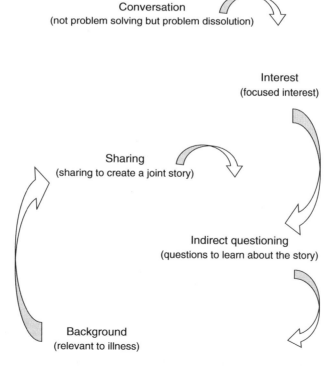

Conversation
(not problem solving but problem dissolution)

Interest
(focused interest)

Sharing
(sharing to create a joint story)

Indirect questioning
(questions to learn about the story)

Background
(relevant to illness)

Figure 2.3 Principles of the narrative process.

Illnesses not only have a biological basis, they also have a social context and, as they are being discussed through conversation, so narratives form part of the consultation. Figure 2.3 illustrates the principles of this process.

Narrative techniques

The following techniques may be used as the illness narrative is developed.

1 Connections – development of a rapport through conversation.
2 Diagnosis/hypothesis – what can it be?
3 Questioning – ranking questions (which is the most/least important).
   a Speculative (what would happen if?).
   b Relational (effect on your family/work).
   c Contextualising (time and place – would it have made any difference?).
   d Difference (what needs to happen?).
   e Worst scenario (supposing nothing changes).
4 Strategy – to meet own need (from learning and experience).
5 Sharing – enablement/empowerment – giving the patient the lead in decision making.
6 Reflection – absorbing facts and renegotiation.
7 Good new story – useful for a patient and acceptable, meaningful.

The benefit of an illness narrative is that it is patient-centred and satisfying to patients and doctors. But the main difficulties are that it is time consuming and objectivity is sacrificed in preference of subjectivity and there is no evidence-based study to confirm the effectiveness of this process in disease and illness outcome.

Towards the end of a consultation comes what Professor Greenhalgh refers to as the '**therapeutic narrative**' – the formulation of a management or action plan of what to do next and so the enactment of that narrative.

Practical point
In a consultation the doctor and patient need to come to a shared understanding about the illness and similarly, as a result of this informed dialogue, a mutual agreement should be made on the decision-making process in relation to that illness.

Narratives are not confined to primary care. In specialties such as psychiatry and family therapy great opportunities exist in dealing with narrative illnesses. In patients with mental health problems, patients are often encouraged to write stories about their illness and express themselves. This is also a recognised form of therapy in psychoanalysis or in terminal illnesses.

What of patients who are referred to hospital outpatient clinics where a diagnosis cannot be made and the patient has multiple symptoms? Is there a role for this new approach and listening again to the patient's story? This should be an opportunity for a person to seek meaning to their experiences. It should be a collaborative search by the doctor and the patient for an acceptable and healing story that the patient 'owns' and understands and takes responsibility for the negotiated plan of action. One of the skills is overcoming the inevitable tension between the patient's complex story and the perceived 'paternalistic' stories of the doctor based on professional knowledge and experiences.

Dr John Launer describes this well in the *BMJ* in 1999:

> The medical consultation becomes an opportunity for dialogue between different stories: the patient's biographical one and the doctor's professional one. The doctor's contributions may come in different forms. The doctor's contribution to the story is valuable not as a truth which has prior and superior validity to the patient's truth but only if the patient finds the doctor's contributions to the plot useful.

We should always be striving for better communication with patients. An American author, Dr Charon, suggests that effective practice requires 'narrative competence, that is, the ability to acknowledge, absorb, interpret, and act on the stories and plights of others'. In consultations, all stories should be integrated – stories of patients and the stories of healthcare workers. These stories commonly expand in direct consultation, face to face, between patient and healthcare worker. Narrative illnesses appear in consultations in a variety of other contexts, including views from families and friends, discussion among professionals or in teaching and training. When better stories do not work, we try to develop another story by exploring and negotiating.

Practical point

In spite of such a vital role of narrative illnesses, doctors should be always aware of the negative aspect of practising narrative therapy in the presence of evidence of serious illnesses, such as an acute stroke, heart attack or injury.

Where evidence of such **serious** illnesses is absent Professor Greenhalgh and Dr Hurwitz (1999b) suggest that: 'The lost tradition of narrative should be revived in the teaching and practice of medicine.'

Conclusion

It can be seen that there are several methods and approaches to taking a medical history. It seems appropriate to end this chapter with the following quotation from the detective Sherlock Holmes:

> We must fall back upon the old axiom that when all other contingencies fail, whatever remains, however improbable, must be the truth. (From *The Adventure of the Bruce-Partington Plans* by Sir Arthur Conan Doyle)

Bibliography

Barry CA, Bradley CP, Britten N, Stevenson FA, Barber N. Patients' unvoiced agendas in general practice consultations: qualitative study. *BMJ.* 2000; **320**: 1246–50.

Campbell EJM. The Diagnosing Mind. *The Lancet.* 1987; **i**: 849–51.

Charon R. Narrative medicine: a model for empathy, reflection, profession and trust. *JAMA.* 2001; **286**: 1897–902.

Coulter A. Editorial: Paternalism or partnership? *BMJ.* 1999; **319**: 719–20.

Durie MH. Editorial: Moving beyond single and dual diagnosis in general practice. *BMJ.* 2003; **326**: 512–14.

Fraser R. *Clinical Method; a general practice approach.* Oxford: Butterworth Heinemann; 2000.

Gale J. Some cognitive components of the diagnostic thinking process. *Br J Educ Psychology.* 1982; **52**: 64–76.

General Medical Council (GMC). *Tomorrow's Doctors.* Recommendations on undergraduate medical education. London: GMC. www.gmc-uk.org

Greenhalgh T. Narrative based medicine in an evidence based world. *BMJ.* 1999a; **318**: 323–5.

Greenhalgh T, Hurwitz B. Why study narrative? *BMJ.* 1999b; **318**: 48–50.

Greenhalgh T, Hurwitz B. *Narrative Based Medicine.* London: BMJ Books; 2000.

Klein JG. Five pitfalls in decisions about diagnosis and prescribing. *BMJ.* 2005; **330**: 781–4.

Launer J. Narrative based medicine: a narrative approach to mental health in general practice. *BMJ.* 1999; **318**: 117–19.

Launer J. *Narrative-based Primary Care: a practical guide.* Oxford: Radcliffe Medical Press; 2002.

Launer J. Editorial: Narrative-based medicine: a passing fad or a giant leap for general practice? *British Journal of General Practice.* 2003; **53**: 91–2.

Levensten JA, McCracken EC, McWhinney IR *et al.* The patient-centred clinical method. 1. A model for the doctor-patient interaction in family medicine. *Family Practice.* 1986; **3**: 24–30.

Marinker M. Whole person medicine. In: Cormack J, Marinker M and Morrell D, editors. *Teaching General Practice.* London: Kluwer Medical; 1981.

Meryn S. Editorial: Improving doctor–patient communication. *BMJ.* 1998; **316**: 1922–30.

McPherson KM, Harwood M, McNaughton HK. Ethnicity, equity and quality: lessons from New Zealand. *BMJ.* 2003; **327**: 443–4.

Pendleton D, Schofield T, Tate P, Havelock P. *The Consultation: an approach to learning and teaching.* Oxford: Oxford University Press; 1984.

Schon DA. *Educating the Reflective Practitioner.* San Francisco: Jossey-Bass Publishers; 1990.

Stewart M. Effective physician–patient communication and health outcomes: a review. *Canadian Medical Association Journal.* 1995; **152**(9): 1423–33.

Tate P. *The Doctor's Communication Handbook.* Oxford: Radcliffe Medical Press; 1994.

Chapter 3

The importance of the 'doctor–patient relationship'

Dr Ryan Prince and Dr Rodger Charlton

Ryan Prince has looked at how rapport and so the doctor–patient relationship is made with patients and he has provided some helpful practical examples. Rodger Charlton has looked at some of the component parts of the doctor–patient relationship and issues of debate such as a doctor's dress and title.

Patients often consult a doctor when they feel ill, anxious and vulnerable. The patient can hold a whole host of worries with an agenda that is sometimes not even clearly known to themselves. It is likely that many have preconceived ideas about their problem(s). The doctor they are most likely to consult is a general practitioner (GP), unless they are referred to a hospital doctor/specialist by the GP.

Doctors have a difficult task to perform; they need to help the patient physically, emotionally and even sometimes socially, often with severely limited resources of both time and services.

This often-fragile understanding of one another can become dysfunctional, especially in the early days of the relationship. Doctors and patients tend to play very complex social games with each other to try (sometimes even unwittingly) to get the other person to understand exactly what they need, but rarely say **exactly** what they are thinking or feeling. However, with some effort on the part of the practitioner, developing a good relationship with their patients can really be the most rewarding side of the job, and make caring for patients much easier once mutual trust has been established.

Communication from doctor to patient is also vital to the consultation and treatment. Good communication benefits both doctor and patient. First, the patient has a better understanding of their problem and treatments available. This in turn promotes better **concordance**. Second, the patients' anxiety in visiting the doctor will be lessened. These factors can make the encounter less stressful for the patient and the doctor.

Practical point

Concordance used to be unwittingly called 'compliance' and it means that the doctor and patient have discussed, negotiated and mutually agreed on a plan of action rather than the patient 'submitting' to the doctor's ideas.

Good communication should start as soon as the patient enters the room. Eye contact should be made and the patient welcomed, setting the tone for the rest of the consultation. It is a common complaint that the doctor continues to look at their computer (the so-called 'third person' in the consultation) while talking to the patient. 'Active listening' should be used to elicit information.

This chapter is divided into the following sections.

- Forming the relationship.
- Bedside manner.
- Before the patient meets the doctor.
- Achieving rapport.
- White coats and dress.
- Addressing patients, respect and titles.
- Balint and rapport with patients.
- Paternalism.
- Empowerment and patient-centred consultations.
- Being patient-centred.
- Forming a partnership in the consultation.
- Patient ideas, concerns and expectations.
- Keys to achieving rapport.

Forming the relationship

The consultation has always been central to medicine as the main point of interaction with patients. It is in the consultation that the doctor–patient relationship is formed. In the past this was often a paternal relationship with the patient expected to undergo whatever the doctor thought 'best'. However, with the recent increase in lay medical knowledge and for many other reasons the doctor–patient relationship has moved towards a true **partnership**, although some patients still prefer a paternalistic approach. For each patient a doctor must judge for him/herself which role a patient wishes to adopt. This can be through a series of questions. For example, the doctor might provide a series of possible investigation/treatment options and ask which one a patient wishes to choose. The patient may choose or may reply, 'I don't know, you tell me, you're the doctor.'

Practical point
In working towards a partnership doctors should try to develop an open relationship with their patients, making sure that they are well informed and involved in any decisions about their treatment.

Within the consultation there are many things which can affect the patient's satisfaction. Research has shown that the doctor's friendliness and courteous behaviour increase patient satisfaction. Satisfaction is also thought to increase with a higher proportion of social conversation in the consultation. Patients in this study preferred a doctor who they liked as a person and whose ability they had faith in (Williams *et al.* 1998). If a patient feels at ease in the consultation then they will be able to 'open their heart'.

Bedside manner

This is a phrase that has perhaps been superseded by the word **professionalism**. However, it is a phrase still quoted by the public and the media and has subtle differences. It derives from the times when patient consultations frequently took place at the hospital or home bedside and doctors wore white coats. Times have changed and are changing, not least the fact that more healthcare takes place in the community and so less frequently at the hospital bed or the bedside in a patient's home. In addition, doctors are now one of many healthcare practitioners whom patients consult with.

Bedside manner is defined in the Oxford English Dictionary as 'the deportment of a medical man towards his patient'. However, a good bedside manner is less easily defined. Aspects of a good bedside manner include a doctor's behaviour and attitudes towards a patient as well as how they communicate both verbally and non-verbally with them. In all, it is being sincere and polite wrapped in the ability to get across to the patient that they have the utmost concern for their welfare.

Practical point

It is important to remember that patients will take their judgements of doctors to the outside world where the doctor's reputation is formed.

Students must be encouraged and inspired to develop a good bedside manner preferably through the example and role-models of others. Universities have also acknowledged the value of bedside manner, with medical courses now emphasising the importance of communication skills training early in their career.

Before the patient meets the doctor

Making the appointment

It might be felt that the initial contact is when a patient meets the doctor. However, rapport will begin through the following:

- the appointment, whether making the appointment face to face, by phone or through the receiving of a letter
- entering the waiting area and letting the receptionist know that you have arrived for an appointment
- reputation of the clinic or doctor.

Waiting room

The waiting room environment is very important as is the building in which it is situated, whether in a hospital or GP surgery. As a doctor, you may have little control over this, but you need to be aware of it. It may give a positive or negative image of the doctor. Imagine entering a busy hospital casualty department which is crowded, someone has vomited on the floor and there are drunk people shouting at each other. The doctor then has an uphill struggle to create a rapport with a patient. In addition, difficulty getting to the clinic with car parking problems may intensify a negative image.

Does the building and the waiting room convey a feeling of caring and one that puts a patient at their ease? What of the waiting room itself? Is it tidy, clean and is there enough space and adequate seating? Is there reading material if a patient has to wait and are the notices displayed relevant? Even issues such as the level of heating, decor and lighting are all important.

A consultation starts with the initial contact which may be the practitioner or a receptionist asking the patient to come into the consulting room. This initial greeting of the patient can be impersonal, e.g. calling the person over a loudspeaker or their name appearing on a neon sign. This can be made worse by having to work out which room it is and then having to knock and wait to be permitted to enter.

Practical point
Make the initial greeting personal: it can be personal by the doctor going out to the waiting room to ask the patient to accompany him or her to the consulting room and at the same time showing the patient the way.

Layout of consulting or clinic room

This is the subject of lengthy articles and the subject cannot be done justice in a paragraph. Rapport may be increased if the patient does not have to sit behind a large desk with the doctor in front. Is the desk a barrier between doctor and patient and what is the size and comfort of the patient's chair compared to that of the doctor?

If the doctor has a comfortable director's style chair on wheels and the patient has an uncomfortable wooden chair it may convey the wrong impression. If the chairs are almost side by side, but the desk can be accessed, e.g. to use the computer, this can be more personal and less threatening. Be aware that some patients value their personal space and do not like you almost sitting on top of them in your attempt to be personable. Or is the position of the computer and the doctor's attention to it such that it has become a 'third' person in the consultation? Is the room tidy and does it look cared for? If not, it may say something about the doctor. Should toys be available in case the patient is accompanied by a child or the patient is a child? It is important to assess the body language of each patient individually in order to assess how to make them feel most comfortable.

Achieving rapport

It may be helpful to show the patient where they can sit, bearing in mind it may be a room they have not been in before. The doctor–patient relationship begins with the greeting and an important issue for the patient and so the doctor is 'the warmth' of the doctor's greeting.

Rapport may also be affected by the time available for the patient to spend with the doctor.

- Do they feel rushed?
- Do they feel that they have had time to talk with the doctor about what is worrying them?

There is no doubt that the longer the consultation the greater the likelihood of patient satisfaction and this has been the subject of considerable research.

Other factors that affect rapport are the dress code adopted by the doctor, the title that they adopt and how they address the patient.

White coats and dress

What doctors wear and how they address patients and how they wish patients to address them are changing. The singer Bob Dylan will be recalled by many for his words: 'The times they are a-changin'.

It used to be that in hospitals most doctors wore white coats and for many years they have been a well-established symbol of the medical profession. Now this seems to be a rarity. However, an Australian study by Harnett in 2001 asked the views of patients attending an oncology clinic whether doctors should wear white coats; 59% thought junior doctors should wear coats and 61% felt that senior doctors should wear white coats.

In hospitals, white coats are a 'rite of passage' and so adopted by new medical students whereas a sign of seniority is seen perhaps by the wearing of a suit but no white coat. However, to confuse matters, many other professions now also wear white coats, such as pharmacists, laboratory technicians and village cricket umpires!

It is even more unusual for GPs in the community to wear white coats. Similarly, doctors may also be found wearing jeans and, in the case of male doctors, an open-neck shirt and no tie.

Practical point
Appearance matters.

During the 20th century, study of the patient–doctor relationship suggests that the white coat may be a possible barrier to effective communication. This has been recognised by many doctors and, in an attempt to overcome this potential barrier, paediatricians, psychiatrists, GPs and doctors in private practice rarely wear a white coat. However, in a busy hospital, a white coat may help the public and patients identify who the doctors are. Van Der Weyden in the Australian Medical Journal in 2001 writes that there is 'now substantive information that adult patients prefer doctors in clinics and hospitals to be traditionally, or at least smartly, dressed; to wear a necktie; to have short hair; and to wear white coats with a name tag'.

On the one hand the white coat is a constant reminder of a doctor's authority and so a barrier to the patient, but without it a degree of professionalism is lost, particularly for the doctor who might adopt jeans, a t-shirt and trainers. A further argument for not wearing a white coat is that it can rapidly become a carrier of bacteria and the same argument can be made for ties.

Addressing patients, respect and titles

Should we address patients by their first name and should patients address doctors by their first name? There is also discussion in the literature as to whether some surgeons now wish to adopt the title 'doctor' and similarly some dentists have adopted the title of doctor. There are also similar arguments whether to call patients 'patients', 'clients', 'consumers' or 'healthcare users'. Given that no one word or title fully defines the terminology used within the complex practitioner–patient relationship, what term or title should be used? Is there a necessity for uniformity? There is no doubt that these are discussions that will continue for the foreseeable future.

Is there a loss of respect or professionalism if patients call doctors by their first name? If first names are used, is this a more patient-centred rather than a doctor-centred approach? There are also arguments around the 'power' of the doctor and empowerment of the patient. As we strive for a global definition of patient-centred care it is the patient who should be the judge of patient-centred care. Cooper in The Lancet writes: 'First names are everywhere and in medicine the use of first names is growing' (Cooper 2000). Cooper goes on to write: 'I prefer patients to call me doctor. A little emotional distance seems helpful when asking personal questions or performing intimate examinations [...] I therefore rarely initiate the use of a patient's first name, unless that person is very young or dying.' Cooper further writes: 'Maybe I haven't changed with the times, but I still find familiarity undignified.'

Perhaps this is an issue for individual doctors and patients. When a doctor meets a patient for the first time there can be no harm in asking how they would like to be addressed, e.g. by the Christian name or by the their title of Mr, Miss, Mrs, etc. If a doctor does not find their preference, the use of first name may offend and be deemed to show a lack of respect, particularly when the patient is senior in years to the doctor.

The title 'Doctor' (Dr)

The primary medical qualification in the UK is the degree of Bachelor of Medicine, denoted by the abbreviation BM or MB and Bachelor of Surgery denoted by abbreviations including, BS, ChB, BCh and BChir depending on the university granting the degrees that a doctor qualifies from. This is a bachelor's level degree but, confusingly, in many countries the title 'doctor' has also come to be used to refer to physicians and is an honorary or a courtesy title as they do not hold a university doctorate degree, such as PhD. To confuse matters further there is a doctor of medicine degree (MD) which is a further qualification obtained by submission and examination of a research thesis or dissertation to a university. The final confusion arises because in the USA and some other countries the bachelor's level degree in medicine is called a doctorate in medicine (MD), but this is in name only. However, this is not a research degree, and is equivalent to the British MB or BM degree. In Latin the word 'doctor' means teacher and so this section could add debate to the discussion as to what title patients should address their doctor/physician by.

Change and the future

It is difficult to be prescriptive and say what is right or wrong and Cohen in an article on the subject in the *New England Journal of Medicine* (2000) writes:

> Change, whether for better or worse, is always difficult. Resistance to change seems hard-wired into our nature as human beings. And when changes come with such speed and ferocity as they do today, it is easy to reject all changes reflexively, without examining their merits.

Similar discussions are raised in relation to mixed-sex, four-bedded bays in hospital wards.

Balint and rapport with patients

This chapter addresses the doctor–patient relationship and what happens in the consultation. One of the greatest influences on this process was the Hungarian psychotherapist Dr Michael Balint, who worked in the Tavistock Clinic, central London, in the 1950s. This was, and still is, a world-famous centre for psychotherapy research and practice, where he worked with a number of general practitioners. He wrote about the doctor–patient relationship extensively, and his writing became so well respected that today there are 'Balint Societies' and people who describe themselves as 'Balint Practitioners'. These comprise practitioners who strongly advocate his approach to interacting effectively with their patients.

Balint tried to dispel the myth that patients take their health problems to a doctor in the same way as one would take a problem watch to the watchmaker when it no longer keeps good time. His classic book, *The Doctor, His Patient, and The Illness* (1957), analysed the doctor–patient relationship in the context of the long-term management of chronic health problems. It is well worth a read, not too thick, and really forms the crux of what we now call 'partnership' between a doctor and a patient or, if you prefer, healthcare provider and user.

The crux of his argument was as follows.

- The doctor and the patient develop an emotional relationship during the consultation.
- Both doctor and patient have the power to influence one another.
- This power could be used for good or detriment.
- Collusion can develop between doctor and patient about which problems will be recognised and which will not.
- Power flows between doctor and patient, i.e. one moment the doctor is steering the consultation, the next minute the patient.

The remainder of this chapter will focus on different aspects of the partnership between the doctor and the patient in the consultation. (Further details of this consultation model appear in Chapter 12.)

Paternalism

The paternalistic doctor

Here is an example of a possible consultation in progress in general practice. Mrs Jones, a 40-year-old management consultant, comes to see Dr Jack Smith, a 32-year-old new partner at a GP practice, and they have never met before. Their private thoughts are in italics underneath.

Mrs Jones: 'Good morning, Doctor.'
(Oh no! A male doctor! And so young! I wonder when he qualified! Still, he looks quite smart and confident; I'll give him the benefit of the doubt for now.)

Dr Smith: 'Good morning, Mrs Jones. Please take a seat. What can I do for you today?'
(Another stressed-looking businesswoman. Smartly dressed and authoritative, yet seems nervous. Best be careful; I had a complaint from someone just like her a year ago. Bet it's irritable bowel syndrome, anxiety or something similar!)

Mrs Jones: 'Well, it's probably nothing, Doctor, but for the last four or five mornings I have noticed some blood on the toilet paper when I wipe myself after I have opened my bowels.'
(I am worried that it's serious, but I don't want him to think I'm a hysterical patient. I'm concerned as my mother died of bowel cancer aged 42. I hope he examines me, but I'd really rather it was a female GP. If he tells me it's just piles and not to worry, I'm not sure what to say next . . .)

Dr Smith: 'Well, this is a very common thing to happen, don't panic! It's probably just a small pile. Let's try some cream for a week or so, but please come back if it doesn't settle.'
(Should I examine her or not? Examining females in this way has always made me feel uncomfortable, and besides which I'm running late and will have to wait 10 minutes or so for Nurse to come in. She won't want me to anyway, I'm sure. She'll be relieved just to have some cream.)

Mrs Jones: 'Well, if you're sure it's not something more serious . . .'
*(**Please** give me a chance to tell you what I'm worried about without sounding foolish! I respect doctors but can you really make a diagnosis that fast? Have you read my notes regarding my family history and my mother?)*

Dr Smith: 'Very unlikely, I assure you. See you in two weeks if it's not stopped. Here's your prescription. Any questions?'
(I'll examine her then if I have to. Odds are it's only a pile anyway. I'd rather she left now as I have that uncomfortable feeling of a dissatisfied patient, but I'm not sure why. Thought she would have been delighted to get away with such a simple treatment. I wonder if she noticed me looking a bit nervous then.)

Mrs Jones: 'Um, I suppose not. See you in a week then.'
(I'll just come back, perhaps see Dr Lewis, the doctor I usually see, in a day or so.)

Dr Smith: 'Two weeks, Mrs Jones, if it's not stopped. Goodbye!'
(Why don't people listen? No wonder I'm always so busy; they never give themselves any time to get better!)

This could be described as a 'paternalistic' or doctor-centred consultation. The doctor decides what is best for the patient, without exploring the patient's ideas of their illness, any major underlying concerns or what their wishes are for a possible plan of treatment.

For those of you who have read any of the 'Doctor' series by Richard Gordon, this is the classic 'Sir Lancelot Spratt approach' to the patient. If you have not, an example would be the scene where Sir Lancelot, an eminent abdominal surgeon, happens to be on a ward round with a huge entourage of nurses, understudies and medical students. The hapless patient has need of a cholecystectomy for gallstones, and the team are all discussing the size of the incision necessary to carry out this procedure. When the medical student suggests a rather conservative-sized cut, Sir Lancelot roars, 'Don't be stupid, boy!', and gestures an incision with his pencil several inches long across the patient's hypochondrium. When the patient shrieks and starts to question this, Sir Lancelot shouts, 'Shut up, man! This is nothing to do with you!'

Practical point

Paternalism is the practice of controlling, like a parent controlling a child. In relation to a patient, it is the doctor providing treatment which they believe is beneficial, but not allowing the patient the freedom of choice or the opportunity to take responsibility for their own illness. This could be described as a **doctor-centred approach**.

Empowerment and patient-centred consultations

A 'patient-centred' consultation would be where the doctor very much takes a more passive role and is directed by the will of the patient where all possible treatment choices have been provided. For example:

Patient: 'I would like you to refer me to my private orthopaedic surgeon for a knee replacement as my arthritis has now become unbearable, despite regular analgesics, physiotherapy and acupuncture.'
(*I really have no interest in your medical opinion, you are too young, my complaint is serious, and besides which Professor Hammer-Drill has always sorted me out in the past!*)

Doctor: 'Fair enough! I'll get my writing pad!'
(*Fine! Off you go then! That was a nice quick one!*)

It is fair to say that both the above styles of consulting do have their place. There are still some people who prefer a more 'old-fashioned' type of consultation, where doctor indeed does know best, and directs the treatment plans. These people often give themselves away with statements such as 'I'm in your hands, doc!' or 'I'll do anything you say, doctor!'.

The most striking illustration of a person who felt this way is the possible example of an elderly gentleman with an enormous laparotomy scar on his abdomen when he was examined for slight constipation. When the doctor enquired why this enormous operation had been performed, he replied, 'I don't know, I never asked!'. The patient who knows exactly what he or she wants and the doctor submits to their request can also indeed be appropriate, as long as the patient's request is reasonable, as was the above patient with the knee pain.

However, in the scenario with the patient with knee arthritis perhaps the doctor should have asked a few more questions to ensure arthritis was the diagnosis and answered any questions that patient might have had about knee replacement surgery.

Being patient-centred

What does it mean? What are the attributes of the patient-centred doctor? Perhaps the following are a few of the attributes that such a doctor might attempt to provide:

- partnership with patients
- informed choice
- empowerment and encouraging patients to take more responsibility
- shared decision making
- dignity in healthcare
- concordance
- health promotion
- expert patients and patient education
- patient advocates
- shared records
- patient participation groups
- helping patients handle uncertainty.

All these pivot on good communication.

Practical point
The more communication improves between patients and healthcare professionals, the more patient-centred consultations will become.

There are certain tasks within consultations which, if undertaken adequately, will enable a doctor to be patient-centred. First and foremost, seeing the patient as a person and being empathetic and so the doctor trying to put him or herself in the predicament of the patient. Being concerned for the whole person and the illness they have and not just disease and parameters of the disease such as blood glucoses in a person with diabetes. This means ascertaining the impact of the psychological, social, emotional, cultural and spiritual factors on their illness (holistic approach).

Furthermore, the doctor should elicit a patient's ideas, concerns and expectations and therefore to be sure that the patient's and doctor's agenda are the same and so finding common ground. Finally, devoting the required amount of time necessary to ensure patient satisfaction, which can be difficult given the present resource and service constraints of the NHS. Little *et al.* (2001), in a survey of 865 consecutive patients, concluded that if doctors do not provide a positive patient-centred approach, patients will be less satisfied, less enabled, and may have a greater symptom burden and higher rates of referral.

Forming a partnership in the consultation

The third style of relationship is probably the most appropriate in most circumstances, and is 'partnership' in decision making. Balint called this state of affairs a 'mutual investment company' between the doctor and the patient. This is where options would be discussed honestly, and the management of the condition negotiated and decided upon together in a collaborative way.

The potential advantage of this situation is:

- concordance of the patient with the agreed treatment plan, and
- hopefully if things do go wrong (which unfortunately will always happen at least once in a doctor's career), the patient would be less likely to instigate a complaints proceedings, as both parties had decided and agreed on the action.

This approach also transfers some of the responsibility of decision making from the doctor to the patient.

Patient ideas, concerns and expectations

Partnerships through meeting a patient's ideas, concerns and expectations (ICE)

Let's re-visit the consultation between Mrs Jones and Dr Smith. This time, Dr Smith will be patient-centred and endeavour to consult 'in partnership' with Mrs Jones and empower her to make an informed decision as to her management.

Mrs Jones: 'Good morning, Doctor.'

Dr Smith: 'Good morning, Mrs Jones. Please take a seat. What can I do for you today?'

Mrs Jones: 'Well, it's probably nothing, Doctor, but for the last four or five mornings I have had some blood on the toilet paper when I opened my bowels.'

Dr Smith: 'You seem rather worried. Would you like to tell me why?'

Mrs Jones: 'I hope you don't think I'm being foolish, but I'm rather worried about bowel cancer.'

Dr Smith: 'Of course you are not being foolish. What makes you think about cancer?'

Mrs Jones: 'My mother died of bowel cancer at about my age, Doctor. I think this is more likely to be piles or similar, as I have not had any weight loss or change in my bowels that my Mother described, and it's only been going on a few days, but, well, you never know.'

Dr Smith: 'I'm sorry to hear about your mother. What were you hoping I could do to help you today?'

Mrs Jones: 'I was rather hoping you could examine me, if it's not too much trouble, and perhaps send me for some tests if you felt it necessary.'
(Dr Smith performs a rectal and abdominal examination with the practice nurse who was between patients and acted as a chaperone with Mrs Jones's agreement. The whole process took about two to three minutes. A small haemorrhoid was found which had recently bled.)
Dr Smith: 'Well, I'm pleased to say you were right about the piles (haemorrhoids) and it would not appear to be anything more sinister at this moment in time.'
Mrs Jones: 'That is a relief. Should I go for some more tests, just to make sure?'
Dr Smith: 'The chance of cancer is very low indeed as I have found a cause for the bleeding. How would you feel about some simple cream to treat the piles first? Tests in hospital can be unpleasant, and have the potential of a slight risk to your health. You could let me know if the bleeding does not stop within the next two weeks, or if you notice any symptoms similar to your late mother developing. Then of course we could organise some further investigations.'
Mrs Jones: 'That sounds sensible, Dr Smith. I'll try the cream first. Goodbye, and thank you for your time!'

Patients' ideas, concerns and expectations

If a patient's ideas, concerns and expectations (ICE) are ascertained during the history as discussed in Chapter 2, they can play a vital part in the mutual sharing, negotiation and agreement of a management plan.
   Dr Smith explored the patient's ICE as follows.

*   Ideas (I) – blood on toilet paper may be due to more than just piles.
*   Concerns (C) – Mrs Jones is worried that she may have bowel cancer which her mother died from.
*   Expectations (E) – physical examination and specialist referral.

In the scenario detailed, Dr Smith has changed from being a doctor-centred paternalistic doctor to a patient-centred doctor, informing and empowering the patient in the decision-making process of the management plan.

Decision making and the management plan

The plan between the doctor and the patient was negotiated, with the doctor being honest about both the risk of cancer and the small risks involved with performing invasive investigations.
   This type of doctor–patient partnership should result in good compliance with treatment, and a satisfied patient.
   Management plans are discussed in depth in Chapter 6.

Keys to achieving rapport

The potential list here is endless. Here are some key points.

- Ensure a good bedside manner by enabling a friendly but professional relationship with patients.
- Pay due regard to the values of medical practice (*see* Chapter 11) and being aware that the values and attitudes of a patient may be different to that of the doctor.
- Be sensitive to the needs of patients through code of dress, communicating professionally with the patient and so addressing them appropriately.
- A doctor should guard against being paternalistic and strive to be patient-centred and so work in partnership with each patient.
- Optimise quality of care through a shared understanding of the health problem and agreeing how it might be managed.
- Chapter 12 will go into depth regarding all the different possible consultation models in relation to optimising the doctor–patient relationship.

Bibliography

Balint M. *The Doctor, His Patient, and The Illness*. Edinburgh: Churchill Livingstone. First published by London: Pitman; 1957.

Bates C. The good doctor. *Clinical Medicine*. 2001; **1**: 128–31.

Cohen JJ. White coats should not have union labels. *New England Journal of Medicine*. 2000; **342**: 431–4.

Cooper C. What do you call yours? *The Lancet*. 2000; **355**: 1566.

Dieppe P, Horne R. Personal view: Soundbites and patient-centred care. *BMJ*. 2002; **325**: 605.

Gordon R. *Doctor in the House*. Novel first published in 1954.

Harnett PR. Should doctors wear white coats? *Medical Journal of Australia*. 2001; **174**: 343–4.

Jeffs SG. Being a good doctor. *Journal of the Royal College of General Practitioners*. 1973; **23**: 683–90.

Little P, Everitt H, Williamson I, Warner G, Moore M, Gould C, Ferrier K, Payne S. Observational study of effect of patient centredness and positive approach on outcomes of general practice consultations. *BMJ*. 2001; **323**: 908–11.

Stewart M. Towards a global definition of patient-centred care. *BMJ*. 2001; **322**: 444–5.

Van Der Weyden MB. Editorial: White coats and the medical profession. *Australian Medical Journal*. 2001; **174**: 324–5.

Williams S, Weinman J, Dale J. Doctor-patient communication and patient satisfaction: a review. *Family Practice*. 1998; **15**: 480–92.

Chapter 4

Physical examination

Dr Rodger Charlton

Rodger Charlton has written this chapter as a vital part of the consultation is a physical examination of the patient and he has attempted to provide some useful hints and principles based on a common area of physical examination: measuring blood pressure. Other issues such as the assessment situation, consent, chaperones, instruments and what to carry in an emergency bag are discussed.

It is often said that the most important part of the consultation in the diagnostic process is the history and a small percentage is attributed to the physical examination and an even smaller proportion to investigations. Nevertheless, the aim of this chapter it to emphasise the importance of physical examination within the consultation and the need to develop competence in the many skills involved, both in their application and interpretation.

This chapter is divided into the following sections.

- An introduction to clinical examination.
- The four rules of clinical examination.
- Measuring blood pressure.
- Assessments and examinations.
- Consent.
- Chaperones.
- Instruments and the doctor's bag.

An introduction to clinical examination

Confirming the diagnosis

Examination traditionally takes place after a history has been taken and may be used to confirm or refute a possible diagnosis.

For example, a patient is complaining of a fever, a severe sore throat, a lump when they swallow and who believes that they have seen white spots at the back of their mouth when they looked in mirror. Examination is likely to reveal a red throat and exudate on the tonsils. In addition, a thermometer may reveal a raised temperature and measurement of the pulse, a tachycardia. A diagnosis of tonsillitis can therefore be confirmed.

Examination as part of the healing process

It is almost an expectation by patients that the doctor will examine them. In this case of a patient with tonsillitis, the patient is reassured that the doctor has used their clinical examination skills to confirm or refute the concern that they have a throat infection, but more than this to make a diagnosis and exclude any other sinister cause.

It may seem far-fetched, but the act of examination in this scenario and palpation to detect lymphadenopathy, a further indication of an associated infection as a result of tonsillitis, is an act of reassurance which may be referred to in healing terminology as the 'laying on of hands'.

A 'good examination'

A comment that some patients make after they return from the hospital is that they had 'a really good examination'. This is often a thorough examination by a junior doctor. For the patient, this signifies that their illness is being taken seriously. The patient is reassured by the care and interest that has been taken. A poor examination, or no examination at all, may lead a patient to a feeling of being 'short changed'.

Why examine patients?

A history is taken to record symptoms. An examination is performed to detect physical signs.

The four rules of clinical examination

In order to detect signs follow four simple traditional rules and adhere to them in this order.

1 Observation using your sight, hearing and smell.
2 Palpation using your hands.
3 Percussion using your fingers.
4 Auscultation using a stethoscope.

Rules for any examination

First and foremost, observe. Do not rush to pull out a stethoscope. The stethoscope has limitations and yet many doctors feel 'naked' without one. The next time you go into a hospital canteen, observe how many doctors have a stethoscope still around their neck or prominently protruding from their pocket.

The trouble with doctors is not that they don't know enough, but that they don't see enough. (Corrigan 1853)

Just by looking at a patient you may notice some important things, e.g.:

• distress, e.g. due to pain
• if they are very pale and possibly anaemic

- jaundice
- cyanosis
- breathlessness
- a rash
- swelling.

Practical point

Observation starts from the minute a patient walks through the door of the consulting room or if you go to see a patient in a hospital ward or in their home.

Examination may involve one of the major organ systems and so undressing a patient – in which case, observe the chest or the abdomen or a particular limb before you do anything else. You may notice a vital sign, e.g. a fast respiratory rate.

Observation and the 'ill' child

Observation is particularly important when consulting with parents and their young children. Many children consult as a result of self-limiting illnesses and a difficult decision to make is to decide when a child is seriously ill and requires specialist treatment. Children usually do not pretend to be ill and so good signs to observe in a young child are that the child is:

- alert
- smiling
- able to walk (over the age of one year)
- running about (over the age of one year)
- talking.

Whereas signs of concern may be the child who is:

- listless and not crying
- pale and floppy
- very irritable
- vomiting.

Vital signs

When asked to see a patient who is acutely unwell it is important to record the following in addition to their overall appearance:

- respiratory rate
- pulse
- blood pressure
- temperature.

Practical point
The purpose of this chapter is not to teach all physical examination skills as there are several books devoted to the subject and referenced at the end of the chapter.

However, there is one generic skill that all doctors will be required to perform regularly and is one that, if conducted incorrectly during an assessment of a practitioner's performance, can be the difference between passing and failing. This is the measurement of a patient's blood pressure.

Measuring blood pressure

Be very familiar with this examination as it is easy to conduct on most patients and lends itself as a basis for assessment. This section is detailed as there is debate over the consensus relating to blood pressure measurement. Knowledge of this topic will provide the basis for defending the approach used to this particular examination. This section details the use of a traditional mercury sphygmomanometer, the technique of which should be learnt prior to using a comparable electronic device.

The blood pressure depends principally on the cardiac output and the peripheral resistance and is traditionally measured using the upper arm. The range of normal varies considerably not only with age but from patient to patient and factors such as the circumference of the arm and the width of the cuff. Other important factors include emotions and recent exercise. The information gained from a single reading can therefore be limited, bearing in mind that most people's blood pressure varies substantially throughout the day. In addition, the diagnosis of hypertension, both systolic and diastolic hypertension, is regularly debated in an attempt to reach a consensus. For these and other reasons, 24-hour blood pressure monitors are being more frequently used in the diagnosis of hypertension.

Which arm?

In 6% of hypertensive patients, there are pressure differences of more than 10 mmHg between the arms. Therefore, in an initial assessment, the blood pressure in both arms should be measured. The arm with the higher pressure should be used subsequently and this is likely to be up to 5 mmHg higher in the dominant arm. If there is a difference greater than 10 mmHg then a cardiovascular cause should be considered.

The cuff

Measurement involves the application of a cuff on the arm of a relaxed patient when relevant clothing has been moved so that the arm is bare above the bifurcation of the brachial artery. Cuffs differ as some are wrapped around the arm and the last part tucked in although many cuffs use Velcro instead.

Be careful to make sure the cuff is applied the correct way round! (The centre of the rubber bag should be over the inner side of the arm.) The standard size is 12 cm, but a smaller cuff may be required in children and a larger cuff in adults who have large arms. This precaution is necessary otherwise the size of cuff will affect the accuracy of the blood pressure reading. (The bladder inside the cuff should encircle 80% of the arm.) Some practitioners even debate whether the tubing from the cuff should point upwards or downwards on the arm. If the tubing lies over or around the brachial artery bifurcation, it may create noise interference when applying a stethoscope. Ideally, the lower edge of the cuff should be 2.5 cm above the antecubital fossa where the stethoscope is to be placed.

The patient's arm should be supported at the level of the heart ('heart height') by an arm rest or by the practitioner. In particular, the midpoint of the upper arm should be at the same level as the heart. The bifurcation of the brachial artery at the elbow will be just below this point.

Inflation of the cuff

The cuff should be inflated until the pressure increases above the systolic pressure in the brachial artery. (The cuff should be inflated rapidly to 70 mmHg and then by 10 mmHg increments while palpating the radial pulse.) At this point, the brachial artery is compressed, so that the radial pulse is obliterated and will become impalpable. (The cuff should be inflated to about 30 mmHg above the systolic pressure as found by palpation.)

Deflation of the cuff

Auscultation should be conducted during slow deflation of the pressure in the cuff of about 2 mmHg per heartbeat.

Blood forces its way past the obstruction artificially created by the cuff when the radial pulse returns and becomes palpable. It is good practice to check the systolic pressure roughly by palpation of the radial artery before applying the stethoscope. Similarly the brachial artery should have been palpated prior the application of the stethoscope.

The bell (low frequency head) of a stethoscope should be applied lightly over the brachial artery and sounds referred to as Korotkov (Korotkoff) sounds can be heard. (Some practitioners will argue for the use of the diaphragm of the stethoscope.) With the pressure continuing to fall slowly and uniformly, the sound increases to its maximum intensity and then decreases at first gradually and later suddenly and then quickly disappears.

Systolic and diastolic readings

Practical point
The systolic pressure is the highest pressure at which successive sounds are heard and is the highest pressure to which blood pressure rises on the walls of the arteries with the contraction of the ventricles.

The pressure or air in the cuff should be allowed to continue to fall slowly while the stethoscope is applied over the brachial artery. The point at which the loud, clear sounds change (fade) abruptly (become suddenly muffled) is considered by some to be the nearest to the diastolic pressure, the so-called fourth-phase Korotkov sound. Very shortly afterwards, these dull and muffled sounds usually disappear altogether and when they are inaudible this is referred to as phase five of Korotkov sounds. However, in a few individuals sounds may be audible until the cuff is fully deflated.

Practical point

The diastolic pressure is the minimum pressure in the artery when the aortic valve is closed and the left ventricle is relaxing.

The second and third Korotkov sounds relate to the intensity and character of the pulse sound and these are now only of historic interest.

Providing systolic and diastolic readings

The systolic reading is the first phase of Korotkov sounds. However, there has always been debate as to the definition of the diastolic. For this reason insurance companies when requesting medical reports often ask for readings at both 'K4 and K5'. Articles cited at the end of this chapter provide a consensus that K5 is the diastolic blood pressure.

Auscultatory gaps

Use of the diaphragm of the stethoscope alone may result in a mistake as Korotkov sounds may not be heard – a so-called 'auscultatory gap'. This is because in some patients with hypertension, the first phase of Korotkov sounds may disappear and then are heard again as the pressure in the cuff is lowered. This is referred to as an auscultatory gap. Similarly, in some subjects sounds disappear during phase 3, then reappear: another potential auscultatory gap leading to a possible erroneous diastolic reading.

Korotkov sounds

At rest, blood flow is laminar and silent. No sounds are usually heard when a stethoscope is placed over the brachial artery although in patients with severe atherosclerosis or with certain heart valve problems the actual diastolic blood pressure may be heard with the cuff fully deflated or lower than one would expect. However, the artery is also silent when the blood flow is stopped by inflating the cuff above the systolic blood pressure.

As blood begins to spurt through the compressed artery, the turbulent flow is audible. The vibrations in the artery walls are called 'Korotkov sounds' and are the sounds that a practitioner listens for with a stethoscope when they are taking blood pressure. They are named after Dr Nikolai Korotkov, a Russian physician who described them in 1905, when he was working at the Imperial Medical Academy in St Petersburg. The sounds are divided into five phases based on the loudness and quality of the sounds.

- Phase 1 – appearance of a pulse sound; loud clear tapping or snapping sounds are heard which grow louder as the cuff is deflated.
- Phase 2 – as the cuff is deflated further, the artery opens and closes, and the flow of blood is turbulent, so a succession of murmurs/sounds are heard. They may disappear during this phase if the cuff is deflated too slowly.
- Phase 3 – the sounds become louder and have a thumping quality similar to phase 1.
- Phase 4 - the point of muffling – the thumping sounds of phase 3 are abruptly replaced by a muffled sound.
- Phase 5 – the disappearance of all sounds. This phase is absent in some people.

When the cuff pressure is less than the diastolic pressure, the artery is open all the time, and the flow of blood is smooth, and all sounds usually disappear.

Repeated readings and discomfort to the patient

The examination should not be repeated frequently or the cuff kept inflated for prolonged periods as it can be quite uncomfortable. In addition, if a reading is initially high, it may be worth repeating after 5 or 10 minutes as some people are apprehensive about having their blood pressure measured which is often referred to as the **'white coat effect'**. This is thought to be a significant influence in at least one fifth of patients, even when the patient is seated in a quiet and calm environment. This can lead to the diagnosis of hypertension being made incorrectly.

When making a diagnosis of hypertension, it is important to review a patient's readings at least on three separate consultations.

Practical point
Measurements can be particularly difficult when an arrhythmia is present and there is variation in blood pressure from beat to beat. Thus, it can be difficult to determine the auscultatory endpoint.

Postural hypotension

To what extent do blood pressure measurements vary depending on position, i.e. sitting, standing, or lying down? Normally, properly taken BP measurements should show only minor variations with changes in position. However, it should be remembered that when the blood pressure is measured, the arm should be at the level of the heart. If the arm is allowed to hang down straight, the BP may be falsely diminished by a few millimetres' mercury below its true value. This is not an issue when the person is lying down, as long as the arm is kept alongside at the level of the body.

When can postural hypotension be diagnosed? This requires measuring the blood pressure when the patient is supine (lying down) and then repeating the reading after they have stood up (erect). If you wait two minutes, this allows for equilibration. In general, the greater the change, the more likely this is to cause symptoms and be of clinical significance. Differences up to 20 mmHg or differences with symptoms such as feeling light-headed or faint would lead a clinician to suspect postural hypotension. In the acute situation this can be due to hypovolaemia and in the clinic setting may be due to, e.g., autonomic nervous system dysfunction in a patient with diabetes who does not generate appropriate arterial vasoconstriction when changing positions. However, there are many possible causes for this and it should be investigated. Usually it will be diagnosed following blood pressure measurements of a patient lying and standing where the condition has been suspected as a result of certain symptoms, e.g. fainting episodes, recurrent dizziness, unsteadiness and falls. The symptoms may result from a temporarily reduced cerebral blood supply. In the early stages this condition may present first thing in the morning when the circulating blood volume is at its lowest.

Which sphygmomanometer?

Which type of sphygmomanometer should be used? This is an area of debate at the present time as the use of mercury sphygmomanometers may be phased out following recommended European legislation and potential hazards of mercury. If a mercury sphygmomanometer is used it must be upright and not tilted. Aneroid sphygmomanometers may need to be recalibrated against mercury ones.

A mercury sphygmomanometer is still seen by many as the 'gold standard' as readings are in millimetres of mercury (mmHg) and care needs to be taken when selecting and using automated devices. All sphygmomanometers need to be regularly serviced and recalibrated. When taking a reading some practitioners round off reading to the nearest 2 or 5 mmHg although this is technically incorrect. It may be that kilopascals are the unit used to measure blood pressure in the future rather than millimetres of mercury.

Common mistakes which interfere with the accuracy of blood pressure measurement

- Use of an inappropriately sized cuff.
- Failure to allow a period of rest before measurement.
- Deflating the cuff too fast.
- Not measuring in both arms.
- Failure to palpate maximal systolic pressure before auscultation.

Diagnosis of hypertension

This is an area of ongoing debate and discussion. There are both local and national consensus guidelines available. In relation to blood pressure measurements it is important to emphasise that a diagnosis of hypertension should not be made on a single reading, but on a series of at least three separate readings. Where there is doubt regarding the diagnosis, 24-hour ambulatory blood pressure monitoring should be considered.

Assessments and examinations

How thorough should an examination be?

It is often not practical to examine every system and to conduct the minutiae of physical examination in every patient. Time in consultations is a limiting factor and a patient who consults with, e.g., acute asthma does not require examination of the foot pulses in the feet as it is very unlikely to have any relevance. Indeed it may be difficult to explain to a patient who is wheezing and having difficulty breathing why you wish to look at their feet. Having said this there are times where examination of the legs may be appropriate in someone with a suspected viral illness to exclude a rash. Therefore, always explain to a patient why you are examining a particular part of the body if it is remote from the site of the symptoms.

For those who are learning examination skills for the first time, it is important to examine the system requested thoroughly and avoid short-cuts. Discrimination and examination of specific aspects of the body will come with experience and the focused examination of the hypothetico-deductive approach. If in doubt, do not skip part of an examination.

Assessments and clinical examinations

Traditionally, the physical examination is a skill that can be observed by a university or Royal College examiner and so assessed against a defined standard. There are, however, slight variations relating to the agreed standards.

In an examination it is likely that a candidate will be asked when presented with a clinical scenario or after they have taken a history: 'What examination would you like to perform and why?'

Think carefully before you answer and do not commit yourself to a complex examination, e.g., of the nervous system, unless it is clinically indicated. Consider a focused examination, e.g. testing power or reflexes in the lower limbs.

Tips in examinations

It may seem obvious, but ensure the following interaction takes place with the patient.

- Wash your hands between patients.
- Greet the patient and introduce yourself.
- Ask their permission to conduct a particular examination.
- Explain what you intend to do and why.
- Suggest that they let you know at any time if they wish you to stop the examination, e.g. if it is uncomfortable.
- Before examining a patient, make sure they are comfortable, e.g. if they are lying on an examination couch.
- Ask them to remove articles of clothing if this is appropriate, e.g. listening to the chest through a shirt will lose you most of your marks.
- Where appropriate seek permission to bring in a chaperone.
- If appropriate and to maintain dignity when undressing a patient, allow them to undress behind a screen and cover up parts of the body that are not essential to the examination and may cause potential embarrassment.

- Be sensitive to a patient's needs and ask them to redress in case they get cold.
- Always seek permission for intimate examinations, e.g. a rectal examination, and conduct such examinations only if they are essential and they will aid the diagnostic process.
- Try and answer questions that a patient may ask as a result of an examination.
- As you conduct the examination, keep talking to the patient and continue to explain what you are doing. If an examiner is present this will reassure them of your competence and ability to maintain a rapport with a patient.

Know when to stop the examination! For example, if you are listening to the lung fields remember that, if the patient is taking regular successive deep breaths, they may start to feel dizzy as a result of hyperventilation. This is particularly the case if they already feel unwell as a result of a chest infection. Allow them to have a rest. If you feel it necessary, repeat the examination, explaining why.

Similarly, measuring the blood pressure repeatedly in the same arm is uncomfortable or leaving the blood pressure cuff at a pressure above the systolic for long periods of time is not a pleasant experience for a patient.

Consent

Before any examination, consent must be obtained and not assumed. For some examinations this involves careful explanation of the various components of the physical examination. Some physical examinations will be highly focused and the patient may be fully clothed; in other cases the patient may be partially or completely unclothed. Doctors have an obligation to respect the dignity of each patient and to conduct each consultation in a manner that strives to provide a comfortable and considerate atmosphere. Where it is necessary to remove clothing or conduct intimate examinations the use of a chaperone should be considered and offered.

Privacy

Give the patient privacy to undress and dress and provide the sensitive use of drapes to maintain the patient's dignity. Also, where appropriate, provide gowns. If possible provide a separate examination room for a patient to undress or ensure a curtain is pulled round the examination couch. Where consultations are being videoed for training, a cap must be placed over the camera lens. Do not assist the patient in removing clothing unless you have clarified with them that your assistance is required.

Where clothing has been removed

UK climate, one feels cold quickly without clothing. Doctors should be ⸱arding this and not prolong examinations and invite the patient to ⸱n as possible.

ut their usual clothing may feel vulnerable and embarrassed.

Patients have clear legal and ethical rights and doctors are likely to be seeing them at a time of illness and therefore considerable stress. There is clear guidance on consent for examination and treatment and the actions doctors must take relating to consent. Similarly, there should be consent for students and doctors in training to see patients as part of their learning (GMC 1998).

Practical point
Consent is the informed choice of a competent patient, freely given.

More complex explanations and the signing of appropriate paperwork (consent forms) is required for consent to treatment for surgical procedures.

Chaperones

Whether a consultation takes place at home, in a general practice surgery, or at an outpatient clinic, the fundamental right of all patients (of either sex or any sexuality) is to maintain their autonomy and to make informed decisions for themselves. This must extend to the presence or absence of a chaperone, and doctors should respect their wishes.

The chaperone may be a relative, patient advocate or an authorised healthcare professional. All must adhere to the confidentiality of the consultation.

Practical point
If a patient falsely accuses you of misconduct during an unchaperoned examination, you will stand alone in court.

Even if you successfully defend yourself or settle the case before trial, the allegation alone will take a significant toll on your reputation and your practice. It almost seems unnecessary to discuss chaperones with adults, but in today's healthcare environment, having a chaperone in the examination room can protect you from potential frivolous legal action. It is probably best if the chaperone is the same sex as the patient.

Offer a chaperone or invite the patient (in advance if possible) to have a relative or friend present. If the patient does not want a chaperone, record that the offer was made and declined. If a chaperone is present, you should record that fact and make a note of the chaperone's identity. If you cannot offer a chaperone, if possible offer to delay the examination until one is available.

The General Medical Council (GMC) regularly receives complaints from patients who feel that doctors have behaved inappropriately during an intimate examination. Intimate examinations, such as examinations of the breasts, genitalia or rectum, can be stressful and embarrassing for patients. When conducting intimate examinations you should:

- explain to the patient why an examination is indicated and give the patient an opportunity to ask questions

- explain what the examination will involve and ensure the patient understands
- obtain the patient's permission/consent
- keep discussion relevant and avoid unnecessary personal comments
- stop the examination if the patient asks you to
- record everything in the patient's records.

Doctors must always be alert to the **patient's** needs. Chaperones should be offered, not inflicted, and it should be borne in mind that chaperones may interfere with the doctor–patient relationship and in some situations may even be perceived as a 'spectator'.

Some patients may also be offended as they see it as a lack of trust in them by a doctor. Patients have a right to an examination without a chaperone being present and it is up to the doctor whether or not to continue with the examination given the discussion above. (This issue is regularly updated on medical websites including the GMC, BMA and some Royal Colleges. These are a useful source of further information.)

Instruments and the doctor's bag

In order to examine a patient adequately and so make a comprehensive clinical assessment, certain instruments should be available and they are the likely equipment to be found in a GP's emergency bag used for conducting home visits. These instruments include a:

- stethoscope
- sphygmomanometer
- torch
- otoscope/ophthalmoscope
- thermometer
- gloves and lubricating jelly
- tendon hammer
- pen!

Other important equipment and items may include:

- urinalysis testing strips
- tongue depressors
- *British National Formulary* (BNF)
- prescriptions.

For a general practitioner performing house visits there are certain other items that may be required which constitute a 'mobile office' including:

- stationery
- booklet of useful emergency numbers
- a mobile phone
- a map or local A–Z.

In emergency situations away from a hospital clinic or GP surgery environment, the following equipment may be useful in a patient's home:

- portable oxygen cylinder
- nebuliser with salbutamol nebules
- syringes, needles and cannulae for intravenous access
- saline drip set
- tourniquet and pressure dressings
- pocket resuscitation mask
- an airway
- blood glucose monitoring laboratory testing sticks/glucometer
- space blanket
- a selection of emergency drugs for oral, rectal and intravenous use, e.g. aspirin, GTN, anti-emetics, opiates, naloxone, frusemide, adrenaline, salbutamol, atropine, dextrose, glucagon, benzyl penicillin and hydrocortisone for IV/IM use, prednisolone, chlorpheniramine, rectal diazepam, chlorpromazine and glycerine suppositories. The list is endless and the medications should be in date and a protocol should be in place to ensure they are regularly checked. Perhaps others, such as antibiotics and paracetamol for use in children, should be considered.

The type of bag used is an individual choice and it should be lockable and have multiple compartments in which to keep the above and not left exposed to extremes of temperature.

Bibliography

Berger A. Oscillatory blood pressure monitoring devices. *BMJ.* 2001; **323**: 919.

Bevers G, Lip G, O'Brien E. ABC of hypertension. Blood pressure measurement. *BMJ.* 2001; **322**: 981–5.

Bignell CJ. Chaperones for genital examination. *BMJ.* 1999; **319**: 137–8 (and associated correspondence – see also GMC website).

Charlton R. Blood glucose testing strips – essential in general practice. *The Practitioner.* 1989; **233**: 1208.

Corrigan DJ. *Lectures on the Nature and Treatment of Fever.* Dublin: Fannin and Co.; 1853.

Epstein O, Perkin GD, Cookson J, de Bono D. *Clinical Examination.* London: Mosby International; 2003.

Fraser R. *Clinical Method: a general practice approach.* 3rd ed. Oxford: Butterworth Heinemann; 1999

General Medical Council (GMC). Seeking patients' consent: the ethical considerations. *Duties of a Doctor.* 1998. Retrieved 15 Dec 2005, from www.gmc-uk.org/guidance/library/confidentiality.asp.

Macleod J. *Clinical Examination.* 6th ed. Edinburgh: Churchill Livingstone; 1983.

McAlister FA, Straus, SE. Measurement of blood pressure: an evidence based review. *BMJ.* 2001; **322**: 908–11.

O'Brien E. Replacing the mercury sphygmomanometer. *BMJ.* 2000; **320**: 815–16.

Swash M, Hutchison R. *Hutchison's Clinical Methods.* Edinburgh: Saunders; 2001.

Toghill P. *Examining Patients: an introduction to clinical medicine.* London: Edward Arnold; 1994.

Chapter 5

Problem solving and the diagnostic process

Dr Ian Ward, Dr Emma Hopgood and Dr Rodger Charlton

Without a diagnosis it is difficult to provide a treatment. Ian Ward and Emma Hopgood look at the problem-solving process in depth. Rodger Charlton looks at the difference between an illness and a disease and the psychosocial factors that influence illness and so problem solving.

To consider reaching a diagnosis as an end point is to miss the point. A simple definition of the term diagnosis is the identification of a disease.

This chapter is divided into the following sections.

- Prior knowledge, presenting complaint and the history.
- Problem solving through diagnostic hypotheses.
- Further enquiry.
- Iterative hypothesis testing.
- Physical examination.

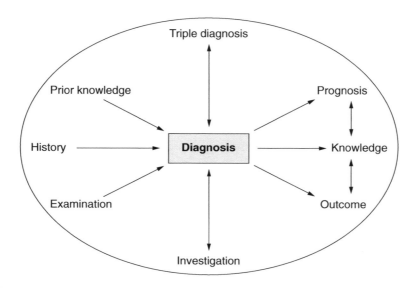

Figure 5.1 'Mind map' for the diagnostic process.

- Health and well-being.
- The bio-psychosocial model and the 'triple diagnosis'.
- Disease or illness?
- Difficult diagnoses.
- Frequent attenders.
- Medically unexplained symptoms.
- The 'difficult' patient.
- Prognosis and outcome.

In reality a diagnosis is a central hub around which numerous issues and activities are taking place in the diagnostic process as illustrated by Figure 5.1.

Prior knowledge, presenting complaint and the history

Even before a patient enters the room, the process of diagnosis is beginning. The clinician will know facts relating to the patient from a variety of sources. This **prior knowledge** may come from the patient's medical record in the form of their:

- age
- sex
- previous consultation notes
- hospital discharge letters
- summaries
- test results.

It may also be from less tangible sources such as personal recollections or information imparted by the patients' family, be it from a consultation regarding a related problem or in a communication from a concerned relative. Additional details may have been acquired from other members of the healthcare team, for example health visitor, district nurse, social services or hospital doctor.

Having greeted the patient and allowed them time to settle, an enquiry into their problem will result in the patient offering a **presenting complaint**, e.g. 'I have come about pain in my chest.'

The process from the presenting complaint through to history taking is described in Chapter 2.

Practical point

It is somewhat artificial to divide a consultation into its component parts, but for the sake of emphasis and learning about the consultation, this is the approach of this book and its division into different chapters.

It may be appropriate to refer to Chapter 2 while reading this chapter in relation to some of the terms that are used.

When the history has been started, diagnostic hypotheses and so the creation of differential diagnoses takes place. There is then a need to test these hypotheses and thus further enquiry and information gathering from the patient is required.

It would be helpful therefore to revise at this point what is meant by 'diagnostic hypotheses' as this is pivotal to the problem-solving process and so making a diagnosis.

Problem solving through diagnostic hypotheses

This is a process of questioning which has resulted from a clinician who has considered the initial history and, following reflection, has formulated a number of possible medical conditions/causes (diagnostic hypotheses)/differential diagnoses for a patient's symptoms or problems. As Figure 5.1 illustrated, hypotheses should take into account other factors contributing to a patient's illness such as age, gender, ethnicity and social circumstances.

In an effort to confirm or refute and thereby reduce the list of potential conditions, selective examination, looking for specific signs to support or reject diagnostic hypotheses, will reduce the list to hopefully limit the number of **working diagnoses to one or two** and certainly less than five. This way of thinking, 'The Diagnosing Mind', arose at McMaster University in Canada and others in the 1970s onwards and has become an important component of the Leicester Assessment Package as detailed in Fraser's *Clinical Method* (2000).

At this point it may be appropriate to instigate selective investigations to substantiate or eliminate one or other of these diagnoses to leave a definitive **diagnosis**. These procedures may vary in complexity from simple practice-based dipstick tests, e.g. of urine, through an array of laboratory-based blood tests to complex investigative procedures such as endoscopy, angiography or a radiological scan. As investigations become more invasive, implications relating to health economics and risks of morbidity and even mortality to the patient increase. It can be appreciated therefore that focused investigation, soundly based on clinical history and examination, is of benefit to patients both individually and collectively.

> When once your point of view is changed, the very thing which was so damning becomes a clue to the truth. (From *The Problem of Thor Bridge* by Sir Arthur Conan Doyle)

Common things are common

This might seem obvious, but it depends on the clinical environment in which a clinician is seeing patients. It is possible to construct a 'symptom pyramid'. Take the example of the symptom of a cough. In general practice it is unlikely that this symptom would indicate a possible lung cancer, but as times passes and the problem does not resolve it becomes more likely that it could be lung cancer when the person consults a doctor in a specialist hospital chest clinic and so the person and their 'problem' moves up the pyramid.

Practical point
Common things are common!

An important lesson is to think of common causes first, before rare more serious causes, particularly when sharing your thoughts with a patient.

Further enquiry

One drawback of an active mind is that one can always conceive alternate explanations which would make our scent a false one. (From *The Problem of Thor Bridge* by Sir Arthur Conan Doyle)

In a case of a person with chest pain creating differential diagnoses/diagnostic hypotheses these might be:

- ischaemic heart disease
- musculoskeletal chest pain
- psychological/stress
- respiratory.

Although ischaemic heart disease is not the commonest cause of chest pain, it is listed first as it is the most important to exclude initially. This leads to the next phase of history taking and so problem solving – further enquiry. The case of a person with chest pain is used as an example to illustrate the problem-solving process of 'further enquiry'.

There is a need now to ascertain which differential diagnosis is the correct one. This is carried out by asking leading and specific questions relating to the list of differential diagnoses and so the process of further enquiry called **hypothetico-deduction**. However, it is necessary to avoid double questions in order to avoid confusion. Examples of double questions are: 'Do you have dizziness or fainting attacks?', 'Do you have pain and numbness in your legs?' The following questions could be posed under the four differential diagnoses/causes raised for a person with chest pain:

- ischaemic heart disease
- musculoskeletal chest pain
- psychological or stress
- respiratory.

Ischaemic heart disease

Ischaemic heart disease would normally present with a central tight/heavy chest pain brought on by physical activity and relieved by rest. Further questions may be:

- 'Do you suffer from diabetes?'
- 'Do you have high blood pressure?'
- 'Do you smoke? If so, how much and for how long?'
- 'Do you have any family history of heart disease?'
- 'Do you have any shortness of breath?' and
- 'Do you have swollen ankles?'

Musculoskeletal chest pain

Musculoskeletal chest pain would be related to chest-wall movement, particularly involving upper body movement. Further questions may be:

- 'Have you had any injury?'
- 'Is there any local tenderness?' and
- 'Is the pain worse on deep breathing, coughing or movement?'

Psychological or stress

Psychological or stress causes of chest pain are likely to come and go in line with periods of stress. It very important to identify other features of anxiety and/or depression. Further questions may be:

- 'Are you happy with your life?'
- 'Do you feel stressed?'
- 'What is your mood like?'
- 'Do you feel depressed?'

If any of these are issues it can be productive to ask around work, rest and leisure compartments of life. Life events analysis could yield interesting information of emotional conflict, unresolved grief as well as ideas and concerns linking their current problems. Relationship problems are a major cause of tension and discontent and need exploration. Thinking about an idea of a family portrait (the nuclear and extended family) set among their community will aid better understanding and direct your enquiry. There is indeed a huge variation from how insular and lonely people can be to the well-connected family and social networks. An open question may be in order.

- 'Who is at home?'
- 'How are you getting on with your partner?'
- 'Is there anybody else around to help with your children?'

Other questions assessing the mental state may be:

- 'Do you sleep well?'
- 'How is your appetite?'

If a deeply depressed picture emerges, then it is vital to enquire about possible self-harm and suicidal intent.

Respiratory

Respiratory causes of chest pain are possible. Symptoms of a chest infection should be excluded. The pain might be localised and you would need supporting evidence and so the following questions may be asked:

- 'Do you smoke?'
- 'Do you have any cough?'
- 'Do you bring anything up when you cough?'

More sinister causes such as cancer or pulmonary embolism may generate questions such as:

- 'Have you ever noticed any blood in the phlegm that you cough up?'
- 'Are you short of breath?'
- 'How is your appetite?'
- 'Are you losing any weight?'

Having gone through a selective systems enquiry, each question will either support or refute a particular differential diagnosis or hypothesis.

Practical point
It is important to appreciate the value of each question with reference to a particular complaint.

In other words, there are sensitivity and specificity issues related to every symptom and its related question. This is largely learned through experience, individual reflection and more importantly through discussion with colleagues.

Iterative hypothesis testing

The testing of hypotheses is part of the hypothetico-deductive way of arriving at a possible diagnosis when taking a history and so attempting to problem solve. The above example of a patient with chest pain illustrates this process well. A paper written by Kassirer on this subject in the *New England Journal of Medicine* in 1983 states that 'by an iterative process, hypotheses are either eliminated or confirmed, and those that survive are made progressively more specific' and so is a method of 'clinical problem solving'.

Using the example above this can form the basis of a teaching seminar where students come with cases they have seen in clinical practice and the only information the rest of the group have is that of a 42-year-old man with chest pain. They ask the student a series of questions, the answers to which can be written by a scribe elected from the group under the following headings:

- prior information, e.g. age, gender, past medical history
- presenting complaint, e.g. chest pain
- pre-diagnostic interpretation
- questions are asked to clarify the presenting complaint, e.g. the severity and location of the chest pain
- specific features, e.g. physical examination and investigations
- a list of diagnostic hypotheses are created (differential diagnosis).

(The prior knowledge of the patient can be 'married' to the presenting complaint formulating a pre-diagnostic interpretation (Fraser 2000). This is a broad-brush assessment to identify affected systems and gives a strategic aim for the history taking. This is detailed earlier in Chapter 2.)

In the paper, Kassirer (1983) refers to the student as a 'data repository' and so substitutes the place of the 'patient' and thus simulates the patient. The information and diagnostic hypotheses are continually refined and reinterpreted through further questions/enquiry in an attempt to confirm or refute a possible hypothesis or diagnosis.

Practical point

By definition iterative means a process that is characterised by repetition.

There is an opportunity for this learning exercise to be extended by the facilitator asking the value of each question asked, its justification and whether it has influenced which is the most likely working hypothesis.

Kassirer suggests that by acting as a simulated patient, 'this proxy eliminates exposure of the patient to a crowd of students who are offering hypotheses to explain his or her illness, rationales for their questions, and – perhaps most threatening – interpretations of the answers'. The approach is based on a sound theory of the cognitive aspects of human problem solving in the clinical setting. The emphasis is on the problem-solving process and not the proxy (the student).

The process of iterative hypothesis testing encourages trainees to **integrate their learning** in basic medical sciences and to process the information they have gained to facilitate problem solving.

Physical examination

At this stage you should be thinking about which system or area of the body you wish to examine. For clinical efficiency, it needs to be focused and appropriate. It should be based on the diagnostic hypotheses that have been generated and so leading a clinician to ask which part of the body they might wish to examine and why.

For each bit of examination you propose, ask yourself what are you looking for and how will it affect your diagnostic thought processes.

Practical point

Examination should further test the diagnostic hypotheses that you have created and so help to confirm or refute them.

Occasionally, doctors 'go through the motions' for the sake of patient expectation/satisfaction but you must weigh the pros and cons of your actions. In the case of the chest pain scenario, it would be appropriate to observe and palpate the chest wall for any areas of tenderness and the apex beat. A simple cardiovascular examination would be required.

It is an expectation by many patients that they will be offered and undergo a physical examination. It can be very reassuring to have a physical examination and there is almost an analogy with the priestly function of 'laying on of hands'. Sometimes where an examination is not indicated, a patient may say, 'Aren't you going to measure my blood pressure while I am here?' Similarly, patients who visit their GP after attending a hospital clinic may say, 'I got a really good examination at the hospital'. Examination for patients can be a very positive experience and part of the 'healing' process.

Physical examination is discussed in depth in Chapter 4. However, bearing in mind the finding that the majority of diagnoses can be made from the history alone, examination is not the most important component of the problem-solving process, but may help to confirm a diagnosis that there is considerable evidence for in the history. There are also occasions where a physical examination may not be indicated and so required, e.g. a patient with a psychiatric problem. Psychiatrists, however, conduct a clinical examination of the patient's mental state.

Health and well-being

To date we have been considering a diagnosis in terms of physical entities. However, a patient's social circumstances, their occupation, housing, family network, financial circumstances and many other factors can interact with any physical condition. Not only may some of these factors contribute to the diagnosis, but also the reverse is true in that the diagnosis will almost certainly have an impact on their social framework. Consider a patient with a simple hernia, which may possibly have occurred at work, through lifting. Not only is the patient now unable to continue his or her job but also surgical repair of the hernia may well require time off work with the possible loss of income. Further reduction in functional capacity through inability to drive and to work post-operatively will also have a social impact.

Similarly a patient's fears and anxieties relating to any given diagnoses has to be taken into consideration. A patient may well have previous experience of a given condition, through a friend or relative, or personal experience of investigation, procedure, or hospitalisation. These anxieties may be unfounded or otherwise but will be very real to the patient and will certainly have an impact. These social and psychological components, taken along with a physical diagnosis, and their mutual interaction affect a person's health and so well-being.

Practical point

The WHO definition of health is a state of complete physical, mental and social well-being and not merely the absence of disease or infirmity.

Marinker, a professor of general practice, wrote in 1987:

At the centre of general practice is the encounter between the doctor and the patient. If we fail to value the uniqueness of the doctor and the patient, the role of feelings and situations in the interpretation of symptoms and findings, we are condemned to be second rate players in a second hand game.

The bio-psychosocial model and the 'triple diagnosis'

Current medical literature supports the use of the **bio-psychosocial model** in assessing patients. This can be a three-way process, as the presenting complaint could originate from one of the three dimensions as well as affecting them (i.e. both cause and effect). A patient presenting with chest pain may have an overwhelming psychological cause, which may affect the physical well-being and capability to do their job. There may be social consequences in terms of loss of income affecting family welfare and social role consequences.

The following diagram illustrates the bio-psychosocial model.

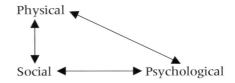

This could be more complex still if further dimensions are considered such as emotional and spiritual.

In contrast, non-specific symptoms like tiredness and lethargy, possibly set against multiple symptomatology or erroneous connections to previous illnesses or life events, may take considerable patience and clinical skill to diagnose. These are short stories set among a far wider story, referring to intercurrent illnesses with a background of chronic illness or multiple pathologies. It needs to be appreciated that patients' stories may be neither well formed or well articulated. Therefore the practitioner's role, in such situations, is to make connections of the different fragments of the story and construct a 'shared' meaning and understanding. The connections of the different fragments of a story to the social situation and relationships needs to be established. This process is referred to as the **bio-psychosocial model**.

The 'triple diagnosis'

If the patient's health beliefs, ideas, concerns and expectations (ICE) and cues to action are sufficiently motivating and he or she believes the benefits outweigh the costs, the decision to consult will be taken. All this before the consultation has begun!

Communication is a two-way process and during the consultation the doctor elicits information to define the physical and social aspects of the patient's problem while trying to ascertain their thoughts and feelings to understand the psychological component. This holistic view of the patient has been referred to as the **'triple diagnosis'**. The process of diagnosis is often complex and involves many variables. Three important factors are physical, social and psychological. In one account of diagnostic method, Marshall Marinker (1981) describes this method of 'triple diagnosis' which requires that physical, social and psychological factors all be taken into account (as appropriate) in every diagnosis. A broad viewpoint such as this helps the doctor to empathise and improves communication.

Practical point
Care should be taken using this phrase as dual or triple diagnoses can also be applied to patients in psychiatric practice who have a mental health problem and substance misuse (dual diagnosis) and HIV (triple diagnosis).

Several studies have found good communication is associated with patients' satisfaction. Indeed, studies have demonstrated that up to half of psychosocial and psychiatric problems are missed and a similar proportion of patient problems and patient concerns are not elicited by the doctor or disclosed by the patient. The psychological component may be volunteered by the patient, partially revealed by body language, or, most frequently, second-guessed by the doctor. Direct questions about the patient's thoughts, worries and hopes can often show even the most experienced doctors how wrong their guesses or assumptions are. A 'dysfunctional' consultation can be remedied by exploring ideas, concerns and expectations when these have not already been addressed. (This is discussed in depth in Chapter 2 with practical examples.)

Disease or illness?

The Royal Colleges of General Practitioners of the UK, Australia and New Zealand have as their College motto – *Cum Scientia Caritas*. This may be defined as: 'Scientific skills with loving-kindness'.

The role of the doctor has been compared to that of both a priest and an engineer. However, with increasing technological advances in medical science the public now perceives the profession more and more as engineers. A greater expectation is therefore put on the scientific aspect of medicine and associated practitioners. Until recently this idea of the doctor as an engineer has been fostered within medical schools where students concentrated on the scientific and technological aspects of medicine rather than the improvement of communication skills and 'bedside manner'.

One stimulus for change has been the discovery that most patient complaints arise out of communication problems, rather than a lack of knowledge or negligence. It is communication that perhaps can be seen as one of the important components of the art of medicine, which is sometimes compromised by the science. Also as most diagnoses arise from the history, good communication skills are essential.

Practical point

Most patient complaints arise out of communication problems, rather than a lack of knowledge or negligence.

Furthermore, the doctor working in primary care should also bear in mind the importance of communication as it has been estimated that many people visiting a GP, and thus perceiving themselves as being ill, have no serious disease (Bass and Murphy 1990). The majority of patients are seen in primary care and it is a role of the primary care practitioner to problem solve when presented with an 'undifferentiated' illness and refer disease which cannot be managed in primary care to specialists in secondary care.

A disease can lead to an impairment of the normal physiological functioning of a patient, often referred to as a pathological condition. In turn, this leads to the characteristic symptoms, 'sickness' and functioning and, thus, an illness.

Similarly an illness can be where a person has symptoms, e.g. due to worry, concern or anxiety, but no disease is present. **Somatising** may therefore be a feature and this is discussed later in the chapter.

Practical point
Illness and disease are therefore not synonymous.

Imagine the scenario where someone says to you: 'You don't look well today. Do you feel OK?' Suddenly, having felt well, you may start to feel ill.

Figure 5.2 illustrates that there are separate entities of disease and illness and that they overlap, but it is not meant to illustrate the likely proportions. The other variable in the equation has been denoted 'life' and so is an extension of the bio-psychosocial model and the concept of the triple diagnosis.

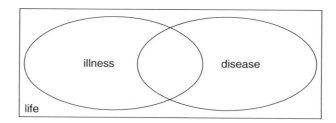

Figure 5.2   Illness or disease?

This concept is well described in a paper in 1981 by Helman who wrote from the perspective of a GP and an anthropologist.

> Illness is what the patient feels when he goes to the doctor and disease is what he has on the way home from the doctor's office. Disease, then, is something an organ has; illness is something a man has. Illness refers to the subjective response of the patient to being unwell; how he, and those around him, perceive the origin and significance of this event; how it affects his behaviour or relationships with other people; and the steps he takes to remedy this situation. It includes not only his experience of ill-health, but the meaning he gives to that experience. Even responses to physical symptoms, such as pain, can be influenced by social and cultural factors; these factors can in turn affect the presentation of the symptoms and the behaviour of the patient and his family.

Furthermore, Helman goes on to say that: 'Illness can occur in the absence of disease.'

Practical point
Illness can occur in the absence of disease.

If a doctor observes a patient from the perspective of an engineer then it may be forgotten that each patient is first and foremost a living being with an illness which is far more important than their disease. Each patient has hopes and fears like any of us and is particularly vulnerable when they come to consult a doctor. Whether or not they have a disease, it is these hopes and fears that can lead to an illness.

An example of a patient who has a disease without an illness is the person who has a high cholesterol where there are no disease symptoms and the person is unaware that they have a high cholesterol. They therefore have a disease, but not an illness. Similarly, a disease such as thyroid disease may have no obvious symptoms. A point in time will be reached, however, where one of these diseases and their eventual associated symptoms will impact on the life of the person and so lead to an illness.

Practical point

A disease will affect individuals in different ways and is likely to present differently in individuals as a clinical 'problem', hence the use of the expression of problem solving.

Much of this section may be seen as semantics and common sense, but it should be remembered that one major role of healthcare and the 'good doctor' is to differentiate in problem solving between disease and illness and to help patients cope in time of illness or disease or both and the associated suffering by guiding them through the complex maze of the medical world as a professional and a friend. This empathetic approach should be based on a definition of empathy.

Practical point

Empathy as a doctor is trying to put yourself in the position of a patient.

Empathy is not a new notion and is defined together with sympathy in the *Journal of the American Medical Association* in 1958:

The act or capacity of entering into or sharing the feelings of another is known as **sympathy**. **Empathy**, on the other hand, not only is an identification of sorts but also connotes an awareness of one's separateness from the observed. One of the most difficult tasks put upon man is reflective commitment to another's problem while maintaining his own identity. The ways in which one person may react to another are infinite. (Aring 1958)

A subtle and significant feature of a happy medical practice is to remain unencumbered by the patient's problem.

Dr Richard Wescott, a GP in Devon, wrote in 2005 that the word 'empathy' is sometimes used as a synonym for sympathy. He further wrote that:

sympathy is feeling with someone; but the stronger empathy is about truly identifying: engaging your own experience and making a real effort to almost become – just for a moment – that other person.

However, a practitioner must also be realistic and remember: 'I can't feel what he is feeling'.

Even when medical science has no more to offer a patient it is still the job of the doctor to continue to care for them. A job of the 'good doctor' is to alleviate the suffering caused by an illness. The philosophy of '**healing**' is often perceived as analogous with curing. However, healing may also be enabling a patient to come to terms with an illness where cure is not possible, e.g. in a terminal illness, and so maintaining an optimum quality of life.

The sections that follow in this chapter describe the importance in differentiating in problem solving between disease and illness and that this is more than a semantic concept and has relevance to clinical practice.

Difficult diagnoses

Any truth is better than indefinite doubt. (From *The Yellow Face* by Sir Arthur Conan Doyle)

Sometimes it can be difficult to make a diagnosis, or a diagnosis may later be found to be incorrect.

C Sidney Burwell, the dean of Harvard Medical School, USA, from 1935 to 1949, said at a Harvard dinner:

My students are dismayed when I say to them, '*Half of what you are taught as medical students will in ten years have been shown to be wrong, and the trouble is, none of your teachers knows which half.*' (*Harvard Medical Alumni Bulletin*, October 1947, p. 4)

Sometimes patients bring multiple symptomatology which may or may not be connected. A particular set of symptoms, such as polyuria, polydipsia and weight loss, would indicate diabetes. If no pattern or meaning emerges, then symptoms will have to be dealt with and explored separately. By negotiating with the patient you may be able to prioritise symptoms/problems that can be tackled on the day. Less important symptoms can be left for another day. Occasionally, the presenting complaint may be vague and ambiguous, e.g. 'I don't feel right', 'I am not a well man' or 'I feel woozy'. The first priority would be to clarify the terms that are used, to shed more light on the problem. For this sort of problem you would require a comprehensive systems analysis, often referred to as an **inductive** method of history taking, detailed in Chapter 2.

History taking is not always a straightforward exercise. For example, patients may come with a **hidden agenda** or a problem unrelated to the presenting complaint. Their reasoning would be to 'test the water' and to see if they felt comfortable enough and 'safe' to disclose the real problem. If the doctor's approach is open and receptive then a patient's disclosure would come both easier and earlier. Sometimes a cycle of frequent and serial consultations develops as the real patient agenda/problem remains undiscovered. Similarly, patients may discuss at length a particular problem and a second problem is thrown in at the end which actually may be much more serious. An example might be of a

65-year-old lady presenting with sore throat and a chesty cough. Before leaving with an antibiotic prescription she introduces a second problem of 'pain in the side of my chest' and pointing into the axilla. Examination reveals a large cancerous gland. Fortunately, this sort of situation is rare but can occur.

Practical point
It may be in some consultations that the patient is deciding whether or not it is 'safe' to tell the doctor why they have really come to consult.

The lady with the large cancerous gland is a good example of this and so the minor physical problem of a sore throat and cough may mask or cover up what is sometimes referred to as the **hidden agenda**. They may also be reluctant to give this information for fear that the doctor may confirm their worry that this might be a sinister disease such as cancer. This may also happen when a patient has what they perceive as an embarrassing request, e.g. for contraception or a sexual problem.

At the end of a consultation or clinical encounter, this possibility of an agenda remaining hidden may be reduced by simply asking: 'Is there anything else you wanted to ask?'

Frequent attenders

The professor of medicine at Manchester in the 1960s, Professor Platt, wrote:

> The first staggering fact about medical education is that after two and a half years of being taught on the assumption that everyone is the same, the student has to find out for himself that everyone is different, which is what his experience has been since infancy. (Platt 1965)

Nick Summerton, a GP in Hull, makes the analogy that symptoms are like unravelling difficult knots. When he was a student it seemed so clear. A patient would describe a symptom or set of symptoms as if he had read an appropriate textbook and would be able to categorise the 'case' into a disease group. The problem is, as Dr Summerton puts it, 'Our patients do not seem to have read the script'. Problem solving is not straightforward as one might imagine and the human body is not one that always lends itself to the problem-solving approach and processes of an engineer. For example, patients and doctors differ in their interpretation of common terms such as diarrhoea, constipation or heartburn. Hopefully, we recognise this with the patient who says that they are 'dizzy' by asking what they mean or understand by dizziness.

Practical point
Ask patients what they understand by commonly used terms such as dizziness, heartburn or tiredness.

The average GP attendance per patient is three to four times a year. What of those who attend more frequently? Clearly those with multiple physical problems need to attend more frequently, but what of those where there is absence of physical disease? This can lead to a high workload, together with increased prescribing and referral rates. In addition studies have shown that entire families and not just individuals may become medically dependent. Sometimes these individuals are referred to as the 'worried well'.

Reasons why a patient might consult frequently:

- fear of what a symptom may represent
- desire for an explanation and symptomatic relief
- pressure from relatives or work
- the wish for medical input rather than self-care
- loneliness or doctor dependence
- medical unexplained symptoms
- other unrecognised issues, e.g. bereavement, depression.

As long ago as 1927, Dr Francis Peabody wrote in the *Journal of the American Medical Association* that perhaps as many as one third of all those attending medical outpatients have symptoms without the presence of disease. He questions the role of holistic care which has been discussed previously and describes doctors as too 'scientific' and writes:

The practice of medicine in its broadest sense includes the whole relationship of the physician with his patient. It is an art, based to an increasing extent on the medical sciences, but comprising much that still remains outside the realm of any science.

He then writes: 'the treatment of the disease may be entirely impersonal; the care of the patient must be completely personal'. He concludes his paper, which is still frequently quoted, 'one of the essential qualities of the clinician is interest in humanity, for the secret of the care of the patient is in caring for the patient'.

When problem solving, a **holistic** approach to care is therefore required. Joshua Freeman, Professor of Family Medicine at the University of Kansas, USA, has written:

We are not doctors for particular diseases, or particular organs, or particular stages in the life cycle – we are doctors for people. People are complex, and live in complex communities in a complex world. All aspects of the world have an impact on the health of the people in it.

A **holistic approach** to medicine therefore deals with health problems in their physical, psychological, social, cultural and existential dimensions (see EURACT – European Academy of Teachers in General Practice: www.euract. org/html/index.shtml). A mission statement of Professor Bill Shannon of the Royal College of Surgeons of Ireland was reported recently in *The Irish Medical Times* as: 'It is often more important for a family doctor to know the person who has the disease than the disease the person has.'

Medically unexplained symptoms

Bearing these comments in mind, papers regularly appear in the literature on the subject of '**medically unexplained symptoms**'. They leave the clinician with a feeling of uncertainty and one result has been the word 'syndrome' in an attempt to explain a collection of non-specific symptoms and signs.

Practical point

A definition of a syndrome can be: 'a complex of signs and symptoms that when occurring together suggest a particular disease'.

Examples are irritable bowel syndrome (IBS) or chronic fatigue syndrome (CFS) where patterns of somatic symptoms are highlighted in relation to particular bodily systems. Sometimes these are referred to as **functional syndromes** which are often transient but in a few people they do not resolve.

In the context of problem solving, one of the difficulties of seeing frequent attenders with medically unexplained symptoms are the array of possible diagnoses that may result, some of which are medical (e.g. fibromylagia) and some psychiatric (e.g. anxiety or depression).

Similarly an illness can be where a person has symptoms, e.g. due to worry, concern or anxiety, but no disease is present – **somatosising** and so physical symptoms may be a feature. Such symptoms of anxiety will be familiar to everyone for their effect on the cardiovascular system, e.g. the heart racing or perhaps 'missing' a beat, and the gastrointestinal tract, e,g. nausea or diarrhoea. *They only become abnormal when they are disabling.*

Practical point

Somatosising is the physical manifestation of psychological problems. It is not the faking or fabrication of physical symptoms. They are real symptoms which the person believes have a medical explanation but where no organic cause is apparent.

Patients with anxiety or depression frequently present with somatic symptoms and symptoms that can resolve with recognition and treatment of the underlying cause. Symptoms should be seen in context. The chances are that the frequent attender without an obvious organic cause may well not have a physical cause of their symptoms. However, that is not always the case and similarly a patient who has not been seen for a long time and has a thin set of patient records may have something serious wrong with them.

It is perhaps helpful to define two further terms that clinicians sometimes use.

Hypochondriasis is the preoccupation with or fear of having a serious illness. This can be a normal process for everyone at least once in their lives, but becomes abnormal when individual patients appear to become 'addicted' to reassurance and have repeatedly normal investigations performed.

Conversion disorder is a syndrome characterised by a loss of function that appears to be due to a physical cause, but is actually a manifestation of unconscious psychological conflict and can be considered the successor to the term 'hysteria'.

In relation to problem solving, the clinician will seek a solution to a patient with medically unexplained symptoms. It may be that psychological and psychiatric factors are overlooked and that the possibility of anxiety or depression should be considered. If this is the case their distress has neither been appropriately identified or addressed.

Practical point

Both doctors and patients are reluctant to explore the 'non-biological' aspects of a person's illness given the continuing stigma associated with mental illness.

For those patients with somatisation disorders, attempted medical 'explanations' may reject the reality of their symptoms whereas identification of underlying psychological issues and the provision of appropriate coping strategies may empower a patient and lead to resolution of their symptoms which may be affecting them at home and their performance at work.

Practical point

Identification of underlying psychological issues and the provision of appropriate coping strategies may empower a patient and lead to resolution of their symptoms which may be affecting them at home and their performance at work.

Problems may be solved in the study which have baffled all those who have sought a solution by the aid of their senses. To carry the art, however, to its highest pitch, it is necessary that the reasoner should be able to utilize all the facts which have come to his knowledge, and this in itself implies, as you will readily see, a possession of all knowledge, which, even in these days of free education and encyclopaedias, is a somewhat rare accomplishment. (From *The Five Orange Pips* by Sir Arthur Conan Doyle)

The 'difficult' patient

A patient could be perceived as 'difficult' as the doctor may not have been able to address a patient's unexplained medical symptoms. They may attend frequently with their symptoms and Professor Tom O'Dowd *et al.* (1988) of Trinity College Dublin in the literature have described such patients as making a doctor's heart 'sink' when they enter the consulting room. They have referred to them as **'heartsink'** patients.

To prevent this scenario from happening it is important to remember that the consultation is a partnership and the doctor should recognise their own emotions and views and so be more **patient-centred**. Chris Pearce (2002), who is a GP in Australia, writes:

Often these consultations degenerate into mutual hopelessness, where the patient feels hopeless as the doctor can 'do nothing' and the doctor feels hopeless for the same reason.

Practical point
Once the doctor and patient recognise this situation they can both agree on achievable goals so the hopelessness may be lifted and so a way of solving the patient's problems may be achieved.

A difficult patient may also be one who is difficult as a result of their behaviour, e.g. a patient who is aggressive or violent. **Antisocial behaviour** is generally on the rise and can surface in consultations. Subtle forms of manipulative behaviours are commonplace, where patients change their roles (child, adult and parent described by Berne, 1964) to suit themselves and their needs. Verbal aggression and body language can shift the power axis within the consulting room, leading to bullying, disturbance of the peace and possible violence. This presents a huge challenge to the therapeutic encounter and it is therefore essential to be perceptive and dampen inflamed attitudes early.

A difficult patient may also be one who is referred to as a '**malingerer**' where disease is simulated for personal gain, e.g. for gaining a sick note to stay off work legitimately.

A rare cause of the difficult patient is a patient with **Munchausen's syndrome**. Munchausen's syndrome is an unusual syndrome first reported by Asher in 1951. Sufferers describe past histories that are dramatic and believable but untrue, and they present with an 'acute illness' which is fictitious. After numerous painful and unnecessary investigations or operations, the many falsehoods in a patient's history may be discovered. At this point a patient may present to a different doctor or hospital, sometimes with a different name. It is usually seen in people with **personality disorders** and may also be induced in a dependent person, e.g. a child, and is referred to as **Munchausen's syndrome by proxy**. These are fortunately rare conditions but in relation to problem solving may be one of a long list of possible differential diagnoses.

Other difficult situations can arise in relation to problem solving in the consultation and these are discussed in later chapters, e.g. **communication difficulties** with patients who speak a different language, may have hearing impairment or have a learning disability.

Ian McWhinney is a professor of family medicine in Canada and he believes we need a 'new clinical method' particularly for 'difficult' patients. He wrote about three aspects of this new **patient-centred clinical method**.

1 At every consultation the doctor should ascertain the patient's understanding of the illness, his feeling about it, especially his fears, its impact on his life, and his expectations about the outcome and about treatment.
2 The doctor should attempt to find a common ground of understanding with the patient.
3 Validation is provided by the patient, who says whether or not they have been given the opportunity to express themselves and whether the doctor has understood them (McWhinney 1993).

An interesting letter appeared in the *Quarterly Journal of Medicine* entitled 'Difficult patients or difficult encounters' (De Marco *et al.* 2005). Focusing solely on difficult patients may influence what is already a complex issue in the doctor–patient relationship. It could be that an observer of a consultation sees not a difficult patient, but a difficult doctor.

Practical point

It could be that an observer of a consultation sees not a difficult patient, but a difficult doctor.

Prognosis and outcome

Establishing a diagnosis allows a clinician to draw on knowledge and experience relating to that specific condition, enabling him or her to predict the natural history or course of the disease and so an extended aspect of problem solving. This is known as the **prognosis**.

Knowledge of the exact diagnosis also allows specific treatment to be brought to bear as part of effective **management**. (Management entails far more then specific medication and will be covered in more detail in the next chapter.) Clearly patient response to management will affect prognosis, and changes in the development of the condition may require alterations to management.

It should be remembered that a diagnosis always carries with it a degree of uncertainty. Clinical history along with examination, supported with appropriate investigations, increase the confidence of a diagnosis. However, it should be remembered that diagnoses are to a certain extent provisional pending a successful **outcome**. As can be seen from Figure 5.1, all these stages interface. An unfavourable outcome requires reassessment of diagnosis through history, examination or investigation, or review of the management plan, which in turn will impact on the triple diagnosis.

In many medical journals there are short sections devoted to personal views. In the *BMJ* they are 'fillers' as well as personal views and in *The Lancet* 'Uses of error'. Many refer to anecdotes and where perhaps problem solving or communication has not been ideal. Kevin Barraclough is a GP who has written a personal view on the diagnostic process in the *BMJ* and its importance. He wrote in 2002:

> All the skills that are rightly revered by the Royal College of General Practitioners – listening, communication, empathy – are seriously devalued if major diagnoses are missed. And are they missed? I have little doubt that they are. My own vicarious experiences, observing the outcome from a distance with family, friends, and colleagues who attend their GPs, have been very mixed. The personal views and fillers in this journal bear witness to the fact that diagnostic accuracy is not necessarily something that you can rely upon in all general practitioners. Nor, of course, in hospital practitioners. None of us gets it right all the time.

Practical point

'None of us gets it right all the time.'

I ask my registrars to try to put down their differential diagnosis with the condition they can't afford to miss as number one. Many of the differential diagnoses may point to the fact that further investigation is unnecessary or undesirable. But they have made that decision with clarity, and not through vagueness or laziness. I try to persuade them that holistic medicine need not be, indeed must not be, woolly and imprecise.

Practical point
'Holistic medicine need not be, indeed must not be, woolly and imprecise.'

This radical suggestion leads to quizzical, raised eyebrows. Am I trying to turn the general practice registrar into a hospital physician? Am I neglecting to keep a reflective diary, neglecting to assess my registrar's ideas, concerns, and expectations? Am I being too dogmatic? Maybe.

But I sit through videos of consultations done to assess competency and have to tick a box about whether the registrar is 'responding to cues'. Surely this is nonsense – an entirely subjective assessment. We seem to be trying to assess something that is important, but manifestly unmeasurable. And we are neglecting something that is at least as important – diagnostic skills – which is eminently measurable.

Practical point
When it comes to assessments and exams, 'diagnostic skills are eminently measurable'.

This is a theme that will appear in another chapter, which reiterates the observation that 'none of us gets it right all of the time', whether undergraduate or postgraduate, student or professor. In other words, we are all lifelong learners and as doctors perhaps the **most important areas of learning are**:

- identification of learning needs
- recognition of our own limitations and
- reflection on critical incidents which result from our ability to problem solve and so make a diagnosis.

Education never ends, Watson. It is a series of lessons, with the greatest for the last. (From *The Adventure of the Red Circle* by Sir Arthur Conan Doyle)

Bibliography

Aring CD. Sympathy and empathy. *JAMA*. 1958; **167**(4): 448–52.
Asher R. Munchausen's syndrome. *The Lancet*. 1951; **260**: 339.
Barraclough K. Actually, making a diagnosis is quite important. *BMJ*. 2002; **324**: 179.
Bass C and Murphy M. Editorial: The chronic somatiser and the Government White Paper. *J Roy Soc Med*. 1990; **83**: 203–5.

Berne E. *Games People Play*. Harmondsworth: Penguin; 1964.

Charlton R. Viewpoint: A shared understanding of cancer. *New Zealand Medical Journal*. 1994; **107**: 245–6.

Charlton R, Smith G, Day A. Munchausen's syndrome manifesting as factitious hypoglycaemia. *Diabetologia*. 2001; **44**: 784–5.

De Marco MA, Nogueira-Martins LA, Yazigi L. Difficult patients or difficult encounters? [Letter.] *Quart J Med* 2005; **98**: 542–3.

Elrington G. Medically unexplained symptoms. *General Practitioner*. 2002; **4 March**: 57–8.

Elstein AS, Schwarz A. Clinical problem solving and diagnostic decision making: selective review of the cognitive literature. *BMJ*. 2002; **324**: 729–32.

Fraser R. *Clinical Method; a general practice approach*. Oxford: Butterworth Heinemann; 2000.

Freeman J. Towards a definition of holism. *Br J Gen Pract*. 2005; **55**: 154–5.

Helman CG. Disease versus illness in general practice. *J Roy Coll Gen Pract*. 1981; **31**: 548–52.

Kassirer JP. Teaching clinical medicine by iterative hypothesis testing. *New England Journal of Medicine*. 1983; **309**: 921–3.

Marinker M. Whole person medicine. In: Cormack J, Marinker M, Morrell D, editors. *Teaching General Practice*. London: Kluwer Medical; 1981.

Marinker M. Journey to the interior: the search for academic general practice. *J Roy Coll Gen Pract*. 1987; **37**: 383–8.

Mayou R, Farmer A. ABC of psychological medicine: functional somatic symptoms and syndromes. *BMJ*. 2002; **325**: 265–8.

McCulloch GL. The James Dundas Simpson Address: Cum Scientia Caritas. *J Roy Coll Gen Pract*. 1969; **18**: 315–20.

McDonald PS, O'Dowd TC. The heartsink patient: a preliminary study. *Family Practice*. 1991; **8**: 112–16.

McWhinney IR. Why we need a new clinical method. *Scand J Prim Health Care*. 1993; **11**: 3–7.

O'Brien MD. Medically unexplained neurological symptoms. *BMJ*. 1998; **316**: 564–5.

O'Dowd TC. Five years of heartsink patients in general practice. *BMJ*. 1988; **297**: 528–30.

Peabody FW. The care of the patient. *JAMA*. 1927; **88**: 877–82.

Pearce C. The difficult patient. *Australian Family Physician*. 2002; **31**(2): 177–81.

Platt R. Thoughts on teaching medicine. *BMJ*. 1965; **ii**: 551–2.

Ring A, Dowrick C, Humphris G, Salmon P. Do patients with unexplained physical symptoms pressurise general practitioners for somatic treatment? A qualitative study. *BMJ*. 2004; **328**: 1057.

Shannon B. *Irish Medical Times*. 2005; **April**.

Summerton N. Making sense of symptoms. *UPDATE*. 2005a; **70**(1): 31–5.

Summerton N. The distinct nature of primary care diagnosis. *UPDATE*. 2005b; **70**(4): 32–5.

Turner J. Editorial: Medical unexplained symptoms in secondary care – consider the possibility of anxiety or depression – or simply distress. *BMJ*. 2001; **322**: 745–6.

Walsh K. How common is common? *BMJ*. 2004; **329**: 397.

Watkins P. Editorial: Medically unexplained symptoms. *Clinical Medicine*. 2002; **2**(5): 389–90.

Wescott R. The power of empathy. *DOCTOR*. 2005; **12 April**: 35.

Wynne-Jones M. Dealing with a frequent consulter. *PULSE*. 2004; **13 September**: 74–5.

Chapter 6

Patient management

Dr Catti Moss, Dr Ryan Prince and Dr Rodger Charlton

In order to resolve an illness and make a patient better a management plan or management plans need to be formulated and agreed with a patient. This chapter is a combined effort by the three authors where treatment is a distinct therapeutic component of the medical management process.

It can be argued which part of the consultation is most important – for example, finding out why the patient has come or making a diagnosis – but, for any of these to have an effect, a diagnosis must be communicated to the patient, and an appropriate agreed plan of action made. Management is that action plan and, defined literally, management is the art or act of managing or skilful treatment.

In a truly patient-centred consultation, successful management is not necessarily what the *doctor* might judge as being 'best for the patient' and this is the theme that this chapter repeatedly explores.

This chapter is divided into the following sections.

- Why have an action plan?
- Reaching a shared understanding.
- Explanation.
- Negotiating a management plan.
- Treatment (medical or surgical).
- Handing over responsibility to the patient.
- Follow-up.
- Conclusion.

Why have an action plan?

For the patient, the management is what they came to the doctor for, and what they take out with them when they go. Traditional medical teaching has laid its emphasis firmly upon the diagnostic process and has tended to include little in the way of management skills. However, a correct diagnosis is of little use if it resides in the mind of the doctor and is not communicated and acted upon.

A plan of action that is not put into practice cannot be very effective, so learning how to transfer the ownership of the plan to the patient is a crucial skill. This process can be called **'formulating a negotiated management plan'**.

Perhaps doctors' poor ability at management is reflected by the many prescriptions given that are not taken to the pharmacy to be dispensed, not to mention those that are started and then stopped. This is the topic of many papers in the literature. There is a difference in patients' and doctors' perceptions concerning the kind and amount of drug information being provided and in 1984 Bartlett reported that for every 100 pills prescribed, only 82 were reported taken. These facts are important as it is estimated that up to two thirds of GP attenders receive a prescription as part of their consultation. Similarly, when, as part of a management plan, a doctor advises a patient to give up smoking, there is less than a 7% chance that they will not be smoking in a year's time according to a recent paper by Grandes *et al.* (2003). However, it is very likely that the other interventions that doctors advise have a better uptake.

Consider the following scenario. With enforced time constraints on consultations, it is all too easy to envisage the common situation that may arise for patients when a friend asks:

'How did you get on at the doctor?'

The patient replies:

'I'm not quite sure, but he said that the problem was in my chest and it would go away if I took these tablets.'

Information is important, as knowledge about the illness provides reassurance and ensures that the correct therapeutic measures are undertaken. Unfortunately, the giving of this information and so management within the consultation which includes **explanation** is a neglected area. While research into the consultation has placed much emphasis on ways of soliciting information from patients, it is has devoted less effort to how informative the consultation should be to the patient.

Practical point
The fact that many patients remember little of what is told to them suggests that methods of explaining problems to them or the amount of information doctors give may be inadequate or inappropriate.

Patients have their own theories about illness and will interpret new information within the framework of their existing ideas. The consultation provides an opportunity for explicit sharing of these ideas. However, there is evidence that patient compliance with management and treatment depends on the information that the doctor provides and the way in which it is communicated.

The role of the doctor should be as an informed professional, being in an advisory rather than managerial position. In other words the doctor should facilitate **patient-centred management** by giving patients the strategies required.

For example, to facilitate effective self-management of the above patient with a chest problem who has actually got influenza the following is required; the patient needs to understand in their own terms what a virus is, its expected course and duration, the appropriate use of combined antipyretic and analgesic preparations and when to seek a further consultation.

So, let us first of all consider what is happening in patient management, and what the process involves.

Delivering a management plan can be divided into three basic stages:

- reaching a shared understanding of the problem
- negotiating a management plan
- handing over responsibility to the patient.

The overall effect is a transfer from doctor to patient: of knowledge, ideas, actions and responsibility.

Reaching a shared understanding

This is the most important part of the whole consultation. In fact, the main aim of any consultation as proposed by Pendleton *et al.* (1984) can be said to be to reach a 'shared understanding' of the problem. Patients often come to a consultation quite late in a long process. They already have definite ideas about their problem, which they will have refined by thought and discussion and reading. They have concerns about the problem that may not be immediately obvious to an outsider, but are very important to the patient, and they come with definite expectations about what they want from the doctor.

Practical point

However, a patient coming to a consultation always expects to gain greater under-standing of the problem from his contact with the doctor, no matter how many other items they may have on the agenda.

Reaching a shared understanding sounds very simple. In practice, it is sometimes easy and sometimes it is difficult. Often the understanding that the patient reaches is not the same as the understanding the doctor wanted to communicate. Often the doctor is unaware of the difference. The information gathered from a patient from the history, examination and investigations should be summarised and related to the patient's own needs and experience.

The better we get at consulting, the more likely we are to be aware of the difficulties, and thus able to respond.

How can we look at the process in a helpful way?

Occasionally when a shared understanding is not reached and the patient disagrees with the doctor, a dispute or complaint may occur. On the whole a doctor–patient consultation is a friendly encounter, but in other walks of life where 'consultations' take place this may not be the case.

Take the example of a strike in a local manufacturing company. Professional negotiators may be called in to help sort out the strike/dispute. The people from the conciliation service will put the representatives from each side in separate rooms to start with, and very carefully work out exactly where each group stands quite independently from the other. They compare notes, and look at where the real differences lie. They then go back to the protagonists (again separately) and find out which areas of difference are possible to get movement on, and which are immoveable. This process gets repeated, until a compromise acceptable to both parties is reached.

In relation to consulting with patients, it can be seen therefore that it is essential to know a patient's **ideas, concerns and expectations** during the first part of the consultation. This is in effect finding out the patient's initial under-standing of the problem. During the process of history taking and examination, the doctor will develop his or her own ideas, concerns and expectations as the working diagnosis is developed. The task is now to identify the differences, and enable the patient to move their understanding to a point acceptable to both parties, so that appropriate action can be chosen.

Thus, if a shared understanding is to be reached, it is essential to know where the patient is coming from. If the ideas, concerns and expectations have been elicited during the history taking, there will be a real feel for what the patient's initial understanding is. It is very easy to ask automatic questions, and fail to get the patient's real reasons for consulting clear. If you have just asked three automatic questions about the ideas, concerns and expectations, the answers you have got will not necessarily reflect the patient's true position. This will make it very difficult to know how to progress with the next step.

Following the model of the professional negotiators, the next part is for the doctor to express their own understanding. First, of course, you must be clear about what your diagnosis is. A diagnosis is not always the name of a single illness. **It is seldom a matter of complete certainty.**

Practical point
Medical science is not an exact science and the way disease presents may differ between individuals. Similarly, a particular treatment may help one individual, but not another with the same disease. It is important to be aware that many of the general public do not have this insight into medical science. Similarly, there is a perception that doctors always cure patients and for many diseases this it not possible.

Even when there is only one pathological entity in your mind, the diagnosis will have elements unique to that patient at that time – physical, social and psychological. Nevertheless, you will not be able to explain it clearly to the patient if you don't have a clear internal concept yourself.

Expressing that understanding in terms that the patient can understand is a skill that improves with practice. Inexperienced consulters often start with:

'From the history you've given, and from the examination I have done, I think you have . . .'

This puts your diagnosis in the context that is familiar to the medical thought process. However, to a non-medical ear, it doesn't sound familiar at all, and probably confuses people who don't recognise the word 'history' for what you meant. More experienced consulters will express the same thing by starting off with lay phrases such as:

'It sounds as if you have . . .'

This conveys to the patient what the first phrase meant to the doctor (an acceptance of the necessary uncertainty associated with any diagnostic thought), without conveying the message that patients often get from the first phrase (I'm not sure of what I'm doing, and I'm trying to justify myself).

Then state your diagnosis as clearly and concisely as possible. There is a conflict here about whether or not to use medical terms. Although it seems better to explain everything in lay terms, thus making things understandable, the evidence shows that patients actually prefer doctors to use medical language – after all that is what they came to the doctor for. However, using medical language means that one must also explain what the words really mean. Take the example of a doctor informing a patient that they have oesophagitis. It may be that the patient does not know what the oesophagus is and it may be appropriate to start using familiar lay terms such as food pipe, gullet and irritation of the lining for inflammation.

Practical point

Medical terminology – Misconceptions can arise, particularly if medical terms are used by the practitioner, who may have assumed the existence of prior knowledge and understanding by a patient. Substantial misconceptions of a broad range of common terms exist and that failure to explain them is a major source of patient dissatisfaction.

Unfortunately, the temptation at this point can be to launch into a detailed explanation of what the diagnosis means without any further ado. The effect that this has in the consultation is rather like the effect that would be produced if the negotiators in our trade union dispute brought a detailed suggested final settlement along with the first statement of position.

Because you cannot know what the diagnosis means to the patient, you cannot explain it in terms that meet their needs. So, straight away, after briefly stating your suggested diagnosis, throw the ball back to the patient, and find out where they stand in relation to it. This is best done by asking a question such as 'What do you know about oesophagitis?' or 'Have you come across oesophagitis before?'.

If the diagnosis is one that you know the patient has not considered in either their ideas or concerns, there may be an even bigger problem to deal with.

You could ask, 'Had you thought about the possibility of oesophagitis?'

Either way, the responsibility is given to the patient, who will tell you what they think or know (and frequently both), allowing you to see where there are areas of difference that need to be breached, ignorance that needs informing/education, and misunderstandings that need specifically to be dealt with.

The very essence of the consultation is **explanation** – explanation through an illness narrative to the doctor by the patient of their illness and then the doctor explaining what the illness is and hopefully the two coming to a 'shared understanding' of the illness. As the Canadian family medicine professor McWhinney (1989) writes, 'the main purpose of our search is to reduce uncertainty', and this can only come through a 'shared understanding' of the problem. Explanation needs to take into account the patient's problems and any hidden agenda (as detailed in Chapter 5) and then to relate it to the patient's own needs and experience.

Explanation

Now you should be in a position to explain the things that need to be explained, at a level that will be appreciated and understood.

Consider the following dialogues with a doctor and patient and a disease referred to as Blogg's disease.

Doctor: 'It sounds as if you might have Blogg's disease. That is a sort of reaction to a viral infection, where your body starts fighting itself, and you get sore inflamed joints and muscles. We'll need to do some blood tests to confirm the diagnosis. Is that all right?'

Patient: 'Oh yes, doctor.'

Or:

Doctor: 'It sounds as if you might have Blogg's disease. You thought it might be that. What do you know about it?'

Patient: 'Well, my grandmother had the first described case of Blogg's disease, and I'm now the tenth member of my family to have it. In fact Blogg was the name of our family doctor in the 1920s '

Or:

Doctor: 'It sounds as if you might have Blogg's disease. You were worried it might be that. What do you know about it?'

Patient: 'My neighbour said it really, I've never heard of it before. She said she read about it on the internet, and it's really serious. You know she says there's this specialist in America who treats it with magnets.'

Or:

Doctor: 'It sounds as if you might have Blogg's disease. You were worried it might be that. What do you know about it?'

Patient: 'I just know it's some sort of reaction to a virus. Don't you have to have blood tests to confirm it? I don't know if I could do that – I've got this awful fear of needles ever since school. Won't it just get better if we leave it well alone?'

Or:

Doctor: 'It sounds as if you might have Blogg's disease. Had you thought of that possibility?'

Patient: 'No, I don't think I've ever even heard the name before. Is it serious?'

Or:

Doctor: 'It sounds as if you might have Blogg's disease. Had you thought of that possibility?'

Patient: 'No, I was worried I had cancer. Can you be sure it isn't cancer?'

Or:

Doctor: 'It sounds as if you might have Blogg's disease. Had you thought of that
          possibility?'
Patient: 'Oh no, isn't that that disease where your blood all goes poisoned and
          you have to have a transfusion?'

Of course, these are hypothetical scenarios, and a mythical illness, but it would be useful to consider what you would say in response to each of the scenarios. Different agendas must be dealt with, but, in theory, you could reach a shared understanding with each, although it wouldn't be the same understanding in any case.

Obviously you would have to check back to find out how successful you had been in achieving an understanding acceptable to you both.

Practical point
Different patients require different pieces of information, explained at different levels.

Sufficient data have now accumulated to prove that problems in doctor-patient communication are common and that they adversely affect patient management. As long ago as 1982, Thompson and Anderson wrote:

Interactions or interviews between doctors and patients are the cornerstone of medical practice.

Much is written on communicating with the patient to discover why they have consulted and to gain information about their illness. However, little is written about information giving to patients and so explanation. An important skill therefore within the consultation is taking the care to give clear explanations, checking the patient's understanding, negotiating a management plan, and checking patients' attention to compliance. Information is important, as knowledge about the illness provides reassurance and ensures that the correct therapeutic measures are being undertaken.

Practical point
It is important not to neglect how informative the consultation can be to the patient.

The fact that many patients remember little of what is told to them suggests that our method of explaining problems to them or the amount of information we give may be inadequate or inappropriate.

How many times have you heard patients say, 'The doctor told me nothing', and yet they have spent 20 minutes in the clinic? Or was it that they didn't understand what the doctor told them? Patients have their own theories about illness and will **interpret new information within the framework of their existing ideas**. The consultation provides an opportunity for explicit sharing of these ideas. However, there is evidence that patient compliance with management and treatment depends on the information that the doctor provides and the way in which it is communicated.

There are different aspects to explanation and these may include:

- explaining the medical terminology that is used.
- explaining about medication prescribed or that it is available over the counter (OTC)
- explanation which provides reassurance
- medical advice concerning the patient's health problem and how the patient may manage it
- health education or preventive medicine, e.g. advising the patient to stop smoking
- explanation as part of informed consent
- breaking bad news.

Breaking bad news

It is sometimes necessary to break bad news within the consultation concerning a serious illness. This must be done sensitively, with sufficient time for discussion and with an explanation that the patient can understand. In such circumstances a patient may remember little of the content of the consultation and it is vital to arrange follow-up for further explanation and support. Imagine the scenario where a lady with a breast lump has a biopsy and the lump is found to be cancer. The 'breaking bad news' consultation is discussed later in the book.

So, to summarise:

- reaching a shared understanding is essential
- enquire of the patient's ideas, concerns and expectations
- confirm what you really think is or may be happening
- state it briefly and clearly
- find out what the patient thinks, and what information they need
- supply the specific information needs through adequate explanation at an appropriate level
- check the patient's understanding again.

Experienced doctors one observes consulting may get this wrong. It is not easy, but just remembering to always get the patient's reaction to the diagnosis will put you in a strong position.

Negotiating a management plan

Once a shared understanding of the problem has been achieved, the next stage is to work out what to do about it. The process of negotiating what is needed will engage the patient actively in the consultation and so contributing to it. The job of the doctor is to make sure that the patient considers all the reasonable potential courses of action and so acts as a resource for the patient to use.

So the first essential is to make sure that all the possible sorts of response have been considered. There are many ways of doing this and some practitioners find a mnemonic useful. For example, the mnemonic RAPRIOP as described by Brian McAvoy in Chapter 4 of the book *Clinical Method* (2000). This mnemonic can be used to remind an individual practitioner of the possible different sorts of response that a management plan might include.

This mnemonic is made up as follows.

- R   Reassurance and explanation.
- A   Advice.
- P   Prescription.
- R   Referral.
- I   Investigation.
- O   Observation.
- P   Prevention.

R: Reassurance and explanation

It is very tempting to take the word reassurance and respond by telling the patient not to worry about the problem if this is appropriate.

In real life one of the most frightening things about health problems **is not understanding them**, and when a shared understanding has been reached, patients are nearly always less worried than when they came in to consult. If the problem is serious, as a result of explaining this to the patient they are likely to be more concerned than when they came in. However, this concern will be lessened if the doctor is able to demonstrate that they will be able to support them through a negotiated management plan. This will be reassuring to a patient. Similarly it should be remembered that if someone has a problem that is life threatening, blind reassurance is not a good idea.

Explanation is the only essential component in an action plan. If you have really reached a shared understanding, you will have covered this element during that process. The rest of the mnemonic is rather like a menu. It details the types of action that you and the patient may consider in response to the problem. **There is no compulsion to choose to consider any of the components of the mnemonic at all.** It is merely an aide mémoire.

Practical point
For many patients, all they have come to the doctor for is to be able to understand what their problem is and what effects it may have on them: no action may be needed at all.

Balint, who is discussed in Chapter 3 and at length in Chapter 12, suggested that **the doctor could act 'as a drug'** through the process of explanation and reassurance. In the 1960s, the concept that physical illnesses and recovery from it had a psychological aspect was revolutionary and perhaps still is. A patient can start to feel better as a result of understanding their illness through a process of explanation and reassurance that something can be done about it or that it will resolve in a given time or that what the patient is describing is normal. In other words, the doctor can be the major 'drug' in getting a patient better. Balint (1957) wrote:

no pharmacology of this important drug exists yet. To put this discovery in terms familiar to doctors, no guidance whatever is contained in any textbook as to the dosage in which the doctor should prescribe himself, in what form, how frequently, what his curative and maintenance doses should be, and so on. Still more disquieting is the lack of any literature on the possible hazards of this kind of medication, on the various allergic conditions met in individual patients which ought to be watched carefully, or on the undesirable side-effects of the drug.

Practical point

Many doctors do not appreciate the impact that their words have on patients and when patients are ill they sometimes 'hang on' to every word that is spoken, particularly when they convey hope and reassurance.

The effect of the doctor as a drug can be more potent than a particular prescribed medication and in certain circumstances this can also be referred to as a '**placebo effect**'. The word 'placebo' can be translated in English as 'I please you', where the pleasing aspect of the doctor–patient relationship is helping the patient feel better.

Practical point

'The physician's belief in the treatment and the patient's faith in the physician exert a mutually reinforcing effect; the result is a powerful remedy that is almost guaranteed to produce an improvement and sometimes a cure' (Skrabanek and McCormick 1990).

In order to reassure any patient, a doctor must first understand their illness. To achieve this, the doctor must find out what the patient's anxieties (ideas and concerns) are. It may therefore be appropriate to ask: 'What was worrying you about your symptoms?'

With this information and a diagnosis, the doctor may be able to reassure the patient by explaining the nature of the patient's symptoms and so illness. Imagine a patient who was worried that their muscular chest pain is due to lung cancer. Explanation that your examination findings verified that the pain is muscular and not cancer will provide reassurance. Hopefully, this will improve patient satisfaction with the consultation playing a part in the healing process.

A: Advice

Many of the ways of acting to resolve a health problem are wholly within the patient's realm. They may be specific actions, such as drinking plenty of fluids when there is a urinary infection. Or they may be bigger lifestyle changes such as taking up an exercise, or changing the food they eat.

As with all the other parts of management, it is very important to find out where the patient is starting from, before presuming to suggest an action. One can easily make a fool of oneself – for example, advising a marathon runner to take more exercise such as a daily walk or advising a vegetarian to eat less fatty meat.

Once you have found out where the patient is in respect of the lifestyle that you want to modify, you can find out if they would consider making a change. Only if the patient is receptive is it worthwhile pursuing a lifestyle suggestion. Then you can find out what sort of change the patient feels would be possible and beneficial.

Health education is often given opportunistically and it is vital that its purpose is well explained. For example, in the case of a young person who has developed a lower respiratory chest infection, it is important to explain the probability of recurrence due to smoking and of its long-term consequences. A doctor can justify this advice, but it is imperative to explain the ways in which the advice can be applied and thus influence patient-centred behaviour.

If medical advice is explained in a manner that a patient can comprehend, it is more likely to promote the facilitation of patient-centred health management. Understanding of advice may be facilitated if three main aspects are addressed;

- the physiological/pathological basis of the illness
- appropriate management
- affirmation of appropriate patient ideas.

For example, in the treatment of hypertension, this understanding may encourage compliance to health education, medication and review.

Example

Imagine the following example where medical advice requires good and sensitive explanation. A young mother with marital and social problems requests a sterilisation. She had already walked out of a consultation with one doctor as she was adamant that she wanted a sterilisation. In order to avoid this scenario of a patient walking out of a consultation in anger, it is important that the patient understands the advice provided and **does not find it offensive or patronising** and that the doctor takes the time to appreciate and understand the patient's views.

P: Prescription

Prescribing medicines is one of the commonest things that doctors do. As compliance is not 100% to prescribed medication, it could be argued that doctors prescribe more drugs than patients want. And yet many doctors think that patients want more prescriptions than they give out. Medicines are frequently taken in a regime that was not recommended. Large numbers of prescriptions cause unwanted effects, and a sizeable proportion of hospital admissions, are caused by problems due to prescription drugs.

If a prescription is clinically indicated, it is important to know before writing the prescription whether or not the patient will consider taking a prescription for their illness. With the exception of perhaps antibiotics, patients seem to prefer to do without drugs if they believe they can. Even patients who came into the doctor expecting a prescription may very well have changed their ideas once they have understood that the condition they have will get better without any treatment. Sharing the understanding of the problem will change the expected prescribing 'solutions' in many cases.

Practical point
Prescribing – Even though you have found out a patient's expectations during the history taking, you need to recheck that they still want a prescription before 'reaching for the prescription pad'.

When you consider any prescription consider the following questions.

- Does the patient want a prescription?
- What is the name, dose and frequency of the drug?
- How long should it be taken for?
- What benefits will this drug give?
- What harm could it do?
- What will happen if the patient doesn't take the drug?
- Is there anything else about this patient that will have an effect on their response to this drug (e.g. allergy, other medication, age, beliefs, etc.).
- Is it going to be difficult for the patient to take this drug, e.g. swallowing capsules?

The patient will need the answers to these questions, and may have some more questions that you hadn't thought of. Be prepared to look up answers in the *British National Formulary*. Patients don't expect you to know everything and are reassured when they know the information they are getting is accurate and has been checked.

R: Referral

A referral is an important part of the management of some patients. A referral is where one healthcare professional is asking for the help and expertise of another. This is so that a patient gets the correct care from the appropriate person in the right place, e.g. a hospital, when it is clinically indicated. By making a referral a doctor is correctly recognising the limits of their own expertise, e.g. a general practitioner asking a specialist to see a patient who has been newly diagnosed with rheumatoid arthritis. Or it may be the limitation of appropriate treatment resources, e.g. a doctor in an accident and emergency department asking a coronary care unit to admit a patient with a myocardial infarction. On many occasions patients do not require referrals. In general practice, most patients are seen and managed by their GP and only a small percentage are referred to an outpatient clinic for a specialist opinion or acutely with the sudden onset of a life-threatening illness such as a cerebrovascular accident.

I: Investigation

When you have finished your history and examination there may still be some areas of uncertainty about the diagnosis. Some of these uncertainties may be resolvable by investigations. Blood tests, urine cultures and x-rays are commonly ordered, but there are many other possible investigations. The temptation is to order every test you can think of so that every possibility is covered, but this isn't good practice, and will not only waste money but will also risk harming the patient – for example, an investigation result that gives a false positive and causes the patient undue anxiety while the test is being repeated. In addition, patients are just as capable of not going and having their blood tests taken as they are of not taking their prescriptions. Also many investigations are unpleasant experiences, e.g. having a sigmoidoscopy.

Before suggesting an investigation consider the following questions.

- What question will be answered by this investigation?
- What difference to the management plan will it make if this test comes back positive?
- What difference will it make if it comes back normal?
- Does it matter to the patient?
- Can I explain clearly what is involved in this test?
- How much difficulty will the patient encounter in order to get this test done?
- Are there any potential harmful effects?
- How can I arrange to discuss the results with the patient in a convenient and timely manner?

O: Observation

Very often one of the most important ways of acting in response to a problem is to 'wait and see'. This involves a clear understanding of what the likely resolution or development of the problem will be like, and choosing an appropriate time to review the problem – either the patient, or the doctor and patient together. It also involves choosing what the appropriate action will be if each scenario happens. As with all the other options, the patient will have an active point of view about this, and should be involved in choosing the timescale and actions.

P: Prevention

This is to remind you that there may be actions that are appropriate that are not directly to do with dealing with the problem itself, but with preventing future other problems. Reminding someone to have an influenza vaccine, to stop smoking or to have their cervical smear repeated may come into this category.

Practical point
RAPRIOP is one of many possible mnemonics to aid the management process and of course there are other possible actions.

It can be seen that treatment is a distinct therapeutic component of the medical management process.

Treatment (medical or surgical)

This would include a surgeon performing an operation or a doctor starting an intravenous infusion or giving cryotherapy to a verruca on the foot. It is important to realise that these possibilities also need to be negotiated, just like treatment through a prescription. It is even more important to the patient's full understanding in these situations so that they can give informed consent for such interventions. Just signing a consent form is not sufficient.

Practical point

Consent is only informed and so valid if the patient has **truly understood** what the intervention involves, what it is trying to achieve, its chances of success, and what could go wrong.

Clinical decision making requires informed consent. This can only evolve if the doctor explains to the patient what the considered diagnosis is and ways in which it may be treated – for example, a laminectomy to alleviate sciatica. If this is the case the doctor needs to use explanation to justify the reasoning behind the options. Through a process of negotiation and a shared understanding, an informed decision can be arrived at.

It seems rather daunting to be considering so many sorts of options. How is it possible to handle such a complex mixture in real practice? The most efficient way of coping is to encourage the patient to be actively involved in the process.

If you have really reached a shared understanding, you will have thrown the ball back into the patient's court, and allowed him or her to tell you what they think about the diagnosis, before starting to talk about the possible management options. With any luck, the patient will naturally go on from there to start to tell you about the action they believe is most appropriate for them and those options that they do not wish to consider.

If this happens, it is relatively easy to allow the discussion to develop naturally, giving more information about the individual options, and allowing the patient to expand his or her horizon and consider extra options.

The next best thing is to learn a standard beginning that will always allow you to get the patient negotiating the plan. A phrase that often works is: 'There are two (or three) things that we can do about this'.

Patients will usually engage with this approach, and if the doctor then gives the options, the patient will often contribute opinions and judgement, and get involved. It is important to realise that, although the number of possible courses of action is large (as defined by the RAPRIOP mnemonic above), in real life there will be a much smaller number of realistic solutions. Sometimes it is difficult to think of more than one thing to do.

However, there is always the **'do nothing' option**, so you can always generate a two-way choice. Bear in mind the embarrassing figures about the take-up of medical options, and you will realise that the 'do nothing' option is often preferred, even when the choice isn't offered. If there seems to be lots of options, restrain yourself from the temptation to list them all and make the patient choose.

Practical point

A choice can only realistically be comprehended between two or three possibilities.

If there really are more than three options, then the only way to cope is to subdivide, and narrow the field down by offering broader choices first or those most likely to be successful.

Example

For example, if a woman has very heavy periods, and you have come to the conclusion that there is no major pathology present, there are large numbers of possible ways of dealing with it:

1   medications such as NSAIDs or the oral contraceptive pill
2   surgical interventions.

You can reduce this to an acceptable set of possibilities by first asking what things she has tried already, then asking, 'Is it causing you enough trouble to be worth considering having an operation?' You will quickly get an idea about which two or three options are in fact worth discussing. If you keep asking the patient for feedback as you go, you will be able to answer the questions that the patient needs to know, and will avoid wasting time telling them things that they already know, or details about something that they would never consider.

Patients will differ in the amount of the decision taking that they will take on, and some patients are very unhappy if pushed into making decisions that they don't feel capable of taking. They might say, 'I don't know, you are the doctor, you tell me.' So it may be a doctor decision, a patient decision, or a joint decision that is actually taken. As long as you have got the patient actively contributing to the understanding of the diagnosis, you can always get enough of a feel to be able to pitch the balance roughly right.

Medical emergencies

If there is a high degree of urgency and seriousness of the condition, it isn't really appropriate to go offering the patient too much in the way of choice, e.g. in the case of an acute myocardial infarction. Obviously, you can't negotiate with a patient who is unconscious in an emergency situation such as a cardiac arrest, but just provide appropriate resuscitation. However, whenever patients are conscious they should be involved as much as possible to allow them to reach an understanding of the diagnosis, and what it means, and the appropriate treatment. It is probably good practice to talk to unconscious patients as they may be able to hear and understand, as sometimes they will tell you all about what they heard when they were 'out'.

Handing over responsibility to the patient

Most consultations however are not emergencies, and the person who will actually carry out most management plans is in fact the patient. So, once a course of action has been chosen, you must give the patient enough information and understanding to **enable** and **empower** them to take it on.

Consider a patient with back pain, having decided that he would benefit from a prescription for a painkiller stronger than the paracetamol that he has been taking. He needs to know quite a lot of information before he will be able to get the drug from the pharmacy:

- frequency of administration
- possible side effects
- what to do if the relief is not sufficient.

Practical point
Very often, there is too much information to get over, and patients cannot absorb it all.

If you watch experienced doctors, they often repeat the important details several times. This can help. The other thing that experienced doctors often do is to give out an **information leaflet**, which a patient can refer to in the future. Or provide the opportunity to ask questions on another occasion.

Follow-up

Arranging follow-up is an important part of handing over responsibility to the patient. Follow-up isn't always necessary, but if you arrange it at all it should be the correct type (closed or open), and at an appropriate time interval.

Closed follow-up

This is when a definite time to come back is suggested. There should be a good reason why the doctor needs to see the patient again, and an indication why a particular timing should be as suggested. An example might be when starting someone on antidepressant drugs. It may be very important to give the patient a definite appointment to come back. Depressed patients may get worse in the first fortnight of taking their drugs, and may lose insight, and so may be becoming suicidal, not take their treatment, or suffer side effects. A definite appointment makes it more likely that they will actually come back, and will inform the doctor that he or she has to chase them up if they don't turn up. A time interval of around the two-week mark for that first follow-up may be appropriate. This is long enough for any initial side effects to be wearing off, short enough to be able to change the treatment if needed, and in the time when they may need extra support before the pills start to work. However, the period may differ in different circumstances and illnesses.

Most hospital follow-up appointments are closed, and frequently cannot be fixed at the time the doctor or the patient would ideally wish. Perhaps it is not surprising that there is such a high non-attendance rate.

Open follow-up

This is when the timing of the follow-up is left to the patient. It is often used in general practice, and GPs often give it the name 'safety netting'. In order for this to work, the patient must clearly understand what should trigger a repeat visit to the doctor or to seek advice, and what timescale would be appropriate. Hospitals similarly operate an 'open access system' for certain conditions.

A typical example is the patient with a cough who comes and is told their lung fields are clear, and they will get better in a few days with only the help of some simple cough linctus as they have most likely got a viral infection. The doctor will suggest that if their chest is not improving in a week or so, or if they suddenly take a turn for the worse, then they should come back, to have their chest checked again. In this way the doctor is allowing the patient sufficient time to improve naturally, but covering the small possibility of a secondary bacterial infection in the convalescent phase.

It is important to get the timescale right – telling the cough patient to come back if it isn't better by tomorrow would just double the workload. However, if you were vaguely worried that a person with abdominal pain might have early appendicitis, but had no positive signs, then a return in four or six hours for clinical review might be indicated.

Practical point

In order to make your follow-up timing appropriate you need to have an understanding of what is likely to happen and over what timescale. In medicine this is called the **prognosis**.

Choosing the time to look again at the problem in order to be able to differentiate between possible outcomes and treatment needs is another area where experiences and knowledge of illness help, but you must also take the patient into account. If too long a follow-up period is given to an anxious patient, they will feel unsupported, and come back sooner, whereas an overconfident patient may fail to come back at all.

Conclusion

We have followed the management process from the making of the diagnosis by the doctor to the point where the patient leaves the room knowing what the problem is, what they are going to do about it, and when and why they should come back. Effective consultations require good communication skills, of which explanation is a primary component. It is important in the development of a 'shared understanding' of a patient's illness and its management between the patient and the doctor. The importance of explanation has implications for education in the recognition of illnesses and their potential for self-management, patient satisfaction and improved compliance to proposed treatment options.

It is all too easy to state what is ideal and, with the enforced time constraints of current clinical practice in the UK, optimal patient management may be compromised. However, constructive self-appraisal is a vital step in the process to continually re-evaluate the effectiveness of one's own performance. Further-more, one's own perception of good communication may not be the same as our patients. Explanation or information giving is often doctor-centred, but should be patient-centred, ensuring a shared understanding of the illness, thus giving the patient the tools to cope with his or her illness. Second, the importance of explanation within the consultation and other communication skills are recognised by many as part of the 'healing' process, but this needs to be proven. Improvements in the quality of care doctors provide will be cost-effective, as their neglect leads to patient dissatisfaction, complaints, a perception of being uncared for and so continued ill health and further consultations. Increased consultation time is important, but so is optimal patient management as outlined in this chapter.

Bibliography

Balint M. *The Doctor, His Patient, and The Illness*. Edinburgh: Churchill Livingstone. First published in London: Pitman; 1957.

Bartlett EE. The effects of physician communications skills on patient satisfaction; recall, and adherence. *Journal of Chronic Disease*. 1984; **37**: 755–64.

Charlton R. Explanation in the consultation. *New Zealand Family Physician*. 1994; **21**(1): 6–9.

Cousins N. *Anatomy of an Illness – as perceived by the patient*. New York: W W Norton and Co.; 1979.

Del Mar CB. Communicating well in general practice. *Medical Journal of Australia*. 1994; **160**: 367–70.

George CF. Editorial: Telling patients about their medicines. *BMJ*. 1987; **294**: 1566–77.

Grandes G, Cortada JM, Arrazola A, Laka JP. Predictors of long-term outcome of a smoking cessation programme in primary care. *British Journal of General Practice*. 2003; **53**: 101–7.

Heath C. What is a good GP? *BMJ*. 1987; **294**: 415–16.

Helman CG. Limits of biomedical explanation. *The Lancet*. 1991; **337**: 1080–3.

McAvoy B. Chapter 4. In: Fraser R, editor. *Clinical Method; a general practice approach*. Oxford: Butterworth Heinemann; 2000.

McWhinney IRA. *Textbook of Family Medicine*. New York and Oxford: Oxford University Press; 1989.

Pendleton D, Schofield T, Tate P, Havelock P. *The Consultation: an approach to learning and teaching*. Oxford: Oxford University Press; 1984.

Roter DL, Hall JA. Strategies for enhancing patient adherence to medical recommendations. *JAMA*. 1994; **271**: 80.

Short D. The importance of words. *British Journal of Hospital Medicine*. 1993; **50**: 548–50.

Simpson M *et al*. Doctor–patient communication; the Toronto consensus statement. *BMJ*. 1991; **303**: 1385–7.

Skrabanek P, McCormick J. *Follies and Fallacies in Medicine*. New York: Prometheus; 1990.

Thompson, JA, Anderson JL. Patient preferences and the bedside manner. *Medical Education*. 1982; **16**: 17–21.

Tuckett D and Williams A. Approaches to the measurement of explanation and information-giving in medical consultations: a review of empirical studies. *Soc Sci Med*. 1984; **18**: 571–80.

Chapter 7

Opportunistic/preventive care and health promotion

Dr Martyn Hull

Healthcare is not just about treating and hopefully curing disease, but it is also about preventing disease and hence the adage, 'Prevention is better than cure'. This is therefore an essential component of 'Learning to Consult' and the principles of preventive care and health promotion are covered by Martyn Hull in this chapter.

Introduction

In medicine, there is a tendency to concentrate on the recognition and cure of established disease, and little emphasis is given to preventing the development of disease in the first place, and to the related subject of health promotion. There are a number of reasons for this.

Governments have, in the past, tended to concentrate their healthcare spending on secondary and tertiary care – hospitals and specialist treatment centres – focusing on the diagnosis and treatment of 'serious' diseases. This spending often leads to a limited clinical gain for a great financial cost. This situation can be contrasted to spending on prevention and health promotion, where great long-term benefits can be gained if this process succeeds, and at significantly less expenditure. It has been estimated that less than 5% of the health spend in the USA is on prevention.[1] This can be put into context by an analysis of the major non-genetic contributors to mortality, which found that 50% were preventable, with 33% attributed to tobacco, diet and activity patterns alone.[2]

At least part of the reason for this bias is the nature of the results gained by therapeutic medicine as opposed to prevention strategies. It is easy to see how policy makers, the wider population, even health professionals and patients themselves, can be impressed by visible life-saving interventions such as chemotherapy, neurosurgery or thrombolysis. These are tangible, almost glamorous ways to attempt to save people's lives. By contrast, there is minimal prestige gained by chatting to a patient about their smoking habit or checking their blood pressure, no scope for plaudits at the potential life saved and rarely any appreciation for your actions from the patient.

The propensity towards secondary care is also pervasive within the medical education system. Traditionally universities have disproportionately taught in great detail on the specialist management of certain diseases, predominantly in hospitals. At the same time, undergraduate medical education has paid little attention to preventive care and health promotion, subjects principally addressed in a community setting. Greater exposure to more teaching in the community will inevitably lead to increased awareness of preventive medicine as a whole.

Despite these obstacles, it is increasingly recognised that preventive medicine – both at individual patient level and at population level – is a significant part of the provision of healthcare.

Practical point

Every healthcare professional must not only be able to diagnose and manage presenting problems, but also recognise opportunities for active health promotion and offer advice and information in order to modify the lifestyle and behaviour of their patients.

In order for this to be achieved, it is important to understand some principles of prevention, and recognise the barriers to its success.

This chapter is divided into the following sections.

- Definitions.
- Obstacles to health promotion.
- Health promotion within the consultation.
- Impetus for health promotion.
- The setting for health promotion.
- How to do it.
- Using smoking as an example.
- Summary.

Definitions

There are three levels of preventive intervention with regard to the natural history of a disease, depending on when the intervention occurs:

- primary prevention
- secondary prevention
- tertiary prevention.

Primary prevention

This refers to the attempt to reduce the risk of a disease developing in the first place. Examples include public health measures such as improved sanitation in the 19th century, or advertising campaigns targeted at stopping people from potentially health-damaging activities such as unprotected sex.

Immunisation programmes are also an example of primary prevention as they prevent individuals from contracting particular diseases, but also offer 'herd immunity' protection to the whole population by decreasing the overall prevalence of the disease in question.

For obvious reasons, primary prevention is the most effective form of prevention: remember the old adage, 'Prevention is better than cure'.

Secondary prevention

This refers to detection of disease before significant damage is done, and relies on this early recognition leading to a better outcome, for example by prompt treatment. Examples of secondary prevention include screening for hypertension, and the subsequent management decreasing the risk of a heart attack or stroke.

Screening – the detection of disease in its presymptomatic phase – is therefore a form of secondary prevention and can be broadly split into two different types: opportunistic case-finding and formal screening.

- **Opportunistic case finding** – looking for a specific attribute in a patient when they attend for something else. A common example is the opportunistic checking of blood pressure. This sort of screening is inexpensive, involves no extra costs, and will reach 90% of a GP's practice population within five years. However, this means that, by definition, not everyone will be screened; indeed it may be the non-attenders who are at most need of the service. Also it takes time and effort in addition to the management of the presenting problem, and the patient may be less receptive to health education when they are presenting either acutely ill or with concerns about other issues.

  Taking into account the resource implications of this approach, it would make sense to concentrate on high-risk patients. For example it is more important to regularly check the blood pressure of a 50-year-old smoker than a 20-year-old non-smoker. It is also imperative to bear in mind the principles of screening, and ensure that the process will not harm the patient.
- **Formal screening programmes** – inviting patients to attend for a particular test, e.g. cervical screening. The advantages of this approach include the fact that there is time set aside specifically for the promotion of health, and as such the attendees tend to be motivated and time can be spent with them. However, it requires considerable organisation and administration, and this can be expensive (and sometimes for debatable clinical gain), and often those that attend are the patients least in need of the service: the so-called 'worried well'.

Practical point
Screening – the detection of disease in its presymptomatic phase.

It is necessary to weigh up the potential costs and benefits of screening for a disease. The potential benefits – improving morbidity and mortality – are obvious, although sometimes the screening process may just discover disease earlier than otherwise, wrongly creating the impression that survival is prolonged. Additionally, not all screening tests are accurate. Falsely positive results can lead to unnecessary and sometimes invasive investigations – for example, prostate biopsy after a raised PSA (prostate specific antigen) blood test – in patients with nothing wrong. These patients may then also experience unnecessary anxiety, even psychological harm, because of the false result, as well as the potential physical harm of the investigation. Falsely negative results incorrectly reassure the patient with a disease that they are free from it, and may delay treatment.

These factors are addressed in the strict criteria that describe a successful screening programme,[3] and the potential pitfalls outlined above help explain why there is currently only formal screening in the UK for cervical cancer and breast cancer. Other diseases are being evaluated, including cancer of the prostate and colon.

Tertiary prevention

Practical point

Tertiary prevention refers to the management of established disease in order to minimise disability and ensure the best possible prognosis.

Examples include the systematic care of a patient with diabetes: regular surveillance aims to promote good control and prevent complications; and regular eye examination, foot care and blood pressure monitoring lead to early identification of potential problems, which in turn can lead to effective treatment. Obviously, this sort of care cannot be efficiently carried out opportunistically, and organised and systematic programmes must be set up. Within this framework, there can also be effective promotion of health – for example, in diabetic clinics, patients can be encouraged to eat healthily and given assistance to stop smoking.

In recent years, this organised management of chronic disease has begun to shift into primary care. Most general practices have disease registers of patients with conditions such as diabetes, coronary heart disease and asthma. Many run specialised clinics concentrating on the care of these patients in a detailed and systematic way, and health promotion plays a significant role within this set-up. In this environment, healthcare professionals are often more successful at delivering the message of health promotion than they would be opportunistically within a consultation for another reason, *but* there are obvious resource implications for primary care with this shift in emphasis.

Health promotion

Health promotion is not simply risk avoidance, rather the active encouragement of individuals to attain their best possible level of well-being. Health promotion can, therefore, operate at any of the three levels described above.

Obstacles to health promotion

Whatever the form that health promotion or disease prevention takes, there are a number of obstacles to its success. These can be broadly divided into patient- and doctor-related barriers.

Patient barriers to success

Some patients:

- are unwilling to sacrifice a habit which is enjoyable or perhaps risky
- believe that the potential health risk won't happen to them
- believe that 'something has to kill you', so why worry?

- believe that the potential risk is so far into the future that it doesn't matter yet
- do not believe what the doctor is saying
- are genuinely ignorant about the health risks of certain behaviours
- rebel, especially in adolescence
- exercise fully-informed personal choice.

Doctor barriers to success

There are a number of potential reasons why doctors do not practice as much health promotion as they might.

- Resource implications:
  - no time to address issues: whenever a doctor does something, by definition, he or she is *not* doing something else
  - shorter consultations have been shown to contain less health promotion[4]
  - financial costs, for example, of setting up formal programmes.
- Frustration at perceived lack of success.
- Requirement of organisation.
- Requirement of enthusiasm.
- Education of doctor: for example, being up to date in order to offer sound advice.
- Stress: less stressed doctors address more preventive issues.[5]
- Communication issues:
  - need to be a good communicator to effectively tailor advice to individual patients
  - the ability to ascertain the motivation of a patient to change behaviour detrimental to their health, and thus knowing when to proffer health-promoting advice.

These are just some of the factors that hinder successful health promotion, and explain why there is still a high prevalence of health detrimental behaviours in our society.

Practical point
Herein lies the challenge facing health professionals, and knowledge of these obstacles is key to the improvement of preventative medicine.

Strategies must be implemented in order to address these obstacles, both individually and at population level.

Health promotion within the consultation

The consultation has been described as 'the central act of medicine',[6] and the role of health promotion within the remit of the consultation is not a new concept. Disease prevention has its roots in the public health measures undertaken in the 19th century. Since then, it has gradually become recognised as an integral part of day-to-day consultations, with the realisation that the key lies with individuals' own understanding and behaviour. Helping patients to take responsibility for their own health must be a fundamental feature of the consultation.

There have been a number of attempts to classify what happens in doctor–patient encounters, and these tend to reflect the role of prevention within the remit of the consultation. For example, Stott and Davis, from the University of Wales, described the consultation as having exceptional potential including the possibility of opportunistic health promotion.[7]

Pendleton *et al.* – a group comprising three GPs and a psychologist based in Oxford[6] – took this principle further in their well-respected model for the consultation. They defined a number of 'tasks' which should be completed within the consultation, and include the task 'to consider other problems: continuing problems, and at-risk factors', thus bringing prevention to the fore of thinking around the role of the consultation.

Impetus for health promotion

In the past, prevention of disease has centred on social measures such as improved sanitation and housing, which resulted in huge improvements in health. Nowadays, however, the majority of mortality and disabling illness in the UK is accounted for by ischaemic heart disease, stroke, cancer and chronic lung disease. These are principally affected by the lifestyle and habits of individuals: smoking, diet and exercise. Consequently, the role of the clinician has become more important and he/she must communicate this information more effectively to his/her patients.

The increasing pressure placed upon clinicians from the above, and the increasing body of evidence of the potential health gain reflects this. The government has made health promotion a priority: in 1990 with *The Health of the Nation* white paper,[8] followed in 1999 by *Our Healthier Nation*.[9] In these documents, the government has identified priority areas – including cardiovascular disease, cancer and accidents – and set targets to tackle these areas. Concurrently, guidelines have been issued specifically addressing areas such as tobacco, alcohol, drugs and sexual health.

Practical point

This represents a significant policy shift from treating sickness to promoting health.

A separate project – the Wanless Report, commissioned by the treasury in 2001 – assessed NHS funding and workload.[10] One of its conclusions was that the future GP '... will concentrate on patient lifestyle, prevention and screening'.

The setting for health promotion

Primary care is ideally suited to the delivery of health promotion:

- Most patients stay with the same GP for many years.
- 90% of people consult their GP at least once every five years, most considerably more than this.

- Surveys consistently show that the family doctor is well respected and their views are trusted.
- This doctor–patient relationship is particularly strong in general practice.
- It is possible to identify patients from the register even if they do not consult.
- The whole primary care team can be involved: receptionist, nurse, health visitor, social worker, midwife and doctor.

Despite this, it is important for every clinician to play a part in the improved delivery of health promotion, and health professionals in secondary care also have an important role to play in preventive medicine. This can be directly relevant to their field, for example advice on healthy diet from a cardiologist to a patient after myocardial infarction. Conversely, it can include health-promoting activities not so obviously linked, such as surgeons offering advice on smoking cessation to a patient due for an appendicectomy. An integrated approach such as this reinforces the message, and increases the likelihood of success. Ideally, there should be a formal integrated programme, for example the surgeon above can identify the smoker receptive to health-promoting advice, and refer them to a local smoking cessation programme where they can be assessed thoroughly.

How to do it

If we agree on the importance of health promotion, and that the GP consultation is ideally suited for its delivery, the questions remain:

- How to do it?
- When to do it?

Time issues

Practical point
One of the obstacles to successful health promotion identified earlier was the time it takes.

It would obviously not be feasible to spend five minutes within every consultation on health-promotion issues, with an average consultation time of less than 10 minutes. Indeed, a recent paper points out that a GP would need to find more than seven hours a day solely on the preventive services recommended by the US task force on the subject.[11] So, patients must be quickly assessed for the appropriateness of health promotion, and then the time spent accordingly with individual patients. Saying that, even lengthening the consultation by one minute on average has been shown to increase the quantity and quality of health-promoting activity.[4] This is one of the reasons behind the movement to decrease the workload of GPs and consequently increase the time available for each consultation.

Patient-centred approach

Health promotion and disease prevention will only succeed if the patient takes it on board. Key to this is the *patient-centred* consultation:

- Patients' reasons for attending are established.
- Patients' ideas and health beliefs are explored.
- Explanations are built on those ideas.
- Reasons for choices are explained, enabling patients to make informed decisions.
- Decision making is shared.
- Support offered is directed at encouraging patients to make their own decisions.

This sort of approach has been shown to be more effective, and means that the patients have *ownership* over their own care. It reflects the fact that it is only possible to influence people's behaviour if one understands their reasons for behaving a certain way.

What to actually do

Accepting that one needs to selectively identify the times that health promotion should be attempted, and that a patient-centred approach should be used, the actual process of effectively communicating the information can now be described. This has been described as four tasks: exploration, explanation, negotiation and support.[10]

Exploration:
- patients' expectations
- nature of their problems and health behaviours
- patients' health beliefs
- social factors.

Explanation:
- reinforce positive ideas, counter negative ideas
- enable the patient to make an informed decision.

Negotiation:
- explore barriers to change
- agree goals to be set.

Support:
- encouragement
- identify and use appropriate resources
- arrange follow-up.

Practical point
By building a relationship with the patient, and using this sort of approach, the patient feels enabled to make their own deicisons regarding their health.

This increases their chances of successfully achieving whatever health-promotion goal is being addressed.

Using smoking as an example

The problem

- Smoking is the single largest cause of premature death in the UK, responsible for 50 000 to 100 000 deaths per year.
- Smoking is the number one preventable cause of ill health according to the WHO, and costs the NHS millions of pounds a year.

Addressing the problem: population level

- Legislation has led to lower tar content of cigarettes and increased use of filters.
- Tobacco advertising has become restricted.
- More public places have been designated non-smoking.

Despite this, almost one third of adults in the UK still smoke, and surveys report that up to 70% of them have tried to give up. This suggests that more can be achieved by focusing on this important area within GP consultations.

A strategy for smoking cessation

Fowler, an Oxford GP, explained the principles of a smoking cessation strategy in his text on prevention in general practice.[10] The basics he described can be applied to other preventive issues within the consultation setting.

Raise the issue

- Especially in respiratory illnesses, pregnant women, etc.

Assess motivation (in this case, to quit)

- 'Have you tried to stop?'
- 'Would you like to stop?'
- 'Do you think smoking affects your health?'
- 'What prevents you from stopping?'
- 'What would be the benefits of you stopping?'

Give information

- Ensure the patient knows the facts.
- Try and increase their motivation to stop (*see* 'cycle of change' below).

Support

- Support a serious quit attempt, e.g. with advice, nicotine replacement, counselling, follow-up appointments.
- Encourage maintenance if successfully stop smoking.

Practical point
The key factor in assessing how to tailor health promotion advice is to assess the motivation of the patient to changing their behaviour.

The advice can then be varied accordingly to the patient's current motivation. One model widely quoted is the *cycle of change* (*see* Figure 7.1).[12]

1 Pre-contemplation – contented smoker, no plans to stop.
2 Early phase of risk awareness – low motivation to stop.
3 Contemplation – moderate motivation to stop.
4 Action – high motivation to stop.
5 Maintenance or relapse.

By enquiring about the smoking status of a patient, and then assessing their motivation to stop, the GP can quickly identify those who are likely to be more receptive to preventive advice or action.

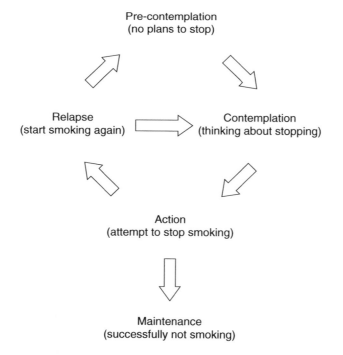

Figure 7.1 The cycle of change.

Example 1

Doctor:	'Do you smoke?'
Patient:	'Yes.'
Doctor:	'How much?'
Patient:	'Twenty a day.'
Doctor:	'Have you thought about stopping?'
Patient:	'Not really.'

This smoker is at phase 1 in the cycle of change: pre-contemplation. They can briefly be reminded of the health risks and given some leaflets, in an attempt to increase their motivation.

Example 2

Doctor:	'Do you smoke?'
Patient:	'Yes, but I know it's bad for me.'
Doctor:	'How much do you smoke?'
Patient:	'I've cut down to 10 a day. I was smoking 20.'
Doctor:	'Have you thought about trying to stop completely?'
Patient:	'I've tried lots of times, but it's too hard!'

This smoker is at phase 4 – action – and is ready to make a serious quit attempt. He/she can be offered more thorough advice on the health issues, including advice on tactics to help quit. They can also be prescribed nicotine replacement, offered follow-up appointments where the smoking cessation can be the reason for the consultation, and referred to local smoking cessation groups.

Patients at levels of motivation between these two extremes can have health-promotion targeted to their motivation at that particular time. The goal is to increase the motivation of the patient towards being ready for a quit attempt, during which they can be offered full support.

By tailoring the health-promoting advice in this way, the clinician increases the chance of success while not spending excessive time on patients who would be less receptive.

Summary

- Prevention and health promotion is increasingly recognised for its important role within medicine as a whole.
- Prevention can occur at three levels – primary, secondary and tertiary – depending on when the intervention occurs.
- Obstacles to successful prevention can be related to patient and doctor factors.
- Every clinician has a responsibility to undertake health promotion and prevention activities; but general practice is its ideal setting.
- Health promotion should be undertaken in a patient-centred approach.
- Within the consultation, clinicians should assess each individual patient and tailor health-promotion advice accordingly.

References

1 Rothenberg R, Masca P, Mikl J *et al.* Cancer. *American Journal of Preventive Medicine.* 1997; **3**(suppl): 30–42.

2 McGinnis JM, Foege WH. Actual causes of death in the United States. *Journal of the American Medical Association.* 1993; **270**: 2207–12.

3 Wilson JMG. In: Teeling-Smith G, editor. *Surveillance and Early Diagnosis in General Practice.* Proceedings of Colloquium. London: Office of Health Economics; 1966. p. 5–10.

4 Wilson A, McDonald P, Hayes L, Cooney J. Health promotion in the general practice consultation: a minute makes a difference. *BMJ.* 1992; **304**: 227–30.

5 Howie JG, Hopton JL, Heaney DJ, Porter AM. Attitudes to medical care, the organisation of work, and stress among general practitioners. *British Journal of General Practice.* 1992; **42**: 181–5.

6 Pendleton D, Schofield T, Tate P, Havelock P. *The Consultation: an approach to learning and teaching.* Oxford: Oxford University Press; 1984.

7 Stott NCH, Davis RH. The exceptional potential in each primary care consultation. *Journal of the Royal College of General Practitioners.* 1979; **29**: 201–5.

8 *The Health of the Nation: a strategy for health in England.* London: HMSO; 1992.

9 *Our Healthier Nation: a contract for health.* London: Stationery Office; 1998.

10 Moore W. Wanless report outlines 'Rolls-Royce' health service for 2002. [News] *BMJ.* 2002; **324**: 998.

11 Yarnall KS, Pollak K, Ostbye T, Krause KM, Michener JL. Primary care: is there enough time for prevention? *Am J Public Health.* 2003: **93**: 635–41.

12 Prochaska JO, DiClemente CC. Stages of change in the modification of problem behaviours. *Progress in Behavior Modification.* 1992; **28**: 183–218.

Chapter 8

Record keeping and referrals

Dr Will Murdoch and Dr Rodger Charlton

Will Murdoch introduces the principles surrounding good note keeping. Rodger Charlton looks at the use of computers and then the writing of referral letters and clinic letters. Will Murdoch then discusses the copying of letters to patients and access to medical records and Rodger Charlton finishes the chapter summarising the issues that relate to email.

Introduction

Keeping notes is an essential part of everyday life for all clinicians regardless of which speciality they work in, whether in training or qualified, and they are an essential part of patient care. They are both a record and a vital tool of communication between members of the healthcare team. The GMC has issued guidance on this in the publication *Good Medical Practice* and that patient notes should be:

- clear
- accurate
- legible
- relevant.

In addition notes should contain:

- the clinical findings
- diagnosis or provisional diagnosis
- investigation results
- patient management
- information and advice given to patients
- treatments including any medication prescribed
- consent forms
- signature in written notes and information on the record to identify the patient.

Entries must also be made for telephone consultations as well as face-to-face consultations.

As an example, GPs are obliged to keep records as part of their terms and services (Paragraph 36 of Schedule 2 to the NHS (General Medical Services) Regulations 1992). They fulfil a number of functions, both practical, as detailed above, and legal.

Practical point

If a complaint is made by a patient the quality of care provided will be judged from the records that have been kept.

This chapter is divided into the following sections.

- Functions of note keeping.
- Use of computers.
- Writing referral letters.
- Clinic letters and discharge summaries.
- Copying letters to patients.
- The use of email.

Functions of note keeping

The reasons for keeping notes are multiple.

- First and foremost, an accurate record of each consultation.
- Legal requirement. This applies to all notes relating to patients throughout the NHS.
- To remind yourself of what you have done in the consultation. This is especially useful in complex cases or when you see someone infrequently.
- To allow others to see what you have done as you may not always be the person attending to any patient. It is essential for others to see what has been done already/planned.
- A historical record should things go wrong. This should not be the primary reason for note keeping but inevitably during your career you will need to rely on the notes that you have made as the result of complaints and or for legal reports.

What should I write?

There are no hard and fast rules about precisely what you should write in any given circumstance. The GMC guidance detailed above should ideally be adhered to. The following is a guide to the type of information that may be important.

Practical point

Remember the only evidence of what you have done will be contained in the words that you write or type.

Perhaps a few other guidelines should also be adopted.

- The date, time and your name.
- Positive *and* negative findings – this applies to the history and the examination. 'NAD' (no abnormality detected) is not adequate. What did you *actually* test that was normal?

- What did you do? Did you perform any investigations? Did you prescribe a medication? How much, how often? Did you warn of side effects?
- Provisional diagnosis – what do you think is happening? Is this diagnosis backed up by your findings?
- Plan – what happened next? Document what you discussed with the patient. 'Usual advice' is not good enough, e.g. 'given head injury advice'.
- Personal facts – if your patient tells you something that may be important later, e.g. worried about housing problems, then write it down.
- In short, **you cannot write enough**. Unfortunately, time is the constraining factor.
- If appropriate in handwritten notes a diagram may also be helpful.

How can I stay out of trouble?

The medical defence organisations publish guidelines to help with good record keeping. Below are a list of suggested dos and don'ts.

- Write legibly.
- Avoid abbreviations.
- Never disguise or alter any entry. If something comes to light at a later date and you wish to amend an entry you may do so but you should make the amendment clear and why, and sign and date the amendment. This is also true of computerised records; all alterations will remain in the audit trail even though the alteration may not be visible.
- Never write anything offensive or humorous.
- Check everything that is written in your name, e.g. hospital letters.
- Never throw records away.
- Ensure that someone in authority understands all of the above.
- Do not record anything you would not be happy for a colleague or the patient to read. (Adapted from the Medical Defence Union.)

Practical point
Clear and unambiguous records are essential to good communication between health-care professionals.

People sometimes joke about the **handwriting** of doctors. This is no excuse for poor records. Your handwriting needs to legible to others so that the record is clear and also that it is not misinterpreted. Similarly, when typing on a computer record, avoid typing errors and re-read your entry before saving it in the patient record.

Other tips worth bearing in mind are as follows.

- Use plain English.
- Avoid jargon.
- Avoid abbreviations and acronyms.
- Stick to the generic names for medications.
- Print your name after your signature.
- When using a computer make sure you have logged in against your own name.

- If you change a duty rota make sure a record of this is kept safely in case it is ever disputed who completed a patient record.

Use of computers

There is great emphasis on the use of computers within the NHS. Some general practices are now 'paperless' and so computers are used entirely for note keeping rather than paper and pen. **However, the rules regarding good note keeping remain exactly the same.** To the computer-literate doctor, computers offer a speedy way to input data and quickly access information from a variety of sources and to audit the healthcare being provided. It can also allow faster communication between health professionals. There are potential problems however.

Advantages to the use of computers

There are many *advantages to the use of computers* and some of these can be summarised as follows:

- a patient record that is legible
- records that are automatically filed
- summaries which are easily available
- patient information that can be transferred immediately
- integration of records to simplify communication between team members
- a record of all prescribing and an efficient repeat prescribing programme
- a system to recall patients for review
- no longer a need to maintain handwritten files and folders or to handwrite letters
- a tool to facilitate audit.

Change in culture to the use of computers

Practical point

To be successful all members of the healthcare team need to embrace the use of computers in the workplace.

This will involve changing culture and working practice and this needs to be addressed sensitively. As the need for data entry becomes apparent this may be a helpful stimulus to see the advantages of such change. The management of patient information in the NHS is one of the keys to both its efficiency and the quality of care that it can provide and ultimately its success. The notion of a paperless NHS has many advantages, but even if the necessary IT (information technology) is available it is no use unless practitioners are adequately trained and confident in its use. NHS trusts will need to work with practitioners to ensure that the necessary funding is available for training.

An issue that should be considered is that of universal patient record software in primary and secondary care, rather than the present situation of different programmes. This may involve practitioners requiring training on several different types of software until a universal package is agreed on.

Disadvantages to the use of computers

- Typing is not a universal skill among doctors and to some it is much slower than writing.
- Most software does not allow drawing which in some circumstances can be very useful, e.g. skin lesions or an abdominal examination.
- Problems with hardware and software.
- Maintaining confidentiality.
- Authorisation and access to patient data.
- Response times for maintenance can be very slow and when a system is 'down' or 'crashes' and this prevents the healthcare team from working normally.
- What happens if the system is infected by a virus?
- Transfer of data to new systems needs to be planned as hardware and software are continually being upgraded.
- Transfer of patient records from practice to practice and in the future to secondary care and vice versa.
- Ease of use of the system by a new employee or locum when consulting.

National Programme for IT (NPfIT)

There have been several recent developments in relation to IT and the NHS that in the future will make it impossible for the NHS to continue without computer systems. First, it is anticipated that in the near future patients will carry a 'smart' card with their medical records which can be recognised and used in all areas of the NHS, e.g. attending an accident and emergency department. The centralisation of patient data and the ability of the NHS to connect with over 30 000 GPs and other members of the healthcare teams in primary and secondary care into a single secure national system is referred to as the 'national data spine'. For a patient this will include details such as health episodes, medications, allergies and much other vital information that is required when a patient is ill. This development is part of the National Care Record Service (NCRS). This change is part of an enormous development that is gathering pace and is referred to as the National Programme for IT (NPfIT).

NPfIT is likely to computerise all aspects of healthcare in the UK over the next 10 years and all communications between every part of the NHS will be electronic. This means that all NHS practitioners will be able to see patient records and associated data when they need to. There are some issues that need to be considered. Perhaps the most important is that most existing software will be integrated or replaced. There is no doubt that we will all need to embrace the use of these technologies. Although constantly dogged by delays the day will come where primary and secondary care are linked via the NHSnet and patients will have their own health records on a NHS smart card.

Practical point

This means that, wherever a patient consults in the NHS, GP or hospital or as a temporary resident away from their own home in the UK, their full health record will be available, both history and a record of prescribed medications.

The transfer of data to a new system has considerable cost implications for the NHS. On the positive side, the proposed use of centralised servers in data warehouses will be beneficial to many NHS trusts as there will be the full-time system administrators available for when problems arise. The issue of increased security of access to information systems cannot be stressed highly enough and methods are being developed to identify the practitioner 'user' who is entitled to have access to this data. This concept is causing some unease among patient groups who are fearful of this step.

If there is to be a transition to a universal NHS software, a smooth transition needs to be facilitated and this will involve training and protected time for staff and it is a task that should not be underestimated. Further training is required, not to mention IT support.

One of the most recent developments is that GPs will soon be able to book patient appointments in secondary care online, thus considerably improving the existing system (referred to as 'Choose and Book'.) However, such a process takes time and time that GPs do not have in 10-minute consultations. If this work is then to be taken on by a clerical member of the primary healthcare team, this has implications for increased resources of staff budgets.

There are further developments in the future that relate to the use of computers:

- the transmission of laboratory results online (already happening in many areas)
- electronic transmission of prescriptions to pharmacies
- protecting patient confidentiality and complying with the Data Protection Act
- the speed at which electronic data can be transferred and the need by the NHS to use methods such as broadband.

With such huge changes in the use of IT likely to happen in the near future there is uncertainty over the funding as it is difficult to be specific about the scale of funding that is required. The impact of computers in the consultation can be debated as practitioners spend greater amounts of time inputting data onto computer templates, e.g. in chronic disease management such as diabetes. However, such technology is the only easy way to both record and audit data and so enable clinicians to demonstrate quality of care.

Writing referral letters

When you write a referral letter it is very easy to forget that you probably know your patient very well. For the person reading your letter it may well be the first time they have met the patient. A referral letter is one healthcare professional asking for the help and expertise of another. The aim of a referral letter is to ensure that a patient gets the correct care from the appropriate person in the right place, e.g. a hospital, and when it is clinically indicated.

Jiwa and Mathers in 2003 write how the referral letter can be 'viewed as a ticket of admission for the patient on their journey into specialist care'. They also write how important it is that referral letters should not entail a 'leap of imagination' for the reader.

Practical point
Always think, 'what would I want to know from a letter if I were meeting this patient for the first time?'

Core details required in a referral letter

- Surgery or clinic name, address and telephone number (may seem obvious until you are on a home visit with a blank sheet of paper).
- Patient's full name, date of birth, hospital number and NHS number.
- Past medical/surgical history.
- Current medications and known allergies.

Practical point
Make it clear what the **reason** for referral is.

Illness details required

- A brief synopsis of the history (remember, what would you want to know?).
- Key examination findings (positive and negative).
- What you have done already (medications tried, etc.).
- Provisional diagnosis (if you have one).
- What you would like to have done/what question are you trying to answer?
- Tell the specialist what you have told the patient so far, e.g. that the ECG shows evidence of a myocardial infarction.
- What does the referrer expect? What does the patient expect?
- Is this a new referral or a re-referral?

Other useful information that should be considered for inclusion

- Age, occupation and any relevant personal information.
- Attach any relevant parts of the medical record, e.g. an ECG.
- Highlight any patient concerns.
- Be clear about the **urgency** of the request and highlight this as appropriate.
- When referring to a specialist, e.g. a knee problem to an orthopaedic surgeon, be sure that this orthopaedic surgeon specialises in knees rather than, say, hips.
- Avoid irrelevant information, e.g. this person's hobby of gardening and recent successes in a gardening competition, unless the information might be relevant, e.g. to an occupational therapist or a psychiatrist.
- For some conditions, e.g. suspected malignant melanoma or other cancer, there may be a rapid access system at a local hospital where a patient may be seen within 14 days.
- Some GP computer systems will print off a summary of the patient's record and a paragraph relating to the referral. Sometimes these can be difficult to read as the computer template does not readily highlight important points and provides a lot of detail that may not be required. However, templates are constantly being improved.

- There is however a role for letter templates – standardised structured letters.
- **All referrals must be logged so that the referring clinician can check if a patient has received an appointment and there is proof that the referral has been sent.**
- Put a copy of the referral letter in the written and computer record.

What to avoid in a referral letter

- Unnecessary information which may mask the message.
- Comments that may distress the reader (specialist or patient).
- Humour.
- Being pompous.

Practical point

The tone of your letter should be formal and polite.

Use of dictaphones

- When dictating, spell out technical terms or drug names.
- Remember to state the patient details first, e.g. name and date of birth.
- Say when you want to start a new sentence or paragraph.
- Check your letter after it has been typed as errors can easily be corrected using a word processor. Similarly, you may wish to alter the letter to clarify your message.
- Ensure that along with your tape is an indication of the patients on the tape otherwise you may be confronted by a note from your secretary saying 'tape inaudible' and no clear record of who the tape was about.

Practical point

It is a brave person who writes, 'Dictated, not signed'.

Writing a referral letter is an educational opportunity

This can be a useful practical exercise for a student, junior doctor or GP to type their own referral letter. This will make the referrer question why they are making the referral, the information that they are including and to recall the history, examination and investigations and think about and reflect on the clinical case in question. In addition, referral letters and their replies can function as a means of education for both parties.

Practical point

Consultation letter writing is an essential skill that cannot be learned simply by reading the letters of others.

A paper appears in 2002 (Keely *et al.*) in the journal, *Medical Teacher*, where it is stated that writing effective consultation letters should be taught in a formal way and provides 12 tips for doing this:

1   Highlight the role of the consultation letter and its potential readers.
2   The essential content of the letter should be readily available to the reader.
3   Trainees should view a referral letter as a powerful educational tool and one where clinical expertise can be demonstrated.
4   Templates should be developed for common clinical problems and the need for an organised approach, e.g. if letters are being dictated.
5   Letters should be clear, succinct and avoid excessive typing.
6   Allow a system where doctors can edit their letters.
7   Format and visual layout of letter is important so that vital information stands out.
8   Make the letter easy to read, with short sentences and confined to a single page.
9   Use a structured workshop to teach the necessary skills.
10 Appraise anonymised referral letters.
11 A system of formative feedback should be in place.
12 This can be assessed using an appropriate devised OSCE (objective structured clinical examination) station.

Practical point
Better writing and improved letters will enhance the referral process and is a core clinical skill.

Several papers have been written following surveys of GPs and consultants **as to what information should appear in a referral letter**. A survey was conducted by Newton *et al.* in Newcastle, UK, in 1992 and reported in the *BMJ* and a similar study repeated in Devon, UK, in 2002 by Campbell *et al.* and also reported in the *BMJ* in 2004 and the two studies compared. The following table summarises the importance of the information to be included in a referral letter from the 2004 survey of 360 GPs and 208 consultants, which had an overall response rate of 84%

However, it should be stated that the information included and the ranking in Table 8.1 does not take into account any deficiencies in the original question-naire. However, it does provide guidance as to a more rational and consistent approach to the possible content of referral letters. Given the variety of clinical conditions and individual details required for each condition it is difficult to be prescriptive and have a standardised structured referral letter.

A Canadian paper by Lingard *et al.* (2004) suggests that a successful referral letter does not just depend on its clinical relevance ('biomedical process of diagnostic reasoning') and content, but also its 'rhetorical relevance' and so the professional processes of asserting reasoned opinions and engaging co-operation.

Table 8.1 What information should appear in a referral letter.

Information	Mean percentage	General practitioners	Consultants
Outline of history	97.5	97	98
Important medical history	96.5	98	95
Management plan	96.5	96	97
Reason for referral	94.5	93	96
Current medication	91.0	95	87
Investigation findings	85.0	90	80
New referral or re-referral	83.0	87	79
Examination findings	83.0	92	74
What GP expects	68.0	76	60
Allergies	61.5	65	58
Psychosocial matters	52.5	46	59
What patient/relative told	44.5	40	49
What patient expects	38.0	38	38
Involvement of patient in decision	34.0	36	32

Practical point
Writing a referral letter is a form of intra-professional communication where doctors need to develop the skills of what to say and what not to say to form a story acceptable for telling in a professional context.

In this Canadian study a grounded theory qualitative research process was undertaken of experienced physicians from the disciplines of family medicine, psychiatry and general surgery and postgraduate trainees. From the results six rhetorical factors were observed to influence doctors' decisions about what material is relevant in a referral letter:

- educational (knowledge and competence of the reader)
- professional (collegial relationships/intra-professional co-operation)
- audience (anticipating readers' strategies and constraints, e.g. time)
- system-institutional (conforming to guidelines/local policies)
- medico-legal (recognising the pros and cons of a particular recommendation)
- evaluative (assessing the knowledge and skill of the writer/referring doctor).

Practical point
A referral letter can provide an insight into a doctor's practice, competence and attitudes.

A study was reported by Jiwa, Walters and Mathers in 2004 of a small study of 'research receptive volunteers' from a local research network of GPs in Sheffield regarding referral letters to colorectal surgeons. A validated instrument was used to score the quality of colorectal referral letters for a six-month period. Following feedback on the quality of these letters, the letters were scored for a further six-month period and 14 GPs in the feedback group were compared to the 24 GPs in a control group. The peer comparison and feedback group demonstrated an influence on medical practice in comparison to the control group whereby the study practitioners were documenting more clinical details that colleagues had previously considered important in relation to colorectal referrals. In the study the majority of the doctors in the feedback group (12) welcomed the feedback and ultimately the improvement of the referral letters.

It can be seen that feedback does positively influence the quality of referral letters and is likely to impact on the clinical performance of the referrers during the clinical encounter and the success of gaining relevant and discriminating symptoms and signs during the history and examination of patients. It would seem reasonable to propose therefore that students and doctors as lifelong learners could usefully receive feedback on referral letters as part of a learning exercise using the criteria outlined in the 2002 Campbell *et al.* paper in the *BMJ*.

Clinic letters and discharge summaries

What should you expect in return?

Practical point

A written reply from the hospital also provides the opportunity for informal feedback on the communication process and facilitates self-reflection on whether communication could be improved through future referral letters.

The survey conducted by Campbell *et al.* in 2002 in Devon, UK, and reported in the *BMJ* in 2004 and Newton *et al.* in Newcastle, UK, also allowed construction of the following table, which summarises **the importance of the information to be included in clinic letters and discharge summaries** from the survey of 360 GPs and 208 consultants.

Table 8.2   **Importance of information to be included in clinic letters and discharge summaries.**

Information	Mean percentage	General practitioners	Consultants
Appraisal of problem/diagnosis where applicable	98.5	98	99
Management plan	96.5	96	97
Investigation findings	92.0	95	89
Who saw the patient	89.5	88	91
Examination findings	88.5	90	87
Time to follow-up appointment	87.5	89	86
What patient has been told	85.0	86	84
Summary of history	81.0	73	89

One should expect to have a reply of an equal standard to the referral letter that was sent. The clinic letter or discharge summary should bring you up to date with the progress with a patient along with any available answers to your questions. The letter should comment on not only the diagnosis, the results to any investigations but also on any new medications, the doses of medications that have been changed or any medications that have been discontinued. There should also be mention of any intended follow up. If the letter does not reach these standards you should approach the relevant professional for clarification in the same way that they approach you for more information if the initial referral letter was not comprehensive.

Practical point

It is never appropriate to be rude about a patient regardless of whether or not they are likely to see the letter.

Perhaps it is appropriate to end this section with a quotation from the GP and writer, Dr Julian Tudor Hart (1980):

The things that ought to have been said in referral letters are not said, letters that ought to have been written are not written, and people go into hospitals without letters and, even more, in the GP's experience, come out without them.

Copying letters to patients

There are plans for all letters between healthcare professionals to be copied to the patient. This notion is referred to in both the NHS Plan and the Kennedy Report of the Public Enquiry at the Bristol Royal Infirmary. It will mean a substantial change in the content of referral letters with more notice being paid to the medical language/terminology used. Implementation should have occurred in 2004 but uptake has been patchy. The plan has a number of potential benefits as well as disadvantages.

Potential benefits

- Increased openness will engender greater trust between patients and doctors.
- Better informed patients.
- Better decision making based on better information.
- Better compliance.
- More accurate records (patients noticing mistakes more readily).
- Health promotion may be reinforced in the letters.
- Clearer letters between healthcare professionals.
- More fact based rather then speculative.

Potential disadvantages

- Having to use lay terms to convey complex concepts, e.g. moderate dyskaryosis.
- Greater time and costs involved with letter writing.

- Potential to increase fear and anxiety.
- Greater conflict between patients and professionals.

There are a minority of circumstances in which copying a letter will not be appropriate. These are:

- where the patient does not want a copy, e.g. for privacy reasons
- where the clinician feels that it may cause harm to the patient, e.g. in mental health or child protection issues
- where the letter contains information about a third party.

Who has access to the records?

Ensure that the records you write are accurate and fair. Remember that the Data Protection Act (DPA) provides a right of access to personal information about everyone held by public authorities and private bodies, regardless of the form in which it is held. This is in contrast to the Freedom of Information (FOI) Act which governs access to all other information held by an organisation, e.g. governance, protocols, etc. Requests for information held that is of a personal nature cannot be made under the FOI Act.

Patients are entitled to see all information relating to their physical or mental health which has been recorded by or on behalf of a 'health professional' in connection with their care. This applies to both paper and computer records regardless of the age of the data.

Practical point
Whatever you record *may* be seen by the person you wrote about.

Patients must apply to the 'data controller'* and they may have to pay a fee:

- £10 to view data solely held on computer
- £10 to view paper records (unless they have been added to in the last 40 days in which case no charge can be levied)
- for any copies up to £10 for records held solely on computer and a reasonable fee of up to £50 for paper records. This must be accompanied by an explanation of any terms which are unintelligible.

Children may apply to view their records provided they are capable of understanding the nature of the request.

There are few situations where access may not be granted:

- the information, if it were to be disclosed, would give rise to serious physical or mental harm
- the information relates to a third party who has not given consent for disclosure of the information

---

*The **Caldicott Guardian** is the person within an NHS organisation who is responsible for the systems that protect patient records and patient data.

- the relatives of a deceased patient have no right of access except where a claim of negligence is being pursued.

If in doubt, check first. Your medical defence organisation and the British Medical Association (BMA) have excellent guidance regarding these matters.

The use of email

Increasingly communication is by electronic mail (email) both locally, nationally and internationally. It might also be said that writing an email is easy and this is true, but if your message is not clear, it can quickly be deleted from the receiver's 'inbox' to their 'trash'. Email can be particularly useful for communication between members of a clinical team and for contact with other disciplines. Information can be passed on quickly and team members kept up to date with any developments or changes. Again comments can be invited from team members regarding the development process and it can save time waiting until all the team can meet as a group as individuals can read and reply to email when they have free time as individuals rather than collectively.

Confidentiality

Unfortunately, many people have a casual approach to writing emails and so there are often typos and grammatical errors. In relation to the NHS, one of the greatest concerns regards confidentiality. An email should be thought of as an open envelope which potentially anyone may be able to read. To protect against this an email should be encrypted. Encryption is the translation of data or a message into a secret code. In relation to patient data this is to protect their confidentiality. Encryption is the most effective way to achieve data security. In order to read an encrypted file, it is necessary to have access to a password that enables you to decrypt it. This is the theory behind NHSnet.

Practical point
Think twice before sending an email with potentially sensitive information.

Similarly, take care that you are sending the email to the person you want to. It is easy to cut and paste the wrong email address – similarly, if you are copying an email to another person. **Check before pressing the 'send' button.**

In relation to the use of email and healthcare, healthcare professionals should be aware of the latest directives under the Data Protection Act and any medico-legal implications. Users should have a clear understanding of its role in healthcare, but also potential pitfalls and limitations of email.

Communicating with patients by email

Over 60% of the population have access to email and the percentage is rising. Furthermore, some patients are keen to communicate with healthcare professionals by email. In two recent *BMJ* papers, Car and Sheikh (2004a, 2004b) describe how electronic communication promises to revolutionise the delivery of healthcare. However, they write that email consultations mark a radical shift from the traditional oral modes of communication and that patients and doctors need education in how to use them safely and effectively. Also there needs to be adequate supporting infrastructure to address security and privacy issues.

Potential advantages of email in healthcare include:

- possible reduction in face-to-face consultations and so costs
- a quick way to obtain advice
- a new way to triage health problems
- convenience for doctor and patient
- a useful way for doctor and patient to pass on information
- benefits for patients living in rural areas where a lot of travel may be necessary to visit a doctor
- monitoring an illness
- an opportunity for a doctor to find answers to a clinical problem
- increased patient satisfaction and access to some individuals
- an easy way to book and cancel appointments or send out reminders.

Potential disadvantages of email in health care include:

- guaranteeing confidentiality
- additional workload for doctors (number and length of emails)
- access may not be uniform to different social groups and disadvantaged members of the community
- it is impersonal unlike face-to-face consultations
- what happens if a response is delayed for a variety of reasons?
- making diagnoses by email is very difficult
- it is not possible to conduct a physical examination
- transmission of computer viruses.

At present there is considerable debate over the use of **'Choose and Book'** in general practice and the potential to use email to send referral letters and similarly 'Choose and Book' appointments is a considerable change in the operation of healthcare. This has further workload implications which need to be researched to ensure successful implementarion.

Practical tips when using email

Practical point
Proofread your email before clicking on the 'send' button!

Sending an email is a form of writing and so for an email to be effective consider the following.

- Who are you writing to (e.g. friend, colleague or patient)?
- Write your email with care and not undue haste.
- Always be polite and not rude or say something you may later regret.

- Once an email has been read by the recipient, it is difficult to retract what you have said.
- Emails may be ambiguous or misinterpreted – take care.
- Remember email is impersonal unlike speaking on the phone or face-to-face.
- You are communicating with another human being and it is also too easy to forget this and use it as a way of avoiding 'human' contact with that person.
- Email is quick and convenient for business contacts.
- Do not underestimate the content of the email. You may have to reveal the contents of an email under the Data Protection Act or the Freedom of Information Act. With this in mind you should consider how you dispose of your emails.

Practical point
If you are annoyed or receive an email that makes you angry, put your reply in the 'draft' box, read and re-read, and wait several hours or until the next day before sending it.

- Be careful when clicking on the 'Reply to All' button as your message can potentially go to a lot of people. Also you may need consent before forwarding on an email from someone else.
- Some people use automatic signatures in their emails that may divulge personal contact details, e.g. mobile telephone number. Beware of inadvertently sending these details to people for whom it may be inappropriate to know your home address, for example.
- Avoid long emails and unnecessary attachments which may not be read or simply deleted.
- Always use virus checking software with your computer.

At first glance email seems straightforward, but great care should be taken when using it with patients and there are times when traditional methods of consulting may be more appropriate and these should always be considered as an alternative.

Summary

This chapter has set out an outline for the contents of the clinical record and how to best go about recording information in a way that is understandable to yourself, your colleagues, patients and perhaps one day a lawyer or even the patient themselves. Good record keeping is a core skill of being a 'good doctor' and should never be thought of as trivial.

Bibliography

Campbell B, Vanslembroek K, Whitehead E, van de Wauwer C, Eifell R, Wyatt M, Campbell J. Views of doctors on clinical correspondence: questionnaire survey and audit of content of letters. *BMJ*. 2004; **328**: 1060–1.

Car J, Sheikh A. Email consultations in health care: 1 – scope and effectiveness. *BMJ*. 2004a; **329**: 435–8.

Car J, Sheikh A. Email consultations in health care: 2 – acceptability and safe application. *BMJ*. 2004b; **329**: 439–42.

Charlton R. Chapter 8, section on 'Computers and IT'. In: *The GP Contract Made Easy*. Oxford: Radcliffe Medical Press; 2005.

Jiwa M, Mathers N. Quality of referral letters. [Letter.] *Br J General Practice*. 2003; **53**: 406.

Jiwa M, Walters S, Mathers N. Referral letters to colorectal surgeons: the impact of peer-mediated feedback. *Br J General Practice*. 2004; **54**: 123–6.

Keely E, Dojeiji S, Myers K. Writing effective consultation letters: 12 tips for teachers. *Medical Teacher*. 2002; **24**(6): 585–9.

Lingard L, Hodges B, Macrae H, Freeman R. Expert and trainee determinations of rhetorical relevance in referral and consultation letters. *Medical Education*. 2004; **38**(2): 168–76.

Mohammed F. Tips on dictating clinic letters. *British Medical Journal Careers Focus*. 2003; **327**: s148.

Naftalin A, Croissant K, Elias L. Email communication with medical trainees – the agony and ecstasy. *British Medical Journal Careers Focus*. 2005; **330**: s140.

Newton J, Eccles M, Hutchinson A. Communication between general practitioners and consultants: what should their letters contain? *BMJ*. 1992; **304**: 821–4.

O'Donovan AE, Ager PM, Davies SJ, Smith PW. An appraisal of the quality of referral letters from general dental practitioners to a temporomandibular disorder clinic. *Primary Dental Care*. 2003; **10**(4): 105–8.

Tudor Hart J. *An Exchange of Letters* (a teaching videotape). Edited by Marshall Marinker. The MSD Foundation.

Westcott R. Make your referral letters work for your patients. *DOCTOR*. 2004; **15 April**: 46–7.

Further reading

Copying letters to patients: http://www.dh.gov.uk/PolicyAndGuidance/OrganisationPolicy/PatientAndPublicInvolvement/CopyingLettersToPatients/fs/en

Data Protection Act: www.bma.org.uk/ap.nsf/Content/accesshealthrecords

General Medical Council. *Good Medical Practice*. London: General Medical Council; 2001.

General Medical Council: www.gmc-uk.org

Medico-legal advice: www.the-mdu.com/gp

NHSnet: www.doctoronline.nhs.uk/masterwebsite/targetpages/nhsNet/NHSNet.htm

Primary care record keeping: Health Service Circular 1998/217 *Preservation, Retention and Destruction of GP General Medical Services Records Relating to Patients*.

Chapter 9

Writing a prescription

Dr Rodger Charlton

Prescribing is one of the central functions of the doctor in society and the right to prescribe is both a professional privilege and a major clinical responsibility. Writing a prescription usually takes place at the end of the consultation. This chapter gives the information needed to write a prescription.

Computers have greatly simplified and increased the efficiency of prescribing in general practice. Legibility is the key to this success with prescriptions that can be easily read by the pharmacist, except where the printer is running out of toner! In addition, there is a permanent record of who prescribed exactly what and when, and computers can warn the prescriber of over- or under-usage and drug interactions.

If you browse through the average pharmacology textbook, few refer to the actual act of writing a prescription. For all doctors, it is a generic 'therapeutic tool'. It is true that there are additional tools. For example, if you are a surgeon, you are taught how to use a scalpel, and if you are an obstetrician, a pair of forceps. But, in addition to these extra tools, a sound knowledge of pharmacology and evidence-based prescribing is required and its application through the act of writing a prescription.

Many prescriptions are typed and printed rather than handwritten, but the principles are the same. Although typed prescriptions overcome legibility problems, doctors still need to know what is meant by the various phrases derived from Latin such as 'prn' and 'tds'.

Practical point
Writing a prescription is not necessarily as straightforward as one might expect and comes after the difficult decision of whether to prescribe or not.

After all, not every patient leaves the consulting room with a prescription. And even when one is written there are two adages that should be considered. First, when you issue an acute prescription, up to 50% of people may not get the medication dispensed and, of those that do, another 50% may not complete the course. Second, although the prescription is written in the patient's name, with the best will in the world, it is difficult to stop a patient offering their medication to another family member with similar symptoms.

Also just because patients are collecting their repeat prescriptions does not mean they are taking their medication and I am sure we have all met someone who has been stockpiling medication rather than taking it, just to 'please their doctor'.

It is perhaps helpful for the reader to distinguish between two words which are commonly used as if they were the same: therapeutics and pharmacology. **Therapeutics** is the branch of medicine that provides remedies for illnesses, but these may be remedies other than drugs, e.g. physiotherapy. **Pharmacology** is the science of the action of drugs, their nature, preparation, administration and effects. This chapter deals with the writing of pharmacological agents (medications) listed in the *British National Formulary* (BNF) as part of the process of prescribing.

This chapter is divided up into the following sections.

- Where are prescriptions written?
- The use of Latin and prescribing.
- Useful guidelines when prescribing.
- The role of the pharmacist.
- Writing a prescription for a controlled drug.
- Classification of controlled drugs.
- Prescribing for addicts.
- Keeping good records.
- Where to find further information.

Where are prescriptions written?

Prescriptions are written in both hospitals and the community. The principles are the same for writing a prescription in either setting, but the paper format is often different.

Practical point

Once a doctor writes a prescription and signs to authorise that prescription and so the giving of medication, they take responsibility for it.

Hence, it is important to have a knowledge of the relevant aspects of pharmacology, possible side effects and interactions – in addition, taking precautions to ascertain whether or not a patient has any allergies and that their progress on a new medication is closely monitored.

A much greater number of prescriptions are written in the community by GPs and the standard NHS prescription form is referred to as an FP10 (*see* Figure 9.1). Prescriptions may be initiated in hospital, often for the first week, and thereafter continued by the GP as appropriate. The route of medication in the community is more often than not oral, whereas in hospital there is a greater likelihood that medications may be given intramuscularly or intravenously. Knowledge of pharmacology in the latter is therefore required and closer monitoring in case of possible adverse reactions. In addition, in hospital a medication that has

Health Service Prescriptions FP10 should be written as follows:

1 Be handwritten in ink or printed.

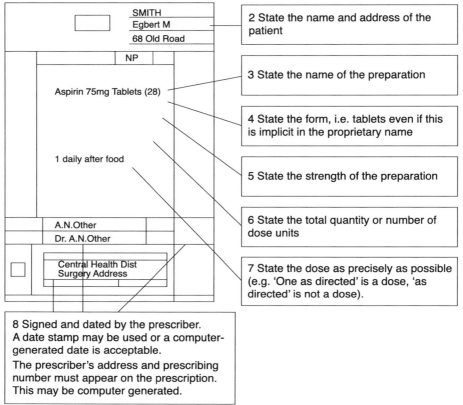

SMITH
Egbert M
68 Old Road

2 State the name and address of the patient

NP

3 State the name of the preparation

Aspirin 75mg Tablets (28)

4 State the form, i.e. tablets even if this is implicit in the proprietary name

5 State the strength of the preparation

1 daily after food

6 State the total quantity or number of dose units

A.N.Other
Dr. A.N.Other

7 State the dose as precisely as possible (e.g. 'One as directed' is a dose, 'as directed' is not a dose).

Central Health Dist
Surgery Address

8 Signed and dated by the prescriber. A date stamp may be used or a computer-generated date is acceptable.
The prescriber's address and prescribing number must appear on the prescription. This may be computer generated.

Figure 9.1   The FP10 prescription form.

been prescribed is often administered by a nurse and double-checked before it is taken by a patient.

Private prescriptions can be done on computer, but are often done by hand. These are for 'blacklisted' drugs where government committees have defined alternative equivalents that can be written on an NHS prescription. An example are some of the branded over-the-counter (OTC) upper respiratory deconge-stants. Private prescriptions should not be used for prescription-only medications which are available on the NHS irrespective of cost. There are few exceptions to this rule, such as sildenafil, for erectile dysfunction.

It should be stated that there some nurses who are authorised to prescribe from a limited list. There are also some medications that may be bought over the counter (OTC) at pharmacies, such as antihistamines, but require the authorisa-tion of a pharmacist and some medications may be bought in shops which do not require authorisation by a pharmacist, nurse or a doctor, e.g. small quantities of paracetamol. Must drugs are prescription only and all drugs in the BNF have a notation defining which category that fall into and whether they are available on the NHS or privately.

The use of Latin and prescribing

Prescriptions were originally written in Latin specifically so that the patient could not understand them. In the era of informed consent and patient-centred medicine this no longer happens, although many of the Latin abbreviations have been retained. Interestingly, until recently FP10s still retained a box labelled 'NP', which if crossed out was an instruction for the pharmacist not to write the name of the drug, but rather 'the tablets' or 'the mixture'. This no longer occurs in practice and as it would make identification of medications difficult. However, it still appears in the BNF and FP10s for handwritten rather than computer-generated FP10s.

Practical point
Directions should preferably be in English without abbreviations.

However, some common Latin abbreviations continue to be used – for example, the frequency with which a medication is to be taken. Abbreviations commonly used are listed with Latin in brackets:

- once daily – od (*omni die*)
- twice daily – bd (*bis die*) or bid
- three times daily – tid (*ter in die*) or tds
- four times daily – qid (*quater in die*) or qds
- as required – prn (*pro re nata*)
- if necessary – sos (*si opus sif*)
- straight away – stat (*statim*).

Similarly, the route of medication:

- orally, by mouth – po (*per os*)
- rectally – pr (*per rectum*)
- vaginally – pv (*per vaginum*)
- intramuscularly – IM
- intravenously – IV
- subcutaneously – sc.

Useful guidelines when prescribing

The best way to think of writing a prescription is to start from scratch with a blank piece of paper as if you were writing a private or non-NHS prescription. Many of the following details appear on a prescription or hospital ward medication sheet or drug chart, but the prescriber should carefully check that they are present.

First, the patient's name and address (and age and date of birth if they are under 12 years of age and over 60 years of age) should be written. (In the under fives, the age is printed in years and months.)

The prescription may start with the symbol Rx, which stands for recipe in Latin, and translates as 'take thou'. The drug is then specified. When prescribing it is essential to know the name of the drug, either by its pharmacological (generic) or by its proprietary (trade) name.

Next the prescriber must ask him or herself the following questions.

- In what form will the drug come (e.g. tablet, elixir, suppository, pessary or injection).
- How often will it be given (as detailed earlier, e.g. tds).
- Endorsement of a prescription – SLS is an English abbreviation for the 'selected list scheme' and prescription of drugs for specified medical conditions, e.g. impotence.
- Why is it being given? Patients understandably like to know why they are taking medication, particularly if they are on more than one drug. For example, on a prescription for paracetamol it might be written, 'If required for pain'.
- How much of the drug should be dispensed? This governs, for example, how many tablets or for how long. The instruction 'to send' in Latin is *'mitte'*. Amounts in the community are often in original packs e.g. 21 amoxycillin 250 mg capsules are for a seven-day course. However, original packs can be split. Continuous medication of a one-month or four-week period, e.g. antihypertensive medication, often comes in calendar packs of 28.

The prescription for an adult might now read:

Rx Paracetamol 500 mg, 2 tablets to be taken by mouth sos, 4 to 6 hourly for pain. Mitte 24 tablets.

The role of the pharmacist

In the community, ideally there should be no more than three items per handwritten FP10 with a line under each item and a diagonal line under the last item by the prescriber to prevent anyone else attempting to make additions. (Computer-generated FP10s can have a maximum of four items per FP10.) For those using a computer, forgery may be avoided by printing the number of items dispensed. All amendments and changes should be initialled.

The prescription is almost complete. The pharmacist will quite rightly not accept it until the prescriber has signed it, provided the date and printed the name of the responsible doctor.

In the community, a GP principal provides his or her prescribing number and prescriptions now have a serial number and to reduce forgery are printed on green patterned paper which is difficult to copy. (There is almost a similarity with the principles used to print bank notes.)

Writing a prescription for a controlled drug

At the present time, prescriptions for most controlled drugs (CDs) should be handwritten. Handwriting CDs is a legal requirement of the 1985 Misuse of Drugs Regulations. However, the Home Office has just amended Regulation 15 to permit the computer generation of such prescriptions, although there is a continuing requirement for doctors to sign and date them.

Practical point
The preparation, the form and strength should be given and the total quantity of the preparation provided in both words and figures and instructions regarding dosage.

Thus, a CD prescription might read:

Morphine sulphate tablets 10 mg
One tablet to be taken four hourly for pain. (28)
(A total of twenty-eight tablets)

The following are the requirements for writing prescriptions for controlled drugs in schedules 2 and 3 (see below) and are that prescriptions should be:

- in indelible ink
- written in the prescriber's own handwriting
- signed and dated by the prescriber.

In addition, prescriptions for controlled drugs should state the:

- name and address of the patient
- name of the preparation
- form of the preparation, e.g. capsules
- strength of the preparation
- total quantity of the preparation (or number of dose units) in both words and figures
- dose, i.e. not to write 'as directed'.

In addition:

- a standard NHS FP10 prescription form should be used containing the name, address and number of the prescriber
- in the case of a registered doctor, e.g. a GP or hospital registrar in training, the practice or hospital address is sufficient, but it is also useful to print your name for the pharmacist.

These are legal requirements and it is an offence to issue an 'incomplete' prescription and also for a pharmacist to dispense an incomplete prescription.

Practical point
One should not take offence if a pharmacist asks for initialled amendments or additions to a prescription for a controlled drug, before a patient receives their medication. It is the law!

Classification of controlled drugs

The Misuse of Drugs Act 1971 and the Misuse of Drugs Regulations 1985 define the basis of control for specific drugs (known as controlled drugs) whose misuse gives rise to social problems. The rights and responsibilities of duly registered medical practitioners are specified by these regulations. For judicial purposes controlled drugs are divided into five schedules, which are sub-divided into three classes, A, B and C, for judicial purposes.

The regulations for each schedule specify the requirements with respect to:

- supply and possession
- storage (safe custody)
- record keeping
- prescription
- destruction.

For most prescribers, it is schedules 2 and 3 that they need to be familiar with. Schedule 2 includes pharmaceutical opioids and amphetamines such as:

- morphine
- diamorphine
- pethidine
- amphetamine
- cocaine.

Schedule 3 includes barbiturates except quinalbarbitone (secobarbital, included in schedule 2) and drugs such as pentazocine, buprenorphine and temazepam.

Schedule 1 covers the most strictly controlled drugs that have no accepted therapeutic use and practitioners have no statutory right of access to them, e.g.:

- cannabis
- hallucinogens, e.g. lysergide, mescaline
- raw opium.

A licence from the Home Secretary is required to possess, produce, supply, offer or administer drugs covered by this schedule.

Schedule 4 includes benzodiazepines.

Schedule 5 includes a number of preparations that contain small quantities of some of the drugs in schedule 2, eg, a cough linctus with codeine or co-proxamol, which contains dextropropoxyphene. This schedule does not relate to any preparations designed for injection.

These requirements do not apply to temazepam and phenobarbitone which may be computer generated, but for the latter medication, it must be dated and signed by the prescriber.

Prescribing for addicts

Writing prescriptions for patients with drug dependence has additional regulations which should be consulted and vary regionally and is a specialist area of practice.

Addicts can be treated at specialist centres or in the community by specially licensed GPs. Rather than prescribing using a standard FP10, a FP10 (MDA) should be used. It is a specialist area and doctors should seek advice if in doubt, before agreeing or attempting to prescribe. It is no longer necessary to notify the Home Office, but doctors are expected to report on a standard form available from their local Drug Misuse Database (DMD) when a patient first presents with a drug problem or one re-presents after a gap of six months. Full details of local DMDs are available from the BNF.

Keeping good records

Although not compulsory, it is good practice to record similar entries in patients' written notes, regarding all prescriptions, their indication, amounts, by whom the drugs are to be administered. This is particularly the case for the prescribing of controlled drugs. An FP10 is valid for six months, except for a CD which is only valid for 13 weeks, and can be dispensed by any pharmacist in the UK. Regulations are constantly changing, so keep up to date.

Practical point
Writing a prescription is a serious business and allows you to give a patient detailed instructions.

If it is done using a computer this may reduce errors through the problems of poor legibility and provide a record where compliance and other details may be checked.

Where to find further information

This is important, but it is surprising how little is written on the subject of the act of prescribing, whereas there is a considerable amount written on therapeutics. This is a neglected area. First, **consult the most up-to-date edition of the BNF**, which contains a wealth of information on all aspects of prescribing and is often neglected and should be referred to if the prescriber is in any doubt. There is also a section at the beginning entitled, 'Controlled drugs and drug dependence', and this is an area even less written about in textbooks!

Bibliography

Banks A, Waller TAN. Chapter 4: Legislation and the GP. In: *Drugs Misuse: a practical handbook for GPs*. Oxford: Blackwell Scientific Publications; 1983.
Charlton R. Writing a prescription is tricky for new doctors. (Medical Education: How to write a prescription.) *New Zealand Doctor Newspaper*. 1992; **21 May**: 29.
Charlton R. Are you using FP10s to their fullest potential? *General Practitioner*. 2000; **16 June**: 65.
Charlton R. Prescribing controlled drugs in general practice. *Prescriber*. 2001; **12**(3): 81–9.
Charlton R, Mucklow J. *Therapeutic Dilemmas for the MRCGP*. Oxford: Butterworth Heinemann; 1998.

Cohen J. Prescribing controlled drugs. *The Practitioner.* 1991; **235**: 452–4.

Gilleghan JD. *Prescribing in General Practice.* Occasional Paper 54. London: RCGP; 1991.

Jolleys JV. Chapter 11: Controlled drugs. In: Harris C, Richards J, editors. *Prescribing in General Practice.* Oxford: Radcliffe Medical Press; 1996.

Morley N. *Controlled Drugs in Primary Care – the Law, Probity and Good Practice.* Northampton: Surelines Pharmaceutical Services; 2003.

Useful websites

British National Formulary (BNF): www.bnf.org

Drug Misuse and Dependence – guidelines on clinical management. Available from website: http://www.dh.gov.uk/PublicationsAndStatistics/Publications/PublicationsPolicy AndGuidance/PublicationsPolicyAndGuidanceArticle/fs/en?CONTENT_ID=4009665& chk=k9LrB5

Surelines Pharmaceutical Services Website on Controlled Drugs: www.controlleddrugs.org

Useful organisations

National Pharmacy Association, Mallinson House, 36–42 St Peter's Street, St Albans, Herts AL1 3NP. Website: www.npa.co.uk

Acknowledgement

Mrs Carolyn Taylor, Pharmacist, Hampton-in-Arden, West Midlands, for checking the accuracy of this chapter.

Chapter 10

Advanced communication skills

Dr Jag Sihota, Dr Abhijit Bhattacharyya, Dr Rodger Charlton and Dr Iram Sattar

---

Jag Sihota has written about consulting with children, adolescents and using interpreters. Abhijit Bhattacharyya has written about the challenges of consulting with people who have a learning disability. Rodger Charlton has written about the topics relating to palliative care and also telephone consultations and Iram Sattar about consultations in emergency situations.

So far in the book we have discussed consultations where there are no additional challenges. However, there are many additional challenges that may present to a doctor when consulting with patients, e.g. communicating with a child or breaking bad news. Several of these challenging situations may arise and this chapter is divided into the following sections.

- Consulting with children.
- Consulting with adolescents.
- People with learning disability.
- Emergency consultations.
- Breaking bad news.
- Breaking bad news of sudden death.
- Religion, spirituality, culture and ethnicity.
- Palliative care – the most challenging of consultations.
- Bereavement.
- Using interpreters.
- Telephone consultations.

Consulting with children

Some doctors believe that the care of children is completely separate from adult medicine. Generally this is not the case and many of the same principles apply. However, when a child is ill they may not wish to communicate with a doctor and so can be tearful, avoid speaking or refuse a clinical examination.

Practical point

Doctors need to engage carefully and patiently with children during consultations. This will require time, consideration, tact, professionalism and above all humane qualities.

Every doctor needs to be perceptive of their own individual consulting style. Here are some tips you may wish to consider or adopt, during such consultations with children (Gada 2003), that could make the encounter more relaxed, enjoyable and productive.

Dos

- Smile (or look saddened) as appropriate. Maintain good eye contact. Being calm shows you are in control.
- Acknowledge and greet the child. Talking to parents or carers first gives the child time and space to relax.
- Observe, wait and listen. Careful observation and attentive listening can provide valuable information and improve co-operation.
- Communication with the child has to be simple, clear and appropriate to their stage of development. Try not to hurry, as this could be counterproductive. Use of 'Mmm', 'I see', 'Yes, go on' will demonstrate your attention and continued interest.
- Act out. Imitating with a doll what you want the child to do can be helpful.
- Giving them choice empowers children. 'Do you want me to "examine" you on mummy's lap or on the "bed" (examination couch)?'
- Play. Adapt yourself to the situation. Children engage better when having fun.
- Distraction. Talk about their interests as displayed by their shirt logos or the toys they may have. Commenting on a football team's results or difficulties may pave the way to a closer relationship.
- Children like to hear positive things about themselves – give enthusiastic praise where possible.
- Acknowledge the child's feelings. They may be feeling ill and possibly in pain. A little caress and empathy may be helpful. Appreciate their struggle to get words out due to illness.
- Always congratulate the child and show your appreciation for their efforts.

Don'ts

- Expect the same things at different ages. Communicate at the child's level.
- Rush. Avoid asking too many questions.
- Express frustration at the lack or speed of response. Avoid blame or criticism.
- Promise things you cannot deliver. Be truthful.

It is obvious that very young children cannot contribute very much to the history. However, every opportunity should be taken to communicate with children. You can usually get toddlers to point to the site of the pain. One can even get an idea of the severity of pain. In cases of earache, one could ask, 'Is it a really bad pain ... or is it little pain?' to differentiate between acute otitis media and perhaps secretory otitis media. The vocabulary must be simple with added animation to generate a dialogue. Even if your attempt is in vain, it will certainly help to build a relationship for future consultations. This process can also confirm the parental history that has been taken and may add some other details.

For older children, your attempt to involve them will give due respect and also values their contribution. This may engender future health awareness, positive self-esteem and a more productive doctor–patient relationship. Direct communication may generate issues which need further exploration, perhaps on a one to one.

Child abuse

A minority of children presenting to healthcare professionals are subject of physical, emotional and/or sexual abuse. This minority is of course substantial, as demonstrated by the access statistics of the ChildLine (www.childline.org.uk) Doctors are under legal obligations of the Children's Act 1989 to act in the best interest of the children that they encounter during consultations. Doctors are in a unique and privileged position to observe behaviours, which may be indicative of abuse and neglect. This requires continued surveillance, a degree of suspicion and a willingness to enquire and corroborate history from different sources.

Working Together to Safeguard Children (1999) expects all agencies and professionals to share concerns in order to promote children's welfare. The confidentiality issue can be forsaken in such circumstances. Information systems within the NHS should alert doctors to any children who are 'under care' or are on an at-risk register of the social services. This can only happen if there is accurate and diligent record keeping across all the 'care' agencies which is regularly updated.

Practical point

All practices should have protocols, which should be followed when one encounters cases of concern in order to avoid problems being swept under the carpet.

Similarly, there needs to be learning from existing cases along the lines of significant event audit. Primary healthcare teams also need to reflect on the high-profile cases reported in the media. Care needs to be taken to substantiate a suspicion of child abuse as it can have such overwhelming and far-reaching consequences for the child and their family and future doctor–patient relationships.

Consulting with adolescents

Teenagers often feel shy of doctor consultations and have huge reservations regarding sexual health problems and confidentiality in general. Nowadays, alcohol, tobacco smoking, and drugs usage are common, particularly in inner city and deprived areas. In addition there are social disorder and crime issues to be thought about when dealing with this age group. There is no way that the health professional can tackle or solve such huge societal problems but they can try to be in a position to appreciate the patient's situation and circumstances.

If a teenager feels comfortable talking to you, then it will be easier to obtain a history, seek their concerns and when it comes to managing their problem to engage them fully in the decision-making process.

Practical point

Use open-ended questions, rather than closed questions requiring a 'yes' or 'no' answer.

It is important to encourage them to talk freely and openly and to listen to what appears to be important to them. One should not interrupt or be condescending. Avoid trying to 'score points', but rather respect their views even though you feel they may be 'wrong'. Try not to show irritation. If you show respect for their opinion, then the chances are that they will listen and respect yours as a doctor and a relationship of openness, confidence and trust will quickly develop with you.

Teenagers tend to use street language. In such encounters we must not be startled or feel intimidated but simply try to understand and communicate effectively.

What happens when a teenager develops a chronic illness?

Being a teenager can be a time of insecurity which is made all the worse by the diagnosis of a chronic disease, such as diabetes. It is a time of considerable change, physically and mentally, with rapidly changing relationships with one's peer group and parents, so imagine what happens if they become ill. Above all they want to be seen as 'normal' with their friends and the need to inject insulin regularly, follow a strict diet and regular blood testing will not help this process. Compliance with a treatment plan may be difficult and sometimes rebelling against doctors and other healthcare workers and their parents is a normal reaction.

In terms of communication, a doctor needs to be patient and understanding and should not expect the same concern and concordance with treatment that they may achieve with an adult. Also one should be aware of the increased likelihood of emotional and behavioural problems which may extend to depression and substance abuse.

Practical point

Most importantly teenagers want to be independent and feel that they are in control.

People with learning disability

A learning disability is a disorder in one or more of the basic psychological processes involved in understanding or in using spoken or written language, which may manifest itself in an imperfect ability to listen, think, speak, read, write, spell, or to do mathematical calculations. (Definition from the Family Education Network, USA.) This is one of several possible definitions.

There are many reasons why learning disability occurs. Impairments which cause or contribute to learning disability can happen before, during or after birth. There may be congenital causes such as Down Syndrome or hypoxia during birth leading to cerebral palsy.

Practical point
Consultation with patients who have learning disability is a challenging process. There are multiple potential barriers to achieving effective patient-centred consultations.

The most important barrier is the lack of confidence or skill in developing a meaningful patient–doctor dialogue. People with learning disability may have difficulties in comprehending an abstract concept, e.g. time, space and emotion. They may lack motivation to interact or communicate. The context, amount of language and the environment may affect their understanding of language. Doctors need to meet these challenges that are posed through identification, understanding and accommodating their individual needs.

Patients with learning difficulty may have the following problems affecting their ability to communicate:

- expressive and receptive language deficit
- difficulties in reading and spelling
- impulsivity
- distractibility and short attention span
- feeling of inferiority
- disorganisation.

People with learning disability may attend for a consultation because of the disability itself or for another unrelated illness.

Challenges

- Late presentation of an illness – inability to express their symptoms earlier.
- Incorrect interpretation of body language by a carer.
- Communication difficulties.
- There may be apprehension towards physical examination.
- Gaining informed consent.
- Management – difficulties offering choice and ensuring patient-centredness, sharing and negotiating a management plan.
- Logistical problems regarding investigation and referral, e.g. refusing blood tests or to wait in a hospital outpatient clinic.
- Knowing the local services and resources.
- Longer consultation time is required.

Health promotion is difficult to implement. It is commonly due to lack of knowledge about their disability and how to approach and educate them at the right level, e.g. lifestyle advice with any chronic disease. Similarly, gaining informed consent for health-promotion activities such as obtaining a sample to perform cervical cytology is fraught with ethical dilemmas.

Practical point
'The practicalities and difficulties of caring for such a special population is usually undertaken by doctors with no special training and no guidance from outcome studies' (Lindsay and Burgess 2006).

Preparation for challenge

Appointments to see a doctor should be at times of the day when they do not have to wait long. A double appointment may be more appropriate than a single appointment as good communication may take time and should not be rushed. Start by putting the person at ease, perhaps by offering to shake their hand and seek agreement for their carer to stay with them. Communication will not just be verbal, but involve gestures or returning gestures such as smiles, laughs or waving. If a physical examination is required, e.g. listening to the chest, it is important to ask the patient if that is all right.

Practical point
Because of the inability to express themselves effectively, a patient may attend late in their illnesses.

They are often infrequent attenders at the GP surgery, so every opportunity should be utilised for a health check when they attend. Interpreting body languages incorrectly can cause doctors to misinterpret the facial expressions and physical movements with the possibility of misdiagnoses and suffering of patients with learning disability. For example, people with Down Syndrome have a high pain threshold and may not exhibit the usual signs of pain if they have a fracture following a fall and refuse physical examination.

Empathy and sensitivity is the first step in the development of the patient–doctor relationship and is the mainstay of successful consultation. During the consultation a doctor should be willing to listen, be aware of his or her emotions – like anger and irritation – and not mind spending additional time. Like doctors, patients with learning disability also feel stress in terms of consulting in a different atmosphere at a strange place, e.g. GP surgery or hospital clinic. They obviously need sensitive handling. An assertive positive attitude can communicate positive feelings in patient's mind. Knowledge of the disability gives the doctor a chance to arrange the necessary equipment for better communication.

> Empathy, compassion and action must be the course which the doctor takes. A kind word can make all the difference and alter the course of another person's life. (Kerr 1998)

The carer

The carer or 'key worker' is in essence a patient advocate, both enabling and empowering a patient with learning disability to have their health needs met. Existence of such a caring relationship directly affects the process of obtaining consent and meaningful decision making in people with learning disabilities.

Practical point
The importance of the presence of a skilled carer or key worker is immense.

The information obtained directly from patients with learning disability may be partial and on occasions may be factually incorrect. This necessitates the following triangulation.

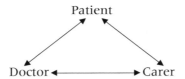

Interacting with people who have learning disability engages them more effectively. There is always a possibility of giving up the effort because of the difficulty in interaction and thus losing the opportunity of engaging with these patients. Another issue is the interpretation of their expressions which takes sensitivity and time, input from the key worker and sometimes relatives.

Doctors should be aware of the local provision and helpful resources for people with learning disability and utilise them where appropriate on behalf of the patient.

Practical point

'The maze through which a carer has to find his or her way in obtaining the appropriate aid or appliance, orthosis or communication aid' is immense (Lindsay and Burgess 2006).

Good consultation skills are needed to respond adequately to people with learning disabilities and this is a challenge in healthcare provision. Various ethical dilemmas and communication barriers make it difficult to optimally provide their health needs. Doctors should be aware of their feelings and be sensitive in dealing with people who have learning disabilities. Poor consulting skills can lead to unintended discrimination in people with learning disability. The intention of the Department of Health is that all patients with a learning disability should agree a Health Action Plan with their doctor from 2005.

It is essential that the 'carer' history is corroborated. It is important to appreciate different perspectives and occasionally these will conflict.

Where there are no relatives available to care for patients with learning disability, care in the community should ensure that it is fully integrated despite a lack of loving family support.

Practical point

These people are truly vulnerable and it is vital that health professionals make special effort to forge relationships and communicate at their level.

This will require lots of consideration and patience.

Emergency consultations

The book has so far described consultations where an instant decision concerning a patient is not required and there is time to explore their ideas, concerns and expectations. However, situations may arise where the clinical skills of a doctor may be necessary to make quick and life-saving decisions. These will be required in acute situations, such as a patient having a heart attack or being involved in a road traffic accident (RTA).

These scenarios are particularly the case for doctors working in secondary care and attending to patients in an accident and emergency department. For those doctors working in the community, an initial assessment may have to be made on the telephone similar to paramedics working in an ambulance control room.

This section does not attempt to instruct the reader how to manage each emergency life-threatening situation, but rather provide some broad principles of how to consult and so communicate in emergency situations.

Practical point
Interestingly, there is much written on the management of emergency situations, but little on how to communicate appropriately and efficiently.

There are many situations in which emergency consultations may take place.

- Face to face with a collapsed patient or a patient who is too ill to talk or the mother of an ill child. This can be in the hospital setting, in a GP's surgery, at the patient's home or at the roadside.
- Over the telephone, directly with the patient or about a patient to another colleague (ambulance service, receptionist, another doctor, nurse).

In each emergency situation, the information to be gathered and exchanged needs to be concise and clear. There are also different levels and types of emergency, from a life-threatening illness to the patient or a parent who may be more worried than ill. In any emergency, it is common and understandable that people will panic, both patients and healthcare workers alike. The most important thing to remember is to stay calm.

Practical point
When we are calm we are more likely to remember what to do and others around us will become calmer too.

In such a situation, the doctor will be expected to take charge. So it is very important for the doctor to look calm and controlled.

Making a rapid assessment

The situation may arise where you are presented with a patient who is unable to communicate what is wrong, e.g. a patient in severe pain and repeatedly vomiting as the result of myocardial ischaemia or a patient who is comatose following a RTA.

Practical point
In both situations every minute counts as you make a decision as to what treatment is required and a history is vital.

The history may be obtained from anyone who has asked you to see the patient or relatives in attendance and their ideas and concerns are important. Similarly, they will have very high expectations of the doctor. These people are likely to be very distressed and it is important to try and remain calm and professional and summon additional help if it is required as quickly as possible.

The assessment also requires a clinical examination remembering the first and most important aspect is **observation**. This will need to take place concurrently with the history although this is not something that students are encouraged to do in routine non-urgent consultations.

It is important to measure the vital signs as they are sometimes referred to:

- pulse rate and rhythm
- blood pressure
- respiratory rate
- temperature.

For example, a patient who is shocked as a result of haemorrhage will have a rapid weak pulse and a low blood pressure. A child who is almost comatose as a result of meningitis with septicaemia may also be shocked, have a fast respiratory rate and a pyrexia.

The next decision to be made is what immediate life-saving treatment is required such as administration of oxygen, application of a tourniquet to a bleeding vessel or insertion of a venflon to commence intravenous fluids and so fluid replacement. Indications for these measures need to be made in seconds.

As soon as any of these decisions are made and acted on to provide basic life support, the decision to seek specialist help must be made on the basis of a possible diagnosis or diagnoses.

However, the situation differs for a patient who is comatose and appears not to be breathing and has no signs of circulation and the patient needs basic life support.

There are five rules for consulting in such an emergency (remember **'BOCHS'**):

1   B – Basic life support
2   O – Observation
3   C – remain Calm and speak clearly
4   H – History taking and help
5   S – Secondary survey.

1   Basic life support (BLS)

There is much written and taught about how to perform basic life support (BLS) for both lay people and healthcare professionals. Basic life support must be given if the patient cannot breathe for themselves or if their heart is not pumping blood effectively around the body.

Practical point
The aim of BLS is to maintain adequate circulation of blood and ventilation until further action can be taken to reverse the underlying cause of the cardiorespiratory arrest.

If the circulation fails for 3–4 minutes this leads to irreversible cerebral damage. The main components of BLS will be outlined here but for full up-to-date instruction please refer to the Resuscitation Council (UK) (www.resus.org.uk).

- First, is the patient **safe** to approach? First and foremost is the safety of both the rescuer and the victim. For example, it is no use rushing across a busy road to help someone and then getting injured as then there will be two patients to look after. Other hazards may include spilt liquids, which could cause you to slip, or live electricity.
- Once the patient has been reached safely, the next step is to shake the patient gently by the shoulders and to ask loudly, '**Are you OK?**' If there is no response, then shout for help and perform the so-called 'ABC' of resuscitation (Airway, Breathing and Circulation):
  - **Airway** – this includes checking that the airway is clear and free from obstruction and applying the 'head tilt' and 'chin lift' manoeuvres to help maintain an airway. However, if spinal cord injury is suspected because of the nature of the accident or injury then care must be taken with movement of the head and neck.
  - **Breathing** – after the airway has been assessed and augmented by the above manoeuvres, the next step is to check for breathing. This is done by 'look, listen and feel'. Hold your ear close to the patient's mouth and look for chest movements, listen for breath sounds from the patient's mouth and feel for air from the patient's mouth on your cheek. Take no more than 10 seconds to do this. If the patient is not breathing then ventilation must be assisted with 'mouth to mouth' or the use of other equipment if in a medical setting (i.e. bag and mask, airway adjuncts, e.g. oropharyngeal airway, nasopharyngeal tube, intubation).
  - **Circulation** – after two effective breaths (i.e. those that cause the chest to visibly rise) have been given or if five attempts have been made at this, then the circulation needs to be assessed. The best place to assess the pulse is at the carotid arteries. If a pulse cannot be felt for more than 10 seconds, move on to 'chest compressions'. The rate of the chest compressions needs to be approximately 100 per minute. The ratio of chest compressions to breaths is 15:2 whether there are one or two people carrying out cardiopulmonary resuscitation (CPR) on an adult.

Get help. It can sometimes be difficult to know when to call for help, especially in an emergency situation. Should the first priority be to perform CPR or to summon further help? With the best will in the world and even the best CPR technique, BLS will only maintain life for a short while.

Practical point

Hence help should be summoned as soon as possible, even as soon as it is established that the patient is not breathing, i.e. before giving rescue breaths.

The only times where you would perform CPR before going for help is if the likely cause of the unconsciousness is a breathing problem – i.e. in drowning, drug or alcohol intoxication, trauma, choking – or if the patient is a child. Remember that in this setting heart problems are more likely in older patients and breathing problems most likely in younger patients. In these cases CPR should be performed for one minute before calling for help. If there is more than one person available to help, then one can be sent to get help, i.e. call an ambulance or another doctor or nurse if in a medical setting, as soon as it is established that the patient is not responding to shaking and 'Are you OK?'

2 Observation

The power of observation should not be underestimated in any clinical situation. For example, before even approaching a patient who has collapsed, one must observe if it is safe to approach. Then apart from the observation skills employed when examining the patient, one must also look for clues about what may have happened to the patient and clues that give more information about a patient's medical history.

- Clues to past medical history – inhalers (asthma or COPD), GTN spray (ischaemic heart disease), oxygen cylinders and nebulisers (more severe breathing problems), medication (recent antibiotics point to infection, regular medication to chronic medical problems). Is the patient wearing a medic-alert badge?
- Clues to what may have happened at the time – where is the patient? Roadside, on the floor (sudden collapse), at home (maybe ill for a while as unable to go out). Is there an inhaler or GTN spray in or near the patient's hand that they may have tried to use before collapsing? Have they been incontinent of urine as in a convulsion? Is there any bleeding or bruising which may point to injuries a patient may have sustained? Are they dressed or still in their pyjamas and is that appropriate for the time of day? Are there lots of empty pill packets that may point to an overdose or empty bottles of alcohol or evidence of illicit drugs?

All of these observations can be made in a matter of seconds and give vital information about the cause of the incident.

3 Calm

Remember to keep calm and speak clearly at all times. This will help you and those around you.

4 History (and help)

History taking and information gathering from others, i.e. relatives, is the next step. Some of the information gathering will de done immediately when you are making observations as you go along.

Practical point
Dealing with and taking details from relatives and bystanders during an emergency situation is difficult as you are dealing with anxious people that may also be in a state of shock.

They may be talking rapidly or not saying much at all. Being calm and clear with your questions is very important in helping them help you. Start with an open question, such as 'Can you tell me what happened?' or 'What did you see?' Allow them to tell their account of the story. At this time it may be excusable to look around for clues and maintain eye contact from time to time with the person you are talking to. Then ask more closed and specific questions as to the presenting problem:

- How was the patient in the last few days?
- Any recent illnesses?
- Any trips to the doctor recently?
- Any recent surgery?
- Any past medical history, drug history, social history and family history.

Keep the questions short and relevant to the present emergency. Questions about the social history and family history can be asked at a later stage when the patient is more stable.

Help – don't forget to ask for help and take equipment with you that may help in the event of an emergency, i.e. injectable drugs (adrenaline, atropine, analgesia, anti-emetic, antibiotics if meningitis suspected), oxygen, a nebuliser, a GTN spray and a defibrillator.

5 Secondary survey

This includes the parts of history and examination that can be done at a later stage, i.e. when the patient is more stable.

Practical point
It also includes the fact-finding that may help further but is not present immediately, i.e. a patient's medication, recent doctor appointment letters.

It also includes assessing the patient after the primary assessment is done, i.e. when the patient is more able to give a history themselves. Further detailed examination can also be done at this stage – i.e. temperature, respiratory rate, blood pressure, pulse rate, pupil reflexes, Glasgow Coma Scale, plantar reflexes, limb movements, response to pain, examination for abdominal distension or tenderness, looking for any bruising or injury on the body, looking for a rash, e.g. in meningococcal disease. As it can be difficult to remember all the parts of examination and amalgamate different system examinations into one big assessment, here are some tips.

Start with vital signs:
- neurological system – is the patient alert, responds to voice, responds to pain, or unresponsive
- cardiovascular system – BP, pulse (rate, rhythm, volume), is the patient cold and clammy (e.g. in a heart attack) or hot (high temperature), colour of patient (cyanosed, pale or normal)
- respiratory system – respiratory rate, use of accessory muscles of respiration, colour of patient (cyanosed or not).

Then examine the rest of the body
Start from the top and work down going through examination of body parts, e.g. head, eyes, lips, chest, abdomen, arms, legs, plantar reflexes (up going in a stroke).

In an emergency do not worry about being too correct with the order of your examination. However, having some sort of system will ensure that you don't miss things. The secondary survey is a stage that may need to be repeated several times as a patient's clinical state changes.

Distressed relatives and friends

When attending to a person who is acutely ill, the relatives or patient's friends may not be foremost in your mind. The relatives may be observing what is happening or they may be in a waiting area anxious for news.

Practical point
It is important to keep them regularly updated with what is happening and be sensitive to the fact that they will be upset.

In addition, appreciate that they may be angry and shouting or screaming or crying uncontrollably.

They may also be feeling guilty that the illness or injury is in some way their fault, leading them to ask, 'If only we had done . . .'. They need to be sensitively reassured.

In acute situations, patients may die despite a doctor's best efforts, an accurate diagnosis and correct treatment. **It is probably best to err on the side of caution and not give false hope and always maintain sensitivity.**

Breaking bad news

One of the difficult things about being a doctor is that on occasions you have to spend time breaking bad news. Much of the time we give good news and watch good things happening, such as a child getting better or a relatively infertile couple conceiving a baby. But there are times when doctors have to deliver bad news and it is a painful process for both the doctor and the patient.

What is bad news? It is assumed that bad news is telling someone that they have got cancer, but there are many other conditions that are bad news such as:

- being told you have diabetes
- breaking a bone
- developing a DVT
- confirming atrial fibrillation
- requiring a termination of pregnancy for a congenital abnormality
- failing a medical examination for a job.

The list is endless, so as well as giving good news, e.g. that test results are normal, doctors often have to give bad news. However, it is all a matter of perspective. Imagine a patient who has lost a lot of weight and is very thirsty at quite a young age. A blood glucose confirms that he has diabetes and he says: 'Thank goodness that is all it is; I thought I had cancer.'

Practical point
We all fear the worst when we are ill and bad news is when our worst fears or nightmares are confirmed.

In the 1950s doctors were seen as paternalistic and thought it was not a good idea to distress patients by delivering bad news that they had illnesses such as cancer and so the patient did not need to be 'troubled' as to the nature of their illness. Relatives might say: 'The doctor knows best'. Times have changed and doctors are open and honest with patients and would not hide the truth from them when they ask what is wrong with them. It should be said though that the literature suggests there are a small percentage of individuals who still prefer not to be told the truth and this is particularly so in some European cultures and countries such as Japan. Doctors need to be aware of this and sensitive to a patient's wishes when they encounter such a situation.

People have a right to know what is wrong with them. They also have a right to choose not to know. But how can we find out what they want to know? Perhaps consider some open-ended questions.

'What is worrying you that is wrong with you?' or
'Before I ask some questions and talk about your results, is there anything you would like to ask?'

Assess how much a patient already knows

Before breaking the news, explore ideas, concerns and expectations. Ask, 'What do you feel the problem is?' or 'What is worrying you might be wrong?' A study in 1976 by McIntosh, on 74 cancer patients, suggested that 28% knew and 60% suspected the diagnosis before having it confirmed.

The all too common scenario is a relative who approaches you, e.g. on the telephone prior to such a consultation, by requesting that you do not tell a patient what is wrong with them as they believe they won't be able to take the news. Going along with this leads to 'a conspiracy of silence' where everyone knows, but no-one is talking, and such collusion would be a breach of confidentiality where everyone is pretending. Indeed you can say, 'I can appreciate what you are saying, but if they ask, I will tell them. I cannot lie.'

One way of overcoming such imposed communication difficulties is suggesting that the patient brings a close relative or friend with them for the consultation. This allows someone else to share the information, but also who may remember a lot of the consultation, of which, because of its painful nature and shock, the patient remembers little after the bad news has been given.

Breaking bad news should not be rushed and if you know in advance that it is going to happen, then make the necessary provision in your appointments. There is no right or wrong way of delivering bad news but as Australian GP Professor Campbell Murdoch (1991) reports:

> That a good telling is possible, is obvious from the fact that some succeeded where others failed.

Ways in which to break bad news

Thurstan Brewin (1991), an oncologist, suggested three possible methods:

1 the blunt and unfeeling way
2 the kind and sad way and
3 the understanding and positive way.

He goes on to state what might seem obvious. Do it privately in a consulting room, not a hospital corridor or on the telephone.

Practical point
Breaking bad news should be considered the basis of a good doctor–patient relationship, not an end, where the doctor makes an empathetic commitment to provide continuity of care to that patient.

There are some ground rules that may be helpful.

- Ensure you are not rushed.
- Advise staff so there are to be no interruptions or organise the consultation outside of a normal clinic.
- Suggest the person brings a relative or friend as previously mentioned.
- If appropriate have someone else present to help console (relative or nurse).
- Listen to concerns and make good use of pauses/silence.
- Find out what the patient understands, knows or suspects.
- Pace the consultation to allow a patient to think and absorb the information.
- Keep summarising and feeding back – 'let's go back a bit'.
- Take one step at a time.

- Provide an information leaflet if available.
- Make patients aware of help-lines and specialist nurses, e.g. mastectomy nurses.
- Avoid jargon and use lay terms.
- If possible allow the patient some time on their own and then a chance later in the day to ask more questions.
- Always provide a review or follow-up consultation soon so the patient can bring a list of questions with them.
- When the patient goes out of the clinic door they should not feel that they are on their own.

Practical point

It is impossible to fit everything a patient needs to know into a single consultation and a further time or appointment should be set aside to see them with relatives as there will be a lot of questions.

How many times have you heard patients say in reply to your question as to how much of the news they were told by the hospital doctor, 'They didn't tell me anything at the hospital'? The chances are that they did, but such was the shock of the bad news, the information was not absorbed, but rather denied and rejected. Each consultation should be seen as a continuum in the breaking bad news process. It is also good practice to make a note of such patients and ensure that you or a colleague continues to follow them up.

Psychological reactions

No matter how good a communicator the doctor is, bad news is devastating and one should be prepared for a series of possible psychological reactions which do not necessarily follow any particular order, so-called **anticipatory grief**:

- anger
- shock
- denial
- bargaining
- depression
- acceptance.

Where the bad news is of a life-threatening illness, acceptance although possible in theory is unlikely in practice and resignation is more realistic enabling a person to prepare for the worst.

Denial is a common reaction and may be prolonged. Initially some of the people who do not wish to know what is wrong with them fit this category. Denial is a natural protective measure and it is possible to go along with this as long as you ask the patient at each meeting, 'Is there anything else you would like to ask?', and so give them the opportunity to move beyond the denial stage. Denial can be a dissociation where, in psychological terms, one half of a person knows what is happening, but the other half prefers not to.

Practical point
We are all complex beings and with time, which may be very short or long, our thinking
changes with what we want or do not want to know.

Or sometimes we just don't know what we want to know. The situation is
seldom clear cut and a sympathetic doctor should bear this in mind and avoid the
'bull in a china shop scenario'.

The 'C' word, where a person is told that they have got cancer, should be used
with care and if possible avoided at the first consultation unless specifically asked.
Substitute words, such as tumour or growth, do not have the same negative and
instant connotations and impact. The word cancer can be devastating for a
patient and can unleash an unpredictable reaction. Taking the consultation
slowly and cautiously may be the key. Some researchers have encouraged
patients to **tape-record** consultations after words such as cancer have been used,
so they have an opportunity to listen and absorb more of the meeting with the
doctor at a later date and so listen when they feel ready.

What if the person cries? Yes, have a box of tissues present, but **should you
touch the patient**? This can show human feelings and be appropriate if
we know the patient well with a good rapport and it is a true and natural
expression of our empathy and feelings. Do what is natural to you and not
something that signifies a sudden change in your personality. But, it can also
be viewed by some as the 'death knell' as the doctor has not touched their
hand before and it can be seen as a non-verbal communication that they have
got cancer. It can also be seen as an invasion of a patient's personal space
from a usually detached paternalistic professional. Give the person space (and
time). It always seems to come more naturally from nurses who tend to get closer
to patients.

Follow-up

What happens after the consultation? When a patient walks out of the consulting room door, they may perceive that they are completely on their own and
if that is the case the doctor has failed. Although the doctor is the bearer of bad
news, they should also be seen as a 'friend', someone the patient can come back
to and is positively encouraged to do so. If we break bad news badly, our words
become a 'scalpel' which will scar an individual and it will be a negative event
they will always remember. Who does the 'mopping up' for the doctors who
deliver bad news in such a way in their zeal and desire and preference to make
people well?

How does it feel for the doctor to break bad news? We are anxious not to upset
patients or unleash an angry reaction or to be seen to have 'failed' when we
cannot cure a patient. It is important that we take care of ourselves and our
colleagues. There should be an opportunity to 'debrief' after such a difficult
consultation. Although this is not a traditional approach for detached professionals expected not to show emotion, times are changing.

Can we give **hope** as well as bad news?

Practical point
In the case of a life-threatening illness, it is important to be clear that although a person cannot be cured, there is a lot that can be done.

The founder of the hospice movement, the late Dame Cicely Saunders, emphasised that patients should be both enabled and empowered to 'live until they die' and so keeping a person as well as we can for as long as we can. Quality of life should be maintained through adequate symptom control and the patient given long-term controlled optimism, rather than being told, 'There is nothing more that can be done'. This is never true or fair on a patient. Healing is both about cure and helping a person come to terms with disease.

We need to become aware of our own feelings and attitudes about death and dying, otherwise we may be influenced to break bad news in a way we would want, without trying to ascertain the patient's wishes.

How much should I tell? Is it all negative?

Bearing this in mind, there is a difference between the truth and the whole truth and not everyone has a need to know everything straight away. Above all, a doctor must emphasise probabilities, rather than absolutes, always leaving room for hope. For example, patients in coronary care units pose the dilemma whether anxiety concerning a cardiovascular complaint may precipitate an acute episode following bad news.

False hope should be avoided, but being positive can give 'a will to live' and a fighting spirit.

Giving a prognosis

How long have I got? The answer is nobody knows. Yes, you can quote five-year survival rates, but some individuals can surprise us and frequently do, such is their '**will to live**'. Researchers have postulated that such a positive and fighting approach can boost the immune system and longevity. It is important to allow a person to prepare for the end by making a will, but encourage them to live one day to the next and make the most of each day and suggest when new problems are encountered that each should be considered and treated appropriately. So it is perhaps better not to commit yourself to time intervals. Yes, it's nice that it you have given a patient a number that they prove you wrong, but it also makes their already difficult life a misery. Prognoses are not easy and predictions are dangerous for all concerned.

Practical point
There is a desire by many doctors and indeed a request of many patients for a prognosis, 'How long have I got, doctor?' This is an impossible question and one which should rarely be quantified, for we invariably get it wrong.

It is probably better to emphasise that it is not possible to make such an estimate and concentrate on the good quality life that they have at present.

Breaking news is often thought of as something that is done in relation to cancer, but the principles outlined are applicable to all diseases and good communication in consultations. Doctors who qualified 25 years ago or longer qualified at a time when there was no teaching on the subject and they learned painfully by witnessing how not to do it, and as medical teachers we are given the challenge to be better role-models. There is no right or wrong way to break bad news, but we have a duty of care to always try to do better. It does not get easier with time as there is a realisation with time that bad news is not something that happens to others; it is something that will happen to you too.

It is a traumatic event, often vividly remembered, that sets the stage for further care. Rob Buckman, a doctor in Canada, has written a book on the subject (1988) and says doctors frequently break bad news badly. Why? He says doctors have a fear of:

- being blamed
- unleashing a reaction
- expressing emotion
- not knowing all the answers and
- a personal fear of illness and death.

'Primum non nocere' – *Above all do no harm.*

- Be empathetic.
- It is a time that a patient will always remember.
- It should be more than five minutes of blunt speaking.
- If handled badly, it will leave lasting scars.
- Being insensitive is unkind and leads to complaints.

Conclusion

Breaking bad news involves significantly more than merely informing the patient. What is not required is the 'naked truth' which may confuse or frighten. Problems in doctor–patient communication are frequent and ones such as these can adversely affect patient management.

Breaking bad news of sudden death

For doctors who have just qualified, the scenario of sudden death in casualty departments and the wards is not an uncommon experience.

Practical point

Death is always unexpected, even for those who are seemingly prepared. Worse still is the grief of dealing with the relatives of a person who dies suddenly without warning.

There is then the unenviable task of having to inform a relative or family. It may occur in the street, the casualty department or during an operation while under anaesthetic and it is something seldom addressed during training. Someone needs to break the news to the next of kin. This should be face-to-face and not on a telephone. It is a time that the relatives will always remember and, if handled badly, may leave lasting scars.

Ways of conducting this difficult consultation of breaking bad news have been suggested earlier. In the situation of sudden death consider:

- seeing the relatives in a private room with another member of staff
- being empathetic
- avoiding technical information
- providing time
- being aware of the need for moments of silence
- dispelling any self-recrimination
- encouraging any reactions such as crying
- appropriate use of touch when communicating bad news.

It is important to review the situation after, say, half an hour and give the family time to be alone together and to facilitate private viewing of the deceased which will confirm the reality of the situation, initiate grieving and allow a chance to say goodbye.

This is reflected in a personal account by a doctor (Awooner-Renner 1991) after the death of her 17-year-old son in a road traffic accident. She describes how the natural reaction of the healthcare professions is to constrain the griever and when they are in contact with the corpse they are advised 'not to do anything silly'. She recalled how she 'desperately needed to hold' her son, 'to look at him' and 'to find out where he was hurting'. She describes the need for the relatives to have time alone with the deceased without restrictions, a situation where verbal communication is perhaps not required.

Sudden death and requesting an autopsy (post-mortem)

In the situation of sudden death, requesting consent from relatives for an autopsy will be required to ascertain the cause of death. In such situations the death is likely to be reported to the coroner and so an autopsy is obligatory and this should be sensitively explained. The requesting doctor must display sensitivity and provide adequate time to counsel distressed relatives.

After an autopsy is performed someone should be available to explain the findings in non-technical terms and organise for a report to go to the GP should the relatives think of further questions in the future. Terms used on the death certificate should be explained, e.g. such as a myocardial infarction. Finally, it is important to arrange for follow-up and explanation of events if the relatives wish, for they will remember little, and a structured arrangement for bereavement counselling may be appropriate and for staff support.

Practical point
It should be remembered that non-verbal communication and listening is probably at least as important as what is said to the relatives and appropriate use of silence is often therapeutic.

Non-verbal skills vary from facial expression, and impression of sincerity, to touch. In this difficult situation organised verbal and non-verbal skills are required.

Religion, spirituality, culture and ethnicity

Every doctor will have their beliefs, values and attitudes of which they need to be aware. There is a good chance in a multicultural society that they may differ from the patients that consult with them and it can occur that these views and ideas are unintentionally imposed on them. Some educators have suggested that a checklist is created of different cultures so that doctors are aware of important differences, but it is not that simple. Within each culture there are differences and variations according to orthodoxy or liberalism and the influence of living in an Anglo-Saxon culture. This section uses many examples that relate to dying, death and bereavement where these issues regularly occur.

Truth disclosure

In the UK, many doctors are under the impression that patients wish to know everything about their illnesses, particularly in the case of terminal illnesses, such as incurable cancer. The information belongs to the patient and it is their right to know and as doctors we feel it is our duty to inform them. But what of the family who wishes not to inform them? For example, some orthodox Jews believe that such full information should not be disclosed as it takes away hope. However, this is not an absolute as not all orthodox Jews may subscribe to this view and you cannot have absolute rules or protocols for individuals.

Healing and palliation

Fifty years ago in the UK, many doctors viewed the inability to cure as 'failure' and palliation was not considered. Similarly, many doctors thought it cruel to inform patients that they were dying. Thinking has changed and healing is not always associated with cure. For some patients with the inner acceptance of their illness and a terminal prognosis and the use of palliation to maintain quality of life, the coming to terms with the illness and caring can be a healing process in itself. Many cultures still hold to the view that a doctor's role is to cure and so expectations vary. There may then be a focus on the family rather than the patient.

Denial and truth disclosure

When treating a patient with a cultural background different to your own, one may feel more comfortable focusing on the family through a perceived lack of knowledge of a particular culture. Even though a family may forbid a patient being told the truth, a doctor may get round this difficult scenario by asking the following at the end of each consultation: 'Is there anything else you would like to ask?'

For those who are going through a phase of denial a repeated opportunity should be given to ask questions. Research suggested that most dying patients know that they are dying even if they have not been told. Most people come to a realisation of what is happening to them and ask: 'Why am I developing more and more symptoms and not getting better?'

Patient-centred practice

In relation to consultations and truth disclosure, there has been a move over the last 50 years from doctor-centred practice and to consider the needs of an individual. Doctors are making less and less assumptions about patients and provide an approach of openness.

What is culture?

It is not just a matter of your ethnic background or the country you are born in.

Practical point

Culture is a complex interaction of ethnicity, background, education and social factors which are in a constant state of flux in existing and new environments.

All these factors impact on the needs of the patient and their family. Within cultures, subcultures develop as cultural thinking moves on, particularly with the experiences of illness and death. Cultures are often associated with particular religions and so doctrines and rituals. But, as time advances, cultures and in particular subcultures lose contact with their religion and its scriptures.

During consultations, it may be appropriate and important to ask what are the requirements of a patient's culture: 'What are the requirements of your culture and what were you hoping we could do for you?'

Cultural sensitivity is necessary to ascertain their ideas, concerns and expectations and this question may need to be phrased differently, thinking of an alternative word for 'culture'.

Religion – what to do at the time of death

Before reading this section it is important to state that it is difficult to be specific as there is variation from orthodox to the non-orthodox between different faiths. In most orthodox religions, when death seems imminent, relatives will want to be present and perform prescribed rituals. After death most religions lay out the body and have different cleansing rituals and the following are a summary of what orthodox believers follow for individual faiths. Certain faiths prefer disposal of the body as quickly as possible. However, registrars of births and deaths, similar to coroners, usually have no weekend or bank holiday service available.

Judaism

As the time of death nears, a Rabbi may be called to join the dying in prayer along with family members and friends. The deceased should not be left alone until collected by the Jewish Burial Society who perform the ritual wash before burial.

Healthcare workers should handle the body as little as possible. The body should be covered with a white sheet. Post-mortems are disliked. Funerals should take place as quickly as possible, preferably on the day of death in a simple coffin. Some non-orthodox Jews allow cremation. Funerals do not take place on the Sabbath or holy days. Although women do nowadays attend funerals, the male mourners recite the prayers and place the coffin in the grave.

Islam

As death approaches, family members and friends usually join the dying person in prayer and the dying person may wish to face towards Mecca (south east). Healthcare workers who are not Muslims and of the opposite sex should refrain from touching the body if possible and ask permission if it is necessary to do so. Keeping the body covered after death is important. Family members, close friends and elders in the community who are of the same sex as the deceased wash and shroud the body in clean white cloth. Post-mortems are disliked but permitted if justified and necessary. Muslim scholars have a difference of opinion on whether organ donation is allowed or not. Cremation is forbidden and Muslims are always buried as quickly as possible, ideally within 24 hours of death. Muslim women usually do not attend the burial. There is a preference for a shroud burial without a coffin which is allowed in some cities. The body is buried with the face towards Mecca. In some cases the body is embalmed and taken back to the country of origin for burial.

Christianity

Some may wish for prayers and for a minister or priest to be present around the time of death. In orthodox practice cremation is forbidden, although there is nothing to prohibit organ donation.

Hinduism

It is believed that the soul is more easily released if the dying person is on the floor on a mattress with his or her head facing north. Around the time of death a priest may be called to perform holy rites. Hindus often wish to die at home. Family members usually wash the body themselves. Jewellery and religious objects should not be removed from the body. Cremation is the usual means of disposal except for children under three who are buried. Post-mortems will be permitted if they are explained sympathetically. During the funeral the chief mourner (usually the eldest son) performs the rituals.

Sikhism

As death approaches, the dying person may wish to recite from the Sikh holy book or a relative or friend may do so. There is no objection to non-Sikhs touching the body. Healthcare workers should not trim the hair or beard and the body should be covered by a plain white cloth. The family may want to wash the body. Cremation should take place as soon as possible.

Buddhism

Ideally death should be peaceful and in a calm state of mind. A monk or another Buddhist may be invited to encourage this by chanting. There are no special requirements relating to care of the body as practices vary depending on the country of origin. The body may be cremated or buried. If other Buddhists are not in attendance, then a monk should be informed of the death as soon as possible. Post-mortems are allowed if necessary. Some want a 'green burial' in their concern for the environment.

Practical point
Traditions and views in relation to post-mortems and methods of disposal vary according to individual faith teachings and beliefs about the journey of the physical body and the soul after death.

Spirituality

This is often associated with religion, but can be quite separate. Religion can be systematised and is linked with the doctrines, acts and rituals of a particular culture. When a clinician thinks holistically, one of the most difficult concepts to explain is that of spirituality. It helps first to recall people you have cared for professionally in the past and where their physical symptoms have been alleviated but they were obviously still suffering with what might be best described as 'spiritual pain'. This may be an issue relating to a religious belief and their reconciliation with God or it may be an unresolved family conflict. Or that they are resigned to the fact that they cannot be cured but have not moved through to the psychological stage of acceptance as described by the late Elizabeth Kubler-Ross. This is not a new concept, but one that the late Dame Cicely Saunders also wrote about nearly 20 years ago and referred to spiritual pain as a part of 'total pain'.

'Spiritual pain' is an unintentionally misunderstood and often unrecognised concept that is therefore usually overlooked when trying to facilitate a 'good death' for patients. Two authors in the USA help to focus one's thinking on this. Bolen (1996) wrote:

> Illness is both soul-shaking and soul-evoking for the patient and for all others for whom the patient matters.

The spirit is the essence or the unique 'being' of a person and is not necessarily about religious faith. Puchalski (1999) wrote:

> Spirituality can be defined as whomever or whatever gives one a *transcendent* meaning in life. This is often expressed as religion or relationship with God, but it can also refer to other things: nature, energy, force, belief in the good of all, belief in the importance of family and community. Spirituality plays an especially prominent role in a patient's experience with terminal illness, the dying process and death.

Spirituality is an area that requires further research on how it should be addressed in the consultation.

Palliative care – the most challenging of consultations

Palliative care is the care of patients with advanced and progressive disease for whom the focus of care is quality of life and in whom the prognosis is limited. It includes consideration of the family's needs before and after the patient's death with bereavement and the care of patients dying with cancer and diseases other than cancer.

Palliative care is the care provided by a multidisciplinary team of doctors, nurses, therapists, social workers, clergy and volunteers and involves much more than the science of symptom control.

Terminal care or palliative care?

The phrase 'terminal care' suggests that the advent of death is felt to be certain and not too far off and so is a negative word. The term 'palliative' has a more positive inference and is about maintaining quality of life and is applicable to the care of anyone who has an incurable life-threatening disease.

Why is palliative care difficult?

It is difficult as not only can a patient not be cured, but they may ask questions like 'Am I dying?' or 'What will it be like?' or say, 'I am frightened'.

If you immerse yourself in such intimate and personal consultations, it is difficult. Why? Because it reminds you of your own mortality. Freud summarised this dilemma:

> Our own death is indeed unimaginable and whenever we make the attempt to imagine it we can perceive that we really survive as spectators ... at bottom no one believes in his own death, or to put the same thing in another way, in the unconscious every one of us is convinced of his own immortality.

No wonder, then, it is difficult to talk to someone about dying.

Illness – a threat to our very being

> As soon as we are ill we fear that our illness is unique. We argue with ourselves and rationalize, but a ghost of the fear remains. And it remains for a very good reason. The illness, as an undefined force, is a potential threat to our very being. (From John Berger's book of a country GP, *A Fortunate Man*.)

Recognising this situation with a patient and helping them try to come to terms with this difficult prospect is the essence of good palliative care.

The need to empathise and become involved

A doctor with testicular cancer in a personal view (*The Lancet.* 1982; **24 July**: 203–5) describes the need to become involved and to empathise. He wrote:

An analogy to living with cancer is solitary confinement: once inside the prison cell you are trapped; you can walk around, examine the furniture, scrutinise the walls until you know every crack in the plaster, and look out the window; sometimes the door will open and fresh air will enter; yet it is impossible to step over the line dividing the cell from the corridor. The most useful people and the best doctors are those prepared to come inside the cell, sit down, and spend some time with you. Doctors often forget that they are also human.

'To live until they die'

These are the words of the late Dame Cicely Saunders, founder of St Christopher's Hospice in London and perhaps too of the hospice movement itself. These words emphasise how our role is to enable someone to carry on living in these situations, where appropriate providing medication to ensure relief of symptoms, such as pain, and maintaining their quality of life until they die.

Symptom control

Practical point
A doctor's role is to enable someone to carry on living who has an incurable disease, where appropriate providing medication to ensure relief of symptoms, such as pain, and maintaining their quality of life until they die.

Four common symptoms are pain, nausea with or without vomiting, constipation and fatigue.

Pain control

Many treatments are available for symptom relief and pain in particular and so there is no excuse for any dying patient to be in pain. Skills are needed in symptom control and to overcome the taboo ideas associated with using morphine and the false notions that in a dying patient there is ceiling dose or potential of addiction to opiates. The task of communication is important, not least in explaining the need for opiates, such as morphine, when the time comes and its implication as perceived by many that it is the end.

Bereavement

Grief is a normal reaction to bereavement, but sometimes it can be severe and overwhelming and the sufferer may need help.

The commonest form results from a death, but bereavement may also present through other losses such as miscarriage, stillbirth and broken relationships, e.g. divorce or redundancy.

According to the WHO definition of health, anything that can impact on the physical, psychological, emotional and social aspects of a person's life can lead to an illness. Bereavement is no exception and it is in this way that bereavement can be considered a 'medical problem'.

Two psychiatrists, Murray-Parkes and Kubler Ross, postulated over 30 years ago that if normal stages of grieving were to be isolated they might be:

- distress
- shock
- denial
- anger
- feeling 'low in spirits'
- depression
- acceptance.

It is now known that people do not necessarily pass through all of these stages or in any particular order.

Practical point

Grieving is no longer 'normal' and so 'pathological' when a person gets 'stuck' in one of the stages described. In this circumstance bereavement is exerting a profound effect and an enduring functional impairment, e.g. depression.

How can a doctor manage or perhaps more appropriately facilitate grieving and so the bereavement process? **Befriending** offers companionship and a listening ear, e.g. through local support groups. **Counselling**, however, is a structured process and can help progression through the psychological stages, the duration of which is unpredictable.

Medication should be avoided unless biological symptoms of depression are present. Tranquillisers or sleeping tablets postpone the outpouring of grief and can lead to dependence. The care of the bereaved may be enhanced by implementing a simple protocol where organised follow-up and monitoring of the care of the bereaved is put in place.

For a small proportion of the population the common event and process of bereavement can effect morbidity and sometimes mortality and so has potential consequences for health. For the majority of the population bereavement is a natural part of the life-cycle with few or no health sequelae and care should be taken not to over-medicalise grief in the majority of people. However, doctors should try to identify the small proportion of the population who are at risk and manage them accordingly.

Using interpreters

It is a fact that Britain is a host to people from all over the world. Bearing in mind migration and those who have not managed to master English the use of translators is necessary. This may be a family member, friend, acquaintance or a 'professional' (in person or online).

The following are some points worth considering in such encounters.

- Primarily, talk to the patient and not the translator.
- Observe the expression of the patient, particularly in response to your questions.

- Appreciate sensitivity of certain questions and their cultural appropriateness.
- There is an effect of such 'sensitivities' on the translator and the translation process.
- The question may subtly but significantly be changed to make it more acceptable. This is particularly important if the translator is a family member where there are further issues of emotional attachment.
- The 'forced' disclosure of information in such encounters may affect the wider family dynamics.
- There is a competency limit of the translator.
- There is interpretation of the patient information before translation occurs (hermeneutics). This is particularly important in mental health symptomatology as translators are not trained to interpret or understand the significance of such symptoms.
- Inadvertently, there will be an attempt to make sense, at lay level, of what is being said before translating the information.

Language

Different cultures are associated with different languages.

Practical point
Communication may involve the use of interpreters and so difficulty in eliciting what a patient wants.

It may be that the head of the family does the talking rather than the individual patient themselves.

Practical point
Health workers need to reflect on their own cultural backgrounds and the nature of power relations (a position derived from historical, social and political processes) in the provision of services to a minority culture by a dominant culture.

This approach is equally applicable to any marginalised population, such as the homeless or the disabled. If these ideas are borne in mind then difference can be appreciated positively and thereby removing additional barriers for ethnic minorities in using mainstream health services.

There are different patterns of illness and its prevalence among various communities which need to be borne in mind.

Telephone consultations

More and more consultations are conducted using a telephone. Often such consultations are for advice in the first instance. Such consultations can be more difficult without the patient in front of you. Furthermore, there is a need for the person answering the telephone to **triage** those calls which need advice and those where a patient needs to be seen at a clinic or GP surgery and those that require a house visit. Imagine what it is like making an assessment without being able to observe the patient and looking for any non-verbal cues.

One's first impression might be that telephone consulting is quick and easy. But it should be emphasised how difficult it is to assess a person's health on a telephone. Also it is difficult to build a rapport in the usual way when the person is not there, 'face-to-face', with the doctor. This is why many organisations have strict protocols, algorithms or guidelines to follow when consulting on the telephone. Within these, there may be **'red flags'** whereby the doctor or nurse taking a telephone call needs to take urgent action – for example, a person who states that they have a crushing chest pain which came on 15 minutes earlier, is making them vomit, sweat and feel breathless. This should alert the doctor or nurse to suspect a possible heart attack and that after taking details of the person's address an ambulance should be summoned while they continue to talk to them and stay on the line until help arrives.

During a telephone consultation accurate notes should be taken in relation to the patient's problem and symptoms. The doctor should try to establish a 'working diagnosis' and the eventual outcome of the call should ensure that it is dealt with safely and is to the satisfaction of the caller and the doctor. In addition, the patient should be given clear information when to call back if they are worried or the onus may be on the doctor or nurse to make a follow-up telephone call at a clinically indicated appropriate interval.

Practical point

Be alert for emotional cues such as crying or audible cues that suggest illness such as difficulty breathing.

Many healthcare organisations will record telephone calls to maintain a record in case of future complaints and also for training purposes. A caller should be made aware of this at the start of a consultation and have the opportunity to state that they do not wish to be recorded.

Situations occur where it is only possible for a patient to consult on the telephone, e.g. if they are in a remote location.

Practical point

It should be remembered that face-to-face contacts are optimal for making many diagnoses.

However, good triage systems can be a useful substitute.

Telemedicine is a useful extension of telephone consulting which is healthcare delivery using a variety of telecommunication technologies, such as digital photographs or video. A good example is sending a dermatologist a picture of a skin lesion asking whether he or she can make a diagnosis from the picture and so save a hospital outpatient appointment.

Telecommunications and associated communication media are rapidly expanding and offer a new dimension to consulting with patients. The advantages of these should be considered, but also balanced against their possible pitfalls.

Acknowledgement

Dr Iram Sattar for her feedback and revisions of the section entitled: 'Religion – what to do at the time of death'.

Bibliography

Awooner-Renner S. I desperately needed to see my son. *BMJ*. 1991; **302**: 356.

Berger J. A Fortunate Man: The Story of a Country Doctor. USA: Random House; 1997.

Bolen JS. *Close to the Bone: life-threatening illness and the search for meaning*. New York: Touchstone; 1996. p.14.

Brewin TB. Three ways of giving bad news. *The Lancet*. 1991; **337**: 1207–9.

Buckman R. Breaking bad news: why is it still so difficult? *BMJ*. 1984; **288**: 1597–9.

Buckman R. *I Don't Know What to Say*. London: Papermac; 1988.

Charlton R. Review paper: Breaking bad news. *Medical Journal of Australia*. 1992; **157**: 615–21.

Charlton R. Autopsy and medical education: a review. *Journal of the Royal Society of Medicine*. 1994; **87**: 232–6.

Charlton R. The preface. *Primary Palliative Care: dying, death and bereavement in the community*. Oxford: Radcliffe Medical Press; 2002.

Children Act 1989 (c.41). London: The Stationery Office.

Freud S. Thoughts for the times on war and death. In: *Collected Papers (Volume IV)*. New York: Basic Books; 1959.

Gada, S. Tips on how to be child friendly. *BMJ* supplement: BMJ careers focus. 2003; 18 October: **327**: s126.

Kerr M. Achieving health gain for people with intellectual disabilities. In: Kerr M, editor. *Innovations in Health Care for People with Intellectual Disabilities*. Chorley: Liseux Hall Publications; 1998.

Kubler-Ross E, Wessler S and Avioli LV. On death and dying. *Journal of the American Medical Association*. 1972; **221**: 174–9.

Lindsay P. Improving care for the learning disabled. *UPDATE*. 2003; **68**(7): 451–4.

Lindsay P, Burgess D. Editorial: Care of patients with intellectual or learning disability in primary care: no more funding so will there be any change? *British Journal of General Practice*. 2006; **56**: 84–6.

Mandl KD, Kohane IS, Brandt, AM. Electronic patient-physician communication: problems and promise. *Annals of Internal Medicine*. 1998; **129**(6): 495–500.

McIntosh J. Patients' awareness and desire for information about diagnosed but undisclosed malignant disease. *The Lancet*. 1976; **ii**: 300–3.

Murdoch JC. Communication of the diagnosis of Down's Syndrome in New Zealand 1972–88. *New Zealand Medical Journal*. 1991; **104**: 361–3.

Puchalski CM. Center to Improve Care of the Dying. *VISION, The George Washington University School of Medicine Magazine*. 1999; October.

Rees W, Lutkins S. Mortality of bereavement. *BMJ*. 1967; **iv**: 13–16.

Saunders C. Spiritual pain. *Journal of Palliative Care*. 1988; **4**(3): 29–32.

Useful websites

Down's Syndrome Association: www.downs-syndrome.org.uk
Handbook on cultural, spiritual and religious beliefs, South Devon
Healthcare NHS trust: www.sdhl.nhs.uk/documents/cultural.html
(accessed 04/05/06).
www.intellectualdisability.info
Religious practices around death, Bristol City Council: www.beaconbristolrace.org.uk/
    social-services/pdf/bcc-religious_practices_death.pdf (accessed 04/05/06).
Working Together to Safeguard Children (1999) (www.dh.gov.uk)

Chapter 11

Bioethics and values in medicine

Dr Rodger Charlton and Dr Gary Smith

Rodger Charlton has written the chapter except for the last section which has been written by Gary Smith who has just qualified as a doctor and has been able to look with a new vision of the attributes of the 'good doctor' and so professionalism.

Learning to consult requires an understanding of the principles of medical ethics and how ethics can be applied practically when consulting. Different phrases are used by different people in relation to ethics, such as: medical ethics, healthcare ethics, bioethics and values in medicine. The first task of this chapter is therefore to define ethics which for many healthcare professionals is a new way of thinking and the importance of which in training has recently been acknowledged and included in medical curricula.

The chapter is divided into the following sections.

- What are ethics?
- Why bother with ethics?
- The four principles.
- Philosophy and ethics.
- Hippocrates.
- Ethics and healing.
- Virtue ethics and values in medicine.
- Professionalism.
- The 'good doctor' and professionalism.

The General Medical Council (GMC) in its publication, *Tomorrow's Doctors*, which was first published in 1993, has emphasised the importance of medical ethics in medical education and awareness of the moral and ethical responsibility of doctors involved in patient care.

What are ethics?

Ethics are regularly talked about. But what are ethics? One of the most helpful definitions I heard was on the *Today Programme* (BBC Radio 4, 5 January 2001) when the Bishop of Oxford described training in ethics as a 'Training in empathy for what another person feels'. Perhaps, too, we should define empathy, which described very simply is trying to put yourself into the position and predicament of a patient.

Another way of defining ethics is that ethics provide a structure to different views and opinions.

It is often asked: what is the difference between ethics and morals? Let's consider some more definitions.

- Morals tend to refer to standards of behaviour held by individuals or groups.
- Ethics refers to the science or study of morals.
- Ethics comes from the Greek and morals from the Latin equivalent.

One might therefore redefine ethics as: 'A system or framework for examining and understanding aspects of the moral life'. For this reason there are three possible approaches to ethics:

- **normative** (presenting standards of right or good action)
- **descriptive** (reflecting the beliefs and actions of groups or societies)
- **analytical** (exploring the concepts and methods of ethics).

Why bother with ethics?

In healthcare there are choices and so a need for decision making which result in:

- dilemmas
- clinical conundrums
- equally unsatisfactory alternatives.

Many people who study medicine and those who comment on the medical profession may have a view that it is an exact science. This is far from the case and it is more than science, but rather the art of the application of the science.

For some, ethics can be viewed as a 'moral toothbrush' where healthcare professionals and patients should discuss together the ethical concerns that choices create as a result of increasing biotechnology. Yes, ethics can raise issues of what can be done, but also of what 'should' be done. Also, with choice comes risk. For example:

- which treatment?
- when should a potential treatment be avoided (e.g. chemotherapy for cancer)?
- which doctor?
- which hospital?
- and much more.

Medical ethics should perhaps then be more correctly referred to as healthcare ethics.

The four principles

Four principles of medical ethics have been defined to help provide a framework for the development of more detailed 'rules', policies and guidelines. The four principles offer objective guidance to a subjective experience. The four principles are:

- autonomy
- beneficence
- non-maleficence
- justice.

These are broad principles to enable clinicians to ask basic questions and so to undertake ethical analyses where there are clinical dilemmas and situations of uncertainty.

Autonomy

This is the right of a person to determine what happens to them – literally, 'self-rule'. As doctors our role should be enablement and so empowerment of a patient, rather than paternalism. In order for a patient to make a decision, they need to be fully informed about their condition (diagnosis and prognosis) and potential treatments in a format that they can understand. In this way, a doctor should be able to gain informed consent for a negotiated therapeutic decision that has been made freely.

Beneficence

Actions of healthcare professionals should always be 'good'. There is an obligation to help those who are ill to meet their legitimate health interests. 'Good' in the sense of 'healing' can be curative or palliative. In relation to palliative care, it is possible to facilitate a patient to have a 'good death' through adequate symptom control. However, achieving pain control in a patient who is dying may raise the issue of the 'doctrine of the double effect'. In a dying patient, morphine is prescribed to alleviate pain. However, in attempting to achieve this good outcome for the beneficence of the patient, an adverse effect of morphine may be respiratory depression and possible death. Before administering the morphine the autonomy of the patient should be respected, enabling them to make a fully informed decision as to what is good for them, given this information.

Non-maleficence

This is referred to as *Primum non nocere* – above all do no harm. As doctors it is therefore important to avoid harm. In addition, there is an obligation not to inflict harm intentionally. An unfortunate and extreme example of this is the serial killer, Harold Shipman, who used to be a GP.

Justice

Actions and treatment decisions should be fair and beneficial to patients and the public. For example, the choice of drugs used should be the best available with the minimal of side effects, avoiding cheap alternatives where there may be side effects. Another aspect of justice might be whether or not we are discriminating fairly in relation to the type of medical care we offer to different individuals.

Tobin, in an editorial (2001), suggests that the 'four principles' approach referred to earlier may exacerbate the very problem it is meant to solve. Indeed on some occasions the principles can sometimes conflict.

Practical point

Clinical conundrums which pose ethical dilemmas may not be resolvable despite the application of these four principles.

However, to further complicate the issue the classical theories of philosophical ethics such as consequentialism, deontology and virtue ethics can be seen by some as even more remote from the practical challenges of clinical medicine. However, all of these theories can assist the reflecting process where the goal of medical ethics is to improve the quality of patient care by identifying, analysing and resolving any ethical issues that may arise. Tobin writes:

> Since doctors, like other people, generally act on what they think they ought to do, it matters that their ethical instincts are transformed into a reasoned, thoughtful ability to choose what to say and what to do.

This last point raises the possibility of new or additional theories or philosophical concepts. The first relates to the internal market as it has been applied to the NHS in the UK and could be:

- prioritisation.

How does a doctor decide who waits for treatment, which is presently available for one patient but not both? Perhaps the principle of Utilitarianism named after the philosophers Jeremy Bentham and John Stuart Mill in the early 1800s, *providing the greatest good for the greatest number,* has a role in this area of discussion.

Further additional concepts might include:

- confidentiality
- communication of risk
- virtue ethics (common values)
- infertility and embryo research.

These are to name but just a few.

Medical ethics and the law

In relation to medical ethics there should be an awareness of the law and its role in defining and limiting clinical judgement and in holding clinicians accountable for their decisions. Ethics not only influence the creation of laws which govern medical practice, but also their interpretation when difficult clinical dilemmas arise. In essence there are a set of laws which dictate what a doctor can and cannot do.

Philosophy and ethics

Ethics is a philosophical subject. But what is philosophy? Philosophy comprises the general laws that furnish the rational explanation of anything. It is also the system of values that are adopted by an individual group. Philosophy is also the study of human behaviour, ethics and morals and, for some, philosophy is calm judgement based on practical experience or wisdom. Philosophical thinking allows an opportunity to think about the great questions that lie at the heart of being human. Philosophy asks:

- What is goodness?
- What is truth?
- What is the nature of right and wrong?
- How do you analyse arguments, reason responsibly and see other points of view?

Why mention philosophy? The reason is simple. Ethics is a subject where there are no 'right' or 'wrong' answers to individual situations, but dilemmas to be recognised and discussed and an informed decision considered and hopefully mutually agreed on.

Practical point
Whatever rules, guidelines or protocols exist in healthcare, they can never be absolute when dealing with individuals who may be ill often in unique situations.

When learning to consult, which is the title of this book, the patient-centred doctor will bear in mind the ethical dilemmas posed by individual patient situations. The doctor who doesn't do this is likely to be doctor-centred, paternalistic and perhaps relatively uncaring.

There are two main philosophical approaches to healthcare ethics that one should be aware of.

1 **Consequentialist ethics.** This involves the principle of Utilitarianism referred to earlier. Any action should have the best consequences, minimal suffering and maximal happiness for all patients. The philosophers that influenced the consequentialist approach were Jeremy Bentham and John Stuart Mill in the early 1800s.
2 **Duty-based ethics.** Deontology is the study of duty and this philosophical approach is named after the philosopher Immanual Kant born in 1724. Deontological ethics are about 'doing the right thing' no matter what the circumstances and can be viewed as a fundamentalist approach. His aim was to make morality a fact like science from a deontological point of view. He says that acting from a sense of duty is good, and acting on that duty is absolutely good – for example, giving a blood transfusion to an unconscious patient who will die without one. However, where difficulties arise are when the patient is a Jehovah's witness and such an action would go against their wishes.

Hippocrates

Hippocrates was a Greek physician who lived in the fifth century BC and after whom was named the first code of ethics. In the mid 1900s doctors used to take a Hippocratic Oath on qualification to follow the six major principles of this code of ethics. However, given the change from a perspective of a moralist to an ethical approach in healthcare there has been a move from duty-based ethics to a more consequentalist way of thinking and application to patient care. As a result doctors usually do not take this oath.

The six principles are:

- reverence to our teachers and consideration towards colleagues
- first, do no harm
- absolute regard for life
- restriction to field of expertise
- abuse of privilege
- respect for privacy

The reasons why doctors might not take this oath might relate to: reverence to teachers. What if you have a bad teacher? Absolute regard for life – there are differing views towards termination of pregnancy. Respect of privacy – does this include a patient who asks for help who admits to being a serial killer? These are just a few examples where modern ethical thinking can go against this first code of ethics.

Ethics and healing

Healing, as mentioned earlier, can be both curing and palliating. In the latter scenario there are often many ethical dilemmas and a dying patient who, over a period of time, is able to accept their eventual demise may find this coming to terms with their fate a 'healing' process. When learning to consult it is important to recognise that not all patients can be cured and that some may go on to die. Palliative care is an occasion where the healing role of a doctor extends beyond that of curing.

Coming to terms with a terminal illness for a patient can be an inner peace and so a healing process and one where doctors have an ethical obligation to play a role. The founder of the hospice movement, the late Dame Cecily Saunders advises that quality of life should be maintained to allow a patient to 'live until they die'. This may enable a patient to have what one might describe as a 'good death'.

Perhaps the greatest dilemma a doctor may face is defining when a patient is no longer curable requiring active therapy and so is in the need of palliative care. Facilitating a good death requires the recognition of the transition point from curative to palliative care. But there is a dilemma as it is difficult to define a point where such a transition occurs from cure to palliation. Furthermore, the simplistic notion of a transition is complex as palliative care to relieve suffering and curative care may be provided at the same time. Indeed some treatments used for cure may also be used in palliation such as chemotherapy and radiotherapy. It may therefore be difficult to define a point where curative treatment stops and palliation begins and also a patient may opt for both.

Practical point

However, the point at which curative treatment becomes futile needs to be recognised by the patient and the clinician, as further treatment aimed at a cure may be futile and in itself cause suffering, e.g. with chemotherapy.

In other words, if curative treatment is continued where there is no prospect of success, there would be the unnecessary prolongation of poor quality life. A management plan needs to be negotiated and informed consent gained for continued curative treatment or agreement that this point has been reached so that it is a smooth transition to ensure palliative care when cure is no longer possible.

The issue of active euthanasia has not been raised as the need for such an action goes against many of the ethical principles discussed and arises purely when palliative care is not adequate.

Virtue ethics and values in medicine

At the start of this chapter ethics was viewed as the *training in empathy for what another person feels*. The final two sections of this chapter focus on the areas where a doctor should be sensitive to the needs of patients and so values in medicine and thus be a person of integrity and so exhibit what might be referred to as professionalism.

In 'virtue theory' it is the character of a doctor that is the focus of moral concern and manifests itself through their sensitive approach and their moral conduct based on accepted professional ethics and so their professionalism as seen by the patient, their family and friends.

Practical point

The term 'virtue ethics' is a relatively recent one and it is a term that incorporates several different theories.

A useful way of looking at the virtues in medical practice is that they are the qualities required to overcome the challenges that doctors encounter with patients. In relation to values in medicine there will be a common core of values or qualities that are essential for a doctor to fulfil particular roles in their clinical practice. For those that are finding the terminology confusing it may be helpful to define the terms value and virtue.

- **Value** – something regarded as desirable, worthy, or right, as a belief or ideal. In clinical practice it is something that is to regard highly and so of considerable worth in estimating the value of a clinician.
- **Virtue** – general moral excellence, uprightness or goodness. Any admirable quality or merit and demonstration of professional integrity. A virtue in clinical practice is not just the demonstration of competence, but that it is borne out in performance as a practitioner.

To quote an author on the subject, Peter Toon: 'All doctors are individuals and there will almost certainly be alternative ways in which doctors can be virtuous.' Values in medicine can therefore provide a regular forum for philosophical debate. Although virtues in medicine tend to be determined from a consensus, they include both questions of fact and value.

Professionalism

This might be defined as a set of values, virtues, behaviours and relationships that underpin the trust that the public has in doctors. There is no doubt that these values evolve for the better with the changes in society both nationally and globally and also the advances in medical science and the increasing treatment options. However, some might argue that there has also been an erosion in professionalism in healthcare.

In 1949 Sir James Spence (professor of child health at Newcastle University) wrote:

> The essential unit of medical practice is the occasion when, in the intimacy of the consulting room or sick room, a person who is ill, or believes himself to be ill, seeks the advice of a doctor whom he trusts. This is a consultation and all else in the practice of medicine derives from it.

Professionalism is all about trust and this is at the heart of Spence's statement. Appraisal in the NHS and so appraising the values of doctors and their professionalism is detailed in the GMC publication, *Good Medical Practice* (3rd edition, May 2001), which covers the following principles that are addressed in an NHS appraisal (http://www.appraisals.nhs.uk).

- Providing good clinical care and being actively involved in clinical governance. As a good doctor one should be familiar/conversant with the GMC's guidance on *Good Medical Practice*, and the conduct and competence expected of a doctor:
  - show appropriate knowledge of medical sciences
  - recognise one's own limitations
  - ensure that a patient is never put at unnecessary risk.
- Maintaining good medical practice, e.g. keeping up to date. A doctor must be able to gain, apply and integrate new knowledge and skills through continuing professional development and thus lifelong learning.
- Ensuring good relationships with patients, e.g. good communication, consent, trust, confidentiality and conduct:
  - understanding the rights of patients
  - communicating with them effectively
  - always respecting the patient and recognising their needs
  - involving patients in decisions regarding their care.
- Working with colleagues within teams.
- Involvement in teaching and training.
- Probity and avoiding conflicts of interest. Being honest in all new areas of practice.
- Maintaining one's health so that it does not compromise fitness to practice. Being aware of health hazards, and of the effect one's own health can have on the ability to practise safely.

Practical point
'Clinical governance is the system through which NHS organisations are accountable for continuously improving the quality of their services and safeguarding high standards of care, by creating an environment in which clinical excellence will flourish' (Department of Health).

In conjunction with this publication, the duties of a doctor registered with the General Medical Council are that patients must be able to trust doctors with their lives and well-being. To justify that trust, the profession has a duty to maintain a good standard of practice and care and to show respect for human life. In particular a doctor must:

- make the care of a patient their first concern
- treat every patient politely and considerately
- respect patients' dignity and privacy
- listen to patients and respect their views
- give patients information in a way they can understand
- respect the rights of patients to be fully involved in decisions about their care
- keep their professional knowledge and skills up to date
- recognise the limits of their professional competence
- be honest and trustworthy
- respect and protect confidential information
- make sure that personal beliefs do not prejudice a patient's care
- act quickly to protect patients from risk if there is good reason to believe that a doctor or a colleague may not be fit to practise
- avoid abusing one's position as a doctor and
- work with colleagues in the ways that best serve patients' interests.

In all these matters a doctor must never discriminate unfairly against their patients or colleagues. And a doctor must always be prepared to justify their actions to them. (Taken from the GMC website: www.gmc-uk.org/guidance/good_medical_practice/index.asp)

Practical point
Medical professionalism is therefore a complex and a constantly changing series of issues.

For some doctors the need to adapt and change may be difficult and sometimes 'painful'. The appraisal process and revalidation are rapidly developing as are defined standards of competence, care and expected conduct. Doctors are also being expected to work in an increasing evidence-based setting and a multidisciplinary partnership following guidelines demonstrating continuous improvement and beneficial healthcare outcomes rather than working as isolated individuals.

Professionalism also relates to caring where professional skills are used to diagnose, treat and cure where this is possible but also **to palliate** where cure is not possible and so to ensure quality of life. Professionalism involves altruism which is greedy of the demands it makes on the individual and so emphasises the point that medicine is a vocation and not just a job. More important than one's reputation with colleagues is the reputation you have with your patients.

Practical point
Altruism is the unselfish devotion to the welfare of others.

The 'good doctor' and professionalism

A general practitioner (GP) is usually the first port of call for many members of the general public when they suffer from any health problems. Most of the public have an inherent trust in 'their' doctor and believe that they will provide them with expert advice and treatment. A GP may refer a patient to a specialist and a similar professional relationship may develop. In order to enhance one's consultation skills, whether as a GP or specialist, it is important to be aware of what constitutes a 'good doctor'. This is an area of debate and the 28 September 2002 issue of the *British Medical Journal* was devoted to addressing this question.

Professionalism is a new term and its attainment could perhaps be equated with the concept of the 'good doctor'. Views on professionalism will differ if you were to survey the public and the following additional attributes to those detailed in the previous section are often seen as being important:

- appropriate dress, e.g. shirt and tie for a male doctor
- politeness
- appearing interested
- displaying concern, sensitivity and empathy
- avoiding confrontation and conflict
- demonstrating appropriate ethical standards
- opinions not influenced by personal or political views
- respecting confidentiality
- admitting mistakes and apologising where appropriate
- availability for emergencies
- does not abuse position
- respected member of the community
- competence.

In a sense the list is endless. A review of the literature on professionalism is also helpful. Ultimately, professionalism forms the basis of medicine's 'contract' with society. In return for 'respect' doctors are expected to:

- show absolute commitment to their patients at all times, and to place the interests of their patients above their own; this altruism aids patient trust
- maintain competency in the appropriate areas of scientific knowledge and skill, and to maintain and develop these through a process of lifelong learning
- maintain high ethical standards, unquestionable integrity, and patient confidentiality; this is vital with the use of electronic data and genetic information
- provide expert advice on healthcare matters

- work as a team player and be prepared to ask others for advice when a problem falls outside one's expertise
- work to improve access and quality of care
- be aware of their individual attitudes.

In being professional, doctors must also be able to acknowledge through **significant event audit** that errors do occur in medical practice and they can be a learning experience and so can be used to prevent future critical incidents and so ensure patient safety. Accountability is essential or the trust of patients and society as a whole may be lost.

Practical point
There is no single factor or set of criteria that defines a 'good doctor' but rather many possible factors which can be debated.

Role-models

Role-models are usually senior doctors with particular attributes. These are commonly a positive attitude towards patients, students and junior doctors and a belief in the importance of a good doctor–patient relationship.

The use of role-models is an integral part of the **informal curriculum** of medical education. It is through role-models that important aspects of medicine such as professional values, attitudes and behaviour have been passed down through generations in the profession.

In an attempt to answer the question, 'What is a good doctor and how can we make one?', the following memory in the Obituary to Dr William L Lamb (1903–2001) was illuminating:

> It was a measure of the respect for him as a good doctor that many colleagues and their families consulted him. (*J R Coll Physicians Edinb.* 2002; **32**: 148–9)

This account continues by defining what the criteria were that led people seek a consultation with him:

> They knew that they would have a thorough assessment of history, a careful physical examination and wise and practical advice. He had the 'holistic' approach long before it became fashionable to use the term.

In addition, as a good doctor he knew his limitations:

> He was never too proud to seek the help of a younger doctor with specialised knowledge.

In addressing the question, 'What is a good doctor and how can we make one?', the past has much to teach us.

However, with the recent changes to the doctor–patient relationship some of these attributes must be updated to stand new doctors in good stead for a career in a 21st-century health service.

Duration of consultations

Time is another major factor in patient satisfaction. Patients want to be able to see their doctor within a reasonable time. They want a consultation where they don't feel hurried, but have time to explain their problem and a consultation where the doctor has time to explain things to them.

There is also the issue of **continuity** of care, where patients usually prefer to consult with the same doctor and so a working doctor–patient relationship with increasing trust develops.

Communication

A vital tool in the consultation is good communication skills. Sometimes, particularly in palliative care situations, it is all the doctor has left to offer. Communication is not as easy as some lead us to believe. There are societal, religious and ethnic factors which are constantly changing, not to mention the variation between the sexes. If you only listen to what your patients say and not **hear** what they say then you may miss some vital cues. More subtle cues can be detected in the manner in which they speak and their body language.

Practical point

A good doctor must be a good listener. This consists of responding to cues from the patient, hearing what they say and exploring their concerns.

The consultation should consist of determining the patients' problems, perceptions, and impact of these problems. This enables the doctor to tailor what information the patient requires and wants to know. Treatment options should be discussed, and decisions made about how to go forward. Doctors should give clear explanations about treatment and diagnosis, and check that the patient has understood. Failure in doing this is shown in the surprisingly high proportion of patients who remember very little about their diagnosis or treatment after a consultation.

Identifying the good doctor through performance indicators

Some of these are as follows:

- keeping up to date (attending postgraduate meetings and courses)
- postgraduate qualifications
- appropriate prescribing
- number of complaints
- meeting healthcare 'targets'
- gaining quality awards in practice.

When a patient is in the consulting room, they usually place their trust in the hands of the doctor. In return the doctor must use his or her good conscience and honesty to help the patient make decisions about their own healthcare in the

absence of certainty. The good doctor is be able to place his or herself in the patients' 'shoes', to understand what it is like to be on the receiving end of their treatment. 'Bedside manner' is very important in forming good relationships with your patients. A doctor must have a repertoire of different 'manners' for the variety of patients, from paternalistic to partnership, transforming as the patients' needs change. Consultation models are discussed in depth in the next chapter.

Practical point

Uncertainty is inevitable in medical consultations, both in making a diagnosis and formulating a management plan, and this should be shared with patients so that they are aware that medicine is not always an exact science with predictable outcomes.

There are many features of care that are impossible to reliably **measure**, such as the ability to comfort, care and console. However, these factors can be accurately described and patients will notice when they are not present. Some of the medical litigation that occurs is because a patient feels that their doctor did not care about them. Patients want to trust the doctor, but this trust must be earned. Patients must be treated as adults, their views heard and their decisions accepted.

In the endeavour to become a good doctor it is important that it is acknowledged that we are only human and cannot achieve perfection. Instead we must continue to strive towards self-improvement and optimising care paying due consideration to the factors that potentially comprise the concept of professionalism.

Bibliography

Alberti G. Professionalism – time for a new look. *Clinical Medicine*. 2002; **2**: 91.

Bates C. The good doctor. *Clinical Medicine*. 2001; **1**: 128–31.

Braithwaite J *et al*. New professionalism in the 21st century. [Letters.] *The Lancet*. 2006; **367**: 645–9.

Campbell A, Gillett G, Jones G. *Practical Medical Ethics*. Oxford: Oxford University Press; 1992.

Chervenak FA, McCullough LB. Professionalism and justice: ethical management guidelines for leaders of academic medical centres. *Academic Medicine*. 2002; **77**: 45–7.

Department of Health. http://www.dh.gov.uk/PolicyAndGuidance/HealthAndSocialCare Topics/ClinicalGovernance/fs/en

Fulford KWM. Moral theory and medical practice. Cambridge: Cambridge University Press; 1989.

General Medical Council (GMC): www.gmc-uk.org

Grayling AC. What's the point of philosophy? *The Independent*. 2006; **17 February**: 8–9.

Irvine D. Doctors in the UK: their new professionalism and its regulatory framework. *The Lancet*. 2001; **358**: 1807–10.

Irvine D. The performance of doctors: the new professionalism. *The Lancet*. 1999; **353**: 1174–7.

Martin J, Dacre J. Professional attitudes: why we should care. *Clinical Medicine*. 2002; **2**: 182–4.

Medical Professionalism Project. Medical professionalism in the new millennium: a physicians' charter. *New Zealand Medical Journal*. 2002; **115**: 203–4.

Spence J. The need for understanding the individual. In: *The Purpose and Practice of Medicine.* Oxford: Oxford University Press; 1960.

Tobin, B. Advancing the field of clinical ethics: particularity and practicality. *Medical Journal of Australia.* 2001; **174**: 269–70.

Toon P. *Towards a Philosophy of General Practice: a study of the virtuous practitioner.* RCGP Occasional Paper 78. London: RCGP; 1999.

Toon P. Defining and cultivating the virtues. *British Journal of General Practice.* 2002; **52**: 782–3.

Watkins P. The perplexed physician and the absence of certainty. *Journal of the Royal College of Physicians of London.* 2000; **34**: 513–14.

Williams S, Weinman J, Dale J. Doctor-patient communication and patient satisfaction: a review. *Family Practice.* 1998; **15**: 480–92.

Chapter 12

Consultation models

*Dr Teresa Pawlikowska, Colonel Jonathan Leach,
Sqn Ldr Peter Lavallee, Dr Rodger Charlton and Dr Jo Piercy*

This chapter has been a labour of love written mainly by Teresa Pawlikowska. It is an area where there has been a vast amount of research and is vital to any book which seeks to instruct its readers in the consultation. It is important to know the history and how the different models have arisen. Jonathan Leach and Peter Lavallee have also contributed to several of the consultation models. Rodger Charlton has written about the Leicester Assessment Package, evidence-based medicine and complexity in the consultation and Jo Piercy has provided a useful conclusion to a long chapter.

Communication skills are unlikely to be perfect and may deteriorate with time for the practising clinician. Effective communication is essential to the current practice of medicine. Over the last 15 years it has been increasingly recognised as a core skill for clinicians. This has had an impact upon their interaction with patients but, of no less importance, it has influenced their contribution to the healthcare team settings in which they work, and the medical community as a whole. A fundamental change in medical culture in this area has been the recognition and acceptance of the fact that the way in which health professionals communicate, on all levels, can be enhanced, irrespective of the innate and learned abilities they already possess. This has been illustrated in the last 10 years with the inclusion of communication skills teaching in all undergraduate education, and a complete change in the educational processes surrounding the teaching and observing of doctor–patient interaction.

> Interactions or interviews between doctors and patients are the cornerstone on medical practice.[1]

The aim of this chapter is to introduce the reader to a patient-centred approach to the consultation by describing various models of the consultation considering the biomedical and psychosocial approaches and how they have evolved. Ultimately everyone will develop their own flexible consulting skills and be able to use elements of these various approaches both when consulting with patients and analysing their interactions.

This chapter is divided into the following sections.

- Definition of the consultation.
- Background to consultation models.

- Individual consultation models:
  - Weiner (1948)
  - Maslow (1954)
  - Balint (1957)
  - Berne (1964)
  - Byrne and Long (1976)
  - Stott and Davis (1979)
  - Helman (1984)
  - Pendleton (1984)
  - Neighbour (1987)
  - Fraser (1994)
  - Stewart *et al.* (1995)
  - Kurtz, Silverman and Draper (1996).
- Other issues and recent influences:
  - empathy, empowerment and enablement
  - evidence-based medicine
  - neuro-linguistic programming
  - narrative
  - complexity and the consultation
  - summary.
- Conclusion.

Definition of the consultation

The medical consultation is a two-way encounter between a doctor or a practitioner and a patient. This may be initiated by a patient when they are ill or by a doctor when instituting preventive medicine or screening. There are many different models and potential structures for these interactions and some of these models are discussed in this chapter.

Practical point

There is no ideal consultation model, but the evolution of the various models over time is of particular interest as a practitioner develops their own unique consulting style.

Background to consultation models

There are several different approaches to the consultation or models. They are all ways of understanding the reality of our experiences. All of the ways of looking at the consultation have their strengths and weaknesses; because of this you will find some more applicable than others when you come to consider a particular type of consultation. For example, a first consultation with a teenager requesting contraception will involve relatively more health promotion than a first meeting with an elderly lady who complains of tiredness and you suspect may be suffering from depression. Take a look at all of the models discussed here before you decide which ones fit best with your natural consulting style. Equally relevant is to consider any unsatisfactory consultations which have made you feel uncomfortable, inadequate or stressed and ask why.

When the human system malfunctions, one will have a biomedical framework, which enables one to hone down on the presenting symptom, e.g. chest pain, to the relevant system (cardiovascular, respiratory, upper gastrointestinal tract, musculoskeletal) by using a structured approach to the patient's history. One may even be able to determine which human system is malfunctioning, but will probably discover little about the individual human condition with this approach and how that condition is affecting them. Evidence is accumulating that, without exploring the latter, a management plan may not be successful or gain the patient's concordance, let alone the chance of them returning to seek your opinion in the future.

> Patients may define success differently from health care professionals, and increasingly the public expects to get its definition of quality and benefit recognised. (Neuberger 1998)[2]

At the beginning of the 20th century the dominant image of a doctor was as a species of 'applied scientist' or engineer.[3] By the end of the 20th century it was evident that science and technology could not always provide a solution to people's problems, and that patients' unquestioning trust in medical professionals had been undermined by enquiries such as the Bristol and Shipman. Social change and the explosion of public access to information and alternatives means that we need to develop a wider view in order to help those who consult us and provide improved access and choice.

The pivotal contribution of the patient's history to the final diagnosis (82%) was pointed out more than a quarter of a century ago.[4] McWhinney in Canada,[5,6] and the growing body of researchers and teachers whose work is discussed in this chapter, have repeatedly drawn attention to the importance of going beyond a biomedical diagnosis to define and address the patient's agenda, and developing a patient-centred clinical method of consultation. By considering different approaches to the consultation, this will help you to reflect on your own experiences so that you can develop an open and flexible method of consulting with patients.

Individual consultation models

The consultation is an exercise in complexity. A number of approaches have been developed to enable us to reflect on the huge variety we routinely encounter in our professional lives. These models of the consultation have been developed by people who bring to their analysis their own experience and vision (e.g. as psychologists or anthropologists), and so the emphasis of each model differs. As a result you may find that a particular model, or group of models, can give you more insight into the analysis of a consultation, e.g. modification of health-seeking behaviour may be important when a usually fit young adult consults with an upper respiratory tract infection wanting antibiotics, but less relevant when a person with diabetes attends for their check-up in a chronic disease clinic.

In comparison with the relatively simple process of written communication, verbal and non-verbal communication is considerably more dynamic and complex, with a cycling of transfer of messages between the two or more parties.

Practical point

These complex situations still reduce down to include the same basic principles once the complex structure of the encounter has been unfolded.

Many authors have written extensively on the structure of the consultation with patients. As you will see these models range from being doctor-centred, such as Byrne and Long (1976),[7] through to the doctor and patient having a 'dialogue' and a greater sharing of responsibilities, such as Pendleton, Schofield, Tate and Havelock (1984).[8] A more in-depth structure to the consultation is provided by the Calgary–Cambridge Guide to the Medical Interview (Kurtz, Silverman and Draper 1998).[9]

Overarching approaches, e.g. Maslow (1954)[10] and Berne (1964),[11] are important as they have a wide application. Balint's work (1957)[12] opened up thinking on consultation dynamics. Contemporary models such as Stewart (1995, 2003)[13,14] Pendleton (2003)[15] and Kurtz (1996)[16] offer detailed frameworks for analysis and quality improvement. Models are not best used as theoretical checklists learned by rote. This can stunt style and the consultation dynamic. Instead, look at the summary table (Table 12.1) and consider which models are most meaningful to you. Greater detail is then provided of each model or you can refer back to the original referenced source if you wish.

The models and approaches included here are not intended to be an exhaustive list. Many of these models have evolved from work in primary care as GPs routinely see people with undifferentiated problems, where consultation skills are key to making a diagnosis and developing a management plan. Individual models and approaches are summarised in tabular form in Table 12.1 and are ordered chronologically.

Weiner (1948)[17]

Communication in its initiation by the sender and interpretation by the receiver is a cognitive process. This means that active reflection on the process of communication is one of the first steps to improving skills. The Shannon Model (1948)[24] which was modified by Weiner (1948), who introduced the feedback loop, is still taught as the basic model of the communication process. Reflecting on this simple model we can identify a number of key stages in improving our communication (*see* Table 12.2) which can be easily applied in the clinical setting.

Maslow: a hierarchy of human needs (1954)[10]

At first glance this may not seem an obvious model for approaching a consultation, but it deals with the fundamental reason of why a patient may feel they need to consult a doctor. Maslow was an American psychologist whose thinking has influenced education, business, social studies and medicine. He recognised

Table 12.1 Individual models of the consultation

Model or approach	Key structure	Comments
Weiner (1948)[17]	Initiation by the sender Interpretation by the receiver	Key steps in improving communication: information source, transmitter, receiver, destination, feedback, clarification, reflection
Maslow (1954)[10]	Hierarchy of human needs	Overarching theory Basic needs (physical, safety, love) must be satisfied before higher level needs can be addressed
Balint (1957)[12]	Doctor–patient relationship	Bio-psychosocial view Doctor as a 'drug' Active listening Hidden agenda Apostolic function of doctor Analysed GP case history dynamics
Berne (1964)[11]	Parent = authority Adult = logic Child = intuitive Transactional analysis Consultation is a 'game' of social interchange	Over-arching theory Simple accessible model Crossed transactions are dysfunctional
Byrne and Long (1976)[7]	Six phases of the consultation: • establishing a relationship with patient • discovering a reason for attendance • verbal and/or physical exam • consider the condition • detail treatment or investigation • terminate consultation	Research based in general practice Doctor = product and prisoner of own medical education Identified many doctor-centred authoritarian styles compared with patient-centred ones
Stott and Davis (1979)[18]	A Management of presenting problems B Modification of help-seeking behaviour C Management of continuing problems D Opportunistic health promotion	Theoretical framework Bio-psychosocial model For GPs in consultation and teaching

Table 12.1 Continued

Model or approach	Key structure	Comments
Helman (1984)[19,20]	1 What has happened? 2 Why has it happened? 3 Why has it happened to me? 4 Why now? 5 What would happen to me if nothing were done about it? 6 What are its likely effects on other people if nothing is done about it? 7 What should I do about it?	Patient-centred and holistic Derived from patient's narrative Illness has social meaning Anthropological viewpoint Holistic approach Lay theories
Pendleton *et al.* (1984, 2003)[8,15]	1 Understand the problem 2 Understand the patient 3 Share understanding 4 Share decisions and responsibility 5 Maintain the relationship	Patient-centred amd partnership model Framework for detailed analysis and feedback Derived from research in GP
Neighbour (1987)[21]	1 Connecting 2 Summarising 3 Handing over 4 Safety netting 5 Housekeeping	Patient-centred Promotes partnership Follows GP consultation flow Links organiser (analysis) with responder (intuition)
Fraser (1994, 1999)[22,23]	1 Interviewing/history taking 2 Physical exam 3 Patient management 4 Problem solving 5 Behaviour and relationship with patients 6 Anticipatory care 7 Record keeping	Patient-centred Addressing patient's ideas, concerns and expectations essential to make progress Unable to reassure or advise if patient's agenda is unexplored Enables detailed assessment of performance, and feedback
Stewart *et al.* (1995, 2003)[13,14]	1 Exploring both the disease and the illness experience 2 Understanding the whole person 3 Finding common ground 4 Incorporating prevention and health promotion 5 Enhancing the patient–doctor relationship 6 Being realistic (time, resources)	'Patient-centred medicine' Holistic, partnership model for clinical method, education and research
Calgary–Cambridge Observation Guide (1996)[16]	Basic stages of a consultation: 1 Initiating the session 2 Gathering information 3 Building the relationship 4 Explanation and planning 5 Closing the session	Patient-centred and collaborative model Underpinned by a detailed framework of skills

Table 12.2 Key steps in improving communication

Step 1	Information Source	Consider what is the purpose of the communication. What is it that needs to be communicated? What is the content of the message to be created?
Step 2	Transmitter	What is the best format for the message to prevent misunderstanding? (The mouth (sound) and body (gesture, writing).) What is the best format for the receiver? Treating a message (spoken or written word) or making a signal.
Step 3	Receiver	Consider the other party in the communication (patient, manager, colleague). What barriers (noise) might you need to overcome to ensure effective receipt of the message (e.g. visual/hearing impairment)?
Step 4	Destination	Considering the other party, what barriers might you need to overcome to ensure correct interpretation of the message (e.g. language, cultural, emotional [depression, fright, stress], hidden agenda, intelligence, recall)? Noise – anything which obscures the message and can act at any stage to prevent the receipt and understanding of the message as intended by the transmitter.
Step 5	Feedback	Monitor for feedback – verbal or physical reaction that indicates understanding (e.g. smile, nodding) or misunderstanding (frown), poor reception (anger, withdrawal), etc.
Step 6	Clarification	Verbal checking that you have correctly interpreted the (non-verbal) feedback, e.g. was there anything about what I said that made you feel unhappy?
Step 7	Reflection	Reflect upon the communication – was it successful? Could it have been improved and, if yes, how?

the importance of a holistic approach: to emphasise the whole person, their culture and environment. He was able to integrate the views of behaviourists (that all things are learned), Freudian analysts (where instinct is paramount) and humanists.

He argued that all humans had needs, which were 'the essence of their lives'. These human needs can be classified as a 'hierarchy of needs' using a pyramidal concept where fundamental needs are at the bottom of the pyramid and must be fulfilled before a person can address fulfilment at the next level:

Self-actualisation
(true to own nature)
Esteem/self-respect
Love/affection/belongingness
Safety (security/stability/reduced anxiety)
Physical needs, for example, air, food and water

In the pyramid model higher needs are later evolutionary developments, and so they can develop later in an individual although their fulfilment creates greater happiness and individual growth and require a better external environment. Lower needs in the pyramid must be fulfilled. For example, a parent in temporary bed and breakfast accommodation who repeatedly presents their child with acute temperatures, coughs and colds (biomedically 'acute minor illness') may be unreceptive to self-management advice (which demands high self-respect and esteem to put into practice) as they are focused on concerns that basic physical needs (adequate food and warmth, etc.) and shelter needs (stable housing and finances) are not being met and may underpin the ill health of their child.

Communication, and consultation in particular, is a complex human interchange and Maslow's theory spans the many threads that make up our humanity. Maslow's hierarchy of needs remains a powerful overarching holistic approach to analysis in many fields, not least that of consulting with patients.

Practical point

Holistic medical care is an approach which considers all aspects of a person's health, including the physical, psychological, emotional, social, spiritual and cultural.

Balint: the doctor, his patient, and the illness (1957)[12]

This was a pioneering approach to the general practice consultation. Balint looked at transference and counter-transference in the consultation. Most importantly Balint commented that doctors have feelings and those feelings have a function in the consultation. He also highlighted that psychological problems are often manifest physically and even physical disease has psychological consequences.

Balint's work changed the landscape for consultation in primary care. He was a Hungarian refugee who worked as a psychoanalyst in London. He felt that a system based solely on biomedical diagnosis was inadequate for the task of the consultation. Balint, together with his wife, worked with a group of 14 GPs. They used case discussion and feedback to enable doctors to work with a dynamic bio-psychosocial view. They also created a training programme to enhance the capability of the GPs for 'practical brief psychotherapy' in consultation.

Balint gave us a better understanding of the emotional content of doctor–patient relationships.

- He emphasised the doctor's pivotal role in trying to make sense of undifferentiated illness (e.g. a patient who says, 'I'm tired all the time …'). Balint stated that, 'Medical history taking means collecting answers to our well tried set of questions' and so '[The doctor] … will always get answers – but hardly anything more', unless the doctor works from a wider **bio-psychosocial perspective**.
- He highlighted the importance of **active listening** (being sensitive to the patient's cues), to enhance understanding of the patient's view.
- The 'ticket of entry', i.e. the reason for attendance, might not be the symptom initially offered, when, with one hand on the door, as the patient is ostensibly leaving, they reveal a second problem which is the real source of their anxiety

('While I'm here, doc ...'). It is the doctor's response to this statement which can allow the patient to reveal their possible '**hidden agenda**'.

- Balint pointed out that advice and reassurance are the two most common forms of psychotherapy used by clinicians in daily practice. However, you can neither advise nor reassure the patient before you have found out what their **real problem** is.

- He described the '**doctor's apostolic function**': an expression of the doctor's individual way of dealing with his/her patients, and their unrealistic expectation of the patient based on their own values. For example, the patient presents with a problem, 'I've been off sick with a cold for a week and I'd like a sick note'. The doctor has a number of possible responses ranging from:

  a 'You can self-certify if you have had a minor illness, and you don't need to see a doctor' to

  b 'Tell me more about what happened and why you need a sick note.'

  In consultation (a) the patient has to accept the doctor's faith and commandments, and be 'converted' (usually superficial), or to reject them and argue, or go to another doctor (b) who is more flexible and will explore the patient's underlying need, instead of merely quoting chapter and verse.

Balint pointed out that avoidance of self-examination and apostolic fervour are often linked. All doctors have limitations and need to be aware of them. No-one is omniscient and the *Good Medical Practice* booklet (General Medical Council 2002) demands that we do not extrapolate beyond the bounds of our capability.

Practical point
How the doctor elicits the reason for a patient's visits and reacts is critical to determining the course of events.

In the 1950s, Balint, to some a prophet, to others the messiah, viewed the '**doctor as a drug**'. He said:

> no pharmacology of this important drug exists yet. No guidance whatever is contained in any textbook as to the dosage in which the doctor should prescribe himself, in what form, how frequently, what his curative and maintenance doses should be.

He went on to say that:

> there is a lack of any literature on the possible hazards of this kind of 'medication', the various 'allergic' reactions an individual may encounter and any undesirable side-effects.

A criticism of Balint's approach is that although it explores the doctor–patient relationship, it remains doctor-centred. Most doctors can identify with elements drawn from the case histories he analysed, and so this framework is of practical help. As students start their consulting career they may be quite doctor-centred and so widening their scope using this approach will be useful.

Balint also recognised that patients can arouse feelings in their doctors (e.g. of anger or despair) and if doctors acknowledge those feelings, they can be used in the consultation dynamic to benefit the patient:

> The patient is in real need of help, the doctor honestly tries his hardest – and still, despite sincere efforts on both sides, things tend obstinately to go wrong.

All patients 'offer' doctors their various needs, and doctors 'respond' to them. Balint's approach is to help doctors become more sensitive to what is going on, consciously or unconsciously, in the consultation. His legacy continues (nationally and internationally) in the form of Balint Groups, which GPs can join locally to explore their consultations using the framework he developed.

Berne: games people play (1964)[11]

This approach continues the application of psychoanalytical principles to the consultation. Berne used the framework of 'transactional analysis' to provide an overview of what is happening in the interaction between doctor and patient. He qualified as a doctor in Canada, and then became interested in psychoanalysis in the United States. He developed a theory of social interchange called **transactional analysis**.

When people meet, the options for interaction are (ordered in terms of increasing complexity):

1 rituals
2 pastimes
3 games
4 intimacy
5 activity (which may support any of the above).

Social interchange e.g. a consultation, usually takes the form of 'games'. The goal of each participant in the interaction is to obtain as many 'satisfactions', gains or advantages as possible from his or her transactions with others. According to Berne's theory the aim of any social contact is to achieve somatic and psychic equilibrium.

Practical point
A person's body language and the quality of conversation relate to a state of mind called an 'ego state': a coherent system of feelings, related to a coherent set of behaviour patterns.

Berne distinguished **three different ego states**, which could be inconsistent.

- Parent – authority figure. Critical and caring, can make some responses reflex but streamlines routine decision making, conserves time and energy.
- Adult – logical, autonomous, objective appraisal of reality. Essential for data processing and risk assessment. Regulates and mediates between the other two states.
- Child – relics of behaviour fixed in childhood: intuition, creativity, spontaneity and enjoyment.

At any instant a person will be acting as one of the above, but he or she will shift through the spectrum of each ego state in time, although individuals differ in their flexibility.

All three states are needed for survival, but problems are due to an imbalance, which can be dealt with by using this analytical model and restoring the equilibrium.

Practical point

At any given moment we think, feel and have attitudes as if we were either a critical or caring Parent, a logical Adult or a spontaneous/dependent Child. Many consultations are conducted with a Parental doctor and a Child-like patient, but this transaction is not always in the best interests of either the patient or doctor.

A conversation, such as a consultation, is a 'transaction' in this model. The person starting the conversation is called the 'agent' and their opening remarks the 'transactional stimulus'. This will provoke the 'transactional response' from the other participant. Using **transactional analysis** you can classify remarks, e.g.:

'Can I have something for my cold, doctor?'
The doctor prescribes.

These transactions are complementary: patient = child (make it go away), doctor = caring parent (fixes it) responses are as expected, and conversations can proceed smoothly, but possibly erroneously!

Conversely communication may be more challenging, when an adult-to-adult transaction occurs, e.g.:

'Can I have something for my cold, doctor?'
'Tell me more about it; what were you expecting from me?'
'I'm worried about re-organisation at work and I need to be on top form for a meeting tomorrow . . .'

The naïve child : parent interaction is transformed by changing the dynamics and asking the patient to give a more adult view of his/her needs, concerns and expectations, resulting in a more balanced adult:adult interchange where self-management and the role of antibiotics can be discussed in context.

Practical point

This analysis of the consultation can be very helpful when you find yourself getting uncomfortable and stressed by a particular type of interchange or patient.

You may assume that as a professional you are going to be the caring parent (on an authoritarian doctor-centred model), or an adult in an exchange of equals (on a patient-centred co-operative model), and it may be uncomfortable to find yourself as the 'naïve' child.

Berne's book offers a thesaurus of 'games people play' – examples from everyday life to the consulting room. The basic principles are easy to remember, and you may use some of them on a daily basis yourself.

Byrne and Long: doctors talking to patients (1976)[7]

Byrne was a professor of general practice at Manchester University; his collaborator Long was an educationalist. They analysed verbal behaviours in tape recordings of doctors in consultation with almost 2500 patients. They concluded that the doctor was 'both a product and a prisoner of his medical education' and authoritarian teaching and role-models fostered a predominance of doctor-centred behaviour, which did not enable doctors to deal with the psychosocial components of patients' problems. In this they echo Balint's findings of the 'Apostolic function' of doctors.

GPs seemed unable to engage with psychological disease or the psychological aspects of disease, and 'worked through a frame of reference which required both patients and illnesses to fit a pre-judged pattern ... which has a great deal to do with the ways with which doctors learn to cope with the diagnosis of organic illness', i.e. working solely from a biomedical model. They commented that few doctors at that time could reflect on the dynamics and process of the consultation: What are you doing? How are you doing it?

The study by Byrne and Long recognised six phases by the doctor in the process of consultation.

I   Establishes a relationship with the patient.
II   Attempts to discover, or actually discovers, the reason for the patient's attendance.
III Conducts a verbal or physical examination or both.
IV   The doctor, the doctor and the patient, or the patient (in that order of probability) consider the condition.
V   The doctor, and occasionally the patient, details further treatment or further investigation.
VI   Ending the consultation.

I   Relating to the patient

Usually this can be completed relatively quickly, e.g. 'Hello, Mrs Biggs, I'm Chris Edwards, a medical student sitting in with Dr Smith ...' Many doctors will use a similar form of words for most patients – you will need to develop your own which is informative, welcoming and professional. e.g. 'Hello, Mrs Baker, I'm Catherine Adams, a medical student working with Dr Holden. He has suggested that I talk to you before you see him – is that all right?'

II   Discovering the reason for the patient's attendance

Variable length: 0–8 minutes.
This is usually preceded by an open question, e.g. 'How are you? How can I help?'
The following variables influence the time a doctor spends in phase II:

• the degree to which the doctor is prepared to accept the first thing a patient says
• the degree of clarity with which the patient presents his or her symptoms

- the number of patients preceding, and waiting
- the degree to which the doctor is weighted towards organic illness
- the doctor's beliefs about him or herself and about his or her patients.

III A verbal or physical examination

This varies according to the type of consultation but is a chance to clarify and enhance bio-psychosocial information, and the patient's ideas, concerns and expectations, flagged up in phase II. Time spent on the physical examination can be used to further the doctor–patient relationship by talking the patient through what you are doing and why.

IV Consideration of the patient condition

This needs to be flexible and patient-centred and reaching a consensus at whatever level the patient requires. It is necessary to place before the patient the information that has been gained in this, and in previous consultations (personal experience or by looking at patient notes and computer records), along with other related information that the doctor may feel important. This will help to establish a consensual approach to the subsequent stages of the consultation and future management of the patient's condition. The study classified this phase as 'optional', i.e. it differed between patient-centred and doctor-centred behaviour.

V Detailing treatment or further investigation

Ensure this is tailored to the patient and takes account of their health beliefs. Look out for the fact that in 8% of consultations this is the point at which the patient reveals their true agenda. 'Thanks for the antibiotics, doc; will they affect my periods as I'm a week late already and I'm worried I might be pregnant . . .', or 'While I'm here . . .'. This can create a feeling of frustration on the part of the doctor, who, just as s/he feels s/he is completing a successful consultation, needs to re-orientate and start again. It helps to be prepared for the inevitable. This phase showed the greatest variation between doctors.

VI Ending the consultation

In 90% the doctor initiated this, e.g. saying goodbye, handing over the prescription and perhaps getting up. Again the doctor usually develops a personal routine.

Practical point

Byrne and Long comment that it was relatively easy to derive these steps but much more difficult to put them in a logical order. This is a common issue with both models and actual consultations. It stems from the natural ebb and flow of human conversation, which is not necessarily linear.

It serves to highlight the reasons why any of these models should not be used in the manner of a sequential checklist, which would lead to a rigid

inflexible consulting style. This chapter is trying to promote a review of potential approaches and adoption of those that feel appropriate and natural for the individual practitioner or lead them to review their present consulting style.

Byrne and Long also made a detailed analysis of consulting styles with transcribed examples, and developed a classification and scoring system for doctor-centred and patient-centred behaviour together with negative (rejecting or closing) behaviours. One should be able to identify with the origins of this framework rooted in the **biomedical model**:

- history taking
- examination
- diagnosis
- treatment.

Practical point

It is worth exploring a model further if you feel that model is one which you can recognise in terms of the way you consult.

> In any consultation there are normally two parties – the doctor and the patient. Although the doctor has special skills and experience, it is wise to remember that the patient also has a unique pattern of knowledge and experience and that any consultation is made up of a mixture of the patient and the doctor.[7]

This detailed study described a logical sequence of medical procedures, and distinguished between 'doctor-centred' and 'patient-centred' styles. It provided the foundation from which later models were developed.

Stott and Davis: the exceptional potential in each primary care consultation (1979)[18]

Building on the theme of widening the brief discussed so far and promoted by evolving wider definitions of general practitioners, Stott and Davis, working in the Department of General Practice at the Welsh National School of Medicine, published a theoretical framework in which they described four areas that could profitably be explored in routine surgery consultations and also used for teaching.

A Management of presenting problems.
B Modification of help-seeking behaviour.
C Management of continuing problems.
D Opportunistic health promotion.

A   Management of presenting problems

This is the main activity, where the doctor seeks to define the 'reason for attendance' formulated in bio-psychosocial terms, the effect on the patient and the patient's ideas, concerns and expectations.

B Modification of help-seeking behaviours

Patients may need advice, information and support in managing some problems themselves, e.g. people with uncomplicated colds, parents with young children who develop acute viral illnesses. Doctors can teach patients 'to be more realistic about what (they) can or cannot treat effectively'. There is also a long-term agenda here of resource management.

C Management of continuing problems

For example, following up obesity and hypertension in a person who has ostensibly become focused on his diabetes.

D Opportunistic health promotion

'Offering advice about diet, exercise, habits or relationships ... to help patients make appropriate lifestyle choices', e.g. discussing contraceptive needs, smoking and diet when a mother comes for her post-natal check, or smoking, weight and cholesterol when checking blood pressure in a hypertensive. Stott and Davis note that this implies mutual adult respect (an 'adult to adult' interaction as in the Berne model, not a 'parent to child' one).

Practical point
Consider how you would broach the subject of smoking cessation using this information.

Stott and Davis recognised that B and D are often areas which are neglected by doctors, and suggested that they could be considered as working in a longer time frame, the end product of multiple consultations or **continuity of care**.

The virtue of this model is that it 'can be easily memorised, understood and used'. It is task-orientated to maximise the opportunity of a consultation to provide comprehensive care.

Helman: culture, health and illness (1984)[19,20]

Cecil Helman is a medical anthropologist and GP who came to the UK from South Africa. His book *Culture, Health and Illness* was first published in 1984 and focused on the contribution of anthropology to understanding health problems and their management in a variety of cultures.

'Doctors and their patients, even if they come from the same social and cultural background, view ill health in very different ways.' The success of the consultation depends on bridging these two positions.

Practical point
Anthropology is the study of human beings and their many different cultures. It is the holistic scientific study of mankind answering the question, 'What is man?'

Helman describes medical school students who are encultured into an applied science; they study the phenomena of sickness and health. Occurrences are subjected to rational objective measurement, and become facts, a 'biomedical consensus statement'. As 'all facts have a cause', the clinician's role is to discover the chain of causal events and so provide a diagnosis, prognosis and management.

Practical point

If this is not possible the problem is labelled **idiopathic** (science underdeveloped and as yet unable to provide an explanation) or **psychogenic** (driven by the mind, not the body, and beyond the remit of such clinicians).

Another layer of complication is that even within the medical profession there are huge differences in emphasis and approach between, e.g., GPs and public health doctors (the individual and the community), surgeons and psychiatrists (the body and the mind). In addition doctors, as members of society, carry with them their own baggage of assumptions, ideas and prejudices from their past personal experience which influence their practice, as discussed by Balint, and Byrne and Long.

Practical point

The **biomedical model** has difficulty accommodating the feelings, beliefs and psychosocial issues (as they are difficult to quantify) which colour the personal experience and meaning of health and illness.

Helman points out that the explosion of technology has made doctors **reductionist**, e.g. focusing on a group of genes that create disease.

Helman states that a patient's view of being **unwell** is more global. **Illness** is the subjective response of an individual and those around him/her to his/her being unwell; particularly how he/she and they interpret the origin and significance of this event. Also how it affects his/her behaviour and his/her relationship with other people; and the various steps he/she takes to remedy the situation. It not only includes his/her experience of ill health, but also the meaning he/she gives to that experience. As this is related to an individual's social and cultural background, together with their personality, the same disease may produce a completely different picture in people whose backgrounds differ.

Helman points out that the individual's response to 'illness' is one of a repertoire of responses to adversity, e.g. a burglary, and so has psychological, moral and social components.

Using this holistic approach, 'a person is defined as being "ill" when there is agreement between his/her perceptions of impaired well-being and the perceptions of those around him/her . . . becoming ill is always a social process'. Contrast this with the narrower biomedical view. The consultation between patient and doctor needs to acknowledge these frames of reference, and the participants need to actively work to build on what they bring to the consultation to produce an integrated individualised outcome: **patient-centred medicine**.

Helman states that each culture will have its own language of distress, which integrates subjective experience, and social acknowledgement of ill health. The doctor needs to recognise the significance of verbal, non-verbal, somatic, or psychological cues within the consultation.

The doctor's way forward is to consider the **patient's story or narrative**, which may cover the following.

1 **What has happened?** The person organises their symptoms and signs into a recognisable pattern, and gives it a name or identity.
2 **Why has it happened?** This explains the cause of the condition.
3 **Why has it happened to me?** Attempts to explain the illness in personal terms, e.g. behaviour, diet, heredity factors.
4 **Why now?** Factual and related to life events, e.g. job loss, the anniversary of a relative's death.
5 **What would happen to me if nothing were done about it?** Considers likely course of events and possible outcomes.
6 **What are its likely effects on other people if nothing is done about it?** Strain on family, implications for work and income.
7 **What should I do about it?** Ranging from self-help, seeking the opinion of family and friend, or consulting a doctor.

Practical point
The pathway to a successful consultation requires negotiation between the patient's and doctor's models of the presenting problem, which provides a consensus on diagnosis, treatment and management.

Using this approach unsatisfactory/dysfunctional consultations can occur when:

- inappropriate emphasis is placed on the individual (when there is an underlying family problem)
- there is misinterpretation of the language of distress (emotion is equated with hypochondria by the doctor)
- patient and doctor models are incompatible
- there is disease without illness (treating a biochemical abnormality in a 'well' person
- there is illness without disease – the patient has ongoing symptoms but 'your tests are all normal'
- there are unrecognised and unresolved differences in terminology, treatment and context between patient and doctor.

Helman suggests the following **strategies for improvement**.

1 **Understanding the patient's meaning of illness** (in contrast to labelling the disease with a diagnostic category).
2 **Improving communication** – recognising the 'language of distress' of your patients.
3 **Increasing reflexivity** – be aware of where you are coming from (your culture, values, prejudices).

4 **Treating illness and disease** and also the patient not just the pathology.
5 **Respecting diversity** (there is usually an alternative model or explanation).
6 **Reflect on the context** – the patient's internal context and the setting of the consultation itself. What are the wider influences and where is the balance of power? Indeed should there be a balance of power?

Practical point

Helman promotes a holistic approach centred on the patient's narrative (see later) and emphasises lay theories of illness, which involve the individual, the natural world, the social world, and even the supernatural world in contrast to a purely medical one.

Pendleton: the tasks of the consultation and cycle of care (1984, 2003)[8,15]

Pendleton is a social psychologist working at the University of Oxford, and together with three GPs (Schofield, Havelock and Tate) have a complementary diversity of interests and experience. Pendleton set out to build on the above approaches, and develop a framework useful for both learning and teaching. This has resonated with advances in technology and teaching by analysis through both video and role-play. Although their work was originally published in 1984,[8] it is ongoing and this is why reference is given to the updated 2003 version[15] for a detailed account.

The 'Pendleton' model of the consultation

The seven '**tasks**' to be achieved in a consultation which originate from the patient's needs and the aims of the doctor are as follows.

- **Understand the problem** and so understand the reason for attendance in terms of the patient's problem and perspective through the doctor and patient having a '**dialogue**'.
  1 To define the reasons for the patient's attendance, including:
     i   the nature and history of the problems
     ii their aetiology
     iii the patient's ideas, concerns and expectations
     iv the effects of the problems.
  2 To consider other problems:
     i   continuing problems
     ii at-risk factors.
  3 To choose with the patient an appropriate action for each problem.
- **Understand the patient**.
  4 To achieve a '**shared understanding**' of the problem with the patient.
- **Share decisions and responsibility.**
  5 To involve the patient in the management and to encourage and **enable** him or her to accept appropriate responsibility. Agree the actions and responsibilities for the doctor and patient in relation to targets, monitoring and follow-up.

6 To use time and resources appropriately (both in the consultation and in the longer term).

7 To establish or **maintain a relationship** with the patient which helps to achieve the other tasks and consider other problems not yet presented (a **'hidden agenda'**), ongoing problems and risk factors.

Practical point

Their original model moved away from an authoritarian biomedical stance, and emphasised that an effective consultation was one in which patient and doctor both worked co-operatively to define problems and their management.

This model has been developed to focus on both patient and doctor dynamics in the consultation. The essence of the consultation was not only to identify and meet patients' needs, but also to enhance their understanding and ability to manage their own health and so **patient enablement**.[25] Each consultation reinforced a **'cycle of care'**.

Doctors are encouraged to assess their own consulting style and develop insight into their feelings, attitudes, strengths and weaknesses – similarly, to be more aware of their mood, health, availability of time and organisational issues which may lead a doctor to react positively or negatively to a patient's issues. There are long-term outcomes for the doctor of job satisfaction, and those of the patient of adherence to a suggested management, satisfaction and a change in health.

To address **the issue that doctors do not always achieve a shared understanding**, Pendleton suggests the following.

1 **Before considering a prescription** always ask, 'Do you want me to give you something for this?'

2 **Before a prescription for an antibiotic** ask, 'What do you feel about taking/giving your child an antibiotic?'

3 **Before giving your diagnosis** ask, 'What thoughts have been running through your mind?'

4 **Before embarking on an explanation** ask, 'What do you understand about ... ?'

Practical point

Since 1984 the development of this work has made a major contribution not only to analysis but also to teaching. Apart from defining the components of a successful consultation this approach explicitly supports a **patient-centred partnership model**.

Neighbour: the inner consultation (1987)[21]

This is a pragmatic holistic model developed by a general practitioner, trainer and examiner. It looks at what is going on within the consultation and doctor behaviours. The five stages are easy to remember and practise as they follow the natural flow of a good consultation.

1   **Connecting** – Have we got rapport? Establishing a rapport and getting on the same wavelength as the patient.
2   **Summarising** – Do I really know why the patient has come? Not only the reason for attending but also the patient's ideas and concerns regarding his/her problem and their expectations of what I can do about it.
3   **Handing over** – Sharing information. Has the patient understood and accepted the management plan we have proposed? Having assessed the problem and formulated a diagnosis (or problem list), and negotiated and agreed a management plan.
4   **Safety netting** – Have I anticipated all the likely outcomes? Manage uncertainty: anticipate likely outcomes and discuss them; look at probabilities and weigh up risks. Organise an appropriate time for follow-up.
5   **Housekeeping** – Am I in good condition for the next patient? Am I stressed? I need to be receptive to the next patient and in a position to offer 'a caring and compassionate state of mind uncontaminated with ... personal preoccupations'. A doctor needs to be psychologically 'fit' for the next consultation and not transfer feelings from the previous one.

Neighbour identifies a pathway to improve your consultation skills by:

- **goal setting** – 'fixing in the mind at the start a clear idea of end point, the outcome, the result you are wanting to achieve'
- **skill building** – 'the process of anticipatory training in the repertoire of component skills you require to achieve the outcome'
- **getting it together** – 'well-intentioned and well-rehearsed, all that is needed is for you to rely on the adequacy of your preparation and give yourself over to the inspiration of the moment, trusting your intuitive and unconscious processes to function appropriately and automatically!'

Practical point
An unfortunate side effect of consultation skills analysis and modelling is to cause a mental distraction. You are trying to focus on the patient, but in parallel you are trying to discern what you should be doing 'in theory'.

Neighbour addresses this 'inner consultation' explicitly with the aim of freeing your intuitive input, to work in parallel with your knowledge to improve the consultation. The image Neighbour uses is of the doctor in consultation as having two heads – one labelled with 'theory', one with 'practice'.

The way that Neighbour's model reflects others can be summarised in a table referred to as the Health Belief Model and this can be viewed in Neighbour's book.

The Inner Consultation is short and easy to use. It provides a basis for understanding the dynamics of the patient–doctor interchange and the resultant internal dynamics of the doctor.

In Neighbour's book he also discusses, at length, how to identify non-verbal cues from patients during the consultation. These cues are certainly worth looking for as they can be the key to identifying the patient's hidden agenda or main reason for attending.

The Leicester Assessment Package (LAP)[22,23]

The LAP is an assessment model with seven prioritised categories of consultation competence as detailed below with the relevant weightings of each.

1 Interviewing/history taking (20%).
2 Physical examination (10%).
3 Patient management (20%).
4 Problem solving (20%).
5 Behaviour/relationship (10%).
6 Anticipatory care (10%).
7 Record keeping (10%).

In the undergraduate setting the LAP utilises the first five categories which have 35 component competences. Fraser *et al.*, who developed the LAP, state that to be able to cope with the varied tasks of a consultation and the associated challenges presented by patients, the clinician needs to master a broad range of skills within these categories.

The assessment of competence can be based on a systematic observation of performance. The seven categories of the LAP as an assessment tool and so a model for teaching and assessing consultation competences has been demonstrated to be valid, reliable and feasible in the setting of general practice (Fraser *et al.* 1994).[22]

This assessment process can be used as a model to teach the consultation through feedback which involves the generation, collection and interpretation of evidence which is compared with valid performance criteria. Such a comparison forms the basis of a judgement which infers competence or otherwise.

The assessment grades for the LAP are as follows.

- A grade – consistently demonstrates mastery of all components (80% or above).
- B grade – consistently demonstrates mastery of most components and capability in all (70–79%)
- C+ grade – consistently demonstrates capability in almost all components to a high standard, and a satisfactory standard in all (60–69%).
- C grade – demonstrates capability in most components to a satisfactory standard: minor omissions and/or defects in some components. Duration of most consultations appropriate (50–59%).
- D grade – demonstrates inadequacies in several components but no major omissions or defects (40–49%).
- E grade – demonstrates several major omissions or defects; clearly unacceptable standard overall. (0–39%).

In relation to calibration of this assessment tool, it can be argued as to what constitutes a 'major omission or defect', as opposed to a 'minor omission'.

The overall aim of the LAP is to help students and doctors further develop the consultation competences required to define and manage the health problems of patients.

Practical point
The LAP seeks to assist students 'to recognise, adopt and develop those clinical skills and values that are fundamental to the practice of rational and humane clinical medicine, whatever the clinical setting'.

For any of the models described they may be adapted for use in assessment and so like the LAP provide feedback to allow the student or doctor to further improve their consultation skills. However, it should be stated that it was Hager *et al.* in 1994 who wrote:

There is no such thing as a process of assessment that is without its critics. Whatever efforts are made to improve assessment someone is bound to be unhappy with the process.[26]

Stewart et al.: *patient-centred medicine (1995, 2003)*[13,14]

This approach has evolved from the ongoing work of the Patient–Doctor Communication Group at the University of Western Ontario, Canada, in 1986. There has been a long history of research by members of the department into the patient–doctor relationship, which has informed the development of the '**patient-centred clinical method**'. McWhinney[5] drew attention to the fact that patients' problems had both breadth (bio-psychosocial elements) and depth (personal meaning). This holistic, patient-centred view is a cornerstone of the model[25] which is also explicitly co-operative. There are six components to the model where component 3 is central to the six components of doctor–patient interactions.[14]

1 **Exploring both the disease and the illness experience:**
    • history, physical, laboratory tests
    • dimensions of illness (feelings, ideas, effects on function and expectations).
2 **Understanding the whole person:**
    • the person (e.g. life history, personal and developmental issues)
    • the proximal context (e.g. family, employment, social support)
    • the distal context (e.g. culture, community, ecosystem).
3 **Finding common ground:**
    • problems and priorities
    • goals of treatment and/or management
    • roles of patient and doctor.
4 **Incorporating prevention and health promotion:**
    • health enhancement
    • risk avoidance
    • risk reduction
    • early identification
    • complication reduction.
5 **Enhancing the patient–doctor relationship:**
    • compassion
    • power

- healing
- self-awareness
- transference and counter-transference.
6 **Being realistic:**
  - time and timing
  - teambuilding and teamwork
  - wise stewardship of resources.

The framework clearly addresses both the patient's agenda and experience of illness and the doctor's agenda (bio-diagnostic) and it has been widely influential in education and research. There are parallels with the Pendleton[15] and the Calgary–Cambridge[16] approaches which are contemporaneous.

The group also highlighted the need to find out why the patient was presenting at that time. Another way the patient-centred model can be summarised is as **ICEE** (Illness Framework) as follows where the doctor explores the:

- patient's **I**deas (I) about what is wrong
- patient's feelings/**C**oncerns about the illness (C)
- impact/**E**ffect of the patient's problems (E)
- patient's **E**xpectations about what should be done (E).

This is the same as ICE referred to throughout the book with an extra 'E' for the Effect or impact of the patient's problems.

Practical point
Patient-centred clinical method – the doctor should elicit and work through the patient's agenda and also be aware and careful of their own agenda and how this can influence the outcome of the consultation.

Kurtz, Silverman and Draper: the Calgary–Cambridge observation guide to the 'Medical Interview' (1996)[16]

This is an approach or structure to teaching and learning communication skills, which was developed jointly at these two universities by experienced educators to support both undergraduates and continuing medical education for qualified practitioners. The emphasis is on core communication skills, which then form a foundation for addressing attitudes and issues encountered in practice.

Riccardi and Kurtz (1983)[27] noted that accuracy, efficiency and supportiveness were goals that doctors attempt to achieve in consultations. Further work by Kurtz (1989)[28] identified generic principles for good communication:

- interactions
- reduce uncertainty
- planned outcomes
- recognise the dynamics of the consultation itself
- mutual interaction of the individuals involved.

The Calgary–Cambridge method is based on '**a patient-centred approach that promotes a collaborative partnership**'.[29] It explicitly seeks to move away from medical paternalism; however, because of the nature of the framework, this model 'concentrates on what doctors can do in the interview to facilitate their patients' involvement'.

There are five main tasks in this framework.

1 Initiating the session.
2 Gathering information.
3 Building the relationship.
4 Explanation and planning.
5 Closing the session.

Seventy individual skills are listed in the guide, but this is a summary of the actions covered in most consultations.

1 **Initiating the session:**
   - establishing initial rapport
   - identifying the reason(s) for the consultation.
2 **Gathering information:**
   - exploration of problems (including active listening, facilitation, and open questioning)
   - understanding the patient's perspective (covering ideas, concerns, expectations and effects on the patient's life)
   - providing structure to the consultation (summarising, sequencing, signposting and timing).
3 **Building the relationship:**
   - developing rapport (empathy, support and sensitivity)
   - involving the patient.
4 **Explanation and planning:**
   - providing the correct amount and type of information
   - aiding accurate recall and understanding
   - achieving a shared understanding incorporating the patient's perspective
   - planning: shared decision making
   - options in explanation and planning if:
     – discussing opinion and significance of problems
     – negotiating mutual plan of action
     – discussing investigations and procedures.
5 **Closing the session:**
   - including summarizing, contracting and 'safety netting' (Neighbour[21]).

The framework builds on previous models from a patient-centred stance. Each skill is discussed in terms of the evidence supporting it, and a variety of words and ways are discussed by which the goal of an effective consultation may be achieved. It is a model which makes the:

- what?
- why?
- how?

of communication with patients explicit.

Practical point
All of these models of approaches to consulting with patients are holistic. They aim to facilitate patient-centredness and partnership. Their structure and emphasis relates to the work and background of their originators.

Other issues and recent influences

More recently shifts in ideas and emphasis have occurred which will increasingly impact on consulting with patients.

Empathy, empowerment and enablement

Without an empathetic doctor none of the models above really work. **Empathy** is the ability to put yourself in the patient's place and act accordingly.

Practical point
Empathy is more than just an intellectual appreciation of the patient's situation; it is a blend of understanding and caring, which is evident to the patient in your actions and words.

Empathy supports the therapeutic relationship between patient and doctor. It is the cognitive and behavioural aspect of compassion and care. There is evidence that patients recognise and respond to empathy, that it improves satisfaction, diagnostic accuracy and outcomes.[30] Empathy involves engaging emotion, difficult when doctors are schooled in the application of objectivity, that can lead to a degree of professional 'detachment'. Empathy can be enhanced by training. It is a key component of a patient-centred approach.

Empowerment is a global movement. In the UK patient empowerment has been embodied in the NHS Plan (2000): '. . . patients will have a real say in the NHS. They will have new powers and more influence over the way the NHS works'. This includes advocacy, more representation, more information for patients and greater patient choice. Moving towards a patient-centred approach from an authoritarian/paternalistic one is required in the 'new' NHS.

Practical point
Most of the approaches above involve seeing a problem through the patient's eyes, addressing their ideas, concerns and expectations and mutually agreeing management.

However, a recent study in the UK shows this is often not achieved:

The sense of powerlessness that characterized many people's experience of the NHS was largely the result of a lack of information and knowledge about how things work. Participants talked of doctors and specialists using an 'alien language'.[31]

A shared understanding requires the use of language that can be understood by the doctor and the patient. A doctor should check that a patient understands the same by a medical term that they do, e.g. a medical term such as 'congestion'.

This study included patients in Europe[31] and reported an equal participation in a dialogue which leads to informed choice difficult to envisage, and there was also 'a reluctance to accept that sometimes there isn't always a straightforward answer ... – but instead a series of choices and trade-offs between less than perfect alternatives'. Doctors need to empower patients to cope with these complex decisions.

Patients consulting healthcare professionals expect to leave their consultation having made progress with their problem. The **Patient Enablement Instrument (PEI)** is a questionnaire that has been developed by Howie and colleagues from a patient-centred approach to reflect the quality of consultation outcome.[32]

Practical point
The theory behind **enablement** is that understanding, adjustment and coping are important influences on outcome for patients.

The enablement questions ask whether, as the result of consulting with the doctor, the patient felt more able to:

- understand their illness better
- cope with illness and life
- be confident about their health
- help themselves, and
- keep themselves healthy.

Enablement increases with a longer consultation time, continuity of care and getting a prescription when one is wanted. Doctors can be distinguished as being 'high' or 'low' enablers.[33] Empathy is strongly correlated with enablement,[30] and enablement shares some characteristics, but is distinct from patient satisfaction.[31] However, as we continue to define and evaluate patient-centredness, the nature of the processes which underpin it are the subject of current research.

Practical point
An **empathetic** doctor can **empower** the patient and **enable** them to 'move on' from their problem productively.

Evidence-based medicine

Development of evidence-based medicine (EBM) is heralded as the way forward. There is an evangelical fervour to convert all doctors to the advantages of this 'explicit and judicious use of current best evidence in making decisions about the care of individual patients' (Sackett 1996).[34] But does this approach always achieve a cure? What of the role of the doctor as a therapeutic agent, once loosely called 'bedside manner'?

Earlier in the chapter, it was discussed how the psychologist Balint viewed the doctor as a drug. Illness and disease are not synonymous and many ill people who consult a GP have no disease, but still have an illness that requires treatment. Thus, the application of EBM has severe limitations. Furthermore it is usually based on randomised controlled trials (RCTs) in secondary care where nearly all subjects have a disease and a different spectrum is seen. For example, only a small percentage of patients in primary care have the type of uncomplicated hypertension that can be managed by standard evidence-based guidelines. So why not have primary care RCTs? Because of ethical and practical concerns, a GP providing continuous personal care to an individual patient may perceive or worry that they are exposing the patient to a medication which is inferior to current treatment. With this come difficulties with recruitment and randomisation. Imagine a double-blind RCT, where the GPs prescribing drugs to patients realise which drug they are giving, and if they do not fully believe in the new product, the outcome will be influenced, whether by verbal or non-verbal cues.

GPs have a dilemma, for they draw on two bodies of knowledge – that of secondary care derived EBM and the insights of their individual experiences. In addition, there is their unmeasured and unrealised therapeutic effect. Hence, their own knowledge, skills and attitudes (or feelings) may have a profound effect on both the process and the outcome of treatment and in some cases an effect greater than any evidence-based treatment. Whether or not a person has a disease or is considered to have a disease, they have an illness.

Practical point

Where appropriate, **reassurance** is a powerful therapeutic tool which can lead to alleviation of an illness and associated symptoms, particularly where there is an absence of disease.

The practice of patient-centred medicine and evidence-based medicine are therefore not mutually exclusive, and should be seen as synergistic. Doctors in consultations should strive to deliver both effective clinical and interpersonal care.

Practical point

'External clinical evidence can inform, but can never replace, individual clinical expertise, and it is this expertise that decides whether the external evidence applies to the individual patient at all and, if so, how it should be integrated into a clinical decision.'[34]

Evidence-based medicine can and should be integrated with patient-centred consultation and care where possible.

The art of medicine is how to apply the science. This is not the mystique of the 'Church of Medicine', but the role of the 'good doctor'.

Neuro-linguistic programming

Many models of consultation are derived from interpretive psychology. In contrast neuro-linguistic programming (NLP) is 'an outcome focused, solution oriented behavioural technology'.[35] It started in the United States in the 1970s with studies into how people change. As such it provides a useful adjunct to the consulting skills models described. Both NLP and patient-centred approaches have the patient's subjective experience at their core. People interpret the world and their experiences uniquely: they have their own *'internal map'*. Every behaviour brings positive gain for the individual. NLP hones our ability to *'read'* people and, in understanding where they are coming from, we can better help them to move on from their problem. It enhances our knowledge and skills to detect and affect thinking patterns.

Narrative

> The effective practice of medicine requires narrative competence, that is the ability to acknowledge, absorb, interpret, and act on the stories and plights of others.[36]

Working with the patient's narrative is implicit in patient-centred approaches. Taking a history starts with actively listening to the patient's story, and understanding its personal meaning. Agreeing on the management of the problem involves exploring the patient's ideas, concerns and expectations. Reassurance, advice and counselling will only be effective if they are framed from the patient's narrative. Launer highlights 'a tension between the complex narrative that a patient brings into the consulting room and a doctor's understanding of what is really going on as formulated in a diagnosis or an idea about pathology'.[37]

A patient's narrative tells us about their personal experience of being unwell. Understanding their narrative can help us to approach their problems holistically, and can point the way to solutions.

> To understand and accept a patient's moral choices, a practitioner must acknowledge that the illness narrative has many potential interpretations but that the patient is the ultimate author of his or her own text.[38]

Narrative is fundamental as it 'deals with experiences, not with propositions'.[36]

> The consultation brings together the human experience of suffering and the paradigms of scientific medicine, with the general practitioner acting as an interpreter at the boundary between illness and disease, and a witness to suffering.[39]

(*See* Chapter 2 for further details.)

Complexity and the consultation

The models above have served to highlight the multi-layered nature of the consultation. A dialogue between a patient and doctor has a dynamic of its own as well as the complexity which the patient and doctor both bring to the interchange. There is a need to differentiate between the consultation models we have considered so far and those that may be aligned to what is referred to as complexity theory. Characteristics of the consultation models so far are:

- appropriate application of a scientific (probabilistic/linear) model
- the traditional scientific clinical method (biomedical medical) model
- pattern recognition or the hypothetico-deductive (probabilistic) model
- application of an often reductionist and perhaps not so patient-centred model
- evidence based (rules)/quantitative approach
- diagnostic certainties – diseases (deductive) model.

Some might say that these models endeavour to provide a scientific objective rigour to simplify what is exceedingly complex. They are based on Newtonian scientific reasoning, which assumes that complex situations may be explained by linear equations. These models may work well for simple situations – for example, myocardial ischaemia producing central crushing angina pain, diagnosed through history and an exercise ECG and treated by drugs reducing preload and afterload on the heart. However, situations such as depression will be more complex with psychological, emotional, social and relational factors which do not fit easily into such a linear framework.

 . . . If things were simple, word would have gotten around. (Derrida 1988)[40]

Characteristics of complexity in the consultation are:

- narrative-based medicine/the illness story
- the unpredictable
- undifferentiated presentation of illness
- patient and illness inseparable – the so-called 'art of medicine'
- illness presentation is unpredictable (within boundaries)
- the approach is holistic appreciating the patient's environment (contextual)
- qualitative (no rules)
- diagnostic uncertainties (illness rather than a distinct disease entity)
- syndromes
- intuitive (heuristic)
- interpretive
- an inductive approach is required to unravel complexity
- outcomes will evolve or emerge over time (a feature of all complex systems)
- the 'butterfly effect' – small events may have vast effects (non-linear chaos).

Practical point
There is an argument to use the rigid structure of models or with experience to use those aspects that complement one's individual and developing consulting style.

Understanding the medical consultation as a complex system allows us to feel more comfortable with the potential **uncertainty** of how it will develop. It helps us understand the role of the doctor, not as an objective external observer, as suggested by traditional medical models of the doctor–patient interaction, but as an enquiring participant who seeks to influence change in a patient's condition for the better and so improving quality of life. This takes into account the WHO definition of health:

Health is a state of complete physical, mental and social well-being and not merely the absence of disease or infirmity. (WHO definition of health)

For many doctors, it is **uncertainty** in relation to problem solving and management that makes consulting with patients difficult and stressful. An excellent series of articles appeared in the *British Medical Journal* on the subject of 'complexity science' in relation to healthcare in 2001. The argument for uncertainty is illustrated by the following statement:

In complex systems, unpredictability and paradox are ever present, and some things will remain unknowable.[41]

How can a medical consultation be considered a complex system? Although many consultations can be successfully considered to only include the doctor and the patient, other influences act as agents within the consultation and will be particularly relevant in complex situations. These include the:

- themes emerging from the patient's narrative
- socio-cultural influences, e.g. religious, social or economic
- physical environment of the waiting room
- consulting room
- organisation of the practice
- constraint of time
- manager
- lawyer
- statistician
- journalist
- computer.

With this diversity of agents acting within a consultation there is the potential for the consultation to develop in many different ways. Free-flowing conversation is a process by which interaction occurs and possibilities can be explored. Structuring a consultation to limit the number of agents influencing the consultation limits potential developments and is insufficiently patient-centred. Complexity theory recognises uncertainty and helps us understand that it is intrinsic to complex systems including individuals and their health.

Human beings can be viewed as composed of and operating within multiple interacting and self adjusting systems (including biochemical, cellular, physiological, psychological, and social systems).[42]

What is a complex system? Take the example of a forest which is formed from many agents including the animals and plants. The agents are diverse in nature, they interact and they co-evolve. Changes emerge over time resulting from **non-linear** interactions, some having a minor and others a major effect on the evolving system. Change is constant resulting both from interactions within the system and external influences from the 'environment', but nevertheless the system can remain relatively stable over long periods of time. However, the state of the system is not entirely predictable in advance.

New conceptual frameworks that incorporate a dynamic, emergent, creative, and intuitive view of the world must replace traditional 'reduce and resolve' approaches to clinical care and service organisation.[41]

In relation to the individual doctor and their training, a skill is acquired to deal with the complexity of each individual encounter (patient consultation) and that is to be able to **integrate, synthesize and apply the knowledge** that they have received from teaching in anatomy, physiology, biochemistry, genetics and many other biomedical sciences and apply it in these clinical situations. (This theme is further explored in the next chapter in relation to Miller's Pyramid of Competence.)

Practical point

If one is to provide optimal and quality healthcare and keep up with the pace of change in the NHS, different consultation models should be considered when analysing the complexity of consultations and improving future performance.

Summary

More than 50 years ago Maslow[10] produced his overarching holistic theory of human need. It has been applied from business to medicine with varying degrees of success because it is difficult to operationalise completely. Through detailed analysis of the process of the consultation the influence of both patient and doctor on dynamics have been explored. The realisation that the application of 'scientific method' cannot always provide the answer to the ill-defined problems which distress people has led to the emergence of a wider perspective which embraces a more holistic approach. The recognition of the relevance of this broader perspective has led to the development of more patient-centred approaches which encourage learning and quality improvement through reflection and consultation analysis.

Practical point

Current views on the complexity of the interplay of influences on the consultation mean that further changes can be expected.

A successful consultation is the customised integration of technical knowledge and skill on the part of the doctor, together with competent interpersonal communication, which enables an understanding, and appropriate engagement of both the consulter and the consulted, to manage the problem.

Having considered these models, the reader will be able to identify approaches which are a better fit with their own intuitive consulting style, and which will help them analyse and build on it. Being a good communicator is not enough, and the latter part of this chapter has drawn attention to other important areas and influences, which one needs to explore and assimilate into professional practice.

Practical point
Models help us navigate a complex reality. They help us distinguish what is important; they increase our understanding, and provide a framework for action.

To reiterate, the WHO definition of health is 'a state of complete physical, mental and social well-being and not merely the absence of disease or infirmity'. Approaches to consultation should utilise this broad bio-psychosocial definition.

Communication is a generic skill, important for all healthcare providers. The GMC in their publication, *Tomorrow's Doctors*, in 1993, identified a range of skills that will be increasingly important to doctors in the future including the ability to work in a team, base decisions on evidence and communicate. Communication skills are an important part of professional expertise. The object of this chapter has been to alert the reader to different approaches to the consultation, and to provide an overview of a variety of models, which can be used to analyse and improve consultations with patients. Flexibility is vital. The consultation dynamic, together with one's professional dynamic, will inevitably undergo change during a lifetime of practice.

Practical point
'The theory and practice of medicine is strongly influenced in any era by the dominant theory of knowledge and by societal values. Medicine is always a child of its time.'[14]

Conclusion

There are very many 'models' of consulting styles. While one should not consult using checklists of tasks, it is important to be familiar with some of these consultation models. They can help to provide a structure and framework for your consultations.

Communication skills can be learned. This is best achieved using experiential learning techniques building on individual style. The following are some suggestions of important skills to incorporate flexibly into consulting with patients that may well aid effective communication. The number of texts written on the consultation is overwhelming as this chapter demonstrates. However, the following general points arise from the many consultation models described.

Establish a rapport

It is important to try and establish a rapport with all patients and develop an ongoing relationship. Try to connect with patients. Greet them with warmth and encourage them to talk early in the consultation. It is important to look interested and avoid stopping the flow in the initial stages.

Questioning style

Appropriate use of open, leading and closed questions. As a general rule, open questions are most appropriate at the start of a consultation followed up by closed/leading questions later. Closed questions tend to increase doctor control and are useful to obtain facts. They are not good at eliciting the patient's beliefs and feelings and are generally answered with 'yes or no' answers.

> Open question: 'Tell me more about ...'. 'What is the pain like?'
> Closed question: 'Have you lost weight?'

Active listening

This is demonstrated by appropriate open body language and verbal/non-verbal prompts (e.g. head nodding, smiling) Good eye contact is essential. Summarising helps demonstrate active listening to patient and aids clarity.

Empathy

This is trying to put yourself into the patient's position. Here are some examples.

> 'I can understand this must be a very difficult time for you.'
> 'This must be devastating news for you ... I am so sorry.'

This is different to sympathy which is less effective

> 'I know how you feel ... the same thing happened to me.'

Summarising

As mentioned in active listening, this can help clarify what the patient has told you. It is particularly useful to clarify the presenting complaint or agreed management plan.

Reflection

Reflect back a phrase or symptom that the patient has mentioned in order to explore it further. This is a good technique to use when trying to 'open' up a patient and again demonstrates active listening.

> Patient: 'I've been feeling a bit out of sorts.'
> Doctor: 'Out of sorts ... tell me what you mean by this.'

Appropriate language

Medical terminology can frustrate and confuse patients. Jargon should be avoided wherever possible and explanations given in the patient's or lay language. It is important to be sensitive to the amount and kinds of words used with people from different social backgrounds and intellectual capacities.

Silence

Try to become comfortable with silence and allow pauses in the consultation. If you wait long enough, the patient will break the silence when they are ready.

Responding to cues

These cues can be verbal or non-verbal. 'You seem very upset/anxious ...' is an example of responding to a non-verbal cue.

Patient's ideas, concerns and expectations

All patients have different health beliefs influenced by personal experience, media information or family/cultural beliefs. It is important to explore these during a consultation to enable a patient-centred consultation.

For example, a 45-year-old man presents with a six-week history of a cough. He seems very concerned and is requesting investigations.

If asked, 'Have you had any thoughts as to what this might be? Are you worried that this might be anything, in particular?':

- patient A might answer, 'TB', because he knows that someone a few doors down from where he lives has recently been diagnosed
- patient B might answer, 'Lung cancer', because he is a heavy smoker
- patient C might answer that he is particularly concerned because he was in Africa two months ago on a working trip and has never felt well since. He is worried he may have picked up some 'rare disease' from there.

Occasionally, if you ask the patient you may get the answer, 'You're the doctor, you tell me'. This should not deter you.

Some patients, at this point, will open up to their deeper fears. This can be the most revealing and important part of the consultation.

Sharing information

Patient-centred consulting means sharing information with patients and agreeing on a shared management plan. This respects that the patient through their experience is the 'expert' in their illness. When sharing information with patients, it is best to actively seek feedback throughout the consultation. Look for non-verbal clues that indicate non-understanding, e.g. facial puzzlement, lack of interest. It is not good enough to deliver all your information and then ask, 'Have you any questions?' It is better to check with the patient after each new piece of information is given. Possible phrases you might use are:

'Have you heard of that before? Does that mean anything to you?'
'How does that come across to you? Do you want to ask me anything about that?'
'I am not sure that I explained that very well. Is there anything you would like me to go over again?'

It is also important to use short words and sentences when delivering information. Give the patient the most important facts first. Do not worry about repeating important information. Check their understanding.

Social and psychological context

Where appropriate, it is necessary to explore these areas to establish a complete picture of the patient's presenting complaint.

For example, if the patient presents with back pain, it is likely to be relevant to ask about occupation; or if the patient is depressed, it is relevant to ask, 'How are things at home?' or 'How are things at work?'

Clinical examination

Some patients may require no examination at all but, if appropriate, clinical examination may help to confirm or refute a possible diagnosis.

Partnership

Consider using plural pronouns to make the patient feel part of a partnership: 'Where shall **we** go from here? What do you think **we** should do now?'

Honesty

Be prepared to admit uncertainty if you don't know exactly what is wrong with the patient.

Safety netting/follow-up

It is important for all patients to know when they should come back if their illness has not improved. This also can provide peace of mind for the doctor, especially in general practice where doctors are often faced with vague symptoms and signs. This is called *'dealing with uncertainty'*. It is often hard to know, when symptoms and signs are soft, whether the patient is presenting with a significant illness but at a very early stage, or whether their symptoms will settle.

By organising appropriate and realistic follow-up this allows you to monitor patients over time which can really aid diagnosis.

Housekeeping

Practical point
This means clearing the mind of the psychological remains of one consultation to ensure it has no detrimental effect on the next.

This might mean, in reality, having a few minutes to yourself to recover from an emotionally draining consultation.

Excellent communication skills alone are not enough

Good communication requires a combination of **knowledge**, **skills** and **attitudes**. It is important to be clinically competent with good diagnostic acumen. A professional attitude is also needed where the clinician is non-judgemental and without prejudice. If these attributes are combined with good generic communication skills, then good doctor–patient consulting can occur.

Communication skills underpin virtually all the factors that either make a consultation successful or alternatively a disaster. While knowledge of a condition or being able to easily refer a patient to another practitioner is very important, this can amount to little, if the communication is poor.

Simple skills to improve communication are available to all clinicians, with a very rewarding outcome for both the patient and clinician in terms of communication, satisfaction and time management in the consultation.

References

1 Thompson JA, Anderson, JL. Patient preferences and the bedside manner. *Medical Education*. 1982; **16**: 17–21.

2 Neuberger J. Patients' priorities. *BMJ*. 1998; **317**: 260–2.

3 Tudor Hart J. *A New Kind of Doctor*. London: Merlin Press; 1988.

4 Hampton JR, Harrison MJB, Mitchell JRA. Relative contributions of history taking, physical examination and laboratory investigation to diagnosis and management of medical outpatients. *BMJ*. 1975; **ii**: 486–9.

5 McWhinney IR. Beyond diagnosis. An approach to the integration of behavioural science and clinical medicine. *New England Journal of Medicine*. 1972; **287**: 384–7.

6 McWhinney IR. Changing models: the impact of Kuhn's theory on medicine. *Family Practice*. 1984; **1**: 3–8.

7 Byrne PS, Long BEL. *Doctors Talking to Patients*. Exeter: The Royal College of General Practitioners; 1984 (first published HMSO; 1976).

8 Pendleton D, Schofield T, Tate P, Havelock P. *The Consultation: an approach to learning and teaching*. Oxford: Oxford University Press; 1984.

9 Kurtz SM, Silverman JD, Draper J. *Teaching and Learning Communication Skills in Medicine*. Oxford: Radcliffe Medical Press; 1998.

10 Maslow AH. *Motivation and Personality*. New York: Harper and Row; 1954.

11 Berne E. *Games People Play*. Harmondsworth: Penguin; 1964.

12 Balint M. *The Doctor, His Patient, and the Illness*. London: Pitman Medical Publishing; 1957.

13 Stewart M, Brown JB, Weston WW, McWhinney IR, McWilliam CL, Freeman TR. *Patient-centred Medicine, Transforming the Clinical Method*. Thousand Oaks, CA: Sage; 1995.

14 Stewart M, Brown JB, Weston WW, McWhinney IR, McWilliam CL, Freeman T. *Patient-centred Medicine, Transforming the Clinical Method*. 2nd ed. Oxford: Radcliffe Medical Press; 2003.

15 Pendleton D, Schofield T, Tate P, Havelock P. *The New Consultation*. Oxford: Oxford University Press; 2003.

16 Kurtz SM, Silverman JD. The Calgary–Cambridge observation guides: an aid to defining the curriculum and organizing the teaching in communication training programmes. *Medical Education*. 1996; **30**: 83–9.

17 Weiner N. *Cybernetics: or control and communication in the animal and the machine*. New York: Wiley; 1948.

18 Stott NCH, Davis RH. The exceptional potential in each primary care consultation. *Journal of the Royal College of General Practitioners*. 1979; **29**: 201–5.

19 Helman CG. *Culture, Health and Illness*. London: Arnold/Heinemann; 2001.

20 Helman CG. The culture of general practice. *British Journal of General Practice*. 2002; **52**: 619–20.

21 Neighbour R. *The Inner Consultation*. Dordrecht/Boston/London: Kluwer Academic Publishers; 1987.

22 Fraser RC, McKinley RK, Mulholland H. Consultation competence in general practice: establishing the face validity of prioritized criteria in the Leicester assessment package. *British Journal of General Practice*. 1994; **44**: 109–13.

23 Fraser R. *Clinical Method; a general practice approach*. Oxford: Butterworth Heinemann; 2000.

24 Shannon CEA. Mathematical theory of communication. *Bell System Technical Journal*. 1948; **27**: 379–423, 623–56 (July and October issues).

25 Levenstein JH, McCracken EC, McWhinney IR, Stewart MA, Brown JB. The patient-centred clinical method. 1. A model for the doctor-patient interaction in family medicine. *Family Practice*. 1986; **3**(1): 24–30.

26 Hager P, Gonszi A, Athanasou J. General issues about assessment of competence. *Assessment and Evaluation in Higher Education*. 1994; **19**: 3–16.

27 Riccardi VM, Kurtz SM. *Communication and Counselling in Health Care*. Springfield, IL: Charles C Thomas; 1983.

28 Kurtz SM. Curriculum structuring to enhance communication skills development. In: Stewart M, Roter D, editors. *Communication with Medical Patients*. Newbury Park, CA: Sage Publications; 1989.

29 Silverman J, Kurtz S, Draper J. *Skills for Communicating with Patients*. Oxford: Radcliffe Medical Press; 1998.

30 Mercer SW, Reynolds WJ. Empathy and quality of care. *British Journal of General Practice*. 2002; **52**: S9–S13.

31 Coulter A, Magee H. *The European Patient of the Future*. Maidenhead: Open University Press; 2003.

32 Howie JGR, Heaney DJ, Maxwell M, Walker JJ, Freeman G, Rai H. *Measuring Quality in General Practice*. Occasional Paper Number 75. London: Royal College of General Practitioners; 1997.

33 Howie JGR, Heaney DJ, Maxwell M, Walker JJ, Freeman G, Rai H. Quality at general practice consultations: cross sectional survey. *BMJ*. 1999; **319**: 738–43.

34 Sackett DL, Rosenberg WM, Gray JA, Haynes RB, Richardson WS. Evidence based medicine: what it is and what it isn't. *BMJ*. 1996; **312**: 71–2.

35 Walker L. *Consulting with NLP*. Oxford: Radcliffe Medical Press; 2002.

36 Charon R. Narrative medicine: a model for empathy, reflection, profession and trust. *Journal of the American Medical Association*; 2001; **286**(15): 1897–1902.

37 Launer J. A narrative approach to mental health in general practice. *BMJ*. 1999; **318**: 117–19.

38 Hudson Jones A. Narrative in medical ethics. *BMJ*. 1999; **318**: 253–6.

39 Heath I. *The Mystery of General Practice*. London: Nuffield Provincial Hospitals Trust; 1995.

40 Derrida J. *Limited Inc*. Evanston, IL: Northwestern University Press; 1988.

41 Plsek PE, Greenhalgh T. The challenge of complexity in health care. *BMJ*. 2001; **323**: 625–8.

42 Wilson T, Holt T, Greenhalgh T. Complexity science: complexity and clinical care. *BMJ*. 2001; **323**: 685–8.

Bibliography

Freed DLJ. Doctors are not scientists but we still need science. [Letter.] *BMJ*. 2004; **329**: 294.

Gorovitz S, MacIntyre A. Toward a theory of medical fallibility. *Journal of Medicine and Philosophy*. 1976; **1**(1): 51–71.

Innes AD, Campion PD, Griffiths FE. Complex consultations and the 'edge of chaos'. *British Journal of General Practice*. 2005; **55**: 47–52.

Latthe M, Charlton R. Cum Scientia Caritas or EBM? *British Journal of General Practice*. 2000; **50**: 852.

The NHS Plan. 2000. www.dh.gov.uk

Sackett DL, Richardson S, Scott W, Rosenberg W, Haynes RB. *How to Practice and Teach Evidence-based Medicine*. 2nd ed. Edinburgh: Elsevier/Churchill Livingstone; 2000.

Silverman JD, Kurtz SM, Draper J. *Skills for Communicating with Patients*. Oxford: Radcliffe Medical Press; 1998.

Sweeney K, Griffiths FE. *Complexity and Health Care: an introduction*. Oxford: Radcliffe Medical Press; 2002.

Tate P. *The Doctor's Communication Handbook*. 3rd ed. Oxford: Radcliffe Medical Press; 2001. www.skillscascade.com

Acknowledgement

Dr Dan Munday, Consultant/Honorary Clinical Senior Lecturer in Palliative Medicine, Warwick Medical School and Coventry PCT, for his review and helpful comments on the section, 'Complexity and the consultation'.

Chapter 13

Aids to learning

Dr Madhu Garala, Liz Winborn, Dr Abhijit Bhattacharyya, Dr Rodger Charlton, Dr Catti Moss, Colonel Jonathan Leach and Sqn Ldr Peter Lavallee

Rodger Charlton defines some of the terms used in medical education, Madhu Garala looks at the different learning environments in medical practice and Catti Moss discusses the video recording of consultations. Jonathan Leach and Peter Lavallee describe the evaluation of consultations. Liz Winborn looks at the importance of feedback by students, and Abhijit Bhattacharyya and Rodger Charlton discuss assessment and how it impacts on learning.

Teaching the consultation can take place in many situations – in hospitals, the community and the university. Teaching may be theoretical or practical using simulated or real patients. Different methods of teaching can be utilised. One skill that is being actively encouraged more frequently for both undergraduates and qualified practitioners is that of lifelong learning.

Although the undergraduate phase of learning finishes with a certification of competence through the awarding of a medical degree, graduates are expected to maintain and improve this standard and so continue their learning as part of their **continuing professional development** (CPD) and keeping evidence of their learning in a **portfolio** or educational diary. Thus, there is a continuum of learning from undergraduate to postgraduate years. The skills of lifelong learning should be acquired in undergraduate years of which the skills of self-directed learning should be a part. A role of the medical teacher is to equip students with these skills and facilitate learning. This chapter is devoted to both different learning styles and different teaching methods.

It is of interest that the Hippocratic Oath which doctors used to promise has a section which relates to medical teaching. The importance of passing on the knowledge of medicine and of ethical practice to the next generation is stressed in the oath and it could be suggested that this is a duty of postgraduates. *Learning to Consult* requires more than self-directed learning. It requires a series of teachers and doctors who facilitate and supervise learning and this chapter focuses on several aspects of teaching and also its evaluation and its success through assessment. Assessment itself has an important contribution to learning.

This chapter is divided up into the following sections.

- Learning and teaching.
- Learning environments.

- Using video in the consultation.
- Personal performance – evaluating consultations.
- Feedback and evaluation.
- Assessments and examinations.
- Summary.

Learning and teaching

Learning in clinical practice can be defined as the cognitive process of acquiring knowledge or clinical skills through study, experience with patients or teaching.
Learning can be classified into three domains:

- 'cognitive' (to do with knowledge)
- 'psychomotor' (to do with skills)
- 'affective' (to do with attitudes, and the resulting behaviour).

Differences between education, training and teaching

Education is:
- transmitting knowledge
- understanding the knowledge you have
- modification by new knowledge
- gaining knowledge and doing things better
- the process by which learning is achieved.

Training is:
- instructing
- the learner taking on new tasks
- doing exercises, gaining competence
- practising (preparation for performance)
- gaining skills/apprenticeship.

Teaching is:
- imparting knowledge (factual information)
- to show/direct/give instruction (skill)
- to inspire/influence attitude (behaviour)
- to demonstrate an art or practice (enable development)
- training in a 'teaching PCT' or 'teaching hospital'
- ongoing – 'maintaining "good doctors"'.

Practical point
It is important to stress that teaching is not necessarily equated with learning.

A teacher's message may be:

- accepted
- modified

- rejected
- ignored.

It should also be asked if the teacher is '**learner-centred**'.

Some practising doctors might recollect their days of medical school teaching where they were '**teacher-centred**' as follows:

- an educational wilderness of didactic, strict, unfriendly teachers
- indigestible textbooks
- rote learning of innumerable facts
- factual knowledge was equated with learning.

Unlike a pure biomedical science, medical practice involves interaction with patients. Following an international conference on medical education in 1991, the GMC in its publication in 1993, *Tomorrow's Doctors*, identified the need to incorporate communication and consulting skills as a part of the core of medical undergraduate curriculums. As a result, during the last decade in medical education there have been great changes in medical teaching methods and undergraduate medical curriculums. There were many recommendations regarding undergraduate medical education and some of the following in the publication had considerable influence on the teaching methods employed and the content of medical curriculums.

Paragraph 8: 'The relationship between the doctor and the patient has changed and there is a clear duty on the doctor to be able and willing to communicate effectively, an attribute that must be developed throughout the undergraduate course and beyond.'

This is the reason for the considerable emphasis in this book and medical curriculums on the development of consultation skills.

Paragraphs 34 and 35 – methods of learning are discussed, and it is suggested that there is a reduced reliance on the 'didactic lecture format' and more on 'learner-centred and problem-orientated approaches'.

In paragraph 40.3 concerning attitudinal objectives there is a need by the end of the course for an 'awareness of the moral and ethical responsibilities involved in individual patient care'.

Paragraph 41 – the advantages of interdisciplinary collaboration in planning courses are discussed.

The GMC advocated changes and so a move from:

- didactic
- unfriendly
- teacher-centred teaching and the use of indigestible textbooks

to

- learner-centred teaching
- involving individual and seminar/small-group worked teaching
- with an emphasis on self-directed and problem-based learning
- gaining the skills of lifelong learning.

A hierarchy of learning can therefore be identified from surface (rote) learning, which is teacher-centred which involves the repetitive process of memorising facts from lectures using a 'prescriptive' curriculum to the **identification of learning needs**. Using modern teaching methods this should facilitate deep learning, thinking, understanding and making sense of facts. As a postgraduate, skills in lifelong learning will encourage a doctor to take responsibility for their own learning and so for it to be self-directed. Adult learning will then occur through curiosity and will be truly learner-centred.

All education is moving very much to the last pedagogical model. (Pedagogy is the art or science of teaching.) It is therefore anticipated that the method of teaching chosen will have the most impact on the learner.

In relation to clinical practice, there is a **hierarchy of learning**, annotated from *Bloom's Taxonomy*, which can be identified as follows.

- **Memory** ('surface learning') (history).
- **Understanding** ('deep learning') (examination and investigating – making sense of the history/consultation).
- **Application** (problem solving/diagnosing).
- **Synthesis** (planning treatment/decision making/medical management).
- **Evaluation** (review) and reflection (audit).

Learning environments

There are wide and varied learning environments. However, these are influenced by the resources that are available, the number of people in the group being taught and the size of the room.

The impact on the learner will also be affected by various factors such as:

- personality
- learning needs
- prior knowledge
- learning styles
- teaching environment
- the learner who attracts attention.

A student may encounter many different learning environments and these are now discussed.

This section is divided as follows:

- lectures
- self-directed learning
- problem-based learning
- small-group teaching
- learning with IT
- the general practice surgery
- hospital clinics
- ward rounds
- simulated patients
- patients as 'teachers'
- e-learning
- multidisciplinary education.

Lectures

A lecture-based programme can work well for the 'nuts and bolts' and, in many universities, lectures are still probably the most common teaching method employed. In using this didactic teaching method, there is a lack of student interaction. It could beneficially be replaced by experiential teaching in small groups where students actively participate, as, at best, lectures achieve passive learning. Some lecturers standing at the front of a lecture theatre may think to themselves:

> 'It's the sea of blank, unresponsive faces; I could just as well be talking in a foreign language.'

We can all recall poor or uninteresting lectures that we have attended and perhaps this is what the lecturers were thinking. A lecture allows one expert to share his or her expertise with a great many learners in a short period of time. It is a cost-effective teaching method for a large number of individuals and a syllabus can be covered quickly and the lecturer can clarify difficult concepts. A lecturer's enthusiasm may be infectious and motivate the learners to find out more.

Practical point
However, lectures are usually a very poor means of changing attitude, inspiring students or inducing positive professional attitude towards the subject.

The three most important points to take into consideration when delivering any lecture should be:

A   length (loss of concentration after 10 minutes)
B   sign posts – being explicit of what you are delivering in a lecture
C   use of audio-visual aids to help emphasise the point and keep learners interested.

Self-directed learning (SDL)

This is a learner-centred process and encourages a student to discover and define his or her own learning needs, explore their own learning styles and evaluate their own development with facilitation as required. Seven factors are associated with successful, self-directed learning outcomes.

1   Openness to learning (enjoyment, enthusiasm motivation).
2   Self-disciplined and organised.
3   Independence.
4   Enjoyment in the exploratory nature of education.
5   Assimilation of new ideas to aid understanding.
6   A desire for continuous improvement.
7   Taking responsibility for one's ongoing learning.

There are several important components of self-directed learning and these include:

- learning through curiosity
- being learner-centred
- planning one's learning
- the individual manages their own learning
- evaluates and reflects upon one's own learning experiences
- assuming responsibility for one's own learning.

Problem-based learning (PBL)

Why distinguish between SDL and PBL? Some medicals schools have a predominantly SDL-based curriculum and some have a predominantly PBL-based curriculum.

PBL involves the learner or groups of learners identifying what problems they face in their working environment and so identifying their learning needs based on these observations and creating the plans necessary to meet these needs. For example, a student realises that they are having a problem making diagnoses of hip problems and how they need to increase their knowledge base, develop a structured diagnostic approach and gain feedback on this approach. The student can also ask which book their tutor recommends and seek tutorials on the subject, review all hip 'cases' and re-assess the situation in a number of weeks.

Important components of problem-based learning are that it is:

- teacher facilitated
- interactive and can involve group collaboration and be fun
- tackling relevant problems, but not necessarily solving them
- exploiting problems for their learning potential.

Small-group teaching

It is difficult to define what a small group is, but ideally it involves about 5–10 students often using a problem-based learning approach. The small group should be a confidential environment where the group builds up a trusting relationship and individuals feel able to interact and are supported by a skilled and impartial facilitator to act as a catalyst and not a critic.

Practical point
It is a valuable environment for open discussion, interaction encouraging active participation and so active learning from the individuals in the group.

Other teaching material may be used within the small groups, including videotape review, which is a powerful educational method, e.g. in relation to consultation skills. This encourages constructive feedback on consulting skills in a supportive and non-threatening atmosphere. Role-plays can also be an effective teaching method in small groups. In issues relating to patients, the small group forum may be used to increase students' awareness of their feelings and of other students' perspectives.

Small groups may also cover a series of topics for postgraduates and in the small group setting or **seminar** the discussion among the members and the teacher replaces a lecture.

Small-group work encourages learners to develop their own ideas and to challenge preconceived beliefs and is often more effective than more passive types of teaching such as lectures, in stimulating learners to think independently, interact, develop ideas and share learning experiences. This type of active learning promotes critical and logical thinking as part of problem solving.

Small-group work is usually based on a task that is wide enough to encourage the learners to own and develop the topic themselves but is focused enough to restrict the ensuing discussions to the matter in hand. The use of a flip chart or white board can be useful tools in this setting to record the discussions.

Dr Bruce Tuckman, an educational psychologist from the USA, published his Forming Storming Norming Performing model in 1965, which is one of the most quoted models of group development. Small groups can evolve through five stages of development in-group dynamics if given sufficient time.

1 Forming – getting to know one another.
2 Norming – the norms, roles and goals of the group worked out through informal discussion.
3 Storming – various ideas are put forward.
4 Performing – decisions reached where a task is agreed with mutual support.
5 Adjourning – group begins to disband as time runs out.

A **workshop** is a short but intensive small-group meeting or course where there is an emphasis on problem solving and with specific learning outcomes, e.g. hand washing in clinical care.

Other ideas to stimulate a small group and encourage active participation can include the following.

a **Talking walls** – group list their perception about a topic on a flip chart displayed on the wall.
b **Active photograph** – the use of photographs can generate in-depth discussion about health issues illustrated in photographs.
c **Goldfish bowl technique** – outer group observes an inner group of two or three people performing a task. The inner group feed back first, followed by the outer group.
d **Trios** – three people make up the small group where they can talk and complete the task set to them.

Learning with information technology (IT)

The learning environment in various settings can use IT to enhance effective learning. A lecturer can make use of audio-visual aids that will enhance the delivery of their material and reinforce their messages and commands the learner's attention including:

- PowerPoint presentation
- overhead slides
- photographic slides
- videotapes
- computer-based learning materials.

The learning environment can vary considerably in various organisations.

The general practice surgery

In this environment most of the educational activity is carried out with either one-to-one teaching or in a very small group setting where initially the qualified GP tutor is observed with questions directed at the students. When the student feels comfortable and confident enough he or she can take the lead role in the consultation with feedback from the observing GP.

This is a very effective form of learning but is time consuming. Consent is obtained from the patient prior to the consultation taking place. The students can observe other members of the primary healthcare team to enhance their consultation skills and knowledge base in primary care. (This may involve sessional attachments to a health visitor, district nurses, midwife, practice manager, community psychiatric nurse and many other members of the team.)

In this environment audio-visual aids can be used to improve skills, e.g. such as the use of video of consultations with appropriate feedback.

Hospital clinics

This is a good opportunity to improve skills in physical examination to aid the diagnostic process and see rare diseases in specialist centres. This is specific to specialties such as cardiology and examination of the cardiovascular system. It is also an opportunity to improve skills in system-based history taking with the observation and input of a specialist. In addition, an understanding of system-specific investigations can be gained, such as:

- electrocardiograms (ECGs)
- ultrasound scans in obstetrics
- a spirometer used in respiratory medicine.

Ward rounds

As more disease is treated in the community, this type of teaching is decreasing, but it is teaching often associated with the training doctors. Ward rounds are usually conducted in a multidisciplinary setting with a patient being present. To benefit maximally from teaching in this situation, it is useful if the student has had an opportunity to become familiar with each patient's case and the disease condition concerned. A student should still benefit even if they have not had an opportunity to prepare.

Various patient cases can help a student to identify their learning needs if the doctor leading the ward round supervises this educational activity constructively. It is helpful if a student can undertake some background reading in the specialty of their attachment to gain some prior theoretical knowledge in the subject. This can be supplemented by attendance at appropriate lectures and seminars. It used to be that ward round teaching was not popular with students, as they were anxious at being put on the spot with their peers being present.

To prevent such a scenario, the doctor or consultant leading the ward round should be sympathetic to students' potential anxiety and relative lack of knowledge and practical experience.

Practical point

Taking a positive approach and providing appropriate feedback in a non-confrontational way with tips and strategies for improvement can greatly benefit a student.

Patients also tend to find ward rounds difficult and can also become quite anxious as their case is discussed with strangers and worrying differential diagnoses are postulated. The doctor in charge should be sensitive to the needs of students and patients alike and ward rounds can be important opportunities to educate both students and patients in a manner from which both parties will benefit. It is also an opportunity to encourage questions and resolve anxieties for the patient through appropriate explanation of their symptoms, investigations and treatments.

Simulated patients

Simulated patients are actors who are trained to act the role of patients based on defined scenarios with carefully written scripts. This is a significant advance from traditional **role-play** where one student assumes the role of a patient and another that of a doctor. They should react as a patient would react and provide a history in terms of their symptoms, but also display any emotions as are deemed appropriate in the script. The learning experience that is induced should be like a real-life consultation. At the present time, simulated patients are used for most parts of a consultation excluding physical examination and investigations. However, the 'doctor' who is consulting can be given the findings on examination and investigation on request having stated what examination and investigations they are feel are indicated in each individual case. It may be possible to train simulated patients to undergo a limited physical examination in the future.

Simulated patients provide a 'safe' environment for students and postgraduates to 'practise' and also to stop a consultation at a particular point or to repeat part of a consultation that did not go well. Simulated patients can also be trained to provide feedback and are an invaluable resource and considerable innovation in medical education. They can also be videoed and this is discussed later in this chapter.

Patients as 'teachers'

A wealth of resources is available to help facilitate teaching through patients themselves. This is an important and practical source of learning for the trainees.

Simulated patients and communications skills training can prepare students for contact with 'real' patients. However, patients are a powerful resource for which there is no ideal substitute. Even for the experienced clinician, encounters with patients continue to facilitate learning whether this is through taking a history, conducting a physical examination, trying to make a diagnosis or to negotiate a possible management plan. A particularly valuable aspect of teaching using patients is following up patients rather than one-off contacts. This might be following up a mother who is pregnant until she gives birth or a patient with a chronic disease or a patient who is dying and requires palliative care.

There is a role for 'expert patients' in the education of trainees and also to help other patients with chronic disease in relation to self-management.

A section in the next chapter entitled 'Work-based learning' describes the role of patient contacts in learning for trainees and practitioners which takes place as a result of individual consultations, feedback from following up consultations in relation to decision making and observing the natural history of diseases.

e-learning

As an aid to learning and teaching, the potential of e-learning is increasing exponentially. Possible e-learning methods are:

- use of CD_ROMs
- online journals
- lectures online (video and audio streaming)
- medical education websites
- interactive software, e.g. to teach anatomy
- discussion forums (interaction with other learners)
- blogs
- virtual learning environments (VLEs)
- learning at a distance and at times convenient to the learner
- an alternative to textbooks
- web conferencing
- simulated consultations
- computer-assisted learning in anatomy
- tutorials
- computer-assisted assessment.

The list is endless and is growing and developing. Students and postgraduates should, however, be cautioned against **plagiarism** given the wealth and quality of material available online for potential assignments.

Practical point

Plagiarism is using the thoughts and writings of others without acknowledging them and the source.

A **blog** is a web log. It is a web page that is accessible by others and is the personal diary or journal of an individual that is regularly updated, perhaps daily. Blogs may also serve as discussion forums. Large institutions may use blogs as communication channels. They can be educational tools. They might contain, e.g. reviews, the sharing of ideas, illustrations or be a collection of ongoing reflections.

Multidisciplinary education

Traditionally, in the UK, education of healthcare professionals has been carried out within single professional disciplines. However, there is an increasing need for multidisciplinary curriculum development in order to improve the teamwork required in the new NHS. Multidisciplinary teamwork is being recognised as essential in the delivery of patient care. It is also being increasingly recognised that team leaders who co-ordinate the care and harness the skills will utilise the contributions of individual professionals within the team to individual patient care. It would seem logical therefore that if delivery of healthcare requires a multidisciplinary team approach to be successful, so does the education of individual members of a future healthcare team.

The teaching methods used need to be flexible in order to accommodate the diversities of knowledge and skills of the students from different disciplines.

Using video in the consultation

Perhaps the most effective way of improving performance is to increase self-awareness and use feedback. Taking a videotape of oneself consulting, and then playing it back to oneself, is the most direct way of giving oneself feedback.

Practical point
Nowadays, the use of videotape in the consultation is becoming commonplace and can also be used in assessment.

Medical students are videoed at several points in their training. Although most student assessments are done with live or simulated patients, and directly observed, it is quite possible that the use of video will increase in under-graduate exams.

When compared with the use of simulated patients or having one's consulting directly observed, the video recording has several big advantages. The video is definitely of a real consultation. It is usually with a real live patient, and the video camera does not change the dynamics of the consultation in the way that a third party does. There is also the wonderful opportunity to stop the tape, giving oneself time to think about what was going on, and what should happen next. One can also rewind, and replay. Thus one can find out exactly what was happening, and what was said at a particular time in a consultation. The third big advantage is that the camera doesn't get distracted, and it continues to watch the patient's face even when you are busy at the computer. It sees and records all the non-verbal communication in the consultation.

Disadvantages in video recordings.

Most of us are not film stars, and get rather uncomfortable when watching ourselves on television. For those with poor self-esteem, watching oneself can be an excruciating experience. Even the more 'hard-boiled' of us will have certain personal characteristics that make us cringe. This embarrassment does nothing to help us improve our performance, and can get in the way of useful feedback.

Pendleton's rules

Because of this, it is essential that video recordings should be watched with the support of someone who is experienced at giving feedback. The rules of feedback (Pendleton's rules) must be followed carefully, and the group of peers that is watching the videos should be supportive.

Practical point
Providing these rules are followed, watching oneself on video can become the most useful way of improving consultation skills.

However, most of us know someone who has been put off using video by an unfortunate experience during his or her training. Pendleton's rules are as follows.

1 The 'doctor' in the consultation should be provided the opportunity to talk first and discuss the positive points raised. It is all too easy to fall into the trap of stating what did not go well. It is therefore essential that the positive points are discussed first.
2 The 'doctor' in the consultation may then voice what they feel would have improved their performance during the consultation.
3 The rest of the observing group are then invited to provide feedback, but again positive points must be raised first.
4 The group can now provide constructive feedback of areas identified for possible improvement of the 'doctor' during future consultations. It is these points that can be taken in a negative fashion and care must be taken by those giving feedback and also the facilitator of the group to ensure they are not destructive.

An opportunity can also be provided for the 'patient' to give feedback in a role-play or where the patient is a simulated patient adopting the same rules.

Pendleton's rules should provide a supportive learning environment and avoid 'teaching by humiliation' which is from a bygone era of medical education and only highlights the limited communication skills of the teacher.

Practical point
Pendleton's rules emphasise the need to give positive feedback before negative feedback. They also offer the 'person in the hot seat' to give feedback first.

Practicalities for video recording consultations

What do we need to enable the video experience to become a positive learning experience? First, the technology should work. We need a video camera, and a means of fixing it in the right position to be able to have both the consulter and patient in view.

In practice this usually means having a good wide-angle lens on the camera, and a wall-bracket to support it in the right position. Consulting rooms are usually too small to allow the use of cameras without wide-angle lenses, and tripods are clumsy and very obvious to the patient. It is worth taking a lot of time experimenting to get the view just right. Ideally both participants should be clearly seen, and the patient's facial expressions should be clearly recorded.

We need lighting that will allow us to see the participants clearly, rather than two dark figures silhouetted against a bright window.

We need a microphone that will pick up the words of the consultation clearly, without being drowned by traffic noise, or e.g. the noise of the water from the patient's toilet next door. Usually the internal camera microphone will cope adequately, providing the camera is sited on a sound-free wall. If this isn't possible, then an external microphone will be needed. The best type may be an omni-directional mike that looks like a flat piece of plastic, and can sit on the desk.

Practical point
Once the hardware is set up satisfactorily, it is often easiest to leave it in place.

The next essential is to have an efficient system for ensuring that patients can choose whether to be filmed or not. The best systems involve telling the patients that this will be a video surgery at the time they book the appointment, so that they can choose a different surgery or time to avoid the possibility of being videoed without having to refuse. The next step is to give the patient a friendly, understandable **information sheet** when they arrive at the surgery. This should say:

- who is videoing
- what the video is for
- who will see the video
- in what circumstances
- who will ensure its safety
- that it is wiped clean.

Practical point
The patient should be given a real choice of whether to be videoed or not, and they should be given the choice of having the video wiped immediately after the consultation without it being seen.

Fortunately, consent forms for videos abound, and they should meet these criteria.

Now you have your consulting room set up, your patients prepared and happy to be videoed, the next step is to have a go. At first both you and the patients will feel very nervous, but very soon, the presence of the camera will be forgotten. Usually the biggest problems are technical.

Once a decent recording has been obtained, it is wise to check that there is a legible signed consent form for every consultation on the tape. Then it is wise to choose which of the consultations you wish to view.

Watching videotapes

This should be done only in safe and secure surroundings. There should be adequate time set aside, without interruptions. At least one experienced person needs to be present, and it is best if all the other people present are either members of an established group, with a good relationship, or have some common ground. Probably the best group for watching videos is small, has been working together on similar work for some weeks, has a skilled leader, and has all the members with a video that they want to watch.

Using Pendleton's rules means that the person showing the video has to think about the positive aspect of their performance first, and then has this reinforced by positive feedback from the other group members. This is not just a means of counteracting the insecurities that we all feel when watching our own performance. The major learning points that we can gain from watching ourselves may very well be from these positive comments. Very often, by recognising where something has gone well, we can make major improvements in our consulting, just by repeating the behaviour and becoming more proficient at it.

The group leader has an important role, in encouraging everyone to be really specific in his or her feedback. It is very little use to say, 'That was lovely', but to say, 'It was lovely when you put your hand out and said, "It must be very difficult"' can be very useful. Similarly, when the third and fourth stages of the Pendleton feedback are reached, it is very important to have feedback in the form of suggestions, not criticisms. The more specific these suggestions are, the more useful they will be. As an aid to this specificity, it is very useful if at least one member of the group writes down, word for word, as much as they can.

With practice, a small group can make watching videos a very supportive and useful experience.

Practical point
Most of us will be able to link some of the major improvements in our consulting with watching videos with the right support.

Videos are rapidly being replaced by DVD recorders, but all the same principles apply.

Personal performance – evaluating consultations

Effective communication is essential to the current practice of medicine. Over the last 15 years it has been increasingly recognised as a core skill for clinicians. This has had an impact upon their interaction with patients but, of no less importance, it has influenced their contribution to the healthcare team settings in which they work, and the medical community as a whole.

Practical point

A fundamental change in medical culture in this area has been the recognition and acceptance of the fact that the way in which health professionals communicate, on all levels, can be enhanced, irrespective of the innate and learned abilities they might already possess.

This has been shown in the last 10 years with the inclusion of communication skills training in undergraduate education, and a complete change in the educational processes surrounding the teaching and observing of doctor–patient interaction.

In comparison with the relatively simple process of written communication, e.g. in a referral letter, verbal and non-verbal communication is considerably more dynamic and complex, with a cycling of transfer of messages between the two or more parties. These complex situations still reduce down to include these same basic principles once the complex structure of the encounter has been unfolded.

Evaluating personal consultations as a springboard to improving performance

A theoretical approach to evaluating communication with a consultation is to consider the attributes of a good consultation and what factors would make a bad consultation. Why not consider two consultations – one which is a great success and one which was a disaster.

- What factors made the consultation a success from both the doctor's and patient's perspective and what would need to change to make it less successful?
- In the second 'disaster' consultation – what factors made it so difficult and what would need to change to improve it? Some factors may be outside of the control of the doctor, but if that is the case, how could the impact of these factors be reduced?

Possible attributes of good and bad consultations

A good consultation

- Patients' physical and mental needs are met.
- Doctor's physical and mental needs are met.
- The consultation runs to time.
- The consultation has a structure: a beginning, middle and a satisfactory closure.
- There is sufficient time.
- There is good rapport between the doctor and patient.
- There is an 'appropriate' end point.
- Both the patient and doctor are happy with the consultation
- Patient is Adult, doctor is Adult (using transactional analysis principles).
- Suitable further care has been arranged (prescription, referral, management plan).

- There is an appropriate safety net for the patient ('If this does not get better in three days, come back and see me').
- Financial aspects dealt with appropriately.

A bad consultation

- Patient needs remain unmet.
- Doctor needs remain unmet.
- Poor administration (no notes, computer not functioning, etc.).
- Failure of understanding (on behalf of doctor or patient).
- There is insufficient time.
- A 'provoking' patient.
- Clash between doctor and patient (either physically or verbally).
- Unreasonable behaviour (on either part).
- Lack of direction within the consultation.
- Inappropriate collusion between doctor and patient.
- Interruptions and distractions.
- 'Helpless doctor' – not able to help, e.g. patient needs a referral but long waiting list.
- Financial aspects dealt with inappropriately.

More practical methods include videotaping your consultations and analysing them following a set format as discussed in the previous section. Useful methods of appraising your performance are described in Tate (2001) and Kurtz, Silverman and Draper (1998) to help you identify further skills you can learn and practise. These include:

- mapping consultations
- self-appraisal proformas
- workbooks
- patient satisfaction questionnaires
- comparing your consultation to a described model.

These can help you to identify further skills that you can learn and practice.

Questions to ask yourself after each consultation (from Tate 2001)

1 Do I know significantly more about this person as a human being than before they came through the door?
2 Was I curious?
3 Did I listen?
4 Did I explore their beliefs?
5 Did I make an acceptable working diagnosis?
6 Did I use their beliefs when I started explaining?
7 Did I share options for investigations or treatment?
8 Did I share in decision making?
9 Did I make some attempt to see that my patient understood?
10 Did I develop the relationship?

Communication skills underpin virtually all the factors that either make a consultation successful or alternatively a 'disaster'. While knowledge of a condition or being able to easily refer a patient to another practitioner are very important, they can amount to little, if the communication is poor. Simple skills to improve communication are available to all clinicians, with a very rewarding outcome for both the patient and clinician in terms of communication and time management in the consultation.

Feedback and evaluation

The increasing significance of quality in education is being recognised in all subject areas of higher education. It is necessary for medical schools to ensure that their current students provide the bulk of the evaluation and feedback process. This will allow development of the curriculum and ensure quality is maintained at the highest standard. The following excerpt is taken from the January 2003 UK Government on Education:

> Student choice will increasingly work to drive up quality, supported by much better information. A comprehensive survey of student views, as well as published external examiners reports and other information about teaching standards, will be pulled together in an easy-to-use Guide to Universities, overseen by the National Union of Students.

Methods of feedback and evaluation

There are two types of feedback that can be acquired.

1 Qualitative feedback is gathered through the use of open-ended questions and will provide more in-depth information. It is usually gathered by conducting an interview or using a questionnaire with open questions, allowing the interviewee to give their views in their own words. An alternative approach is to hold group discussions or focus groups, which has the advantage of being more interactive.
2 Quantitative feedback is obtained through the use of closed questions and provides numerical data which can be analysed and reproduced in statistical form. This information is gathered using a questionnaire which is designed to generate responses such as 'strongly agree' or 'strongly disagree'.

Qualitative versus quantitative

Most feedback received from students is obtained using a questionnaire with closed questions. The information received can be summarised as a set of statistics which may quickly identify problem areas. However, these questionnaires are generally completed at the end of a course, thus not allowing for any immediate changes that benefit the group of students who have participated in answering the questionnaires.

Practical point
A more dynamic and intersting approach should be developed to obtain qualitative feedback through the use of group discussion.

The discussion can be at the mid point and end of clinical attachments and all students encouraged to participate. Holding the discussion at the mid point allows for any urgent issues to be raised and hopefully resolved during the placement, and allows planning and changes for the next attachment.

Such a discussion group needs to be run, e.g., by an Administrative Officer who is viewed by the students as neutral and runs the discussion with no teaching staff present. The students work together and this provides information which is collectively agreed upon. A report is formed from this discussion process which ensures confidentiality by not naming individuals and is made up of action points. All teaching and administrative staff can then work to make changes immediately or over a longer period.

Advantages of this process are that it ensures working with students and allows the students to feel valued. It also allows for any misunderstandings or misconceptions to be discussed at that particular point in time; this in itself can sometimes resolve perceived issues. On the other hand, this method does require a significant investment of time on the part of the person running the discussion group.

There are merits in using each of these types of methods of gaining feedback, individually or as a combination, and they enable teaching and support staff to identify areas for change, and thus contribute towards an improved learning experience for the students. Where changes are made they should form part of a 'feedback loop' so that students and staff can re-evaluate them during subsequent clinical attachments.

It is important that learners are made aware that, whichever method of feedback is implemented, they can be the driving force behind change. Encouraging them to take part in completion of questionnaires and/or group discussions is an important part of their educational experience. It is also important that staff act upon the information received in a positive way.

In an ideal world, evaluation of a course or a curriculum requires a triangular process taking into account the views of the teachers, the students and the outcomes of the assessments. In relation to assessment the view of patients can also be sought.

Assessments and examinations

Medical education should be trainee or **learner-centred**, where learners are encouraged to take responsibility of their own learning and so develop the skills of lifelong learning in preparation for their transition to qualified practitioners.

Practical point
Assessment can be an important stimulus for self-directed learning and this method of learning not only enables individuals to pass examinations, but assists when they are faced with a future similar clinical problem or just curiosity.

In addition, it is an opportunity for the student to gain feedback and for teachers to ascertain the success of their teaching.

Whatever assessment procedure is employed it should be judged in relation to its fairness, suitability and role in promoting learning through feedback. All assessments should be modified through the views of the teachers, trainees and a peer reference group such as the General Medical Council (GMC). Assessments should not be a unilateral, faculty-driven process. Trainees value a fair assessment process for:

- a route to gaining feedback
- evaluation of the curriculum
- as a guide to their learning
- increasing their confidence
- motivating further learning.

A valid and reliable assessment process should also be an indicator of their performance in future.

This section covers the following:

- defining assessment
- purpose of assessment
- the skills that should be assessed
- formative assessment and learning
- summative assessment
- continuous assessment
- assessment of attitude
- visual assessment methods
- OSCE (objective structured clinical examination)
- competence and performance.

Defining assessment

Assessment is the measurement of achievement of learning outcomes following education and training. In medical practice this may be through the sampling of behaviours, drawing inferences and making estimates of worth. Assessments should provide evidence of learning (knowledge gained) and evidence of the effectiveness of training demonstrated through competence and performance which is calibrated summatively.

Assessment of consultations considers the process of collecting, synthesising and interpreting information by trainees and how this impacts on their decision making in relation to diagnosis and management.

The results of an assessment process or tool should be:

- valid (accurate)
- reliable (consistent)
- feasible (in relation to resources and practicality).

In this way conclusions about a trainee's knowledge can be made and whether their training has helped them meet the educational aims of the curriculum through observation of the outcomes.

Purpose of assessment

The process of assessment has two purposes:

- accountability
- education.

Accountability

Ideally, an efficient assessment should provide patients and communities with reassurance of the quality of education and training of future doctors. In essence, an assessment procedure should calibrate important professional attributes such as knowledge, understanding, clinical examination skills and problem solving. Students should demonstrate attainment of defined standards and thus competence. To facilitate this process, assessment strategies should ensure equity and uniformity.

Education

The feedback that the person being assessed receives enables them to learn and focus or areas where they have strengths and limitations.

Assessment seeks to:

- help students to improve their learning
- provide certification of competence
- contribute to quality assurance.

The skills that should be assessed

To ensure that doctors are 'safe', both communication and consulting skills as well as biomedical knowledge need to be assessed, together with the application of biomedical knowledge. An assessment should determine if the **learning outcomes** of a curriculum have been met.

Consultation skills assessment looks at an individual student's performance compared to specific learning objectives or performance standards. The learning objective of consultation skills is to develop the practical skills needed to work as a medical practitioner with the required competence and the personal attributes to develop successful working relationships with patients.

One of the tasks of this book has been to detail the many potential consulting skills necessary to become a 'good' doctor.

Practical point
The attributes of a 'good' doctor are regularly debated and a consensus can be difficult to achieve, particularly as views of doctors and patients may differ.

An assessment tool therefore needs to be able to test a wide range of clinical skills and knowledge which enable a trainee to perform satisfactorily during consultations with patients.

Formative assessment and learning

Feedback is two dimensional; there is a necessity to know what you are good at and then areas where you can improve. Trainees therefore appreciate and benefit from the feedback of formative assessment.

Formative assessment is intended to give students feedback on their learning progress. It also allows the teacher to evaluate their teaching by identifying the areas the trainees have mastered and where they are having difficulties and so their learning needs. It should not be used to assign marks or grades summatively. The learning needs identified are the outcomes of the formative assessment process and can be used to direct both the teacher and the learner.

Important components of formative assessment are that it:

- is subjective
- is learner-centred
- requires an 'educational appraisal'
- identifies learning needs
- provides feedback to 'trainee' and trainer.

Practical point
Formative assessment is an educational tool and can be regarded as a learning aid, thus fulfilling the requirement of an assessment being motivating and influencing education.

Through this process teachers and learners can determine the progress that has been achieved in meeting the learning objectives and can determine what remains to be learned in the future. There is good evidence that implementing formative assessment and **learning contracts** helps to improve students' performance and presentation. A student can be aided to identify their strengths and weaknesses and thereby become motivated to learn and perform better by enhancing their strengths and increasing knowledge and skills in the areas required for improvement, in respect of their consultation performance.

Practical point
A **learning contract** is an individual agreement between a learner and a teacher and the responsibility is put on the student for their learning and culminates in a mutually agreed assessment.

Formative assessment helps students prepare for summative assessment.

Summative assessment

Summative assessment is an end-point assessment at the conclusion of a module or course. It is an objective method to assign marks or grades that determine whether the student passes or fails the course. Similarly it can be used to evaluate the teaching.

Important components of summative assessment are that it:

- is objective
- is assessor/teacher-centred
- details a summary of learning/training
- gives a 'pass'/'fail' grade.

The advantages of summative assessment are that it:

- assesses attitude and knowledge
- standardises training
- is educationally valuable
- is easier to justify if extra training is needed.

Disadvantages of summative assessment are that it:

- may not involve clinical/patient contacts
- focuses students learning on passing the assessment.

Continuous assessment

Assessment is not an end point in learning, but defines a standard attained at one point in time. In this way it fulfils a role in accountability, but also a method of identifying where learning needs are and so where educational improvement can take place. Traditionally in medical training, higher education assessments have been at the end of a course, where the student crams the learning of knowledge to pass a test. Most medical courses now employ a process of regular assessments during each module or part of the course or 'continual assessment', some of which may be ongoing work on a project. It is the first step in a **continual learning cycle**.

Continuous assessment is a process that can be supplemented if the student maintains a **portfolio** and so collects evidence of learning. A portfolio comprises a collection of items rather than a single piece of work. Students typically collect from various sources the learning experience pertinent to their evaluation – clinical record, audit, diaries, log or assessment by patients and peers. There should be guidance regarding the collection of data, otherwise only those data will be collected in areas which student likes the most and the student may not concentrate on their areas of weaknesses. Continuous or portfolio assessments are widely used in undergraduate and postgraduate medical education to assess the performance of students.

Continual assessment should be looked on as an opportunity to reflect on what has been learned and what further learning is required. A wealth of information can be gained and retained in a continuous assessment programme. Effective continuous, portfolio assessment requires a high level of trust between assessors and students, provided the structure matches the learning objectives.

Practical point
Trainees welcome assessment methods which provide meaningful feedback.

Assessment of attitude

Attitude is important for development of professional behaviour and expertise. Attitudes of future doctors may affect their relationship with patients and can influence the outcome of the consultation process. Assessment of attitude is thus a part of the assessment process in medical education.

Practical point

An attitude is a mixture of belief, thoughts and feelings that predispose a person to respond in a positive or negative way to other people, institution or objects.

Attitudes sum up the past, but influence the future. Past performance is no guarantee to future performance. Likewise attitudes can also change. They may change under the influence of:

- personal experience
- group activity
- social and cultural activity
- professional identity.

Change in attitude may not be reflected in behaviour. A successful consultation requires the student to be non-judgemental, be able to show empathy and can be assessed by direct observation. A continuous or portfolio assessment may be more useful as a formative tool in assessing attitude. While assessing attitude one should ensure explicit criteria and an adequate sample of behaviours with regular reflection on the methods used.

Visual assessment methods

Visual assessment gives us the opportunity to observe the performance of a student against set criteria. Consultation assessment can be expanded to look at knowledge as well as common consultation skills like history taking, clinical reasoning, management style and interpersonal skills.

Practical point

The advantage of watching a real patient consultation is that the assessor can judge the actual performance in real life and thus assessing performance rather than competence.

However, it is difficult to standardise the core content of the assessment for all students, but the standardisation of simulated patients may make this achievable. Standardisation means a more reliable, reproducible assessment with greater face validity. With real patients the assessment process has no control over the patient. Direct observation is a better measure of clinical performance than indirect methods – such as modified essay questions and/or a clinical viva.

Organising such assessment processes can be substantial with problems of fatigue, problems of repetition and predictability. Although a trainee student may perform well in one consultation, they may not do so well in another. Assessing multiple consultations will help to overcome the problem. However, time constraints may not allow for too many consultations to be assessed. A valid assessment will require a minimum number of consultations to be assessed.

Audio or video taping of a consultation is an alternative method of assessing the consultation.

OSCE (objective structured clinical examination)

An assessment looks at an individual's performance compared to the specific learning objectives or performance standards. Criterion-referenced assessment tells us how well students are performing on specific goals or standards, e.g. an objective structured clinical examination (OSCE) rather than telling how their performance compares with a standard group of students (norm-referenced). Furthermore, OSCEs can be used to assess the adequacy of curriculums.

The use of OSCEs is viewed by many as a useful technique for assessing students' abilities and communication skills. The OSCE consists of a circuit of 'stations' which tests a range of skills and learning and thus can be used to assess a candidate's performance in a standardised way. In addition, the OSCE can be used to judge the quality of training as it can serve to identify areas of weakness in the curriculum or the teaching methods employed. A variety of evaluative methods are used to assess a student's competence and an emphasis is placed on those methods which encourage the learning of clinical skills.

Practical point
The OSCE can be used to assess many fundamental clinical skills in a rigorous way.

The OSCE can not only be used to assess core interpersonal skills such as history taking, clinical examination, and the ability to explain things to patients, but also to integrate the examination of important skills relating to the choice of appropriate investigations and appropriate responses to test results.

Multiple OSCE stations can cover a wide range of the curriculum and thus allow the student to be assessed thoroughly. In particular they help to show a student's ability to integrate knowledge and skill with the clinical problem presented to them and particularly how they manage the problem.

However, a major impediment to the use of the OSCE is that it is labour intensive and a costly form of assessment. Costs are related to the development, production, administration and post-examination reporting and analysis.

Limitations of OSCEs:

- very short and isolated aspects of clinical problems are dealt with
- students' thinking needs to agree with a predetermined checklist of the clinical problem decided by the examiners
- there is minimal content and there is no scope of showing further knowledge
- summative rather than formative.

Competence and performance

Competence can be defined in many ways. In relation to clinical practice it represents the clusters of skills, abilities and knowledge needed to perform different tasks to a certain or expected defined threshold and so be 'qualified' to undertake a particular set of clinical tasks. Important components of competence are:

- the knowledge/skills/attitudes required to perform
- 'passed' assessment/gain qualification
- demonstrating potential 'fitness' to practise
- being able to undertake independent practice without supervision
- does not necessarily confirm ability to perform
- 'poor performers' can be competent.

Performance can also be defined in many ways and the act of performing something successfully requires not only knowledge, but using or applying that knowledge to a defined standard as distinguished from merely possessing it.

Practical point
The argument for revalidation is that past performance does not guarantee future performance.

Important components of performance are:

- competence in practice although adequate performance does not always ensure underlying competence
- able to conduct clinical duties
- fulfils tasks
- meets expectation of patient and clinical team/seniors/peers
- succeeds in independent practice.

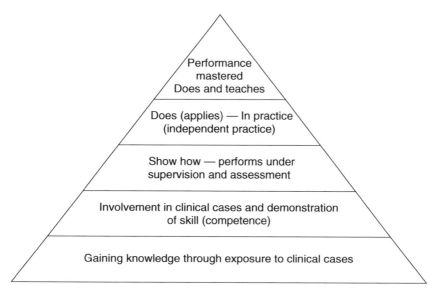

Figure 13.1   Miller's Pyramid of Competence.

When assessing competence and performance, norm referencing provides a relative standard whereas criterion referencing provides an absolute standard.

USA professor of education George Miller (1990) has described a **Pyramid of Competence** which arrays competencies from 'Knows' (the base) to 'Does' (the apex) and the pyramid shown in Figure 13.1 is an annotation of how this conceptual model relates to clinical practice.

Competence shows that a skill has been learned by acquiring knowledge and demonstrating skill. Performance also demonstrates the same, but also what happens in real life and so its application is the 'does' in Miller's Pyramid. Essentially it includes the effects of other factors like feeling nervous, taking responsibility and other related emotions in interacting with patients.

Miller has suggested no single assessment method can provide all the data required for judgement of anything so complex as the delivery of professional services by a successful physician.

Practical point
In essence there is no ideal assessment.

Assessment can serve many purposes that might vary throughout a course or period of study such as:

- selection of candidates for educational or career opportunities
- maintenance of standards
- motivation of students
- providing feedback to students and identification of learning needs
- obtaining data for curriculum evaluation

Summary

Effective teaching in medicine requires flexibility, energy and commitment amid a busy background of clinical care. Successful medical teaching requires the teacher to be able to address the learner's needs and understand the variation in learning styles and approaches. Teachers can accomplish these requirements while creating an optimal teaching-learning environment by utilising a variety of teaching methods and teaching styles.

Bibliography

Department for Education and Skills. The future of higher education; Chapter 4. *Teaching and Learning: delivering excellence*. White Paper 2003.

Duffield KE, Spencer JA. A survey of medical students' views about the purposes and fairness of assessment. *Medical Education*. 2002; **36**: 879–86.

General Medical Council (GMC). *Tomorrow's Doctors. Recommendations on undergraduate medical education*. London: GMC; 1993.

Kirkpatrick DI. Evaluation of training. In: Craig R, Bittel I, editors. *Training and Development Handbook*. New York: McGraw-Hill; 1967.

Kurtz SM, Silverman JD, Draper J. *Teaching and Learning Communication Skills in Medicine.* Oxford: Radcliffe Medical Press; 1998.

Miller GE. The assessment of clinical skills, competence and performance. *Academic Medicine.* 1990; **65**: S63–7.

Paradigms of learning: http://bmj.bmjjournals.com/cgi/content/full/318/7193/0/DC1

Silverman JD, Kurtz SM, Draper J. *Skills for Communicating with Patients.* Oxford: Radcliffe Medical Press; 1998.

Tate P. *The Doctor's Communication Handbook.* 3rd ed. Oxford: Radcliffe Medical Press; 2001.

Useful website

www.skillscascade.com

Chapter 14

CPD, lifelong learning and preparing for examinations

Colonel Jonathan Leach, Sqn Ldr Peter Lavallee and Dr Rodger Charlton

---

Rodger Charlton has written extensively in relation to CPD and describes why it is important for trainees to gain skills in lifelong learning. Jonathan Leach and Peter Lavallee provide some very helpful tips in preparing for medical examinations.

Hopefully this book dispels the notion that attaining a medical degree or Royal College membership is an end point or continuing licence for life to practice. All doctors, whether in training or qualified are learners and throughout their lifetime of professional practice, should be supported and encouraged to stay up-to-date. This is through a process of continuing professional development (CPD) and lifelong learning (LLL). In essence this is an acknowledgement of the need to maintain, develop and broaden expertise and personal qualities to be able to cope with the professional work challenges of the future in an increasingly competitive world – also a health service with a relentless process of innovation, care provision, change in structure and increasing technology.

This chapter is divided into the following sections.

- CPD and lifelong learning.
- Appraisal and PDPs.
- Preparing for assessments and examinations.

A record of self-directed learning in the form of a **portfolio** can form the basis of revalidation for a qualified practitioner.

CPD and lifelong learning

CPD is both a philosophy and a process, which should be built on the culture of LLL. Thus a medical degree or attaining a college membership is not an end point, but the attainment of a standard. There is a rapidly developing new culture in medical training of self-directed problem-based learning. In 1993, the GMC's publication *Tomorrow's Doctors* recommended that undergraduate curricular change also provided a focus on students' professional careers, LLL and establishing a 'lifelong curriculum'. Furthermore, the following skills and attitudes should be established from the start as an undergraduate in relation to CPD thus removing the traditional gap between undergraduates and postgraduates and so emphasising the continuum of learning:

- critical appraisal
- healthcare ethics and the law
- self-directed problem-based learning
- communication skills
- IT skills.

One should also bear in mind the need for skills in teaching, research, management, interviewing and committee work.

All trainees should seek advice from an educationalist to help identify their own individual learning styles and also to consider new ways of learning. In order to ascend Miller's Pyramid of Competence referred to at the end of the last chapter, gaining new skills in learning and how to integrate knowledge of basic medical sciences in relation to clinical scenarios will greatly help clinicians in problem solving and patient management.

Professionalism

Professionalism is the maintenance of high standards to meet the best interests of patients. It is interwoven with CPD and, with this change of learning culture, accountability should be demonstrated externally and poorly performing doctors identified. Royal Colleges should lead in the provision of CPD and maintenance of standards of their members. It is therefore necessary for doctors to keep a **portfolio**.

Practical point

A portfolio may be described as 'the collection and storage of evidence gathered by an individual in his or her role as a learner' and is a useful method to record learning.

This process of **portfolio-based learning** is an opportunity to demonstrate learning and a tool to recognise learning needs. Such evidence of LLL may form the basis of a doctor's **revalidation** and this should become an everyday part of their clinical practice. This may also form the basis of evidence of performance (what the doctor does) and so competence (what the doctor is capable of doing) and therefore demonstrate accountability through the process of **quality assurance**. Furthermore, this can form a part of **clinical governance**.

Clinical governance can be defined as a system through which the NHS organisations are externally accountable for continuously improving the quality of their services and safeguarding high standards of care by creating an environment in which excellence in clinical care will flourish.

The difference between CME and CPD

Continuing medical education (CME) is viewed by some as collecting 'points' for attending a postgraduate meeting where there has been little strategic planning into identifying learning needs and meeting them. CPD is a more systematic and coherent approach to education than the limited effectiveness of opportunistic and poor attendance at didactic lectures.

CPD is a conscious move from the unstructured traditional CME for doctors by a transition to the accreditation of structured personal learning plans (PLPs). These are more correctly referred to as personal development plans (PDPs), where learning may be both knowledge (education) and gaining a new skill (training) which enhances CPD through the identification and meeting of professional development needs in terms of new knowledge and skills. The goal of CPD is the promotion and development of doctors who retain a curiosity about their subject which is a stimulant for the philosophy of lifelong learning, which may be formal or informal. Additional elements include learning by reflective practice, portfolio development, professional self-awareness and multidisciplinary involvement.

This is illustrated in Figure 14.1.

PDPs appear to have evolved from industry and the teaching profession, although the terminology used may be different. Department of Health (DoH) papers in 1998 on CPD suggested a move from unstructured CME by transition to the accreditation of structured PDPs following an 'educational appraisal' and appropriate mentoring, e.g. by a clinical tutor. The next three sections consider learning that takes place as a result of patient contacts.

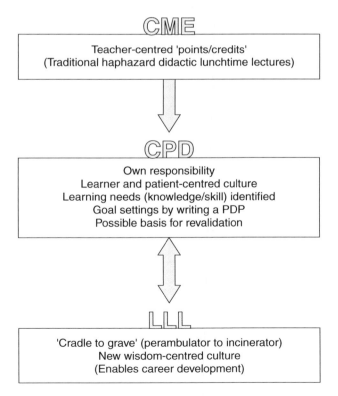

Figure 14.1 Continuing medical education, continuing professional development and lifelong learning.

Work-based learning (WBL)

Attending lectures and clinical update are important ways of learning, but the apprentice learning model for students and other learning strategies should not be forgotten. Perhaps the most important area of learning for postgraduates and one that is taken for granted and so largely goes unrecognised and unquantified is work-based learning as a result of daily clinical contacts. Doctors have many different learning strategies. Imagine two new products that have been released on the market or, for example, preparing for the National Service Framework (NSF) in relation to coronary heart disease. Yes, doctors know about these things, but how did they find out about them? Here are a few possibilities for individual doctors' learning strategies or WBL:

- reading a journal or professional magazine
- a mailing
- attending a postgraduate meeting
- patient correspondence
- talking to a colleague over coffee
- listening to a student or registrar
- a request from a patient
- asking the pharmacist
- letter from a specialist
- watching the television
- seeing a pharmaceutical company representative
- ringing an NHS Trust
- patient investigation results
- viewing a website
- PUNs and DENs (*see* below).

The list is endless. Each of us may use one, some or all of these and other strategies. But we all have our own individual and unique learning strategies, although we may not know what they are. Everyone has a preferred learning style, as demonstrated by Honey and Mumford (1992), which may be one or a combination of the following characteristics; Activist, Reflector, Theorist and Pragmatist. Appraisal and educational mentorship through an appraiser or tutor can help develop this and other learning strategies as a part of LLL and CPD.

PUNs and DENs

There has been a considerable increase in the number of acronyms and two important ones which may be viewed as both patient-centred and doctor-centred are PUNs (Patients' Unmet Needs) and DENs (Doctors' Educational Needs).

These can be applied to any consultation when you reflect on how the consultation went with questions such as: 'Could the consultation have been conducted better?' This might be in terms of meeting the needs of the patient or where there are areas of education that the doctor should address should he or she meet the same issues in a future consultation. The concept was described and patented by Dr Richard Eve (2000), a GP Tutor in West Somerset. Ultimately, they enable doctors to address areas of learning needs and should be logged.

These can be logged on the NHS Appraisals toolkit website (www.appraisals. nhs.uk) under 'Learning activities'.

The following appears on the NHS Appraisals toolkit website:

During consultations we are commonly aware of gaps in our ability, gaps in the 'in-house' systems or attitudinal problems. You need to focus on the patients' needs to identify these. The doctor, not the patient, will decide whether the patients' needs have been met. Recognition of deficiencies leads to the discovery of Doctors' Educational Needs.

Practical point

If one is to provide optimal and quality healthcare and keep up with the pace of change in the NHS, such acronyms or models should be considered when analysing consultations and improving future performance.

This is a further important potential for work-based learning.

Risk management

Competence and performance are distinct constructs where competence is an important determinant of performance, but many motivational and situational factors are involved, e.g. personality, health, professional ethics, standard of premises, equipment, support staff, workload and time of day. Just as competence may differ from performance, medical error may be related to neither, as all doctors are human and make mistakes. New systems and procedures need to be put in place to maintain the health and safety of patients through informed consent, measuring performance where practical, the recording of critical incident events, preventing the recurrence of risk and making services safer. **Significant event audit meetings** for teams of healthcare professionals can aid learning and the adoption of the findings from critical incidents to ensure more robust protocols to protect patients and practitioners.

Practical point

Critical incidents should stimulate learning and the approach to revisit decisions or judgments that are made during consultations where there has been a feeling of uncertainty in relation to the diagnosis and subsequent management.

Appraisal and PDPs

It is important to define what is meant by appraisal as perceptions and interpretations differ widely. Appraisal if correctly applied is not an assessment, but a method to value quality, e.g. through evidence of good performance in clinical practice. Appraisal should be formative rather than summative and should be thought provoking and where possible challenging through the identification of learning needs and so the basis for a PDP. It should be aimed at development, not assessment, otherwise it is not an appraisal, but a performance management tool.

Practical point
Appraisal is a formal and structured process which allows an individual to reflect on their clinical work, valuing good areas of performance and identifying areas where with support other areas of clinical care may be further optimised in a constructive way, e.g. through a personal development plan (PDP).

When a practitioner meets with an educational appraiser, a potential PDP should be discussed on the basis of perceived learning needs. An action plan should be considered and mutually agreed on to implement that PDP and so relate to professional development in the future.

A PDP is a tool to encourage LLL and identify any areas for further development. We are all learners from 'cradle to grave'. At secondary school through to undergraduate years there is a transition from 'teacher-centred' learning of a carefully defined curriculum to self-directed learning. The latter is the learner's responsibility and doctors are usually curious to know more and gain new skills in this way. A PDP also gives a doctor an opportunity to look at their overall learning by reflecting on their career so far and also mapping their aspirations and challenges for the future.

Doctors' individual educational needs and how they influence service delivery should be co-ordinated in with team development plans, so-called **practice professional development plans (PPDPs)**.

It is often asked, for example, how a PDP relates to concepts of clinical governance. Ultimately, the processes of CPD, LLL, appraisal, clinical governance and revalidation inform PDPs and overlap. This is illustrated in Figure 14.2.

Encouraging doctors to maintain portfolios will help them provide evidence for fulfilling these processes and requirements.

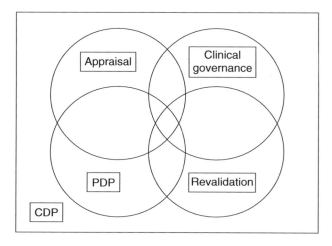

Figure 14.2 Venn diagram of CPD.

Table 14.1 Common postgraduate examinations

Examination	Body	Comments
Membership	Royal Colleges	There are several diplomas of which the following are a few examples: MRCP, MRCS, MRCGP and MRCOG.
Diploma (DRCOG)	Royal College of Obstetricians and Gynaecologists	Aimed at general practitioners wishing to provide obstetrics and gynaecology.
Diploma in Family Planning (DFFP)	Royal College of Obstetricians and Gynaecologists	For practitioners with an interest in sexual and reproductive health.
Diploma in Geriatric Medicine (DGM)	Royal College of Physicians of London	For general practitioner vocational trainees, clinical assistants and others working in non-consultant career posts in Departments of Geriatric Medicine, and other doctors with interests in or responsibilities for the care of elderly people.
Diploma in Ophthalmology (DRCOphth)	Royal College of Ophthalmologists	For those not wishing to pursue a career as a consultant ophthalmologist in the United Kingdom.
Diploma in Dermatology (Dip Derm)	Various institutions	Available as a distance-learning course for those wishing to improve skills in dermatology.
Diploma in Child Health (DCH)	Royal College of Paediatrics and Child Health	Two-stage examination with written examination followed by clinical to increase skills in paediatrics.
Diploma in Occupational Medicine (Dip OccMed)	Faculty of Occupational Medicine of Royal College of Physicians of London	Basic qualification in occupational medicine and is awarded by the Faculty of Occupational Medicine (FOM) of the Royal College of Physicians, London. It is intended primarily for GPs or other physicians who have an interest in it or are working part-time.
Diploma in Palliative Care	Various institutions	For individuals with an interest in palliative care.
Diploma in Medical Education	Various institutions but University of Dundee in particular	For individuals with an interest in medical education.
Diploma in Immediate Care (Dip IMC)	Royal College of Surgeons of Edinburgh	For individuals with an interest in providing pre-hospital immediate care.

Practical point
The appraisal process, if used formatively as designed rather than inappropriately as a management tool, can be used to identify qualities and learning needs, to encourage and aid rather than threaten development.

Preparing for assessments and examinations

Examinations and assessments are a fact of life and it does not matter which discipline you choose, examinations will continue after graduation for several years for most health professionals. The reasons for taking examinations range from 'mandatory' (professional requirement or career development) to personal, where the individual wishes to demonstrate that they have satisfactorily studied in an area to a recognised standard.

Examinations come in all shapes and sizes, with a very large range of subjects available. If you can think of a discipline there will be an additional postgraduate examination available. Table 14.1 lists a selection of the postgraduate examinations relevant to general practice.

Choosing: which examination?

Considering the range of examinations available, and that a number of institutions provide high-quality taught courses, some of which are available as distance-learning packages, there are some fundamental questions to consider before embarking upon a particular course of study for an examination. We shall briefly consider these in turn.

1 **Why do I want to take an examination in this SUBJECT AREA?**
    Is a qualification in this area essential as part of your personal development plan and subsequent appraisal? Will it provide the necessary skill or knowledge for either your personal advancement or improving patient care? If so, are there alternative qualifications in this you could consider? For example, to provide a family planning service within a family planning clinic, the Diploma in Family Planning (DFFP) is the minimum essential qualification in many cases. However, to improve resuscitation skills there are a range of courses from the Advanced Life Support Group (ALSG) which could be appropriate (from intermediate life support to advanced trauma life support) depending on your aim. In addition there are other course providers to consider (such as the British Association for Immediate Care, BASICS). Before committing yourself to any particular examination it is worth considering the alternatives by gathering the relevant details concerning the curriculum to see if they are applicable to the learning need you have identified.
2 **Why do I want to take THIS examination?**
    Having identified alternatives, or decided on a particular course, it is worth considering the following questions.
    a Is this qualification the most relevant to your learning needs?
        Write down your aims for doing the course or qualification and compare them with the published syllabus and its learning outcomes. Alternatively

discuss with colleagues who have undertaken the study or course tutors. Is there sufficient overlap between what you wish to gain from the course and what the course aims to deliver? Do you find the syllabus interesting? Is this qualification most likely to be of immediate use in your clinical practice?

b Is this qualification the most feasible to complete within the time you have available?

All qualifications require a period of study and frequently intensive revising prior to the examination – do you have sufficient time for the course, taking into account current work and personal life commitments? What would you need to stop doing to free up sufficient time for the course? Are there clinical components to the course you will need to timetable?

c Can I afford the course or examination fees or find suitable sponsorship?

Consider both direct course costs, which may vary from a few hundred to a few thousand pounds, but also any indirect costs such as any reduced income or travel costs necessary to attend courses or undertake study. While in some cases, bursaries or funding may be available to assist in paying the costs of courses, it is rare that they cover the whole cost.

3 **WHERE do I want to take this examination?**
For any accredited course, e.g. the diploma in dermatology, there may be a number of institutions who are course providers. Choosing the right institution may be straightforward after considering the syllabus or location (a local institution will make attendance and support much easier). For some qualifications, you may need to consider the location of the relevant examination centres.

Summary – key questions before embarking upon study for an examination

1 **Why do I want to take an examination in this SUBJECT AREA?**
   a Is it 'mandatory' or desirable for personal reasons?
   b Do you need the qualification?
   c Are there alternative qualifications you could consider?
2 **Why do I want to take THIS examination?**
   a Is this qualification the most relevant to your learning needs?
   b Is this qualification the most feasible to complete within the time you have available?
   c Is this qualification the most interesting to you?
   d Is this qualification most likely to be of immediate use in your clinical practice?
   e Can I afford the course or examination fees or find suitable sponsorship?
3 **WHERE do I want to take this examination?**
   a Local/distant course provider.
   b Local/distant examination centre.

The preparation process

There are various factors worth considering when beginning to plan your preparation for an assessment or an examination. They fall roughly into two groups – the methods of assessment used in the examination (examination factors) and how you best prepare as an individual (individual factors).

Examination factors

A wide range of examination techniques are used, ranging from the traditional written paper, MCQ, MEQ and clinical examination, to the slightly more innovative such as video or the submission of written work (assignment, essay or portfolio). *See* Table 14.2 for a summary of the main examination methods used.

Individual factors

Planning your time
A minimum six months' preparation time is frequently recommended for Royal College Membership Examinations. For examinations that have a simpler or more 'traditional' format, three months' study may be sufficient. Developing a structured learning plan is recommended in most cases (*see* Table 14.3).

Identifying your learning style
Making the information retrievable is the most important. Individual factors are key here as individuals learn and memorise in different ways. Consider the best way you learn – is it by drawing, by reading aloud, making short notes, key points or asking questions about it? It does not matter which method is used, as long as the methods used are helpful. All tend to need repetition. Other ways that have been found helpful are breaking key words by suffix or prefix or using memory tricks (linking a subject to a patient, mnemonics, making up silly rhymes or using humour). Others have found that using flashcards or discussing and using tutors in the learning process or going on preparation courses very helpful.

Practical point
Application of learning to patient case studies may help to **apply and integrate the learning**.

Practising technique
Prior to sitting an examination, it is essential that the requirements are fully understood. Many written examinations require candidates to answer in short answer form, giving key points. For example, in the MRCGP written examination, the questions test the ability to integrate and apply theoretical knowledge and professional values in primary care. Experience shows that few marks are gained in the last few minutes, but missing out a whole question significantly reduces the overall scoring potential. Answers should be in short note format as they score better (and can be marked more easily). It is recommended that candidates think laterally about the question and about as many aspects that can reasonably be considered. Think as broadly as possible. For example, a 46-year-old patient with a history of alcoholism, who is unemployed, presents to you for

Table 14.2 Summary of the main examination methods used

Format	Notes	Preparation hints
Multiple-choice question paper (MCQ)	Common method of testing knowledge. Many examinations do not now use multiple true/false questions, but have moved to extended matching questions and single best answer.	Practise, practise, practise, preferably past papers or published samples if available. Ensure you understand the format the paper will take before attending.
Written paper	Common method, but in most cases short answers using key points rather than an essay is recommended.	Write legibly; practise timed examples. Maintain a logical outline. Prepare in groups.
MEQ (modified essay question)	Seeks integration of factual and practical knowledge to enable problem solving and decision making.	Agreed method of checking understanding and whether you have encountered a scenario clinically.
Oral examinations	Continues as a part of many examinations, despite concerns about its reliability.	
Video	Video of consultations needed for most candidates sitting MRCGP examination.	Ensure you have a clear idea of the range of examples you need, and the type of criteria the examiners are looking for.
Simulated surgery or clinic	Candidate is asked to consult standardised patients who are portrayed by role-players.	Find out what equipment you will be required to take with you on the day. Practise timings.
Objective structured clinical examination (OSCE)	A number of time-limited activities (a 'station') that each student completes. Each station may comprise a patient scenario or situation devised to assess particular skills. A range of tasks may need to be performed, e.g. demonstrate a skill.	Keep answer brief and to the point.
Projected material	Pictures or slides projected onto a screen; candidates are then expected to answer questions regarding the subject.	Many books and atlases are available for revision in relevant areas, e.g. dermatology.
Clinical examinations	Short and/or long cases.	Regular contact with patients.
Practical demonstration of skills	For example, cardio-pulmonary resuscitation	Practise in groups.

Table 14.3 Developing a structured learning plan

Step 1: Gathering information	Obtain the syllabus and specific revision aids or articles, discuss with colleagues who have taken the examination and plan the areas of academic work that need to be covered. Write the areas as headings. What do you need to learn/refresh in each area?
Step 2: Identify learning style	Consider the ways that you have found best to learn in the past. Have they worked, or how could you improve?
Step 3: Identify exam technique	Consider the assessment methods of the examination. What skills are needed (e.g. critical appraisal) or tested (e.g. clinical examinations)? What skills do I already have? Where is there room for improvement? How can these skills be learned/refined?
Step 4: Work in groups	Work with other candidates to identify areas of learning, refine knowledge and solve problems. Present topic areas to each other and share the burden of researching answers.
Step 5: Practise skills	Practise questions, practise exam techniques in groups/pairs.
Step 6: Attend a preparation course	Closer to the exam, a preparation course can help you focus on outstanding learning requirements, and refine necessary exam techniques in a focused way. Often such courses are tutored by examiners who can give individual feedback.
Step 7: Plan final revision	Prioritise likely topics, clarify areas of uncertainty in a strategic manner.
Step 8: Take the examination	Record a few areas that you can remember after the examination where you need to improve in case you are required to sit the examination again and as areas of learning need for the future.

an HGV medical examination. What issues does this raise? The issues could be for doctor, patient and family, medico-legal, society, employment law or DVLA. Consider each in turn, as described above. Most candidates benefit from practising answering questions as it assists in breaking a question into manageable areas and formulating an answer.

In terms of examination elements that are designed to show an element of skill (such as a simulated surgery or OSCE), consider two important questions.

- What are the elements or themes that the examiners are looking for that will allow a candidate to pass (or gain most marks)?
- What are the commonest reasons for candidates to fail?

By considering both ends of the scale, it will allow for higher marks to be gained without gaining penalty points. For example in the Diploma in Immediate Care, safety and the safe use of a cardiac defibrillator are paramount; incorrect or unsafe use gives an immediate fail, whereas the confident and correct demonstration with a patient with a simulated cardiac arrest gains high marks.

Practical point

By reading articles on how to pass an examination, discussing the examination with past candidates, course tutors and if possible examiners for the exam, a view can be gained on what is required, what is not and what are the penalty areas.

Preparation courses

Courses can assist in the preparation very considerably, but consider when the best time to go on the course is. Some courses are designed as 'pre-exam cramming', whereas others try to guide an individual's learning plan, giving time for further preparation. What they should do, however, is provide focused time on the examination, guide learning and provide a network of individuals who can assist (either course participants or tutors).

Conclusion

Examinations are a fact of life. Many consider that taking additional qualifications may enhance their professional life, lead to improved job prospects and improve patient care. When considering whether to take additional qualifications the two most important questions to consider are 'Why do I want the qualification?' and 'Do I need it?'. Having extra qualifications can be very advantageous, but there are potential drawbacks in terms of time, effort and the costs associated with the preparation and taking of examinations. However, investing in the conscious process of preparing for an exam should significantly improve your performance on the day. Ultimately, gaining your qualification will be your reward.

Bibliography

Charlton R. Continuing professional development (CPD) and training. *BMJ*. 2001; **323**: Career Focus, s2–3.

Charlton R. Personal development plans (PDPs). *BMJ*. 2002; **325**: Career Focus, s36–37.

Charlton R. Work-based learning (WBL). [Letter.] *Medical Education*. 2001; **35**: 709.

Charlton R, Prince R. *Be Open to Personal Learning: writing a PDP*. Solihull: Hampton-in-Arden Publishing; 2003.

Eve R. Learning with PUNs and DENs – a method for determining educational needs and the evaluation of its use in primary care. *Education for General Practice*. 2000; **11**(1): 73–9.

Honey P and Mumford A. *The Manual of Learning Styles*. Maidenhead: Peter Honey; 1992.

Chapter 15

Prescribing for common conditions

Dr Ryan Prince

Ryan Prince has made a valiant effort in this chapter to give students and trainees a taste of some of the more frequently prescribed agents for common conditions. This is an absolutely vast topic and it is very difficult to give a user-friendly guide in a short chapter. One of the principal sources referred to in this chapter is the website: www.gpnotebook.co.uk.

Rather than give long lists of treatment regimens, the aim is to give a feeling for the **rationale** behind effective prescribing for common conditions, again taking as primary importance the patient's expectations of therapy (or not) from the doctor, and the effects on the patient day-to-day of their condition. The list is by no means exhaustive, and dosages are not included as they can vary with age, weight and presence of co-morbidities such as renal failure. Advances in thinking and new guidelines were being considered as this chapter was being written and should be consulted as guidelines change.

Always look up or check medications and their dosages as you go along. It is easier to build up your experience in this way. Even very experienced doctors regularly consult the *British National Formulary* (BNF). It is far better to be safe with prescribing than to guess.

Infection

This is one of the commonest presentations to any doctor. Since the advent of antimicrobial therapy, infections are a few of the only conditions that are truly curable in modern medicine. Most diseases such as asthma, diabetes and hypertension are not, and are chronic rather than acute. The treatment of infection can thus produce feelings of immense achievement in the doctor, especially when one has truly saved a young life, e.g. from cellulitis or septicaemia. Any part of the human body can be infected, from the brain to the big toe nail.

Practical point

The principle of empirical antimicrobial prescribing is to think of the most common pathogens that tend to cause disease in a tissue or organ of the body, then to use the antimicrobial agent that is most effective.

This can be done regardless of expense, in life-threatening or serious situations, or alternatively one can use an agent that is the most cost-effective in more trivial disorders. For example, ciprofloxacin will eradicate nearly 100% of *Escherichia coli* that cause simple urinary tract infections, but costs about 15 times as much as trimethoprim, which eradicates about 75%. One could thus try the trimethoprim first and move on to an alternate therapy if it fails, provided the patient was not bacteraemic on presentation.

The other aspect one must consider is the prevention of emergence of **antibiotic resistance**. Thus some antibiotics for more serious infections would be used only rarely, perhaps in some hospital settings needing to be prescribed by a consultant or on the advice of a microbiologist only.

It is always worth remembering that many minor bacterial infections have conservative treatments that can be advised before needing formal therapy. The types listed in Table 15.1 are all available over the counter (OTC) in the UK. To decide whether to use antibiotic therapy in these areas has been a dilemma, especially for the GP, for many years! It is best to check with the current evidence base before prescribing in these circumstances and negotiating therapy in conjunction with the patient's health beliefs, social circumstances and expectations as discussed in Chapter 6 on patient management.

Table 15.1 Treatments for bacterial infections.

Condition	Conservative treatment	1st-line treatment	2nd-line treatment
Eyes (conjunctivitis)	Bathe with boiled, cooled water	Fucidic acid eye drops	Chloramphenicol eye drops
Tonsillitis	Paracetamol/ ibuprofen	Penicillin V	Erythromycin
Otitis media	Paracetamol/ ibuprofen	Amoxycillin	Erythromycin
Otitis externa	Acetic acid spray	Gentamycin + hydrocortisone drops	Neomycin + hydrocortisone drops
Lower respiratory tract infection	Paracetamol/ ibuprofen	Amoxycillin	Erythromycin
Urinary tract infection	Cranberry juice, increase fluid intake	Trimethoprim	Cephalexin
Skin (abscess/cellulitis)	Topical antiseptics	Flucloxacillin (+/−) penicillin V	Erythromycin
Meningitis	Inappropriate	Intravenous benzyl penicillin	Intravenous chloramphenicol
Sinusitis	Decongestion	Doxycycline	Cefaclor

Practical point

Before prescribing an antibiotic always enquire about possible allergies, e.g. to penicillin, to avoid possible anaphylactic reactions.

Local antimicrobial policy is always changing. For the most up-to-date advice consult the BNF, or your local hospital NHS trust/primary care organisation guidelines.

Delayed prescriptions

This may be necessary in the case of antibiotics, particularly when it is the patient's expectation to be prescribed antibiotics. Simply explain to the patient that you can understand their concern and reiterate the possible problems with taking antibiotics if they are not absolutely necessary. Write a prescription for antibiotics and suggest to the patient that they do not go immediately to the pharmacy to get it dispensed, but perhaps wait a few days and see if things persist or deteriorate. The doctor can inform the patient of the sort of problems that can arise as a result of their illness and what they should look out for if it were to get worse for which they should perhaps start taking the course of antibiotics.

In this way the patient is:

- listened to
- empowered
- given the responsibility in managing their illness and
- their view and expectation is acknowledged.

It seems to be an innovation that many GPs have developed without realising it or labelling it as 'delayed prescribing'. Recent evidence also suggests that less 'delayed prescriptions' are actually dispensed if the patient needs to return to the GP surgery to collect them a few days later.

Practical point

The patient becomes a real partner in the doctor–patient encounter and the consultation is truly patient-centred.

Prior to this innovation, this seemingly straightforward consultation had the potential to lead to confrontation if antibiotic was refused as it was not clinically indicated.

Pain and inflammation

It is best always to adopt the 'analgesic ladder' approach with any prescription for analgesia. In a nutshell, this means starting with the lowest dose of the least potent drugs and working upwards until effective analgesia is attained.

In prescribing for chronic pain, as for any chronic condition, the golden rule of 'do no harm first' certainly applies.

For example, consider an 80-year-old lady admitted with haematemesis who is found to have been regularly taking the NSAID (non-steroidal anti-inflammatory

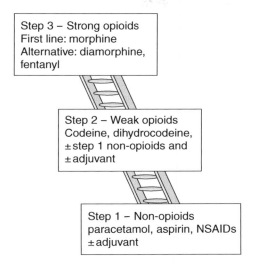

Figure 15.1   World Health Organization (WHO) analgesic ladder.

drug) diclofenac for her mild and generalised osteoarthritis for five years. Her urea and electrolytes on admission showed her to be in chronic renal failure also. How could these two notorious side effects have been prevented? Maybe by using a safer, yet less potent drug such as paracetamol. This has a much better safety profile and rarely causes the two complications that the lady above had the misfortune to encounter from her chronic NSAID ingestion.

One of the most important aspects of analgesia for chronic pain is to keep the circulating levels constant – i.e. regular rather than sporadic dosing during the duration of the pain. As mentioned before, even simple paracetamol can be a highly effective painkiller if taken to the maximum daily dose for body weight.

An example of a potential 'analgesic ladder' is now provided for chronic pain.

Analgesics may be divided into three categories:

- non-opioid
- weak opioid
- strong opioid.

The World Health Organization 'analgesic ladder' (*see* Figure 15.1) is widely accepted as a sound basis for pharmacological intervention to pain control. It describes how treatment should progress through the three categories of analgesics according to the type and severity of pain. The step of the ladder chosen should be decided according to objective pain assessment and one's own judgement.

Skin disorders

Skin disorders present vast diagnostic difficulties. There are a myriad of skin rashes, and it is nearly impossible even for a very experienced specialist to be able to recognise them all merely by inspection. The *history* of the rash or anomaly may well be the key to working out what it is most likely to be and so the cause.

Practical point
It is usually easier to use your basic principles of anatomy, physiology and pathology to work out what the underlying cause could be, rather than wading through tomes of dermatology atlases.

Remember also: 'Common things occur commonly'. Eczema is common whereas *Mycosis fungoides* is not.

For example, Medical Student X is confronted by a 3 cm by 3 cm isolated red patch on the forearm in a 19-year-old lady. She has never seen this before, so thus the first inclination is to announce to her medical teacher that she does not know what it is. But, being a good problem solver, her mind starts to work out what this could be rather than depending on pattern recognition.

1 The patch is red and erythematous thus inflammation of the skin or **dermatitis** is present. Student X knows that dermatitis can have many causes, including allergy, autoimmune disorders, infection and neoplasia.
2 The lady has no history of atopy or asthma personally or in her family, the rash is very localised and she has had no contact with jewellery or new laundry washing powder so it is less likely to have an **allergic** cause.
3 She also has no history of **psoriasis** and the patch does not have a silvery scaly surface.
4 It is in a non-sun-exposed area, and the patient is reasonably young, thus a malignancy or pre-malignancy such as Bowen's Disease is less likely.
5 The patch is itchy, sore and has a yellowy crust overlying. The student presumes that thus the dermatitis possibly has an **infective** cause, and decided that a topical antibiotic is necessary, without actually knowing the name of the condition, and is probably right.

Acne vulgaris

Acne vulgaris is a very common skin disorder most usually found in early teens to early adulthood, although it can occur at any time of life. It is characterised by the formation of whiteheads or comedones, which become colonised by the bacterium *Propionobacterium* acnes. This has very low pathenogenic activity, but its waste products seem to set up an inflammatory reaction within the skin, resulting in the well-known red, inflamed pustules.

Practical point
The treatment of this condition is thus aimed at two parts of the process, the excess sebum production that result in the comedones, and the resulting infection that causes the inflammation.

It is often the case that a young person presents to the doctor complaining most bitterly of their acne ruining their life and confidence as they perceive it is compromising their appearance. It is wise never to underestimate the profound psychological effect that even seemingly trivial acne can have on the patient, and the area needs to be dealt with with some sensitivity. Always ask the patient how the condition is affecting their life; you may well be surprised by the answer. One may have come across the not-uncommon scenario of a person who consults with seemingly 'invisible' acne, and divulged that she was in danger of losing her job at a well-known company with a particular 'public' image as they (probably illegally) insisted that the employees had a near-perfect complexion.

Somewhat like the treatment of pain, the treatment of acne can be a 'treatment ladder', starting with simple therapies and increasing in cost and complexity if the simpler ones fail.

It is useful to look at the skin to see if infection/pustules or simple comedones are the predominant feature. Most acne is a combination so, in all but the most trivial acne, a combined approach with anticomedonals and antibacterials is often necessary.

It is also essential to warn the patient that, whatever treatment is tried, it will take some months to achieve a noticeable difference, and that a degree of perseverance and commitment is necessary on the part of the patient.

Again, Table 15.2 is just a suggestion of a treatment progression; please consult the BNF regularly as advances in treatment are common.

Table 15.2 Suggested treatment progression for acne.

Treatment line	Comedonal acne	Infective acne
1st line	Benzoyl peroxide gel, starting at 2.5% and increasing slowly to 10% if necessary. Anticomedonal – available over the counter, applied at night as causes photosensitivity. Warn patients about transient reddening and drying of the skin on commencement.	Topical antibiotic, e.g. erythromycin solution
2nd line	Retinoid cream, e.g. adapalene. Vitamin A analogue, anticomedonal, same application and potential side effects as benzoyl peroxide. Prescription only. One should be aware that even topical retinoids are potentially teratogenic and contraceptive advice is also required in females.	Topical antibiotic with zinc – added anti-inflammatory effect
3rd line	Oral retinoid therapy, e.g. isotretinoin. Consultant dermatologist prescription only. Need to check LFTs and serum cholesterol before initiation and monitor at regular intervals.	Oral antibiotic therapy, e.g. oxytetracycline (which should be avoided in pregnancy)

Eczema/dermatitis

Generally, start with and continue emollients (moisturisers), as invariably the skin is dry and cracked. The more 'user friendly' the moisturiser, i.e. the easier it goes on and gets absorbed, the less effective it can be. The list below are generic preparations which start with these thinner types and progress to thicker, greasier preparations which are fabulous to treat dry dermatitis but not user friendly. Prescribe the thickest preparation that you feel the condition warrants, in collaboration with the patient as to what they will tolerate. This list demonstrates increasing thickness or viscosity.

- E45 cream
- aqueous cream
- oily cream
- emulsifying ointment (useful as soap substitute)
- white soft paraffin/liquid paraffin mix.

Sometimes in the treatment of dermatitis it is necessary to use a steroid preparation to act as a direct anti-inflammatory on the skin.

Practical point
When using a topical steroid, the rule is to use the least potent preparation for the shortest time possible.

If this rule is adhered to, these ointments and creams are relatively safe if used sensibly and have minimal systemic absorption. If a more potent therapy is used, it is important to 'step down' to avoid rebound dermatitis. For example, if particularly bad eczema needs treatment with Betnovate, on improvement it would be wise to finish off the therapy with Eumovate. Ointments are generally preferable to creams as they have less allergenic properties, and are less likely to harbour bacterial contamination.

An example of steroids preparations in order of potency (least potent first) is:

- hydrocortisone*
- clobetasone butyrate – 'Eumovate'
- betamethasone valerate – 'Betnovate'
- clobetasol propionate – 'Dermovate'.

Trimovate cream is a moderately potent steroid treatment that also contains antibiotic and antifungal components – useful where mild/moderate eczema is infected in areas such as the groin. There are also steroid/antibiotic preparations (hydrocortisone and fusidic acid) that are recommended only if treatment with steroid alone is not working – sometimes *Staphylococcus aureus* can prevent resolution if it is colonising the eczema. Many authorities are not keen on using these steroid/antibiotic combinations, claiming they can cause bacterial resistance. In all but the mildest cases it may be prudent therefore to consider oral antibiotic therapy alongside the steroid.

---

* One should be aware that the preparation hydrocortisone *butyrate* is potent, not mild like hydrocortisone acetate.

Psoriasis

An immune mediated disease that causes hyperkeratosis (scaling) of the skin, classically in plaques on the extensor surfaces of limbs but not always so.

- Emollients can also be useful but not quite as much as in eczema.
- Coal tar solutions are a reasonable first-line treatment for guttate psoriasis (i.e. widespread 'teardrops' of psoriasis).
- Calcipotriol for plaque psoriasis (vitamin D analogue which slows down cellular turnover). There is also a betamethasone/calcipotriol mix available for red inflamed plaques.
- Referral is sometimes necessary for higher strength tars in hospital, or ultraviolet light therapy.

Depression

Anxiety and depression are disorders that affect a significant proportion of people at some time in their life. They are thought to be a variant of the same family of neurotransmitter disorders in which low brain levels of serotonin and mono-amines can cause symptoms. Thus, part of the treatment regimen for endogenous depression where there is no obvious cause can be the use of serotonin specific reuptake inhibitors (SSRIs), or other drugs that increase the available levels of other neurotransmitters such as noradrenalin. **Endogenous** depression appears independently of adverse external stimuli. Other well-recognised and evidence-based treatments include counselling, and cognitive behavioural therapy (CBT) and depression relates to life circumstances (**exogenous** depression), such as adverse events in a person's life, e.g. bereavement, chronic stress at work or a divorce. This is called **reactive** depression.

The ICD (International Classification of Diseases) classifications are useful in defining depressive and anxiety disorders; please refer to them for full details. However, a good rule of thumb for screening for **depression** is to ask about the classic triad of:

1 anhedonia – the loss of enjoyment of previously pleasant aspects of life
2 anergia – or loss of motivation and energy, a feeling of chronic tiredness and poor will to achieve goals
3 persistent low mood – often accompanied by bleak feelings about the future and even thoughts of suicide.

When would you prescribe a pharmacological agent? It depends on the classification of the illness into major or minor depression. There is evidence that prescribing benefits major depression.

Major depression

Five of the following biological symptoms of depression, including one or both of the first two, should have been present almost every day for more than two weeks. The disorder must not be caused by bereavement or organic disease.

1 Depressed mood for most of the day.
2 Anhedonia.

3   Significant weight changes or marked alteration in appetite.
4   Sleep disturbance.
5   Agitation or retardation.
6   Fatigue.
7   Excessive guilt or worthlessness.
8   Inability to concentrate, indecisiveness.
9   Recurrent thoughts of death or suicide

Mild depression

Generally the symptoms will be of recent onset, not satisfying the above criteria, often associated with anxiety symptoms, adjustment disorders or bereavement.

The British Association for Psychopharmacology recommendations regarding indications for antidepressants are as follows.

- In cases of major depression, antidepressants are a first-line treatment irrespective of environmental factors.
- In acute milder depression at initial presentation, treatment with antidepressants is not indicated, but support, education and simple problem-solving techniques are. Cognitive behavioural therapy (CBT) may be tried. The patient should be monitored for persistence or the emergence of major depression, and then antidepressants may be needed.

Practical point

Below are some of the common agents used in the above conditions. Generally, older tricyclic antidepressants are falling from favour as they have increased side effects and serious potential sequelae in overdose.

Serotonin specific reuptake inhibitors (SSRIs)

Below is a selection of some of the commonly prescribed agents. It is worth warning the patient that:

1   it is common to have early side effects such as nausea, headache and anxiety but these are generally transient if the patient perseveres
2   they take at least two weeks to start working and perhaps up to 6–8 weeks to reach their full therapeutic effect
3   they can be difficult to stop as patients can experience what is referred to as 'discontinuation syndrome'.

- Paroxetine – has some sedative properties and can be useful for agitation.
- Fluoxetine – has some stimulating properties and can be useful for lethargy.
- Sertraline – neutral effect on energy.

Anxiety disorders

Anxiety is a normal response to an unusual or stressful event; it is the psychological component of the 'fight or flight' response.

Anxiety is considered to be abnormal when:

- it is excessively severe or prolonged
- it occurs in the absence of a stressful event
- it impairs social, physical or occupational functioning.

There are many variants on anxiety disorder, which again cannot be covered properly in a short chapter. These include phobic disorders, panic disorder, neuroses and obsessive-compulsive disorders.

Like depression, there are both effective pharmacological and psychological treatments e.g. cognitive behavioural therapy. Possible drug treatments are as follows:

Tranquillisers, such as the benzodiazepine **diazepam** – where possible these should be avoided and not used in a prolonged manner due to the potential for dependency, but can be useful during the very initial crisis.

Beta-blockers, e.g. **propranolol**, can be particularly useful if palpitations are a problem. They are absolutely contraindicated in people known to have a history of asthma.

SSRIs can have a role if it is severe anxiety.

Hypertension

The term hypertension literally means high pressure. Hypertension can occur in the systemic, pulmonary and portal circulations. The term hypertension is often used synonymously with systemic arterial hypertension.

The definition of hypertension is difficult, being based on an arbitrary blood pressure above which there is a significant increase in complications such as myocardial infarction and cerebrovascular accidents.

There is a customary division of hypertension into two categories.

- The majority of patients (95%) will have essential hypertension, which means of unknown aetiology.
- The remainder have secondary hypertension, where the cause is determined, e.g. renal artery stenosis.

Practical point
Screening of the population for hypertension should be a priority because the condition is common, asymptomatic and has potentially devastating complications as its prevalence increases with age.

The use of non-pharmacological measures should be used in all hypertensive and borderline hypertensive people regardless of initial blood pressure. These include:

- exercise
- weight loss if necessary

- reduction of salt intake
- restriction of excessive alcohol intake
- reduction of stress.

The British Hypertensive Society Guidelines at present state:

- Therapeutic targets – for blood pressure measurements in clinic:
  - optimal <140/85 (no diabetes), <140/80 (diabetes)
  - audit standard <150/90 (no diabetes), <140/85 (diabetes).
- Therapeutic targets – for mean daytime ambulatory blood pressure monitoring or home measurement:
  - optimal <130/80 (no diabetes), <130/75 (diabetes)
  - audit standard <140/85 (no diabetes), <140/80 (diabetes).

Antihypertensive drug treatment should be initiated in patients with sustained systolic blood pressure >=160 mmHg or sustained diastolic blood pressure >=100 mmHg.

In people with sustained systolic 140–159 mmHg or sustained diastolic 90–99 mmHg then the decision on treatment or not is according to the absence or presence of target organ damage, cardiovascular disease, or a 10-year coronary heart disease (CHD) risk of >=15% according to the Joint British Societies CHD risk assessment programme/risk chart.

The guidance regarding combination treatment of systemic hypertension has been recently updated.

This guidance suggests that essential hypertension and its treatment fall into two main categories.

1 Younger Caucasians usually have renin-dependent hypertension that responds well to:
   - angiotensin-converting-enzyme inhibition or angiotensin receptor blockade (A) or beta blockade (B)*
   - A and B inhibitor specifically block the renin-angiotensin system – younger white hypertensive patients tend to have higher levels of renin and angiotensin II.
2 Older patients (>=55 years old) and black patients – these patients, in general, have low-renin hypertension that responds better to:
   - calcium channel blockade (C) or diuretics (D)
   - these drugs lower blood pressure independent of the renin-angiotensin system, and cause a reflex activation of this system – thus rendering patients responsive to the addition of renin suppressive therapy.
- The majority of patients require a combination of drugs in order to achieve a blood pressure target of 140/85 mmHg (140/80 mmHg in people with diabetes).
- Coincidence of the initials of these main drug classes with the first four letters of the alphabet permits an AB/CD rule, according to which recommended combinations are one drug from each of the 'AB' and 'CD' categories of drugs.

---

*Beta-blockers are contra-indicated in patients with asthma.

- Changes in treatment depend on the tolerability and efficacy of the first drug.
  - If the first drug is ineffective (e.g. systolic fall in BP < 5mmHg) then patient should be switched from a drug from one category to another, e.g. beta-blocker to calcium antagonist.
  - If blood pressure falls but is not controlled then a drug should be added from the other category.
  - If a patient responds to the first drug but does not tolerate it then change to another drug within the same category.
  - This is neatly summarised in a handy table from the British Hypertension Society; see www.bhsoc.org/images/abcd_bhsis_version.jpg.
- Other drugs that lead to a reduction in cardiovascular risk, e.g. statins and aspirin, should be used in those hypertensive patients where additional benefits have been shown – similarly, smoking cessation where it is applicable.

Hypertension is a constantly changing area as a result of ongoing research such as the ASCOT (Anglo–Scandinavian Cardiac Outcomes Trial) study.

Practical point
New guidelines are constantly being developed in hypertension and the reader must seek the latest research in relation to hypertension.

Diabetes

The two main types of diabetes mellitus are:

- type I Diabetes
- type II Diabetes.

The distinction between type I and type II diabetes is clinical.

- If insulin therapy is required to prevent ketoacidosis the patient has type I diabetes.
- If insulin therapy is not required to prevent ketoacidosis then the patient has type II diabetes.
- If the patient has type II diabetes but insulin is required to maintain acceptable glycaemic control then the patient has insulin-treated type II diabetes.

When managing diabetes there are two aims:

- to maintain blood glucose as near to normal levels as possible without unacceptable risk of iatrogenic hypoglycaemia
- to prevent/treat as necessary the long-term micro- and macro-vascular complications of diabetes, such as cardiovascular disease, neuropathy, nephropathy and retinopathy.

Practical point
Thus in both types of diabetes, a great part of the aim of treatment is to achieve good glycaemic control as demonstrated by glycated haemoglobin (HbA1c) levels below 7.5%.

Type I diabetes

Typically a young patient will present with a short history of polydipsia, polyuria, weight loss and malaise. Polyuria is due to the osmotic diuretic effect of glucose and there are ketone bodies in the urine. Weight loss is due to the combined effects of dehydration and catabolism. There may be associated features such as:

- infections:
  - often bacterial and fungal skin infections
  - urinary tract infections
  - candidial genital and sometimes mouth infections.

Some patients will present with overt diabetic ketoacidosis, which is characterised by nausea and vomiting, acidotic breathing, and ketones on the breath.

Type I diabetes presents different management difficulties from type II diabetes, mainly in the form of recurrent acute crises which are much more common. These include diabetic ketoacidosis during times of physiological stress, e.g. infections and hypoglycaemia.

As well as the current nutrition advice dealt with below, all type I diabetes patients require insulin replacement treatment.

At present, injections of insulin are administered subcutaneously by patients with diabetes, usually with metered 'pen devices'. The technique is taught by diabetes specialist nurses and, depending on the insulin or insulins prescribed, nurses can teach patients how to adjust their insulin dosage depending on their blood glucose measurements.

Type II diabetes

The agents below are used when dietary treatment has failed.
Types of oral agents include the following.

- Sulphonylureas, e.g. gliclazide and glimepiride, work by increasing beta cell secretion from the pancreas thus increasing insulin release.
- Metformin, a biguanide, works primarily by augmentation of glucose uptake by muscles, reducing gluconeogenesis and intestinal glucose absorption. Its great advantage is that it does not cause hypoglycaemia although rarely it can lead to lactic acidosis. It cannot be used in patients with renal failure, and must be discontinued if the patient's creatinine reaches 150 μmol/l. Lactic acidosis also occurs at times of physical stress, e.g. operations or infections, and unwell patients may need conversion to insulin temporarily under these circumstances.
- Glitazones – these are a class of drugs which reduce the insulin resistance seen in type II diabetes. There are currently two licensed drugs in this class, rosiglitazone and pioglitazone. The effect of the thiazolidinediones is mediated by the activation of a transcription regulator called peroxisome proliferator-activated receptor gamma (PPAR-gamma). This action modulates adipogenesis and carbohydrate metabolism in adipocytes and skeletal muscle. They can improve sensitivity to insulin in the liver and so removal of glucose.
- Alpha-glucosidase inhibitors reversibly antagonise and slow the action of sucrase within the intestinal tract. This hinders the production of absorbable

monosaccharidases and so reduces the postprandial blood glucose concentration. They are rarely used because of their gastrointestinal side effects.
- Meglitinides, e.g. repaglinide, nateglinide, lower blood glucose by stimulation of insulin release from the pancreas.

The role of both alpha-glucosidase inhibitors and repaglinide in treatment of type II diabetes is unclear.

Practical point
Diet is an essential component of managing diabetes, particularly as medications such as sulphonylureas and insulin can lead to weight gain.

The nutritional recommendations for patients with both types of diabetes are currently as follows.

- Energy:
  – must be enough to maintain or achieve an ideal weight. Even a slight weight loss can result in a fall in insulin resistance, raised hepatic gluconeogenesis, a fall in blood pressure and a more favourable lipid profile.
- Carbohydrate:
  – should provide about 50% of the total daily energy intake Although the diabetic diet should be high in complex carbohydrate with a low glycaemic index, there is no need to insist upon a complete restriction on sugars in diabetics. A diabetic diet is viewed nowadays as a 'healthy' diet where fatty and sugary treats are taken very occasionally.
- Fat:
  – should provide about 30–35% of the total daily energy intake
  – saturated fatty acids should provide less than 10% of this.
- Protein:
  – should provide 10–15% of daily energy intake
  – protein intake should be higher in the elderly, pregnancy and children, and lower in patients with microalbuminaemia.
- Alcohol:
  – should be consumed in moderation in all people with diabetes due to its 'empty calorie' effect.

These recommendations are designed to provide all essential nutrients whilst minimising obesity, hyperinsulinaemia, hypertension and dyslipoproteinaemia.

Commonly encountered gastroenterological conditions

GORD and peptic ulcer disease

Gastro-oesophageal reflux disease (GORD) is defined as symptoms of heartburn or mucosal damage (oesophagitis) resulting from the exposure of the distal oesophagus to gastric contents. However, endoscopy and histology findings correlate poorly to the degree of symptoms experienced by patients.

It is quite difficult in some situations to decide when it is abnormal. Pressure and acid manometry studies often show that gastro-oesophageal reflux occurs in normal situations, such as belching.

Practical point

'Alarm symptoms'

Where a patient presents with new symptoms suggestive of GORD, or symptoms of 'food sticking' in their oesophagus when eating or weight loss, further investigation is often indicated to exclude more sinister pathology.

This condition may be investigated by endoscopy, barium swallow or by 24-hour pH monitoring.

Proton pump inhibitors (PPIs) in gastro-oesophageal reflux disease

- Current guidelines would suggest that a 'healing' (e.g. high) dose of a proton pump inhibitor should be prescribed for at least one to two months in patients with abnormal histology (Barrett's oesophagus) or ulcers.
- The dose should then be reduced to the lowest that prevents recurrence of symptoms, and tailed off if possible. The higher dose must be restarted if there is a recurrence of symptoms.
- Latest British Society of Gastroenterology guidelines would suggest a 'test and treat' policy for the infection *Helicobacter pylori* (H. pylori) for anyone presenting without 'alarm symptoms' but with reflux or dyspepsia. The rationale is that many become symptom-free after its eradication.
- In cases of complicated oesophagitis (e.g. haemorrhage, stricture) the higher healing dose should be maintained.
- In patients who do not have proven pathology/mild symptoms of GORD then often alternative therapies to PPIs can be used in management, e.g. alginates, antacids, histamine 2 (H2) receptor antagonists.
- In severe cases a H2-antagonist may be used in addition.
- In some patients, gastric motility stimulants may be effective, by increasing the rate of gastric emptying and hence reducing the opportunity for reflux. Metoclopramide and domperidone may be of use in stimulation of gastric emptying, particularly in patients with systemic sclerosis, diabetes mellitus, and autonomic neuropathy.

The general management of **peptic ulcer disease** involves advising the patient to stop smoking, avoid NSAIDs and reduce stress where possible.

In patients with a proven duodenal or gastric ulcer, the British Society of Gastroenterology also advise *Helicobacter pylori* eradication therapy (triple therapy) because of the high prevalence of H. pylori in patients with these conditions (duodenal ulcer – 95% patients H. pylori positive; gastric ulcer – 70% H. pylori positive). They have outlined three alternative one-week therapies.

- Omeprazole 20 mg bd or lansoprazole 30 mg bd with either:
  - amoxicillin 500 mg tds, metronidazole 400 mg tds (eradication 84–90%)
  - clarithromycin 500 mg bd, tinidazole 500 mg bd (eradication 90%)
  - amoxicillin 1 g bd, clarithromycin 500 mg bd (eradication 90%).

The treatment of reflux oesophagitis with omeprazole in patients who are *H. pylori* positive increases the risk of atrophic gastritis.

Some patients may require maintenance therapy of a PPI for the rest of their lives.

Irritable bowel syndrome (IBS)

Irritable bowel syndrome is a common functional bowel disorder.

The typical complaints are of abdominal bloating, multiple areas of abdominal pain which is often relieved on defecation. There may be changes in the bowel habit.

It used to be known as a 'diagnosis of exclusion', meaning it was advised to investigate people with symptoms and label them with IBS if the results came back negative. Recent guidelines suggest it is all right to diagnose IBS if the clinical history and examination seem to fit, and there is nothing to suggest cancer or inflammatory bowel disease.

The cause is not known; an organic trigger, such as bacterial gastroenteritis, is seen in some patients. However, there is undoubtedly a psychological component.

Explanation and symptomatic relief help 75% of patients.

The fibre content of the diet should be gradually increased. Soluble fibre has been shown to be beneficial. Soluble fibre such as isphaghula found in some proprietary fibre products may be of benefit in up to 40% of patients. Trials with bran supplements have shown that bran is no better than placebo.

Drug therapy is directed towards symptomatic relief.

- Antispasmodics, especially mebeverine hydrochloride, have long usage and their antimuscarinic actions may relieve pain by moderating smooth-muscle contractions.
- Peppermint oil 0.2–0.4 ml tds 30 minutes before meals may be of benefit with colonic spasm and symptoms of bloating.
- Anticholinergic effect of a tricyclic antidepressant may be of help – there is evidence that antidepressants seem effective for patients with IBS.
- Bulk-forming agents for constipation; occasionally constipation-predominant IBS may also require treatment with an osmotic laxative.
- Drugs such as loperamide may be of benefit for diarrhoea once other pathology has been excluded.
- Hypnotherapy – a small randomised controlled trial has shown that hypnotherapy can be of benefit in the treatment of symptoms of IBS
- Cognitive behaviour therapy – this may be effective in certain circumstances.

An exclusion diet may be considered, e.g. exclusion in turn from a diet of wheat flour, dairy produce, tea, coffee, citrus fruits, nuts, chocolate, and food colourings and additives, to see if any of the above precipitate symptoms.

Practical point

IBS can be a difficult diagnosis to make. Where the symptoms change or there is a history of blood loss with defecation, weight loss or symptoms that wake a person from their sleep, or doubt in the mind of clinician and patient, further investigation is indicated.

With respect to trial evidence, smooth-muscle relaxants are effective for relieving abdominal pain, and loperamide is effective for reducing diarrhoea. However, data are inconclusive for other drug treatments for IBS.

Asthma

Asthma is a syndrome of variable reversible airflow obstruction characterised by symptoms such as:

- cough
- chest tightness
- wheeze.

Pathologically there is bronchial inflammation with a prominent eosinophilic infiltrate.

Asthma is common particularly in developed countries where up to 10% of children have the disease.

The disease has many variants. The management is different for adults and children, and whether the doctor is dealing with the acute attack or long-term control. Only the treatment of chronic asthma in adults is dealt with in this chapter.

Each step is ascended if control is not adequate. The guidelines are dynamic and regular monitoring of the asthma is essential as patients often move from one step to another as the disease waxes and wanes.

Treatment of chronic asthma in adults – British Thoracic Society (BTS) guidelines

- STEP 1: Start with inhaled bronchodilators, e.g. salbutamol prn.
- STEP 2: Add inhaled steroid, e.g. beclomethasone 200–800 micrograms daily if using salbutamol more than once daily.
- STEP 3: add long-acting bronchodilator (LAB), e.g. salmetorol. If no improvement, stop LAB and increase inhaled steroid. If partial improvement, continue and increase inhaled steroid.
- STEP 4: increase strength of inhaled steroid to up to 2000 micrograms daily; consider fourth drug such as oral leucotriene receptor antagonist or Xanthine.
- STEP 5: introduction of daily oral steroids at minimum dose needed to obtain control.

The diagnosis of COPD requires spirometry testing.

Practical point

For many of the conditions listed in this chapter there are specialist societies which issues guidelines and also NICE (the National Institute for Health and Clinical Excellence) who develop series of national clinical guidelines and these should be regularly consulted for changes based on evidence-based medicine, e.g. in relation to recent new advice regarding the use of beta blockers in hypertension.

A course of oral steroids can also be used at any time as a rescue step for rapid deterioration.

Acknowledgement

With special thanks to Dr Jim McMorran and colleagues for reference to the website www.gpnotebook.co.uk and for kind permission to use information from the website for this chapter. For up-to-date information please refer to the website: www.gpnotebook. co.uk.

Bibliography

Arroll B, Kenealy T, Kerse N. Do delayed prescriptions reduce antibiotic use in respiratory tract infections? A systematic review. *British Journal of General Practice.* 2003; **53**: 871–7.

British National Formulary: www.bnf.org

Charlton R, Smith G. Pain concepts and pain control in palliative care. Chapter 17.2: Volume 2. *Oxford Textbook of Primary Medical Care.* Oxford: Oxford University Press; 2003. p. 1277–83.

Drugs and Therapeutics Bulletin for independent reviews of medical treatments: www.dtb.org.uk

National Institute for Health and Clinical Excellence: www.nice.org.uk

Index

Page numbers in italic refer to figures or tables.

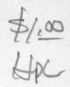

Susurros de pasión

books4pocket

Karyn Monk

Susurros de pasión

Traducción de Marta Torent López de Lamadrid

EDICIONES URANO

Argentina - Chile - Colombia - España
Estados Unidos - México - Perú - Uruguay - Venezuela

Título original: *Every Whispered Word*
Copyright © 2005 by Karyn Monk

© de la traducción: Marta Torent López de Lamadrid
© 2006 by Ediciones Urano
          Aribau, 142, pral. – 08036 Barcelona
          www.edicionesurano.com
          www.books4pocket.com

1ª edición en Books4pocket septiembre 2010

Diseño de la colección: Opalworks
Imagen de portada: Alan Ayers
Diseño de portada: Epica Prima

Impreso por Novoprint, S.A.
Energía 53
Sant Andreu de la Barca (Barcelona)

Fotocomposición: books4pocket

ISBN: 978-84-92801-55-8
Depósito legal: B-25.295-2010

Impreso en España – *Printed in Spain*

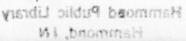

A Genevieve,
con todo mi amor

PRIMERA PARTE

El lenguaje del corazón

Capítulo 1

Marzo de 1885, Londres, Inglaterra

¡Qué condenadamente bien le habría ido tener la piqueta a mano!

En su defecto, le propinó frustrada una patada a la puerta y soltó una palabrota cuando el dolor le recorrió el pie.

«¡Odio este maldito lugar!»

La puerta chirrió y se abrió ligeramente, mostrando una parte del vestíbulo que había detrás de ésta. Miró un momento fijamente mientras analizaba a toda prisa sus opciones.

Sin duda, lo correcto sería cerrar la puerta. Seguro que en Londres la gente no esperaba que alguien abriera la puerta de su casa de una patada y a plena luz del día, pensó, sobre todo tratándose de una mujer joven y de aspecto relativamente respetable. Pero ¿y si el señor Kent estaba en casa y no le había oído llamar? Quizás estuviese atareado en alguna parte de la casa desde donde fuese difícil oír a alguien que aporreaba incesantemente la puerta. Claro que lo más probable, reflexionó, era que un hombre de su nivel social tuviese mayordomo. Entonces ¿por qué el criado no le abría?

Porque debía de ser viejo y estar sordo como una tapia, especuló enseguida. O tal vez bebiese a escondidas y se hubiese desplomado sobre la cama, completamente beodo. O acababa de sufrir algún ataque terrible y estaba tumbado en el suelo, indefenso, demasiado débil para pedir auxilio. ¡Sería una tragedia que ella se limitase a cerrar fríamente la puerta y marcharse, dejando que el pobre anciano y sordo mayordomo sufriera en soledad y muriera!

—¡Hola! —gritó, abriendo la puerta del todo—. ¿Señor Kent? ¿Está en casa?

Se oyó un fuerte golpe procedente de algún punto de la casa. Era evidente por qué nadie había contestado a su llamada a la puerta. Con semejante estruendo tenía que haber alguien en el interior de la casa, aunque, quienquiera que fuese, apenas podía imaginarse qué estaría haciendo.

—¿Señor Kent? —Entró en el vestíbulo—. ¿Puedo pasar?

Curiosamente, en el recibidor no había ningún mueble, como si el propietario se acabase de instalar. En un lateral de la entrada había un taburete desvencijado y *spindly-legged* sobre el que se erguía una inestable montaña de libros y papeles puestos de cualquier manera. Por el suelo y la escalera había esparcidos más montones desordenados de notas y volúmenes de gastadas tapas de cuero, que le obligaron a pisar con cuidado mientras se abría paso por el vestíbulo.

—Señor Kent —volvió a gritar, intentando que la oyeran a pesar del ruido—, ¿está usted bien?

—¡Eso es! —exclamó alguien, triunfalmente—. ¡Lo sabía! ¡Lo sabía!

La voz procedía de la cocina, en el piso de abajo, lo que le dio a entender que no se trataba del señor Kent, sino de alguno de sus criados. En realidad, era mejor. Un criado podría decirle si el señor Kent estaba en casa. De ser así, Camelia podría ser conducida al cuarto de estar, donde esperaría mientras el criado la anunciaba formalmente. Era preferible una presentación formal a que el renombrado Simon Kent se encontrara de pronto en su casa con una desconocida en medio de su desorden de libros y papeles personales.

Repitiéndose a sí misma que socialmente estaba actuando del modo más aceptable, cerró la puerta principal. A continuación se enderezó el sombrero y se frotó las manos enguantadas en la tela de rayas de color marfil y esmeralda de su falda. No había ningún espejo a mano para comprobar el estado de su pelo, pero la multitud de horquillas que se había puesto torpemente ya empezaban a soltarse, por lo que el tosco moño colgaba sobre su nuca. Seguramente Zareb tenía razón, pensó con resignación. Si se quedaba en Londres mucho tiempo más, es probable que tuviese que acabar contratando una doncella; aunque la idea de tan frívolo gasto le irritaba. Se puso bien unas cuantas horquillas, cruzó una puerta que había en el recibidor y bajó el estrecho tramo de escaleras que conducía a la cocina.

—¡Sí, sí, eso es! ¡Eso está mejor! —chilló la voz grave, extática—. ¡Sí, señor, ya está!

Un hombre de estatura considerable estaba de pie en medio de la cocina, de espaldas a ella. Llevaba unos sencillos pantalones oscuros y una camisa blanca de lino arremangada informalmente hasta los codos, empapada y pegada al cuerpo. Lo que no era de extrañar, dado el extraordinario calor y humedad que inundaba la cocina. Un vaho fino y suave flotaba en el aire, proporcionando a la habitación un aspecto ligeramente etéreo. Era un poco parecido a estar en la selva después de una copiosa lluvia veraniega, pensó Camelia, deseando no ir vestida con tantas capas sofocantes de ropa femenina que rápidamente perdían volumen.

Un fuerte ruido y un rugido salieron de la enorme máquina que había junto al hombre. «Es un motor de vapor», pensó ella, sintiendo una ola de excitación. Estaba girando una gran manivela que facilitaba el movimiento de una serie de discos rotatorios. Estos discos eran parte de una compleja estructura que estaba conectada a un gran barreño de madera, pero Camelia no lograba entender para qué servía el extraordinario aparato.

—Ahora espera, espera un poco, tranquila, tranquila; no tan rápido, ¡poco a poco! —decía el hombre con paciencia, hablándole al artefacto como si fuese un niño que aprende alguna nueva habilidad.

Apoyó sus delgados y musculosos brazos en el borde del cubo de madera y clavó los ojos en su interior, intensamente concentrado en lo que sea que estuviese ocurriendo.

—¡Un poco más, un poco más! ¡Eso es! ¡Sí! ¡Genial!

Intrigada, Camelia se acercó sorteando el laberinto de largas mesas repletas de extraños aparatos mecánicos. Había pilas de libros por todas partes, y las mesas, el suelo y las paredes de la cocina estaban cubiertas de complicados bocetos y notas.

—Un poco más deprisa —instó el hombre, excitado—. ¡No, no, no! —ordenó, pasándose la mano por los rizos húmedos de su pelo cobrizo. Empezó rápidamente a ajustar una serie de palancas y válvulas del motor de vapor—. ¡Un poco más, un poco más! ¡Venga! Ya casi lo tenemos, ¡eso es!

Se produjo una explosión ensordecedora de vapor caliente. La manivela del aparato comenzó a girar más deprisa, lo que provocó que los discos rotaran cada vez con mayor velocidad.

—¡Eso es! —chilló exaltado—. ¡Perfecto! ¡Magnífico! ¡Maravilloso!

El barreño de madera empezó a vibrar y a temblar. El agua se derramó por sus bordes y cayó al suelo.

—Demasiado rápido. —Sacudiendo la cabeza, rectificó desesperado los ajustes que le había hecho al motor de vapor—. Ahora espera, más despacio. He dicho más despacio, ¿me oyes?

Cada vez más preocupada, Camelia observó cómo el enorme barreño temblaba y enviaba olas de agua jabonosa por el aire. Fuese cual fuese el objetivo de la máquina, estaba claro que no tenía que haber duchado por completo a la persona que la estaba manejando, que era lo que acababa de suceder.

—¡Para, espera, para! ¿Me oyes? —ordenó el hombre con los ojos llenos de agua mientras se esforzaba en reajustar los mandos del aparato.

La manivela y las ruedas giraban ahora a una velocidad alarmante y el gran barreño temblaba y se agitaba como si fuese a romperse.

—¡He dicho que pares! —gritó el hombre, golpeando el recalcitrante artefacto con la llave inglesa—. ¡Para de una vez antes de que te parta en dos con un hacha!

De pronto, del barreño empezó a salir ropa empapada en todas direcciones. Un par de calzoncillos mojados aterrizaron con fuerza en la cara de Camelia, que se tambaleó hacia atrás, momentáneamente cegada. La mesa que estaba a sus espaldas se movió y tiró la que tenía detrás. Un terrible estrépito inundó la habitación y Camelia se cayó al suelo de espaldas.

—¡Para, chatarra inútil! —gruñó el hombre, que, desesperado, seguía intentando controlar el artefacto—. ¡Ya basta!

Camelia se sacó los calzoncillos de la cara y justo entonces vio cómo la máquina exhalaba su último y desafiante resoplido. El hombre estaba frente a ella, chorreando, con las piernas separadas y empuñando la llave inglesa como si fuese una amenazadora espada. Llevaba la camisa desabrochada casi hasta la cintura, dejando al descubierto el firme contorno de su pecho y vientre, y la considerable anchura de sus hombros era más que perceptible debajo de la tela de lino prácticamente transparente. Camelia pensó que parecía un fornido guerrero listo para la batalla, excepto por el lánguido calcetín que colgaba sobre su cabeza.

El hombre esperó un buen rato, respirando con dificultad, por si la máquina volvía a darle más problemas. Visiblemente satisfecho de que no fuese así, bajó la llave inglesa despacio y se volvió, cabeceando indignado. Recorrió con la mirada la escena: mesas volcadas, el revoltillo de inventos hechos añicos y el desorden de notas y libros esparcidos por el suelo mojado.

Al fin, sus penetrantes ojos detectaron a Camelia.

—¿Qué demonios se cree que está haciendo? —inquirió sorprendido.

—Intentar levantarme —contestó ella, apresurándose a taparse las piernas con la falda. Recuperada parcialmente su dignidad herida, alargó el brazo y lo miró expectante.

—Me refería a qué diantres hace aquí —aclaró, haciendo caso omiso de su brazo extendido—. ¿Tiene por costumbre entrar en las casas de la gente sin ser invitada?

Ella trató de mantener un aire de correcta formalidad, lo que era tremendamente difícil, teniendo en cuenta que estaba repanchingada en el suelo y el hombre la miraba furioso, como si fuese un vulgar ladrón.

—He llamado —se defendió ella con decoro—, pero nadie me ha abierto la puerta...

—¿Y por eso ha decidido forzarla?

—Le aseguro que no he forzado la puerta. —A la vista de que carecía de los modales elementales incluso del más inexperto de los mayordomos, decidió que su interlocutor debía de ser uno de los ayudantes del señor Kent. Entendía que pudiese resultar difícil encontrar ayudantes dignos de confianza que tuvieran los conocimientos matemáticos y científicos necesarios, pero eso no justificaba la absoluta descortesía de este hombre—. Estaba abierta.

Él se sacó el calcetín mojado de la cabeza y lo dejó a un lado.

—¿Y eso le hizo pensar que podía entrar a hurtadillas y espiarme?

Como era evidente que no iba a ayudarle a levantarse, se puso sola de pie con la mayor dignidad de que fue capaz, dado el reto que suponían el polisón, la enagua, el ridículo y el sombrero incómodamente ladeado. Una vez levantada, lo miró a los ojos con frío desdén.

—Le aseguro, señor, que no he entrado a hurtadillas, sino más bien andando tras pasar varios largos minutos llamando a la puerta y anunciar mi presencia en voz alta. La puerta estaba abierta, como ya le he mencionado, un descuido que estoy convencida de que, si se lo comunicase, su jefe no aprobaría.

El hombre abrió los ojos desmesuradamente.

«¡Bien! —pensó Camelia con satisfacción—. He captado su atención.»

—Da la casualidad de que esta tarde tengo una cita con el señor Kent —prosiguió resuelta, dándose aires.

Sólo estaba disfrazando un poco la verdad, dijo para sí. Lo cierto es que había escrito cinco veces al señor Kent para pedirle que le diera cita, pero, lamentablemente, no había contestado a ninguna de sus cartas. Aunque algunos miembros de la sociedad londinense ya le habían advertido de que el respetable inventor era un tanto excéntrico y en ocasiones desaparecía durante semanas sin que nadie lo viese y sin contestar el correo. De modo que en lugar de esperar a que el señor Kent le respondiese, había decidido actuar y escribirle una nota anunciándole que iría a verlo concretamente ese día y a esa misma hora.

—Así que tiene una cita con el señor Kent. —El hombre arqueó las cejas, escéptico, lo que aumentó aún más la irritación de Camelia.

—¡Pues sí! —le aseguró Camelia con rotundidad. Obviamente el señor Kent no estaba en casa, de lo contrario a estas alturas ya habría corrido a la cocina para averiguar a qué era debido el tremendo alboroto del laboratorio—. Y es para un tema de suma importancia.

—¿En serio? —Impasible, él cruzó los brazos delante del pecho—. ¿De qué se trata?

—Disculpe, señor, pero no es de su incumbencia. Si me dice cuándo puedo encontrar mañana en casa al señor Kent, vendré a verlo entonces.

Había decidido que sería mejor no esperar a que llegase el inventor. No había ningún espejo en la cocina, pero estaba segura de que los calzoncillos mojados que se habían estrellado en su cara no habían producido un efecto estimable. Notaba el enorme sombrero peligrosamente inclinado hacia un lado y la cabellera colgando por debajo de éste en una maraña húmeda. En cuanto al selecto atuendo que ella y Zareb tanto se habían esmerado en planchar hasta dejarlo en un estado de absoluta perfección, ahora era un empapado y arrugado desastre.

Si quería que el señor Kent se tomara en serio su propuesta, no podía aparecer ante él con aspecto de vagabunda azotada por un vendaval.

—Yo soy el señor Kent —le informó el hombre con brusquedad.

Camelia lo miró atónita.

—No, no lo es.

—¿No soy como se había imaginado?

—Para empezar es usted demasiado joven.

Él frunció las cejas.

—No sé si sentirme halagado u ofendido. ¿Demasiado joven para qué?

La descarada ironía de su mirada le dejó claro a Camelia que se estaba burlando de ella. Pues bien, con ella no se jugaba.

—Demasiado joven para haber obtenido diversas licenciaturas en matemáticas y ciencia por la University of St. Andrews y el St. John´s College de Cambridge —señaló Camelia—. Y para haber dado numerosas conferencias sobre Mecanismos y Mecánica aplicada, haber escrito dos o más docenas de artículos publicados por la Academia Nacional de Ciencias y haber registrado las patentes de unos doscientos setenta inventos. Y, obviamente, demasiado joven para ser responsable de todo esto —concluyó con un gesto que abarcaba la actividad científica que inundaba la habitación.

Él estaba impasible, pero ella pudo ver que le habían sorprendido sus conocimientos sobre los logros de su jefe. «¡Bien!», pensó, perversamente contenta de haber conseguido pararle los pies.

—Dados los desastrosos resultados del experimento, de los que acaba usted de ser testigo, me temo que he dañado para siempre la excesivamente generosa opinión que tiene usted de mí. Sin embargo, como ha irrumpido en mi laboratorio sin ser invitada ni anunciada, supongo que no puede culpárseme de ello. No acostumbro a dejar que nadie vea en lo que estoy trabajando hasta que estoy relativamente seguro de que no explotará y empezará a arrojar prendas de ropa en todas direcciones.

Camelia lo miró fijamente; se había quedado sin habla. Al fin y al cabo, no era tan joven, reflexionó, notando de pronto las arrugas que tenía en la frente y el entrecejo, que indicaban la cantidad de horas que se había pasado estudiando y deliberando. Sin duda, tendría treinta y cinco años o quizás incluso uno o dos más. Si bien era joven para haber hecho cuanto ella acababa de mencionar, no era imposible. No, si el hombre en cuestión era excepcionalmente inteligente, disciplinado y trabajador. Se le cayó el alma a los pies al percatarse de que acababa de insultar al hombre que tan desesperadamente había querido impresionar con su visita.

—Discúlpeme, señor Kent —se excusó, deseando que la tierra se la tragase—. No era mi intención molestarle. Es que tenía muchas ganas de hablar con usted.

Él ladeó la cabeza con expresión circunspecta.

—¿Por qué? ¿Ha venido a entrevistarme para uno de esos irritantes periodicuchos que encuentran un placer inestimable en tacharme de inventor demente?

Su tono era sarcástico, pero Camelia detectó una pizca de vulnerabilidad que le dio a entender que semejante descripción no le había dejado indiferente.

—No, nada de eso —le aseguró ella—. No soy escritora.

—No es escritora, y no es una espía. Eso son dos tantos a su favor. ¿Quién es usted, entonces?

—Soy lady Camelia Marshall —respondió mientras sujetaba el sombrero, que empezaba a resbalar por su cabeza—. Una gran admiradora de su trabajo, señor Kent —añadió con seriedad, apresurándose a evitar que el recargado adorno floral le cayera sobre la cara—. He leído varios de sus artículos, y me han parecido de lo más fascinantes.

—¿De veras?

Si le había sorprendido el hecho de que una mujer hubiese leído algunos de sus escritos o le hubiesen parecido fascinantes, no dio muestras de ello. Se limitó a caminar y a levantar la primera de las mesas que Camelia tenía a sus espaldas y había tirado.

—¡Esto es un maldito desastre! —murmuró mientras se agachaba para recoger algunas de las docenas de herramientas, piezas de metal y blocs que había esparcidos por el suelo mojado.

—Siento muchísimo haberle tirado las mesas —se disculpó Camelia—. Espero no haber roto nada —añadió, inclinándose para ayudarle.

Simon observó cómo cogía con dificultad una pequeña caja metálica. La sujetó con una mano enguantada y sucia mientras con la otra agarraba rápidamente la enorme monstruosidad de su sombrero fláccido. Entonces empezó a levantarse. Por desgracia, el gran peso de su polisón mojado comprometió su equilibrio. Sacó la mano del sombrero y la agitó en el aire con cara de repentino horror, aunque el invento metálico siguió estando a salvo contra su pecho.

Simon alargó el brazo y la sujetó mientras el sombrero y sus rosas marchitas caían sobre su rostro. Al aterrizar sobre él, el aroma de Camelia le embriagó; una extraordinaria fragancia distinta a todas las que había olido. Era exótica, pero le resultaba vagamente familiar, una esencia ligera y fresca que le recordaba los paseos por el bosque en la finca de su padre durante una lluvia veraniega. La agarró, inhalando su perfume y percibiendo con intensidad la delicada estructura de su espalda, sus suaves jadeos y las agitadas subidas y bajadas de su pecho, que latía contra el lino húmedo que se le había pegado a su propio cuerpo.

—¡Cuánto lo siento! —Tremendamente avergonzada, Camelia se apartó enérgicamente el sombrero de la cara. Al fin liberado de las horquillas, el tocado traicionero fue a parar al suelo, llevándose consigo lo que aún quedara de peinado, hasta que su pelo cayó sobre su espalda en una irremediable maraña.

Simon la miró con fijeza, contemplando la ahumada intensidad de sus ojos, muy abiertos y llenos de frustración. Eran del color de la salvia, observó, de ese tono verde suave que tenía la salvia de la selva, que crecía en los brezales secos y umbríos de Escocia. Un tenue abanico de arrugas rodeaba sus pestañas inferiores, poniendo de manifiesto que rebasaba de sobras la aniñada lozanía de la veintena. Su piel estaba atípicamente bronceada y salpicada de pecas, y su cabello de color miel veteado de hilos de un suave dorado, lo que indicaba que estaba acostumbrada al sol. Algo que, a juzgar por la calidad de su atuendo, sorprendió a Simon. Había notado que la mayoría de inglesas de buena cuna preferían protegerse del sol en sus casas o a la sombra. Claro que, reflexionó, la mayoría de las mujeres de buena cuna no tenía la osadía de entrar en casa de un hombre, sin invitación y sin ser acompañada. De algún modo sabía que Camelia ya no seguía necesitando su ayuda para ponerse de pie, pero era extrañamente reacio a soltarle la mano.

—Estoy bien, gracias. —Camelia se preguntó si la consideraría incapaz de mantenerse derecha durante más de tres minutos. Aunque tampoco le había dado motivos para pensar lo contrario, pensó con tristeza—. Supongo que no estoy acostumbrada a llevar sombreros tan grandes —añadió, creyendo que él necesitaría algún tipo de explicación respecto a su incapacidad para mantener el detestable adorno encima de la cabeza. Evitó mencionar que un par de calzoncillos mojados se habían estrellado contra su cara, desafiando la integridad de sus horquillas torpemente puestas.

Simon no sabía qué decirle. Se imaginaba que lo propio de un caballero sería asegurarle que el sombrero le sentaba de maravilla, pero es que el puñetero adorno le parecía ridículo. Desde luego estaba mucho más guapa sin él, especialmente ahora que los rizos dorados de su melena colgaban sobre sus hombros.

—Tenga —le dijo Simon, que cogió el sombrero y se lo devolvió.

—Gracias.

Él se volvió, sintiendo la súbita necesidad de separarse de ella.

—Entonces, dígame, lady Camelia —empezó a decir, intentando concentrarse en el desastre de su laboratorio—, ¿de verdad teníamos hoy una cita que yo ignoraba?

—Sí, sin ninguna duda —contestó Camelia con rotundidad—. Seguro que sí. —Tosió suavemente—. En cierto modo, sí.

Simon arqueó las cejas.

—¿Y eso qué significa exactamente?

—Significa exactamente que nuestra cita no ha sido confirmada. Aunque fue anunciada, de eso no hay duda.

—Ya veo. —Simon no tenía ni idea de qué estaba hablando—. Disculpe mi torpeza, pero ¿cómo se acordó la cita exactamente?

—Le escribí varias cartas pidiéndole una cita, pero, por desgracia, nunca me contestó —le explicó Camelia—. Y en la última me tomé la libertad de informarle de que vendría a verlo hoy a esta hora. Supongo que fue un atrevimiento por mi parte.

—Me temo que eso no es nada comparado con entrar en casa de un hombre sola y sin ser anunciada —puntualizó Simon, tirando un montón de papeles mojados sobre la mesa—. ¿Saben sus padres que va por Londres sin dama de compañía?

—No necesito ninguna dama de compañía, señor Kent.

—Discúlpeme, no me había dado cuenta de que estaba usted casada.

—No lo estoy. Pero tengo veintiocho años, mi presentación en sociedad fue hace años y no tengo el tiempo ni las ganas de estar constantemente ocupándome de que un ama de llaves vieja y charlatana me siga a todas partes. Con un cochero tengo suficiente.

—¿No le preocupa su reputación?

—No especialmente.

—¿Y eso por qué?

—Porque si viviese mi vida conforme a los dictámenes de la sociedad londinense, nunca haría nada.

—Ya veo. —Arrojó sobre la mesa un palo de madera con un accesorio metálico.

—¿Qué es eso? —preguntó Camelia, que miraba el objeto con curiosidad.

—Un nuevo sistema para fregar el suelo —respondió con indiferencia mientras se agachaba para recoger algo más.

Ella se acercó para examinar el extraño aparato.

—¿Cómo funciona?

Simon la miró titubeante, no acababa de creerse que le interesase realmente. Eran pocas las mujeres que se habían atrevido a entrar en su laboratorio y de ellas sólo las pertenecientes a su familia habían demostrado un reconocimiento auténtico de sus ideas a menudo extravagantes. Sin embargo, había algo en la expresión de lady Camelia, que estaba ahí de pie, que mitigó su impulso inicial de limitarse a obviar la pregunta. Miraba atentamente con esos ojos verdes del color de la salvia, como si la curiosa herramienta que tenía delante fuese un misterio que quisiese a toda costa resolver.

—He sujetado una gran abrazadera en el extremo del palo de un friegasuelos, que es accionado por esta palanca —comenzó su explicación mientras cogía el objeto para enseñárselo—. La palanca mueve esta varilla, que tensa este muelle y hace que la abrazadera se cierre firmemente. La idea es escurrir la bayeta de la base del mango sin tocarla ni tenerse que agachar.

—¡Muy ingenioso!

—Tengo que seguir trabajando en ello —comentó, encogiéndose de hombros—. Me está costando obtener la tensión adecuada del muelle para que estruje suficientemente la bayeta sin romper la palanca. —Dejó el invento en la mesa.

—¿Y esto qué es? —Camelia señaló la caja metálica que sostenía en las manos.

—Un exprimidor de limones.

Lo miró intrigada.

—No se parece a ninguno de los que he visto hasta ahora. —Lo abrió y vio un cono acanalado de madera rodeado por un anillo con agujeros—. ¿Cómo funciona?

—Se pone medio limón sobre el cono, luego se cierra la tapa y se presiona con fuerza, usando la palanca para ejercer todavía más presión —explicó Simon—. El hueco que hay en la tapa aprieta el limón contra el cono, extrayendo el zumo sin necesidad de girarlo. El zumo cae por los agujeros en la cubeta que hay debajo sin las pepitas ni la pulpa, que se quedan en el anillo superior. Después se extrae este pequeño recipiente y ya tenemos el zumo.

—¡Qué maravilla! ¿Ha pensado en fabricarlo?

Simon cabeceó.

—Lo he hecho para mi familia; siempre intento encontrar formas de aliviarles un poco el trabajo. Me imagino que a la gente le parecería una tontería de aparato.

—Pues yo creo que a la mayoría de las mujeres les encantaría cualquier cosa que aligerara las tareas del hogar —repuso Camelia—. ¿Ha registrado al menos la patente? ¿O la del friegasuelos?

—Si me dedicase a patentar todo lo que se me ocurre, me pasaría la vida tramitando papeles.

—Pero tiene unas doscientas setenta patentes.

—Eso es porque, con la mejor intención, algunos miembros de mi familia decidieron ocuparse de llevar mis dibujos y mis notas sobre esos inventos en concreto, y presentar los documentos y el dinero necesarios a la oficina de patentes. No tengo ni idea de lo que ha sido registrado y lo que no. Y, francamente, tampoco me interesa.

Ella lo miró con incredulidad.

—¿No quiere saber que sus ideas han sido debidamente registradas, para que pueda obtener el reconocimiento merecido?

—Yo no invento cosas para que me sean reconocidas, lady Camelia. Si alguien más quiere hacer suya una de mis ideas, mejorarla e invertir el tiempo y el capital necesario para producirla, por mí no hay problema. Si todos los científicos guardaran sus teorías y descubrimientos como si fuese oro, la ciencia y la tecnología nunca avanzarían.

Levantó la segunda mesa y empezó a amontonar sobre ella más papeles mojados, herramientas y diversos inventos que se habían caído al suelo.

—Y dígame, lady Camelia —dijo mientras escurría el agua de una maraña de alambres—, ¿a qué se debe que me haya escrito todas esas cartas pidiendo verme?

Camelia vaciló. Se había imaginado dirigir su encuentro con el señor Kent desde una sala de estar llena de suntuoso terciopelo, donde pudiese disertar con calma sobre la importancia de la arqueología y la evolución del hombre, tal vez mientras algún criado convenientemente respetuoso le servía un té en un juego de plata. Aunque, dados los numerosos montones de platos grasientos apilados junto al hornillo y en el fregadero que había en el otro lado de la cocina, le había quedado clarísimo que el señor Kent no tenía criados. Pensó en sugerirle que volvería otro día, cuando él no tuviese que ocuparse de devolverle al laboratorio un aire de ordenado, pero desechó la idea de inmediato.

El tiempo no se detenía.

—Estoy muy interesada en su trabajo con los motores de vapor —contestó, agachándose para recoger unos cuantos objetos más del suelo—. He leído uno de sus artículos al respecto en el que exponía los enormes beneficios de la energía de vapor aplicada a las bombas utilizadas para minas de carbón. Su tesis acerca de que la energía de vapor todavía no se utiliza eficazmente me pareció absolutamente fascinante.

Simon no podía creerse que hablara en serio. De todas las posibles explicaciones de su presencia allí, habría jurado que el tema de los motores de vapor y las minas de carbón era el más improbable.

—¿Le interesan los motores de vapor?

—Me interesan en su aplicación al desafío de la excavación y el bombeo —matizó Camelia—. Soy arqueóloga, señor Kent, como mi padre, el difunto Earl de Stamford. Seguro que habrá oído hablar de él.

Sus ojos brillaron de esperanza, y por alguna razón Simon detestaba tener que desilusionarla. Sin embargo, no quiso mentirle.

—Lamentablemente, lady Camelia, no estoy muy familiarizado con el campo de la arqueología y no suelo asistir a la clase de eventos en los que quizás hubiese tenido el placer de conocer a su padre. —Su tono era de disculpa.

Camelia asintió. Supuso que tampoco podía realmente esperar que conociese a su padre. Después de todo lo que había oído decir sobre el señor Kent, saltaba a la vista que pasaba la mayor parte de su tiempo encerrado en su laboratorio.

—Mi padre dedicó su vida al estudio de las riquezas arqueológicas de África en una época en que el mundo está casi exclusivamente interesado en el arte y los objetos de los egipcios, romanos y griegos. Desde un punto de vista científico se tienen muy pocos datos de la historia de los africanos.

—Pues me temo que yo no sé gran cosa sobre África, lady Camelia. Según tengo entendido su población se compone básicamente de tribus nómadas que llevan miles de años viviendo con muchísima sencillez. Nunca se me ha ocurrido que pudiesen tener algo valioso, excepto los diamantes, claro.

—África no tiene la abundancia de edificios antiguos y arte que ha sido descubierto en otros lugares del planeta —concedió Camelia—. Y de ser así, aún no los hemos encontrado. Pero mi padre creía que en África vivieron civilizaciones mucho más antiguas que las existentes en cualquier otra parte del mundo. Cuando Charles Darwin propuso su teoría de que a lo mejor los seres humanos descendían del mono, el mundo entero se burló de él. Sin embargo, lo que eso hizo fue reforzar la convicción de mi padre acerca de la singular relevancia de África en la evolución de la humanidad.

—¿Y todo eso qué tiene que ver con mis motores de vapor?

—Hace veinte años mi padre descubrió un terreno en Suráfrica que presentaba numerosos indicios de que en el pasado había vivido allí una antigua tribu. Compró unas ciento veinte hectáreas y empezó a excavar, hallando muchos objetos apasionantes. Ahora yo continúo la labor de mi padre y necesito su bomba de vapor.

—Pensaba que las excavaciones arqueológicas se realizaban básicamente con una pala, un cubo y un cepillo.

—Y así es, pero excavar en Suráfrica supone un reto constante. Una vez traspasada la primera capa de tierra relativamente blanda, la corteza se vuelve durísima y difícil de romper. Luego está el problema del agua, que se cuela en el agujero a medida que uno se acerca al nivel freático. Y, además, está la estación lluviosa, que puede durar desde diciembre hasta marzo. En este momento mi excavación está completamente inundada, por lo que a mis trabajadores les es imposible continuar.

—Seguro que en Suráfrica habrá bombas de vapor disponibles —sugirió Simon.

—La verdad es que no son fáciles de conseguir.

Camelia procuró hablar con serenidad. No quería que Simon supiese los tremendos obstáculos que se había encontrado al intentar obtener una bomba para su terreno. Si él se enteraba de que le habían saboteado el equipo anterior o de que creía que la De Beers Company había dado orden a las empresas de bombas de que no le alquilaran más maquinaria, tal vez le pareciese demasiado arriesgado suministrarle la única bomba que tenía.

—Las bombas de agua están monopolizadas por la De Beers Mining Company —prosiguió—, y su prioridad, lógicamente, es el suministro de servicios para el bombeo de las minas de diamantes. Debido a eso no puedo comprar ni alquilar una bomba, y mi excavación ha llegado a un punto muerto. Pero tras leer su artículo, me convencí de que su bomba era muy superior a las empleadas actualmente en Suráfrica. Por eso he venido a verlo.

—¿Y qué le hace pensar que mi bomba es mejor?

—En su artículo tacha las turbinas de vapor actuales de extremadamente ineficientes. Propone que se aprovecharía mucha más energía si el vapor pudiese expandirse de forma gradual en lugar de hacerlo de golpe, permitiendo que la turbina se moviese a gran velocidad, lo que, a su vez, haría que la bomba actuase con más fuerza y rapidez. Como una prolongada exposición al agua puede dañar los objetos que excavo y estoy tremendamente ansiosa por hacer progresos en mi trabajo, creo que su nueva bomba de vapor es la mejor solución para extraer el agua de mi terreno.

De modo que era cierto que había leído el artículo, reflexionó Simon. Y lo que era más sorprendente, parecía que lo había entendido. Se pasó las manos por el pelo y echó un vistazo a su alrededor, tratando de recordar dónde había puesto sus notas y dibujos de los motores de vapor. Empezó a rebuscar en varios montones de bocetos que había esparcidos por el suelo, y después se acercó a una de las mesas que no había ido a parar al suelo a consecuencia de la espectacular caída de lady Camelia y continuó buscando.

—¿Por qué ha hecho que este motor agitase el cubo? —inquirió Camelia mientras él buscaba.

—No pretendía que el motor hiciese eso. Se suponía que tenía que hacer girar la hélice que hay en el interior del barreño para que, a su vez, ésta forzase que el agua mojara la ropa. Lamentablemente, no ha funcionado tan bien como yo esperaba.

Camelia miró asombrada el enorme artefacto.

—¿Me está diciendo que esto es una lavadora gigante?

—Es un prototipo —contestó Simon—. Las máquinas actuales utilizan un cubo de madera y una hélice que es accionada por una manivela. Estoy intentando crear una máquina que funcione con energía de vapor para librar a las mujeres del agotador trabajo que supone girar la manivela a mano.

Pese a que su experiencia lavando ropa era limitada, Camelia comprendía, sin duda, que para una mujer a cargo de toda la colada de una casa una máquina de vapor supondría una gran ayuda.

—Es una idea maravillosa.

—Me faltan muchas horas de trabajo —reconoció, lanzando una mirada de indignación a las prendas de ropa empapadas que había esparcidas por la cocina—. Es difícil fabricar un motor de vapor; me está costando obtener una rotación buena y regular. Además, es demasiado grande, y caro. Otra opción es hacerlo con gas, pero muy pocas casas lo tienen. Igual que la electricidad, que aún no llega a la mayoría de las casas. —Comenzó a buscar debajo de un montón de platos sucios, que daba la impresión de que en cualquier momento se le caerían sobre la cabeza—. Aquí está —anunció al tiempo que sacaba un arrugado dibujo de debajo de una sartén.

Camelia se acercó mientras él despejaba un poco una de las mesas e intentaba alisar el papel sumamente arrugado y manchado.

—Un motor de vapor se basa en la premisa de que somete el vapor a una enorme presión, permitiendo que se expanda y cree una fuerza susceptible de ser convertida en movimiento —comenzó Simon—. Utilizando un pistón y un cilindro, se crea el efecto de bombeo, que puede usarse para muchas cosas, incluido el bombeo de agua de minas de carbón y pozos. Lo que he intentado es mejorar la eficacia del motor haciendo que el vapor se expanda en varias fases, por lo que su presión aumenta significativamente.

—¿Y lo ha conseguido?

—He logrado fraccionar el movimiento del vapor e intensificar su presión. Pero, por desgracia, no ha sido suficiente para producir una diferencia sustancial en lo que a la eficacia de la bomba se refiere.

Camelia se llevó un desengaño.

—Pero ¿la bomba que ha construido funciona bastante bien para extraer agua de un hoyo?

—Por supuesto —le aseguró Simon—. Le hice una serie de ajustes para que funcionase mejor de lo que lo hacen la mayoría de las bombas, aunque no fue suficiente para garantizar la fabricación a gran escala. Los materiales que empleé son más caros que los usados habitualmente y se tarda más en montar la máquina, lo que significa que ningún fabricante consideraría que el diseño es económicamente viable.

Camelia pensó que una bomba un tanto perfeccionada era mejor que nada.

—¿Estaría dispuesto a alquilármela?

—Lamentablemente, no hay nada que alquilar. La desmonté casi entera porque necesitaba las piezas para otras cosas.

Ella lo miró fijamente, abatida.

—¿Cuánto tardaría en construir otra?

—Más tiempo del que dispongo ahora mismo —respondió Simon—. En este momento estoy enfrascado en muchísimos proyectos. Además, esa máquina tenía una serie de problemas que, al parecer, no he sabido solucionar.

—Pero eso es lo que debería impulsarle a invertir más tiempo en ella —repuso Camelia—. Como científico, deberían motivarle los desafíos.

—Mire a su alrededor, lady Camelia. ¿Cree honestamente que no tengo suficientes desafíos que requieran mi atención?

—No estoy diciendo que los demás inventos en los que trabaja no sean importantes —le aseguró Camelia—, pero no compare un exprimidor de limones y una lavadora con algo que me ayudará a desenterrar un episodio vital de la historia de la humanidad.

—Eso es muy subjetivo —replicó Simon—. Para la gente que cae rendida en la cama cada noche exhausta por las angustiosas cargas de sus quehaceres diarios, cualquier invento que facilite la ejecución de una tarea supone una mejora en sus vidas. Mejorar potencialmente las vidas de miles de personas me parece mucho más importante que desenterrar unos cuantos huesos descompuestos y reliquias rotas de los páramos africanos.

—Esos huesos descompuestos y todas esas reliquias nos dan información acerca de quiénes somos y de dónde venimos —protestó Camelia, enfurecida por la forma en que Simon despreciaba su trabajo—. El descubrimiento de nuestra historia tiene una importancia crucial para todos nosotros.

—Me temo que me interesa más dedicar mi tiempo a unos inventos que mejorarán el presente y el futuro. Si bien respeto el campo de la arqueología, lady Camelia, es una profesión que interesa principalmente a una minoría, a unos cuantos académicos privilegiados. No creo que vaya usted a descubrir nada que mejore la vida de miles de personas. Y dado que dispongo de muy poco tiempo y ya estoy embarcado en bastantes más proyectos de los que puedo manejar, me temo que no podré ayudarle. —Empezó a coger más inventos y papeles que había esparcidos por el suelo.

—Le pagaré.

Simon se detuvo y la miró con curiosidad. Su rostro estaba impasible, pero sus manos sujetaban el ridículo con tanta fuerza que en la zona de los nudillos la tela de los guantes estaba tensa. No había duda de que proseguir la labor de su padre significaba mucho para ella.

—¿En serio? ¿Cuánto?

—Mucho —contestó ella—. Generosamente.

—Disculpe si le parezco grosero, pero me temo que tendrá que ser un poco más precisa en su respuesta. ¿Cuánto es con exactitud «generosamente»?

Camelia vaciló. Sus recursos financieros eran realmente escasos. Apenas tenía fondos suficientes en el banco para pagar durante los dos próximos meses al puñado de leales trabajadores que se habían quedado en el terreno. Pero el señor

Kent no tenía por qué saberlo. A juzgar por su hogar modesto y escasamente amueblado, y su aparente imposibilidad de contratar a alguien que le ayudara, ya fuera con sus inventos o con la avalancha de ollas sucias y platos grasientos apilados por el hornillo y el fregadero, daba la impresión de que el hombre desaliñado que estaba frente a ella también pasaba por dificultades económicas.

—Señor Kent, si me fabrica una bomba de inmediato, estoy dispuesta a ofrecerle el cinco por ciento de los beneficios que obtenga en los dos próximos años. Supongo que convendrá conmigo en que la cantidad es muy generosa.

Simon frunció las cejas.

—Lo siento, lady Camelia, pero no entiendo qué ha querido decir con eso. ¿De qué beneficios habla exactamente?

—De los que obtenga de lo que sea que encuentre durante la excavación.

—No sabía que hubiese un mercado floreciente de fragmentos de huesos y vasijas rotas.

—Lo hay, si son arqueológicamente relevantes. En cuanto haya estudiado y documentado las piezas, se las venderé al Museo Británico para su colección con la condición de que pueda tener libre acceso a ellas cuando así lo desee.

—Ya veo. ¿Y cuánto han ganado con este proyecto en los últimos cinco años?

—Lo que mi padre y yo ganáramos en el pasado no importa ahora —repuso con firmeza—. Hace seis meses, cuando falleció, mi padre estaba a punto de realizar un descubrimiento sumamente importante. Lamentablemente, la lluvia y las filtraciones de agua han inundado el terreno de manera muy gradual, y mis trabajadores no han podido avanzar gran cosa.

De hecho, la mayoría de ellos estaban convencidos de que había caído una maldición sobre el terreno y habían huido, pero no había por qué compartir ese detalle con él.

—Con la ayuda de su bomba de vapor —prosiguió ella—, podré excavar el terreno cien veces más deprisa de lo que lo haría usando sólo mano de obra para extraer el agua y el barro. Así podré desenterrar, al fin, lo que mi padre pasó tantos años buscando.

—¿Y qué era?

Camelia titubeó. Desde el inicio sus trabajadores habían tenido miedo de lo que ella buscaba, pero tras los accidentes ocurridos el miedo se había convertido en un pánico exacerbado. Claro que Simon Kent era un instruido científico que probablemente no creía en las maldiciones y los espíritus vengativos.

Aun así, cuanto menos supiese mejor.

—Mi padre buscaba objetos pertenecientes a una antigua tribu que habitó en la zona que ocupa nuestro terreno hace unos dos mil años. —Sin duda, eso era cierto, se dijo para sí, aunque no era toda la verdad.

Simon no parecía nada impresionado.

—¿Unos cuantos trozos rotos de unos objetos pertenecientes a una antigua tribu? ¿Nada de cámaras ocultas con oro o diamantes ni antiguas fuerzas misteriosas atrapadas en un cofre con piedras preciosas incrustadas?

—El valor de estas reliquias será enorme. —Camelia se esforzó por controlar su rabia—. Mi padre se pasó los últimos veinte años de su vida a punto de hacer un importante descubrimiento científico, que, sin duda, abrirá la puerta a un área completamente nueva de estudio arqueológico.

—O sea, que a la vista de que usted y su padre hasta ahora aún no han dado con este «significativo descubrimiento», como usted lo llama, lo que me está ofreciendo es esencialmente el cinco por ciento de nada —le espetó Simon. Empezó a recoger la ropa empapada que había esparcida por la cocina y la metió de nuevo en la lavadora—. Le pido disculpas, si le parezco un desagradecido, lady Camelia, pero por realmente tentadora que sea su oferta, me temo que tendré que declinarla.

Camelia lo miró fijamente, desalentada. Simon Kent no era en absoluto como se había esperado. Se había imaginado que era un refinado anciano de ciencias y letras, dominado, como su padre, por una sed insaciable de conocimiento. Creía que el señor Kent valoraría la extraordinaria oportunidad que suponía participar en su exploración, en la que uno de sus inventos sería utilizado para ayudar a que el mundo entendiese mejor sus propios orígenes. Se había autoconvencido de que no sería como el resto de británicos que había conocido a su regreso a Inglaterra, la mayoría de los cuales consideraba, al parecer, que Suráfrica no era más que un polvoriento terreno lleno de maleza habitado por bárbaros, una tierra simplemente a la espera de que saquearan sus diamantes y su oro.

—Está bien, el diez por ciento de los dos próximos años —ofreció Camelia con frialdad mientras él seguía metiendo prendas de ropa en su detestable lavadora. Odiaba necesitar su ayuda con tanta desesperación—. ¿Le parece mejor?

—No se trata únicamente de dinero. —Simon estaba impresionado por su manifiesta determinación. Desde luego su deseo de honrar la labor vital realizada por su padre y de triunfar donde él había fracasado era admirable—. Aunque construyese otra bomba de vapor para usted, lo que como mínimo me llevaría unas cuantas semanas, ¿quién la manejaría una vez llegase en barco a Suráfrica? Ya me ha hablado de los grandes desafíos que plantean la geografía y el clima. La bomba que yo construiría sería diferente de las que se usan actualmente. Y debería adaptarse para afrontar los problemas que, sin duda, surgirían. Habría que enseñar a alguien a manejarla y mantenerla; de lo contrario, acabaría usted cargando con una máquina completamente inútil.

Camelia se dio cuenta de que tenía razón. El único motor de vapor que había conseguido alquilar para su excavación justo tras la muerte de su padre había sufrido un sinfín de averías durante los pocos días que, en realidad, estuvo en funcionamiento. Después se cayó al suelo de forma misteriosa y los engranajes se hicieron añicos, quedando por completo destruida. La empresa que se la había alquilado le exigió que pagase la máquina rota y luego se negó a alquilarle nada más.

La máquina del señor Kent no le serviría de nada a menos que contratase alguien con los conocimientos pertinentes sobre semejante aparato para poderlo hacer funcionar.

—¿Estaría usted dispuesto a venir a Suráfrica y enseñarle a alguien a usarla? Serían sólo una o dos semanas —se apresuró a asegurarle Camelia—. Justo el tiempo necesario para enseñarle cómo va la máquina y que se familiarice con su mantenimiento.

—Es posible dominar su manejo en dos semanas, pero se tardarían semanas e incluso meses en aprender a mantenerla y repararla —señaló Simon—. Me temo que no tengo ni el tiempo ni las ganas de viajar hasta África para hacer eso; ahora mismo tengo muchos otros proyectos que requieren mi atención.

—Por supuesto que incrementaría mi oferta para compensarle por su tiempo —agregó Camelia—. Aumentaría sus ganancias a un diez por ciento de los beneficios que obtenga durante los próximos cinco años, seguro que eso compensará el tiempo que le pido que invierta.

—Lady Camelia, me parece que no comparto su fascinación por excavar en tierras africanas. Espero que lo comprenda.

Camelia apretó los labios. ¡Menudo desastre! Se había pasado dos semanas estudiando sus artículos en *The Journal of Science and Mechanics* a la vez que le había escrito una carta detrás de otra, pidiéndole educadamente una cita. Durante esos días se había autoconvencido de que podría persuadir al brillante y con fama de excéntrico Simon Kent de que le suministrara la bomba de vapor que con tanta desesperación necesitaba. Dos preciosas semanas perdidas para no conseguir absolutamente nada. Le inundó el pánico.

Clavó los ojos en el grasiento dibujo que había encima de la mesa que había frente a ella.

—¡Claro que lo entiendo! —repuso con tranquilidad—. Espero que pueda disculparme por haber entrado en su casa sin ser anunciada, señor Kent, y gracias por su tiempo. —Se puso el enorme sombrero en la cabeza—. ¡Oh, Dios mío! —exclamó mientras palpaba en vano la parte posterior del mismo—. Creo que he perdido mi pasador de perlas. Debe de habérseme caído al suelo, ¿lo ve en alguna parte?

Simon escudriñó el desorden de cosas que había por el suelo.

—Aquí hay algunas horquillas —constató, agachándose para recoger media docena de pasadores metálicos que había entre el revoltijo—, pero me temo que...

—¡Oh, aquí está! Lo tenía enganchado aquí encima del sombrero. —Se puso el pasador en la enredada melena y avanzó airosa hacia las escalera que conducían a la planta baja.

—La acompañaré a la puerta —se ofreció Simon.

—Eso no será necesario —le aseguró Camelia con indiferencia, subiendo los peldaños tan rápido como le permitían la falda y el polisón húmedos y pesados. Cruzó el vestíbulo a zancadas y abrió la puerta principal—. Espero no haberle estropeado el día entero, señor Kent.

Le dedicó su sonrisa más dulce, luego se volvió, y se dispuso a bajar los escalones de piedra que había hasta la calle.

Simon la observó mientras se alejaba precipitadamente por la acera en dirección a un elegante carruaje negro estacionado, la arrugada falda crujía con fuerza y su melena rubia caía en una cascada de rizos debajo de las mustias rosas de su absurdo sombrero. Se preguntó por qué el cochero no la había esperado con el carruaje justo frente de su puerta. Tal vez le había ordenado que se detuviese un poco más adelante para poder disfrutar de un breve paseo. Fuera por la razón que fuera, su paso era rápido y decidido, y su ridículo con abalorios pendía oscilante de su muñeca enguantada. Los colores malva y añil del atardecer se arremolinaban a su alrededor formando un velo crepuscular y cuando llegó al carruaje, se volvió y se despidió con la mano.

Entonces abrió la puerta del vehículo y se subió a él, tan manifiestamente ansiosa por marcharse que no esperó a que el cochero bajase para ayudarle.

Simon cerró la puerta y permaneció unos instantes de pie en el vestíbulo. La luz plúmbea bañaba la habitación apenas amueblada, proporcionándole un inusual aspecto agobiante y melancólico. Se le ocurrió encender la lámpara de gas que había en la pared, pero decidió no hacerlo. De todas formas, raras veces salía de su laboratorio antes de medianoche y con todo lo que aún quedaba por recoger probablemente estaría ahí abajo hasta el amanecer. Mientras regresaba a la cocina se percató de que sus pantalones estaban mojados y se le pegaban a las piernas, y de que llevaba la camisa empapada y abierta casi hasta la cintura.

«¡Genial!», pensó con ironía. Ahora además de ser etiquetado de ermitaño, distraído y tremendamente excéntrico, podía añadir un calificativo más a la lista: exhibicionista. A lady Camelia no parecía haberle importado su estado de semidesnudez, reflexionó, y de ser así, había disimulado de maravilla su desconcierto. Tal vez el tiempo que había pasado en la selva surafricana le había insensibilizado a los cánones sociales de Inglaterra. Dudaba mucho que sus empleados nativos trabajasen bajo el sol sofocante con una camisa almidonada, chaleco y americana.

Cogió de la mesa su fregona experimental y se dispuso a limpiar el suelo, esforzándose por no pensar en sus ojos verdes del color de la salvia ni en la delicia de su suavidad y calidez durante el instante dolorosamente breve en que la había tocado.

—Disculpe, señora, pero ¿qué está haciendo? —le preguntó el hombre de rostro rollizo que miraba fijamente a Camelia desde el otro lado del carruaje—. ¡Éste no es su coche!

—¿Ah, no? —Con fingida sorpresa, Camelia echó un vistazo al interior de terciopelo granate del carruaje—. Pues, sin duda, se parece al mío, las cortinas son iguales. ¿Está usted seguro de que no se ha subido al coche equivocado?

—Absolutamente —replicó el hombre con obstinación—, acabo de regresar del campo y no me he movido de este asiento en las últimas tres horas. Justo cuando usted ha subido yo me disponía a bajar.

Miró con discreción por la ventanilla y vio que Simon entraba de nuevo en su casa y cerraba la puerta.

—En ese caso le ruego que me disculpe, señor —le dijo, abriendo la puerta—. Le he dicho a mi cochero que me esperase aquí, pero, al parecer, debe de haber estacionado un poco más lejos. Lamento haberle causado molestias. —Salió del vehículo y se apresuró calle abajo, sujetando con fuerza el ridículo.

El corazón le latía con fuerza contra las costillas mientras corría, temerosa de que en cualquier momento el señor Kent descubriese que le había robado su dibujo y fuese tras ella. Una embriagadora mezcla de júbilo y miedo mantenía su respiración jadeante y su paso rápido. Quizá no pudiese contar con la novedosa bomba de vapor del señor Kent, pero tenía un dibujo extremadamente detallado. Ya encontraría a alguien que se la construyese, alguien que compartiera su visión de hacer avanzar el campo de la arqueología. Había más inventores en Londres; hombres interesados en objetivos más nobles que intentar utilizar la energía de vapor para lavar ropa interior o extraer la última gota de zumo de un limón.

Llegó al final de la calle y cruzó, después se deslizó por una callejuela situada detrás de una hilera de casas, en dirección al lugar donde había dejado a Zareb con el carruaje. Su amigo africano había discutido vehementemente con ella cuando le había insistido en que no la dejara delante de casa del señor Kent, pero, al fin, había cedido. No podían permitirse llamar la atención, y debido a su apariencia Zareb fascinaba a la gente dondequiera que fuese.

Cogió el sombrero con una mano y con la otra apretó el ridículo contra su pecho, ignorando lo mucho que le apretaba el corsé y la engorrosa opresión del polisón y la enagua. ¡Qué placer cuando por fin volviese a África y pudiese deshacerse de ambos! Seguro que dentro de mil años los arqueólogos los considerarían instrumentos de tortura.

—¡Hola, preciosa! —Un hombre corpulento apareció de pronto, bloqueándole el paso—. ¿Adónde vamos con tantas prisas?

Antes de que pudiese responder una mano gigantesca le tapó la boca con brusquedad, ahogando la enfurecida protesta de su garganta.

Capítulo 2

—Stanley, ¿quieres sujetarla con fuerza para que no chille? —El hombre robusto y bajo que estaba frente a Camelia miraba exasperado al gigante que la había agarrado por la espalda—. No tengo ganas de recibir un puñetazo en el ojo.

—Está bastante asustada, Bert —le explicó Stanley en tono de disculpa mientras intentaba sujetar los agitados brazos de Camelia al tiempo que le seguía tapando la boca—. Creo que tiene miedo.

—¡Pues claro que está asustada, tonto de remate! —le espetó Bert—. ¡Tiene que estarlo! —se apresuró a añadir mientras fruncía amenazadoramente sus oscuras y gruesas cejas al tiempo que se aproximaba a Camelia—. Una dama como ésta no está acostumbrada a tratar con un par de peligrosos asesinos como nosotros, ¿verdad que no, preciosa?

Camelia le propinó una patada en la espinilla con todas sus fuerzas.

—¡Maldita sea! —gritó Bert saltando sobre un pie—. ¡Joder! ¿Has visto eso? Me ha dado una patada justo en la espinilla, tendré suerte si no sangro. —Se agachó para frotarse con cuidado la pierna que le dolía—. ¿No puedes sujetarla mejor, Stanley, o necesitas que lo haga yo?

—Lo siento, Bert —se disculpó Stanley, procurando con valentía mantener a Camelia quieta mientras su enorme sombrero se caía al suelo—. No puedo sujetarle los brazos y taparle la boca, y encima impedirle que mueva los pies. ¿Qué hago, le saco la mano de la boca?

—No, no saques la mano de su boca, maldita cabeza de chorlito. ¿No querrás que se ponga a chillar y se presente aquí medio Londres?

—Tal vez no grite, si le pedimos que no lo haga.

—¡Oh, sí! ¡Qué buena idea! —se burló Bert, que, exasperado, puso los ojos en blanco—. ¡Claro, Stanley! Saca la mano de su boca y pídele por favor a la señora que no chille.

Stanley empezó a retirar la mano de la boca de Camelia.

—¡Para, gusano inútil! —gritó Bert, agitando los brazos como un pollo histérico—. ¡No lo decía en serio!

—Entonces ¿por qué lo has dicho? —inquirió Stanley, confuso.

—Estaba siendo irónico, ya sabes, cuando se expresa una cosa diciendo lo contrario.

Stanley cabeceó perplejo.

—¿Diciendo lo contrario? Entonces ¿cómo sabré cuándo hablas en serio o no?

—¡Dios! Te avisaré, Stanley, ¿de acuerdo?

—Pero ¿lo harás antes o después de decir algo irónico? —insistió Stanley, preocupado—. Porque quiero estar seguro de si hablas en serio o en broma.

—¡Por el amor de...! Te lo diré después, ¿vale? ¿Te parece bien?

—Preferiría que me lo dijeras antes —declaró Stanley—. Así me aseguraré de no hacer lo que me digas, porque en realidad será una broma.

—Muy bien, pues te lo diré antes. Te diré: «Stanley, ahora no me hagas caso porque voy a decir algo irónico», ¿vale?

Stanley sacudió la cabeza, completamente confundido.

—Pero si no quieres que haga algo, entonces ¿por qué lo dices?

—¡Jesús, María y José! ¡Está bien! —Bert tenía los ojos fuera de las órbitas—. No diré nada de nada, ¿de acuerdo? Y ahora, si no es mucha molestia, ¿podemos seguir con lo que estábamos?

—¡Por supuesto, Bert! —exclamó Stanley con amabilidad—. ¿Qué quieres que haga?

—Simplemente sujétala bien para que no pueda volver a darme una patada en la pierna —ordenó Bert mientras le dirigía a Camelia una mirada feroz.

—Pero es que no puedo sujetarle las piernas si no suelto otra cosa —explicó Stanley.

—Entonces rodéala con una pierna, para que no pueda mover los pies.

—Eso no está bien, Bert —le dijo un Stanley sensato—. ¿Por qué no te alejas un poco de ella para que no pueda alcanzarte con el pie?

—Porque quiero esa bolsa que tiene debajo del brazo.

—Ya la cojo yo.

Camelia forcejeó con fuerza, luchando por no despegar el brazo firmemente apretado contra su cuerpo, pero no era un rival para su enorme captor. Manteniendo una manaza sobre su boca, Stanley usó el resto de su enorme brazo para sujetarla con rapidez mientras le quitaba el ridículo de la muñeca y se lo tiraba a Bert.

—Vaya, vaya, ¿a ver qué tenemos aquí? —dijo Bert, chascando la lengua. Extrajo el dibujo arrugado que Camelia había apretujado apresuradamente en su bolsa y lo examinó—. ¡Ajá! Le brillaban los ojos cuando, victorioso, levantó la vista del valioso papel—. Por casualidad no estará este dibujo relacionado con su magnífica excavación en África, ¿verdad, señora? ¿No se lo habrá dado el gilipollas ése amigo suyo, el inventor?

Camelia lo miró con tranquilidad, como si no le importara lo más mínimo que le quitasen o no esa hoja de papel.

—Me lo temía —continuó Bert, que se introdujo el dibujo en el bolsillo—. A ver qué más tenemos aquí... —musitó, escudriñando la bolsa—. ¿Tiene pasta?

—Él no ha dicho nada de trincarle la pasta, Bert —objetó Stanley.

—Tampoco ha dicho que no se la trinquemos —señaló Bert pragmático mientras sacaba del ridículo de Camelia un pequeño monedero de piel y se apresuraba a contar las monedas que había en su interior—. Hemos hecho un gran trabajo y tenemos derecho a una parte del botín; así se hacen los buenos negocios —declaró, metiéndose el monedero en el bolsillo.

—¿Ya hemos terminado? —Stanley ejerció menos fuerza sobre Camelia; ahora que había dejado de forcejear no quería sujetarla más fuerte de lo necesario.

—No del todo. Tengo un mensaje para usted, señora —dijo Bert recalcando las palabras y acercándose a Camelia—. Aléjese de África —susurró mientras sacaba una pistola del abrigo— si no quiere ver cómo la palma el resto de sus magníficos trabajadores. Le aseguro que sobre su terreno ha caído una maldición; lo mejor que puede hacer una dama como usted es mantenerse alejada de él; de lo contrario, usted también la palmará, ¿entendido?

—Disculpen, caballeros. —De pronto, desde el otro extremo de la callejuela, se oyó una voz que arrastraba las palabras—. ¿Alguno de ustedes podría decirme por dónde se va a Blind Pig?

—¡No! —le espetó Bert, mirando ceñudo al borracho que se tambaleaba por la calle—. Y, ahora, ¡lárguese de aquí, jodido borracho!

—Es una taberna —explicó el hombre con voz indistinta, como si ese detalle pudiese ayudarles a orientarle mejor—. Van las mejores prostitutas de esta zona de Londres. Una de ellas es una auténtica joya; la llaman Millie la Magnífica, y no me avergüenza decir que le he entregado mi corazón, mi alma ¡y también la mayor parte de mi dinero! —Hipó con fuerza.

Bert lo apuntó con la pistola.

—Lárguese, pirado, o le agujerearé el culo.

—Disculpen... —El hombre se tambaleó hacia ellos—, creo que voy a vomitar. —Se agachó y apoyó las manos en las rodillas.

—¡Por el amor de Dios! —musitó Bert con una mueca de disgusto mientras el hombre comenzaba a tener horribles arcadas—. ¡Al menos podría hacerlo hacia el otro lado! —protestó bajando la pistola.

—No se encuentra bien, Bert —apuntó Stanley compasivamente—. A lo mejor se ha comido algo en mal estado.

Aprovechando el caos reinante, Camelia profirió lo que esperaba fuese un grito de desvanecimiento convincente y cayó en los brazos de Stanley.

—¿Y ahora qué pasa? —preguntó Bert, alarmado—. ¿Qué demonios le has hecho, Stanley?

—Yo no he hecho nada —se defendió Stanley mientras intentaba torpemente que Camelia no fuese a parar al suelo sucio—. Debe de haberse asustado y se ha desmayado, ¡ya te he dicho que estaba asustada, Bert! Y tú venga a hablar de palmarla. ¡A las señoras no se les habla así!

Doblada como una muñeca de trapo, Camelia sacó la navaja que llevaba enfundada en la bota mientras sus captores discutían acerca de quién era el causante de su desmayo. Una buena puñalada en el muslo de Stanley forzaría al gigante a soltarla. Luego arrancaría la navaja de su pierna y se la tiraría a Bert, haciendo que se le cayese el arma mientras ella huía.

«Uno... dos... tres...»

Una atronadora explosión atravesó el aire, seguida de otras dos. A su alrededor estallaron bolas de fuego.

—¡Socorro! —gritó Bert, corriendo calle abajo tan rápido como sus gruesas y cortas piernas se lo permitían—. ¡Nos están disparando! ¡Venga, Stanley, corre!

—Señora, hay que irse de aquí. —Stanley levantó a Camelia y la protegió con su cuerpo—. ¡Ese borracho se ha vuelto loco!

—¡Bájeme! —Desechó la idea de apuñalarlo al percatarse de que, al parecer, el gigante intentaba salvarla.

—¡Suéltela —ordenó Simon— o le cortaré en pedazos tan pequeños que las ratas se pasarán una semana entera comiéndose los restos! —Lanzó varios petardos más a sus huidizas siluetas, que explosionaron en una bola de fuego roja, verde y naranja.

—¡Maldita sea, esto parece un jodido ejército! —gritó Stanley que protegía a Camelia con su cuerpo mientras avanzaba pesadamente, ajeno al hecho de que ella tenía ahora una navaja en la mano.

—¡Por Dios, Stanley, déjala en el suelo! —instruyó Bert, jadeante—. ¡Es a ella a quien quieren, no a nosotros!

—Intentan salvarme, Stanley —le explicó Camelia tratando de separarse de su enorme pecho—. Déjame en el suelo.

Stanley frunció las cejas, preocupado.

—¿Seguro que se encuentra bien, señora? ¿No volverá a desmayarse?

—Estoy bien —le tranquilizó ella.

—Entonces, de acuerdo. —La plantó bruscamente en el suelo y la sujetó unos instantes hasta que estuvo seguro de que se aguantaba sola.

Otra serie de explosiones tronaron por la callejuela.

—¡Por Dios, Stanley, venga, corre! —chilló Bert.

Complaciente, Stanley corrió a paso largo por la calle para reunirse con su amedrentado compañero.

—¡A por ellos! —gritó Simon con dramatismo mientras alcanzaba a Camelia—. ¡Que no se escapen! —Siguió lanzando petardos hacia Stanley y Bert hasta que sus aterrorizadas siluetas llegaron al extremo de la callejuela y desaparecieron. Finalmente, se volvió a Camelia.

—Señor Kent —dijo jadeando, sorprendida—, ¿qué diablos hace aquí?

Simon la miró fijamente, reparando de inmediato en las manchas negras de su rostro, su despeinada melena sin sombrero, el roto en su vestido, sobre el hombro, y trató de controlar la rabia que sentía. Al llegar a la callejuela y ver a ese monstruo sujetando a Camelia mientras esa bola inmunda la amenazaba, se llenó de una ira distinta a cuantas había conocido hasta entonces. Por suerte, su sensatez habitual hizo que se pusiese a correr como un idiota. Estaba solo, desarmado, y era consciente de que él solo no podía enfrentarse con un gigante como Stanley, sobre todo si el enano de Bert lo apuntaba con una pistola.

Entonces recordó que llevaba unos petardos en el abrigo que se había puesto al salir de casa.

—Pues de pronto se me ha ocurrido, lady Camelia, que el coche en el que se ha subido lleva el escudo de lord Hibbert, que casualmente es uno de mis vecinos. Y me ha sorprendido un poco, sobre todo cuando he vuelto a asomarme y he visto que el carruaje seguía ahí, al parecer, esperando a llevar a lady Hibbert a visitar a una de sus amigas. Lord Hibbert me ha dicho que se ha subido usted por error en su carruaje y que luego ha salido disparada calle abajo; lo que ha despertado mi curiosidad lo suficiente para decidir ir en su busca, sólo para averiguar si, al fin, había logrado dar con su coche. —Enarcó las cejas con expresión burlona.

—Agradezco su preocupación, aunque le aseguro que habría podido lidiar yo sola con esos dos ladrones. —Camelia se levantó el borde de la falta e introdujo la navaja de nuevo en su bota.

—¿Acostumbra a ir con un cuchillo en la bota?

—Londres puede ser una ciudad muy peligrosa —observó—. Ésa es una de las razones por las que mi padre acabó cogiéndole tanta aversión; hay ladrones en todas partes.

—No me ha dado la impresión de que esos tipos fueran unos ladrones comunes.

—¡Claro que lo eran! —insistió Camelia. Como no sabía en qué momento de la escena había llegado Simon, decidió que lo mejor era minimizar el incidente—. Lo único que querían era mi bolsa, ¡y eso se han llevado!

—¿Es ahí donde había escondido el dibujo que me ha robado? —inquirió él con rostro impasible.

—Sólo lo he tomado prestado. Pensé que no le importaría; de todas formas tampoco iba a usarlo. Pretendía devolvérselo.

—¿Cuándo? ¿Después de dárselo a alguien más para que lo copiara y lo utilizara como base para construir su bomba de vapor? Estoy convencido de que la ley dictaminaría que es un robo sacar un dibujo de mi casa sin mi consentimiento, lady Camelia, por mucho que quiera llamarlo de otra manera.

—Pero usted me ha dicho que no le interesaba proteger sus ideas e inventos; que la ciencia y la tecnología no progresarían nunca si los científicos se guardaban para sí sus descubrimientos —replicó Camelia—. Y dado que no disponía de tiempo para invertirlo en esa bomba de vapor, he pensado que no hacía daño a nadie tomando prestado el dibujo sólo temporalmente. Pero me lo han robado, ¡es terrible!

—Por si le sirve de consuelo, la verdad es que no necesito el dibujo; me sé de memoria el diseño de ese motor.

—Pero ¡ahora saben que estoy en Londres para conseguir una bomba de vapor!

—¿Quiénes?

—Esos dos rufianes —se apresuró a contestar. No quería que Simon supiese que estaba siendo vigilada—. Me preocupa que le vendan su invento a algún otro científico, que lo construirá, se llevará el reconocimiento y ganará una fortuna a costa de su esfuerzo.

—Me conmueve su preocupación —declaró Simon con escepticismo—. Lo que no entiendo es por qué sus encantadores amigos, Stanley y Bert, tienen tanto interés en sus movimientos y por qué se sube usted en carruajes que no son suyos, y se escurre por callejuelas oscuras y desiertas con un dibujo robado y una navaja de quince centímetros oculta en su bota. ¿Le espera realmente un coche en algún lugar, lady Camelia, o es sólo otra de sus fascinantes mentiras?

—Mi cochero me espera en Great Russell Street, frente al museo —se sinceró Camelia—. Pensé que lo mejor era que me esperase allí.

—Déjeme adivinar... Le ordenó que estacionara ahí y entró en el museo, fingiendo que estaría en su interior varias horas; una forma perfectamente creíble de pasar la tarde para la hija de un respetado arqueólogo durante su estancia en Londres. Después salió discretamente del museo por otra puerta y anduvo hasta mi casa, creyendo que nadie sospecharía que había abandonado el museo sin usar su vehículo.

—Era un buen plan.

—Supongo que sí, hasta que aparecieron sus amigos Stanley y Bert. Es evidente que no son tan fáciles de engañar como usted pensaba. La cuestión es, ¿por qué tienen tantas ganas de que no regrese a África? ¿Hay algo en su excavación que les fascine especialmente?

—Como le dije, estoy a punto de realizar un descubrimiento muy importante. Hay un montón de arqueólogos por ahí a los que les encantaría quitarme la excavación y obtener el reconocimiento de lo que hallasen en ella.

—No creo que esos tipos fueran arqueólogos precisamente.

—¡Por supuesto que no! No son más que unos ladrones a sueldo de alguien que les ha dado la orden de seguir de cerca mis movimientos e intentar intimidarme.

—No tenía ni idea de que en el campo de la arqueología hubiera tanta rivalidad. ¿Se le ocurre quién puede ser este arqueólogo enemigo?

—No. En principio, a todos los miembros de la Sociedad Arqueológica Británica les parece absurdo que pueda haber nada relevante en Suráfrica, pero yo creo que hay alguno que sí comprende la magnitud del hallazgo que estoy a punto de realizar. Piensan que si logran asustarme, estaré dispuesta a vender mi terreno a cualquier precio al primer comprador que se presente. Y se equivocan. Jamás me iré de África. Y jamás dejaré mi excavación hasta haber desenterrado todas las reliquias que haya por desenterrar.

—Admiro su determinación.

Una pizca de esperanza iluminó los ojos de Camelia.

—¿Quiere eso decir que me ayudará?

—No, estoy tan comprometido con la consecución de mis inventos como usted con encontrar sus reliquias africanas, lady Camelia. Sin embargo, la acompañaré hasta su carruaje. —Zanqueó por la callejuela y recuperó su sombrero.

—No necesito que me acompañe —le informó Camelia con decisión, molesta de que siguiese negándose a ayudarle—. Le aseguro que soy perfectamente capaz de llegar yo sola a mi vehículo; siempre lo hago.

—Concédame ese placer —suplicó Simon mientras le entregaba el sombrero—. ¿No cree que es lo mínimo que puede hacer después de haberme robado el dibujo?

—Usted mismo ha reconocido que no lo necesitaba —Camelia se puso el laxo y sucio sombrero en la cabeza—; que se lo sabía de memoria.

—Entonces deje que la acompañe en agradecimiento por haberla salvado galantemente cuando estaba en apuros —propuso Simon—. Le confieso que mi actuación de borracho enamorado me ha parecido especialmente brillante.

—Agradezco su interés, señor Kent, pero lo cierto es que no necesitaba su ayuda. Tenía la situación controlada.

—Supongo que si llama controlada a estar inmovilizada por un gigante de dos metros de estatura mientras otro individuo amenaza con matarla, apuntándole a la cara con una pistola, entonces sí, admito que tenía la situación absolutamente controlada.

—Estaba a punto de asestarle un navajazo a ese monstruo en el muslo cuando apareció usted tambaleándose por la calle.

—¿En serio? ¿Ha hecho alguna vez algo así?

—He cazado y ayudado a matar animales grandes en un sinfín de ocasiones. Estoy convencida de que podría acuchillar los músculos de la pierna de un hombre sin ningún problema.

—Gracias por la advertencia —dijo Simon ofreciéndole su brazo.

—Disculpe, señor Kent, pero ¿no le preocupa que lo vean prácticamente a medio vestir? Por lo visto ha olvidado ponerse el sombrero y la corbata, y lleva la camisa desabrochada.

—He salido de casa con bastante prisa. —A Simon le hacía gracia su repentino decoro—. Aunque me temo que es habitual en mí salir de casa indebidamente vestido; es una de las consecuencias de estar casi siempre absorto. ¿Le molesta que vaya sin sombrero?

Camelia lo observó mientras se abotonaba la arrugada camisa sobre su musculoso pecho.

—En absoluto —contestó, mirándolo a los ojos con naturalidad—. Estoy acostumbrada a ver hombres sin sombrero.

—De acuerdo; entonces no tendrá inconveniente en que la acompañe hasta su carruaje. —Con la camisa correctamente abrochada hasta el cuello, le ofreció su brazo una vez más.

Ella suspiró.

—Dejaré que me acompañe, si eso le hace sentir mejor, señor Kent. —Posó la mano con suavidad sobre la fina tela de la manga de su abrigo. Su brazo era sorprendentemente duro y el calor penetró su guante de algodón, haciendo que sintiera un cosquilleo en la palma de la mano.

Caminaron en un agradable silencio, cambiando la humedad y la oscuridad de la callejuela por la luz plomiza de las calles. Hombres y mujeres con elegantes trajes y vestidos de noche paseaban a pie y en sus carruajes en dirección a alguna fiesta, cena o al teatro. Camelia sabía que Simon y ella formaban una pareja extraña: ella con su vestido de día penosamente desplanchado, despeinada y con el sombrero ladeado, y Simon con sus pantalones húmedos y abrigo arrugado. La gente les lanzaba miradas reprobadoras, sin duda pensando que no tenían derecho a andar entre la clase alta o, lo que era peor, dando por sentado que planeaban alguna fechoría como robar. Le irritaban sus miradas de censura. Miró a Simon de reojo, preguntándose si también le molestaría cómo llamaban la atención.

Para su sorpresa, su expresión era casi alegre mientras paseaban el uno al lado del otro. O no se daba cuenta del recelo con que los miraba la gente o no le importaba lo más mínimo.

—Había olvidado lo sumamente agradable que puede llegar a ser un paseo al atardecer —comentó—. Tengo que intentar esforzarme por salir un poco más de mi laboratorio.

—¿Cómo ha hecho esas explosiones en la callejuela? —inquirió Camelia con curiosidad.

—He utilizado unos cuantos petardos que había fabricado para entretener a mis hermanos pequeños y me había dejado en los bolsillos del abrigo. Tenía pensado hacerlos estallar la próxima vez que fuese a visitarlos.

—¿Esas enormes bolas de fuego eran simples petardos? Parecían disparos.

—Me gusta que mis petardos hagan mucho ruido y sean espectaculares —le confesó Simon—. Les añado sales metálicas y polvo clorinado para intensificar los colores y hacer que las explosiones sean más vistosas. Mi madre teme que algún día vuele algo por los aires, pero a mis hermanos les parecen geniales.

—¿Cuántos hermanos tiene?

—En total somos nueve, pero sólo hay tres todavía lo bastante pequeños para que les impresione un hermano mayor capaz de fabricar petardos. El resto tienen recuerdos de todos los incendios que estuve a punto de provocar cuando era un adolescente e intentaba averiguar cuánta pólvora se necesitaba para hacer saltar la tapa de una cazuela o ver cuánta luz podía generar una lámpara de aceite con cinco mechas en lugar de una sola.

—¿Y provocó algún incendio?

—Unos cuantos —admitió Simon, encogiéndose de hombros. Desembocaron en la calle del Museo Británico, frente al que había una media docena de carruajes esperando. Había un grupo de niños y adultos apiñados delante de uno de ellos, que se reían y señalaban algo—. Pero, afortunadamente, y pese a que Oliver, nuestro mayordomo, estaba convencido de que lo haría, nunca incendié la casa.

—Ése es mi coche —dijo Camelia señalando el vehículo negro de tamaño mediano en torno al que estaban los niños agrupados.

—¿Qué están mirando esos niños?

—A mi cochero. Suele llamar bastante la atención dondequiera que vaya.

Simon se acercó junto a Camelia al carruaje para ver qué tenía ese hombre que los niños encontraban tan fascinante.

Sentado en el banco del cochero había un africano delgado de unos cincuenta años o más. Su piel era oscura como el café y tenía profundas arrugas tras años de exposición al intenso sol africano. Tenía la mandíbula cuadrada, la frente ancha, los pómulos marcados, pero mejillas ligeramente hundidas, lo que indicaba que en algún momento de su vida la comida había escaseado. Estaba sentado con la espalda recta y la cabeza erguida, mirando al frente, su porte altivo, casi arrogante, revelando una nobleza y fortaleza de espíritu que a Simon le pareció inmensamente convincente. Estaba envuelto en una serie de magníficas túnicas, tejidas con intensos colores escarlata, zafiro y esmeralda. Sobre la cabeza llevaba un sencillo sombrero de piel de alas anchas, que no armonizaba con el resto de su exótico atuendo, pero que era mucho más práctico que los sofisticados sombreros de fieltro que la moda dictaba que debían llevar los caballeros londinenses. Su soberbia piel oscura, sus impresionantes túnicas y extraño sombrero habrían sido más que suficientes para despertar la curiosidad de todos los transeúntes, pero no era ninguna de esas cosas la causante de los gritos y carcajadas del grupo de niños.

Era el mono que subía y bajaba de su cabeza, y les tiraba cerezas.

—Zareb, te pedí que no dejaras salir a Oscar del vehículo —le reprendió Camelia.

—Quería ver a los niños —se defendió Zareb.

—Yo más bien diría que quería darles de comer —musitó Camelia. Alargó los brazos en dirección al mono, que gritó contento de verla y bajó de un salto de la cabeza de Zareb para aterrizar tranquilamente en sus brazos—. En serio, Oscar, si quieres que te lleve conmigo tendrás que aprender a quedarte dentro del carruaje.

Oscar soltó un grito de protesta y rodeó el cuello de Camelia con uno de sus delgados y peludos brazos.

Zareb miró a Camelia con sus ojos de color pasa, reparando rápidamente en su aspecto desaliñado. A continuación miró a Simon fijamente un buen rato, como si tratase de ver más allá de su aspecto igualmente desarreglado. Al fin, centró su atención de nuevo en Camelia.

—¿Podemos volver ya?

—Podemos volver a casa —contestó Camelia, consciente de que Zareb no se refería a eso. Se volvió a Simon.

—Gracias por acompañarme hasta el carruaje, señor Kent, y por haber acudido en mi ayuda. Le pido disculpas por haberle causado tantas molestias y por haber perdido su dibujo.

—No es necesario que se disculpe. —Una vez más había llegado el momento de decir adiós y, de nuevo, Simon estaba curiosamente reacio a despedirse de ella—. ¿Está segura de que estará bien?

—¡Por supuesto! —repuso Camelia, intentando impedir que Oscar le sacase las últimas horquillas de su pelo dorado—. Estaré bien. Si por cualquier motivo cambia de opinión, señor Kent, vivo en Berkeley Square número veintisiete. Me quedaré aquí unas cuantas semanas más antes de regresar a Suráfrica.

Simon titubeó. No estaba muy seguro de cómo debía despedirse de ella. Un caballero le besaría la mano, pero dado que tenía las dos manos ocupadas para evitar que el mono jugara con su pelo, la cosa estaba un tanto difícil.

—Está bien, pues, ya nos veremos, lady Camelia —logró decir, como si creyese que algún día tropezaría con ella por la calle. Le abrió la puerta del carruaje y le ofreció la mano para ayudarle a subir.

Oscar trepó por su brazo y se subió en su cabeza, sobresaltándolo.

—¡Oscar, baja de ahí inmediatamente! —ordenó Camelia.

El animal protestó con insolencia y sacudió la cabeza, agarrándose del pelo de Simon.

—¡Oscar, baja ahora mismo —exclamó Camelia en tono de advertencia— o no te daré galletas de jengibre después de cenar!

El mono le dedicó una descarada sonrisa, provocando las risas de la multitud que seguía aglomerada alrededor del vehículo.

—¡Oscar, baja! —intervino Zareb—. ¡Qué paciencia!

Oscar vaciló, como si estuviese pensando qué hacer. Después le dio unas palmadas a Simon en la cabeza y saltó sobre el gastado terciopelo del asiento del carruaje.

—Lo siento —se disculpó Camelia—. Normalmente no hace eso; suele portarse bastante bien. —No era ni remotamente cierto, pero Simon no tenía por qué saberlo.

—No pasa nada. ¿Siempre lo lleva con usted?

—No siempre, pero me temo que en esta casa se agobia un poco. Está acostumbrado a tener mucha más libertad en África, pero no puedo dejar que pasee solo por Londres. Debería quedarse en el interior del vehículo cuando salimos, pero no le gusta. No está habituado a permanecer encerrado.

—Lo comprendo. —Simon le ayudó a subirse al carruaje y cerró la puerta.

Camelia lo miró esperanzada.

—¿Cree que es posible que reconsidere mi oferta, señor Kent?

Simon titubeó, conmovido por sus implorantes ojos extraordinariamente verdes. Durante unos instantes estuvo tentado de decirle que sí. Aunque, por desgracia, era muy consciente de sus obligaciones. Le había jurado a su hermano Jack, propietario de una floreciente empresa naviera, que dedicaría todo el tiempo posible a desarrollar un motor mejor de propulsión marina. Jack quería que la North Star Shipping presumiese de tener los barcos más rápidos del mundo, y Simon estaba decidido a hacer que eso sucediese. Luego estaba la miríada de inventos en los que estaba trabajando, incluida su lavadora, que tenía que estar lista en sólo seis semanas para mostrarla en la feria de la Sociedad para el Avance Tecnológico Industrial. Por mucho que le disgustase la parte financiera de su profesión, por desgracia había asuntos financieros que no podían ser ignorados. Si bien hasta el momento algunos de sus inventos habían sido fabricados en pequeña escala, eso no había generado suficientes ingresos para que pudiese continuar trabajando.

Aunque quisiese dejarlo todo e irse a África con lady Camelia, simplemente, no podía permitírselo.

—Haré indagaciones para ver si encuentro a alguien que pueda ayudarle —le ofreció Simon—. Estoy convencido de que hay algún fabricante de bombas en Londres dispuesto a alquilarle una y enviársela en barco a Suráfrica.

Camelia asintió, intentando ocultar su decepción. Ya se había puesto discretamente en contacto con todos los fabricantes de bombas que había en Londres, y todos habían rehusado su petición, alegando escasez de maquinaria disponible o que ella no pudiera pagarles. Pero Camelia sabía que no era ése el motivo por el que la rechazaban.

Como proveedores del monopolio que controlaba el mercado de bombas de Suráfrica, habían recibido instrucciones de no suministrarle una bomba a menos que quisieran rescindir sus contratos.

—Gracias, es usted muy amable.

Zareb sacudió las riendas y el carruaje empezó a avanzar. Oscar se levantó de un brinco para gritarle a Simon, lo que provocó más risas entre la multitud todavía apiñada junto al vehículo.

Simon observó cómo el coche se alejaba tranquilamente por la calle antes de torcer y ser engullido por las sombras cada vez más frías de la noche. Al fin, con una extraña sensación de soledad, se volvió y comenzó a andar a paso lento hacia su casa.

Olió el humo antes de verlo.

Volvió la esquina de su calle y vio a un montón de gente arremolinada frente a su casa, contemplando con horror las refulgentes llamas naranjas que bailaban tras las ventanas.

«¡Dios mío!»

Le inundó el pánico. Apenas si oía el eco de las campanas a lo lejos, que indicaba que los caballos que arrastraban las bombas aspirantes del Cuerpo de Bomberos Metropolitano estaban en camino. Se había formado una fila de más o menos veinte hombres que rápidamente se pasaban unos a otros cubos llenos de agua, que el hombre fornido del extremo de la hilera arrojaba con valentía a la casa. Pero el agua salpicaba en vano la fachada sin llegar al humo y las llamas que se extendían por las habitaciones del interior.

—¡Déjenme paso! —gritó Simon, tratando de abrirse paso entre la multitud de espectadores fascinados que bloqueaban la calle llena de humo—. ¡Es mi casa! ¡Déjenme pasar!

—¡Es él! —exclamó alguien—. ¡Es Kent, el inventor! ¡No está dentro de la vivienda!

Atónita, la muchedumbre se disgregó formando un estrecho sendero para que Simon pudiese llegar a su casa.

—Siempre he sabido que acabaría quemando la maldita casa entera —murmuró alguien más cuando él pasó por delante—. Eso pasa por inventar tantas tonterías.

—Pues tendremos suerte si sólo se quema su casa —añadió otro espectador.

—Si el viento empieza a soplar, el fuego se propagará por toda la calle —soltó otra persona—. Miren qué altas son las llamas.

—¡Deberíamos haberlo expulsado del barrio! —gritó furiosa una mujer—. En mi opinión, la ley tendría que prohibir estas cosas.

Simon la ignoró, concentrado en la escena de su casa en llamas. Siempre había sabido que a sus vecinos no les gustaba que un inventor viviese entre ellos; sobre todo un inventor con un pasado no precisamente inmaculado. El calor era ahora más intenso y el aire, denso por el humo y las cenizas. Una irrespirable columna negra salió por la puerta principal abierta, pero el vestíbulo y las escaleras que había tras ésta estaban a oscuras, lo que significaba que las llamas aún no habían llegado hasta allí. Simon se quitó de pronto el abrigo, cubriéndose la cara con él mientras corría hacia las escaleras que comunicaban la calle con la entrada de servicio de la cocina.

—¡No intente entrar! —le advirtió uno de los hombres que ayudaba a pasar cubos de agua—. ¡No vale la pena arriesgarse por un montón de chatarra!

Simon apenas lo oyó mientras miraba por las ventanas y veía cómo se quemaba su laboratorio. Con los ojos entornados debido al bochornoso calor y al humo, vio los restos de casi once años de trabajo esparcidos por el suelo. Todos sus libros y papeles se estaban quemando y todas las mesas, sobre las que había un sinfín de prototipos, proyectos en marcha y más de una ilusión, se habían caído. Su magnífica lavadora, que habría supuesto que en tan sólo un par de meses revolucionaría el sistema de lavado de la ropa, estaba volcada sobre un costado, inservible. El enorme barreño de agua se había salido de su estructura y había caído rodando, dejando que las llamas lamieran la construcción de acero de su motor de vapor.

—Lo lamento, señor, pero será mejor que salga de aquí —dijo una voz—. Es peligroso que esté tan cerca; los cristales podrían estallar en cualquier momento. Ya no puede usted hacer nada.

Simon se volvió y vio a un joven y serio bombero de pie, a sus espaldas. Los caballos habían traído tres bombas y unos treinta bomberos pertrechados empezaron a rociar la casa con agua. Pese a que se movían con rapidez, Simon era consciente de que no había absolutamente ninguna esperanza de que salvasen su casa, excepto tal vez la fachada. Lo único que podían hacer era tratar de impedir que las llamas se propagasen a las casas colindantes.

—¿Ha visto alguna vez un incendio en el que el fuego vuelque mesas y un artefacto que pesa más de doscientos veinticinco kilos?

El bombero lo miró confuso.

—No, señor. No, a menos que se haya producido algún tipo de explosión.

Simon lanzó una última y dolorosa mirada a su laboratorio en ruinas, esforzándose por controlar la impotencia y la rabia que le invadía.

—Yo tampoco.

Capítulo 3

Zareb anduvo despacio hasta el comedor sosteniendo el preciado sobre en su curtida y oscura mano.

El sobre había viajado desde Suráfrica y tenía marcas, manchas y arrugas que ponían de manifiesto su largo y arduo trayecto. Había venido a caballo, en tren y en barco, había viajado casi cuatro semanas surcando el encrespado océano para estar cada vez más cerca de ellos. Lo apretó fuerte, deseando sentir su calor originario. Añoraba las liberadoras caricias del cálido sol africano, que brillaba como un magnífico círculo de oro fundido en contraste con la extensión intensamente azul del cielo. En Londres el cielo solía estar encapotado y un perpetuo velo de repugnante y hediondo humo flotaba en todas partes, como resultado de decenas de miles de lumbres que ardían de la mañana a la noche. Daba la impresión de que las casas estaban construidas unas encima de otras, formando bloques de ladrillo y piedra que a Zareb le recordaban una prisión, y en su interior la gente se recluía en habitaciones oscuras atestadas de gruesas telas y recargados muebles. No había espacio, ni aire ni luz, y por lo que había visto, tampoco había alegría en esta ciudad llamada Londres.

Cuanto antes se llevase a Camelia a casa, mejor.

La encontró sentada frente a la mesa del comedor, con la cabeza inclinada y las cejas fruncidas, concentrada en la carta que estaba escribiendo. Oscar estaba sentado a su lado, en la mesa, mientras comía cacahuetes con avidez y llenaba la mesa y la alfombra de cáscaras rotas. Desde su llegada a Londres, el animal poco podía hacer aparte de comer y meterse en líos. Y Zareb pensó que, si comía, eso al menos significaba que no estaba haciendo ninguna travesura. Aunque esperaba que su pequeño amigo no se empachase o engordase tanto que no pudiese moverse con su habitual agilidad. El turaco unicolor de Camelia, una espectacular y presumida hembra de pájaro llamada Harriet, se había posado sobre el respaldo de una de las sillas del comedor y se contemplaba en el espejo ovalado que Camelia había colgado de la lámpara de araña para que se entretuviese. Cuando Zareb entró, el ave graznó y batió las alas anunciando su presencia.

—Tienes carta, Tisha —le dijo Zareb a Camelia, llamándola por el nombre africano que él le había puesto de pequeña—. Es del señor Trafford. —Hizo una breve pausa para saber si quería saber más.

—¿Y?

—Sopla un viento oscuro. —No se lo habría dicho, si no se lo hubiese preguntado. Le disgustaba agobiarla con más cosas—. Es cuanto percibo.

Camelia asintió. ¡Naturalmente que soplaba un viento oscuro! En su opinión, llevaban meses así, de modo que ¿por qué iba a cambiar hoy? Suspiró y dejó la pluma. Tal vez Zareb se equivocase. La verdad es que no recordaba que se hubiese equivocado nunca, pero en ocasiones lo que decía era lo bastante impreciso para que pudiese hacerse una libre interpretación. Soplaba un viento oscuro. «muy bien», pensó, reprimiendo la ansiedad que le oprimía el pecho. Cogió el sobre que Zareb le dio y lo abrió. «A ver qué me trae hoy este viento.»

—Ha habido otro accidente en la excavación —declaró en voz baja, repasando rápidamente el contenido de la carta del señor Trafford, su capataz—. Han intentado sacar el agua a mano, pero el terreno está inundado y los muros que construimos en el margen sureste se han vuelto inestables. Uno de ellos se derrumbó de pronto, matando a Moswen e hiriendo a otros cuatro hombres. Se han ido nueve trabajadores más.

Dejó la carta encima de la mesa y tragó saliva. Moswen era un buen hombre. Sólo llevaba dos meses trabajando para ella, pero era fuerte y voluntarioso, y le había parecido que se alegraba de verdad cada vez que encontraban una nueva reliquia. Y ahora había muerto por su culpa. Y otros cuatro estaban heridos. El señor Trafford no mencionaba nada acerca de la gravedad de las heridas, pero Camelia suponía que el hundimiento de un muro podía causar daños terribles. Se llevó los dedos al pinchazo que acababa de darle en la sien.

—Hay más —dedujo Zareb. No era una pregunta, sino una afirmación.

Camelia asintió.

—Ahora los trabajadores restantes están aún más convencidos de que hay una maldición sobre el terreno. Le han dicho al señor Trafford que se irán a menos que yo les suba el suelo para compensarles por el peligro que corren ellos, y sus familias por extensión, trabajando en un área maldita. Les ha prometido más dinero para mantenerlos tranquilos hasta que tenga noticias mías. Quiere saber qué debe hacer.

Zareb esperó.

—Le escribiré para decirle que le ofrezca a cada uno un quince por ciento más que les pagaré cuando finalicen sus contratos.

—Eso no les satisfará, Tisha —objetó él en voz baja—. Sólo son hombres y están asustados. Temen morir antes de que terminen sus contratos. Debes darles algo ahora, para demostrarles que tienes fe en ellos. Debes recordarles que su lealtad será recompensada.

—Pero ¿cómo voy a pagarles más ahora, si ni siquiera tengo dinero para pagarles lo que aún les debo?

—El dinero llegará. Está en camino.

—¿Cuándo? ¿Cómo?

—Llegará —insistió Zareb—. Lo obtendrás; lo sé.

Camelia suspiró.

—Agradezco tu confianza en mí, Zareb, pero hasta el momento no he conseguido apalabrar la financiación que necesitamos para continuar el proyecto. Los amigos de la edad de mi padre se han negado a invertir más dinero, porque ahora que él ha fallecido no creen que yo tenga la capacidad de triunfar donde él no lo hizo. Ningún fabricante de bombas de la ciudad ha accedido a suministrarme maquinaria; me dijeron que no era solvente o que no tenían máquinas disponibles, pero yo sé que en realidad es porque la De Brees Company les ha dicho que no negocien conmigo. Mi última esperanza era el señor Kent y también me ha negado su ayuda.

De hecho, su última esperanza había sido el dibujo de Simon, pero incluso ésta se había desvanecido. No conocía a nadie más en Londres que pudiese construir una bomba de vapor y que todavía no hubiese sido contratado por uno de los fabricantes que se negaban a tener tratos con ella. Camelia no le había dicho a Zareb que le había robado un dibujo a Simon; Zareb era un hombre intachable.

Por mucho que quisiese a Camelia y deseuse su éxito, no aprobaría que para obtenerlo recurriese a un vulgar robo.

—El señor Kent te ha ayudado —repuso Zareb—. Te ayudó en la callejuela.

—No necesitaba su ayuda —protestó Camelia—; tenía la situación bajo control.

Había vuelto al carruaje en tan lamentable estado que no había tenido otra opción que explicarle a Zareb lo sucedido con los dos hombres que el día anterior habían intentado amedrentarla. Le describió el incidente como un simple robo a manos de dos miserables ineptos. Le aseguró que la habían sobresaltado únicamente por no haber sido suficientemente cauta mientras andaba; un error que no volvería a cometer. No podía dejar que Zareb creyese que estaba en peligro. Bastante se preocupaba ya por ella su viejo amigo, que para empezar no la había dejado viajar sola a Inglaterra. No le habría gustado enterarse de que alguien había contratado un par de matones para forzarle a abandonar su excavación.

Londres ya le parecía bastante sucio, incivilizado y atestado de bárbaros.

—El señor Kent volverá —insistió Zareb—. No quiere, pero lo hará.

Camelia lo miró con escepticismo.

—¿Cómo lo sabes?

—Lo sé.

Ella suspiró. Sabía que no podía hacerle más preguntas sin correr el riesgo de insultarlo. Cuando Zareb aseguraba que sabía algo, se aferraba a ello con la tozudez de un león que protege su *kill*.

De repente alguien aporreó la puerta principal, haciendo que Harriet graznase asustada y revoloteasé sobre la mesa del comedor. Sobresaltado, Oscar saltó al hombro de Camelia, volcando de paso el tintero.

—¡Oh, no, mi carta! —Cogió rápidamente la carta que había estado escribiendo y observó con desespero cómo las gotitas negras se deslizaban por ella y caían en la rayada superficie de la mesa—. Se ha echado a perder.

Oscar soltó una serie de gritos acusatorios a Harriet y luego apoyó la cara con docilidad en el cuello de Camelia.

—Oscar no está a gusto aquí —comentó Zareb—. Le falta espacio. —Las maravillosas túnicas de colores que llevaba crujieron mientras salía de la habitación para ir a abrir la puerta.

—No pasa nada, Oscar —musitó Camelia, acariciando el lomo del mono arrepentido. Dejó la estropeada carta encima de la mesa, extrajo un arrugado pañuelo de lino de su manga y se puso a absorber enérgicamente la tinta para que no gotease sobre la alfombra—. Ha sido sin querer.

—Ha venido lord Wickham, mi lady —anunció Zareb con solemnidad.

Un hombre joven, alto, guapo, de pelo de color arena y ojos de color miel apareció en el comedor.

—¡Elliott! ¡Cómo me alegro de verte! —Camelia corrió hasta él y cogió ansiosamente sus brazos alargados—. ¡Oh, no! —se lamentó, mirando con horror las huellas negras que sus dedos manchados de tinta habían dejado en la piel de Elliott—. ¡Cuánto lo siento!

—No te preocupes, Camelia. —Elliott sacó enseguida un pañuelo de lino blanco perfectamente doblado del bolsillo de su actual abrigo hecho a medida y se limpió la tinta de las manos lo mejor que pudo, hasta que su piel pasó de ser negra a sólo de color gris sucio—. Ya está, ¿lo ves? Esta vez venía preparado —dijo medio en broma.

Aún agarrado al cuello de Camelia, Oscar le gritó malhumorado.

Elliott frunció las cejas.

—Veo que sigo sin caerle bien a Oscar.

—Lo cierto es que no le cae bien casi nadie —replicó Camelia, tratando de sacarse al animal de encima—. Y aquí aún está peor; todo le resulta extraño.

—Hace muchos años que me conoce, Camelia, tendría que resultarle familiar.

—Bueno, es que me parece que no le gusta pasar la mayor parte del tiempo encerrado en esta casa —continuó Camelia, que hizo una mueca de dolor cuando Oscar le hundió obstinadamente sus pequeños dedos en el hombro—. ¡Ya basta, Oscar! —le reprendió mientras lo apartaba de sí y se lo daba a Zareb—. Vete con Zareb.

Elliott miró a Zareb expectante, esperando a que el criado se ausentase.

Pero Zareb le devolvió tranquilamente la mirada y se quedó donde estaba.

—Quizá podríamos tomar un té, Zareb —sugirió Elliott.

—Gracias, lord Wickham, pero no tengo sed.

Elliott apretó ligeramente los labios.

—No me refería a usted, Zareb, sino a lady Camelia y a mí.

Zareb se volvió a Camelia.

—¿Te apetece un té, Tisha?

Camelia reprimió un suspiro. La tensión entre ambos hombres arrancaba desde que ella tenía trece años, cuando fue por primera vez a Suráfrica para trabajar junto a su padre.

—Sí, Zareb, si no te importa prepararlo, te lo agradecería.

—Muy bien, Tisha. —Zareb se dirigió entonces a Elliott—. ¿Y usted, mi lord, quiere un té también?

Camelia vio que Elliott asentía, manifiestamente satisfecho de que Zareb obedeciese. El pobre no entendía el comportamiento de Zareb, por lo que no había podido darse cuenta de que, en realidad, Zareb acababa de ofrecerle un té a Elliott en calidad de anfitrión en lugar de criado. La diferencia era sutil.

Pero para Zareb era crucial.

—Tendrías que haberme hecho caso y haberlo dejado en África —comentó Elliot cuando Zareb salió del comedor—. Ya te advertí que Londres no era un buen sitio para ese viejo criado. No sabe comportarse.

—Zareb no es mi criado, Elliott —recalcó Camelia—. Era amigo de mi padre y ha dedicado su vida entera a cuidar de mí. Jamás me habría dejado venir sola a Londres.

—Era el criado nativo de tu padre —repuso Elliott con énfasis—. El hecho de que a lo largo de los años tu padre y él establecieran cierta clase de extraña amistad no cambia las cosas. Entiendo que sienta cariño por ti, Camelia, pero no tiene derecho a influir en tus decisiones. No deberías haberlo traído, igual que a ese ridículo mono y, ya puestos, a ese pájaro tampoco. La gente no hace más que hablar y detesto enormemente lo que dicen.

—No me importa lo que la gente diga de mí —confesó Camelia—. No podía dejar a Zareb allí. Y, como no sabía cuánto tiempo estaríamos en Londres y era imposible hacerle entender al pobre Oscar que volveríamos, no tuve más opción que traerlo también. Si lo hubiese dejado en África, habría intentado seguirme y se habría acabado perdiendo.

—¡Por el amor de Dios, Camelia! ¡Es un mono! ¿Cómo diantres va perderse en África?

—Hasta los monos tienen un hogar, Elliott. El hogar de Oscar está con Zareb y conmigo. Si lo hubiéramos dejado allí, se habría sentido abandonado y habría hecho todo lo posible por encontrarnos. —Clavó los ojos en la alfombra y después miró de nuevo a Elliott—. ¿Por qué no vamos a la sala de estar —sugirió con repentino optimismo, agarrándole del brazo— y nos sentamos mientras esperamos el té?

Perplejo, Elliott miró hacia el suelo.

—¡Dios! —exclamó, dando un respingo y alejándose de la serpiente naranja y negra que se deslizaba por su bota—. ¡Camelia, no te acerques, podría ser venenosa!

—Sólo un poco. —Camelia se agachó para coger el animal de ochenta centímetros de largo—. Rupert es una serpiente tigre, por lo que su veneno no es especialmente peligroso para las personas. Supongo que tus botas le han llamado la atención, porque suele estar escondida.

Elliott la miró con incredulidad.

—¡No me digas que también te la has traído de África!

—La verdad es que no pretendía traerla, pero se escondió en uno de mis baúles mientras hacía las maletas. Cuando me di cuenta ya estábamos en alta mar. Aunque no me ha ocasionado ningún problema. Siempre y cuando esté bien alimentada y tenga un lugar caliente donde enroscarse, está más que satisfecha.

—Me alegra oír eso —logró decir Elliott, que miraba a la serpiente con recelo.

—¡A ver, Rupert! Quédate aquí con Harriet y pórtate bien —ordenó Camelia mientras dejaba la serpiente de ojos protuberantes sobre el gastado terciopelo de una de las sillas del comedor—. Volveré dentro de un rato y te daré de comer. —Cerró las puertas del comedor al salir y luego condujo a Elliott a la sala de estar, en el piso de arriba.

—Me preocupas, Camelia —empezó a decir a Elliott mientras ella se sentaba en el sofá—. Esto no puede seguir así mucho más tiempo.

—¿El qué?

—No puedes vivir sola en esta casa con esos animales salvajes. La gente habla y no me gusta lo que dice.

—En primer lugar, no vivo sola, vivo con Zareb.

—Lo que de por sí ya es problemático. Como mujer soltera no deberías estar viviendo aquí con un hombre, aunque sea sólo tu criado. No es correcto.

Camelia se abstuvo de repetir que Zareb no era su criado.

—Sea o no sea correcto, éstas son mis circunstancias. Sabes que Zareb ha cuidado de mí desde que era pequeña, Elliott, y me sorprende que creas que es indecoroso el hecho de que siga viviendo conmigo después de todos estos años. Las cosas no han cambiado.

—Tu padre ha muerto, y eso lo cambia todo —insistió Elliott—. Sé que te cuesta entenderlo, Camelia. Te has pasado la mayor parte de tu vida siguiendo a tu padre en sus excavaciones sin una institutriz o dama de compañía que te cuide como Dios manda. Y aunque tu padre quiso complacerte dejando que te quedaras con él y vivieras una vida sin duda inapropiada para una niña de tu edad, ahora que ha fallecido es importante que pienses en tu reputación.

—La única reputación que me interesa son mis logros como arqueóloga. Si la gente quiere hablar de mí, debería hacerlo de mi trabajo y no de con quién vivo o de qué animales me he traído de África. De verdad, no comprendo qué les importan esas cosas.

—Lo que la gente debería hacer y lo que hace en realidad son dos cosas completamente diferentes. Te guste o no, tu reputación como mujer soltera también afecta a tu reputación como arqueóloga. Estás aquí para recaudar más fondos para tu expedición ¿no? Y qué, ¿has tenido éxito?

—Algo he conseguido, pero aún no he terminado.

No quería que Elliott se enterase de las tremendas dificultades que tenía para obtener el dinero necesario para continuar la excavación. Desde que su padre falleció, Elliott había estado intentando persuadir a Camelia de que abandonase el terreno y lo vendiera. Él mismo había estado allí quince años, trabajando al lado de su padre, y aunque su amor por África y su lealtad hacia lord Stamford lo retuvieron en el continente durante años, se fue convenciendo gradualmente de que en ese lugar no había nada valioso. El profundo cariño que Elliott sentía por Camelia le llevaba a protegerla, y Camelia sabía que él no quería ver cómo se gastaba el poco dinero que le había dejado su padre y dedicaba al proyecto a lo mejor muchos años de su vida para fracasar, igual que había hecho su padre.

—¿Cuánto dinero has logrado recaudar? —inquirió él.

—Suficiente para seguir funcionando un tiempo —contestó ella sin precisar. Pero no podrían continuar mucho más tiempo si tenía que pagarle más dinero a sus trabajadores para evitar que se marchasen, aunque no era necesario que Elliott lo supiese—. Pero en breve obtendré más. He pensado en abordar a los socios de la Sociedad Arqueológica Británica en el baile que se celebrará esta misma semana para hablarles de mi excavación. Estoy segura de que en cuanto oigan hablar de las extraordinarias pinturas rupestres que encontramos el pasado mes de octubre estarán ansiosos por darnos su apoyo.

—Las pinturas rupestres no pueden ser trasladadas a un museo británico —recalcó Elliott—. Y a los socios de la sociedad les interesa más financiar empresas que compensen con creces su inversión; en otras palabras, les interesan los objetos que puedan traer aquí y vender a una colección.

—Estoy convencida de que los encontraremos en cuanto consigamos sacar el agua y seguir excavando.

—¿Has conseguido una bomba?

—La conseguiré.

—¿Has tenido noticias de Trafford?

—He recibido una carta suya esta mañana. Siguen intentando sacar el agua a mano.

—¿Es todo lo que te ha contado?

—Por desgracia, se ha derrumbado un muro y ha matado a uno de los trabajadores; un hombre joven, encantador y muy trabajador llamado Moswen. Cuatro más han resultado heridos.

Elliott sacudió la cabeza con pesar.

—Ahora los demás trabajadores estarán todavía más convencidos de que ha caído una maldición sobre el terreno.

—Cosa que tú y yo sabemos que es absurda. No hay ninguna maldición.

—Da igual lo que tú y yo creamos, Camelia, lo que importa es lo que crean los nativos. Si todos abandonan la excavación, ese terreno no valdrá prácticamente nada —observó con serenidad—. Deberías considerar en serio la oferta de compra de la De Beers Company, Camelia. Teniendo en cuenta que el terreno aún no ha demostrado poseer valor alguno, te han hecho una oferta muy razonable.

—A mí me parece que el terreno posee un valor extraordinario, Elliott.

—Tu padre no encontró un solo diamante en veinte años.

—Mi padre no buscaba diamantes.

—Sólo te digo que, dada tu actual situación financiera, tienes suerte de que la De Beers Company esté interesada en adquirirlo simplemente porque quiera ampliar sus posesiones alrededor de Kimberley.

—Elliott, ya te he dicho que nunca le venderé a De Beers el terreno para que lo acabe destrozando en busca de diamantes, sea el año que viene o dentro de cincuenta años. Ese terreno es una valiosa ventana al pasado y es preciso protegerla. Por eso tengo que volver allí lo antes posible. Cuando estoy yo los trabajadores no tienen tanto miedo; supongo que cuando ven a una mujer blanca dispuesta a excavar, su orgullo masculino les obliga a ser al menos igual de valientes.

—El orgullo no tiene nada que ver con esto. Sé que detestas oír esto, Camelia, pero los kaffirs* te consideran una fuente económica, nada más. Cuando se acabe el dinero, abandonarán la excavación y te quedarás sola.

—Entonces excavaré yo misma —insistió Camelia—; tarde los años que tarde.

—Eres tan tozuda y orgullosa como tu padre.

—Tienes razón, lo soy.

Él suspiró.

—Muy bien, Camelia. Haz lo que quieras. Yo también tenía pensado asistir al baile de la Sociedad Arqueológica, así que te acompañaré.

—Eres muy amable, Elliott, pero no es necesario, de verdad. Zareb me llevará.

—Zareb levantará rumores —repuso Elliott—. Con esas extravagantes túnicas africanas que lleva, cada vez que va a algún sitio la gente se acerca a tu carruaje atraída por su ridículo aspecto. No deberías consentirlo, Camelia, deberías ordenarle que llevase algo más acorde con su condición de criado, al menos durante el tiempo que permanezca aquí.

—La ropa inglesa es para los ingleses.

Camelia y Elliott se volvieron y vieron a Zareb en la puerta. Su rostro estaba impasible, pero sus labios apretados le indicaron a Camelia que había oído que Elliott le había llamado criado.

—Yo no cometo el error de pensar que soy inglés por estar en Inglaterra —intervino Zareb—, de la misma manera que estar en África no lo convierte a usted en africano, señor. —Dejó la bandeja que llevaba encima de la mesa que había delante del sofá—. Tu té, Tisha.

—Gracias, Zareb. —Camelia dudaba que Elliott hubiese entendido que Zareb acababa de insultarlo; ni se le pasaba por la cabeza que un blanco quisiese parecerse a un africano.

Oscar saltó sobre la mesa y cogió una galleta de jengibre del plato, tirando al suelo una jarra de leche.

—¡Oh, Oscar! —exclamó Camelia, que cogió al mono en brazos y le secó el líquido de las patas con una servilleta de lino—. ¿No podrías estarte quieto?

Contento de estar en sus brazos, Oscar empezó a devorar su galleta.

—Bueno, yo me tengo que ir, Camelia —le informó Elliott—. Espero que reconsideres mi ofrecimiento de acompañarte al baile.

—Te lo agradezco, Elliott, pero la verdad es que preferiría ir en mi coche —le aseguró Camelia—. Sé que te gustan este tipo de eventos, pero a mí me resultan aburridos y no quisiera que por mi culpa tuvieras que retirarte temprano. Seguro que estarás ansioso por contarles a los socios tu nuevo negocio de importación.

Una pizca de desengaño ensombreció su elegante rostro de facciones marcadas. Aunque le hubiese gustado seguir hablando con ella del tema, Camelia sabía que no lo haría delante de Zareb. Pese a haber pasado muchos años en Suráfrica, Elliott seguía concediendo mucho valor a las normas de la sociedad británica.

No había que discutir delante de los criados. Jamás.

—Muy bien. Nos veremos allí.

Elliott inclinó el cuerpo con la intención de besar la mano de Camelia, pero estaba todavía manchada de tinta y ahora también húmeda debido a las peludas patas de Oscar, que se habían mojado de leche; de modo que optó por un leve y formal movimiento de cabeza y a continuación siguió a Zareb escaleras abajo hasta la puerta principal.

Zareb puso la mano sobre el pesado pomo de cobre y notó que ardía. El calor traspasó la palma de su mano y sus dedos rígidos, que no habían dejado de dolerle desde su llegada a la desagradable humedad de Inglaterra. Estaba a punto de ocurrir algo, pensó. Algo significativo.

Abrió la puerta lentamente.

—Buenas tardes, Zareb —saludó Simon silabeando—. He venido a ver a lady Camelia.

Zareb lo observó con calma, valorando la percepción de la ira que emanaba de él. Era fuerte, pero no suficientemente intensa para explicar el calor que sentía en la mano. La energía que irradiaba el hombre blanco y desaliñado que estaba frente a él no era atribuible a su furia apenas refrenable. Había otra fuerza que emergía de este inventor de aspecto peculiar, que hablaba como un caballero, pero cuyo atuendo y modales mostraban que era indiferente a la estética de su clase.

—Por supuesto, señor —repuso Zareb abriendo más la puerta—. Pase, por favor.

Simon entró en el vestíbulo.

Elliott le echó un vistazo a su chaqueta y camisa arrugadas, y a sus pantalones y dedujo que se trataba de algún repartidor.

—Disculpe —dijo en tono educado pero inequívocamente condescendiente—, pero los repartos no suelen hacerse por la puerta principal.

Simon lo miró con curiosidad. El hombre que tenía delante era increíblemente guapo e iba impecablemente vestido, dos atributos que por alguna extraña razón sólo sirvieron para irritarle.

—Lo tendré en cuenta la próxima vez que venga a traer algo.

Elliott arqueó las cejas.

—Me debo de haber equivocado. Le pido disculpas. Soy lord Elliott Wickham —se presentó en un intento por arreglar su desliz—, ¿y usted, señor, es...?

—Simon Kent.

Elliott lo miró sorprendido.

—¿El inventor?

En ese momento Oscar, que daba gritos de alegría, apareció dando saltos por el pasillo y se encaramó a Simon, plantando con decisión su pequeño y huesudo trasero sobre su cabeza.

Simon frunció las cejas.

—¡Señor Kent! —Camelia miró a Simon extrañada mientras bajaba las escaleras. Estaba serio, lo que era comprensible, teniendo en cuenta que Oscar le había empezado a revolver el pelo rojizo en una afanosa búsqueda de piojos—. No esperaba verlo tan pronto.

Simon la miró fijamente; durante unos instantes se quedó sin habla. Camelia llevaba un sencillo vestido de día de seda verde pálido que acentuaba el extraordinario color salvia de sus ojos. El vestido se pegaba a las curvas de sus pechos y caderas como la lluvia que cae sobre las flexibles formas de un helecho, y un delicado volante de encaje de color marfil adornaba su provocativo y pronunciado escote. No llevaba polisón, lo que daba a entender que no le gustaba soportar la forzosa incomodidad de los atuendos femeninos cuando no estaba en público, y el cabello con mechas de color miel colgaba suelto, lo que le proporcionaba un aspecto encantadoramente dulce y desaliñado. Su aroma le embriagó una vez más; esa fragancia fresca y veraniega que olía a dulce hierba y a limón. Cuando sus miradas se encontraron y ella lo miró con esos ojos grandes y de un verde transparente, el calor creció en el interior de Simon, haciendo que se excitara y se sintiera extrañamente mareado.

¿Qué demonios le ocurría?

—Tenemos que hablar, lady Camelia —anunció, firmemente decidido a salir de su aturdimiento—. Ahora.

—¿De qué? —inquirió Elliott.

—El señor Kent es inventor, Elliott —le explicó Camelia—. Ayer fui a verlo para discutir un asunto de negocios.

Elliott observó a Simon con interés.

—¿Pretende venderle una bomba a lady Camelia?

Simon lo examinó de nuevo y llegó a la misma conclusión que la vez anterior. Elliott era un magnífico ejemplo del género de hombre conocido como caballero inglés engreído, desde el ángulo patricio de sus cejas enarcadas hasta el tremendo brillo de sus costosas botas marrones de cuero hechas a medida. Simon sintió una brutal e inmediata antipatía hacia él, lo que parecía un tanto injusto, teniendo en cuenta que aparte de haberlo confundido con un repartidor, el hombre no había hecho nada para fomentar su aversión.

—Lo lamento, Wickhip, pero es un asunto que nos concierne a lady Camelia y a mí. —Simon desvió la vista y miró a Camelia.

—Me llamo Wickham —le corrigió Elliott con suavidad—. Y estoy seguro de que, dado que soy uno de sus más antiguos amigos, lady Camelia no tendrá inconveniente en hablar en mi presencia de lo que sea que haya usted venido a hablar aquí.

—Eso lo dudo. —Los ojos azules de Simon lo miraron con dureza, penetrantes, haciendo que Camelia se sintiese violenta y entre dos aguas—. Sin embargo, si insiste...

—Lo cierto es que lord Wickham ya se iba —le interrumpió Camelia.

No podía imaginarse por qué Simon parecía tan enfadado con ella; al fin y al cabo, estaba al tanto de que le había robado el dibujo. Tal vez había roto algo muy importante al caerse contra las mesas de su laboratorio la tarde anterior.

—Nos veremos a lo largo de la semana, Elliott —se despidió ella colocando una mano sobre su brazo y conduciéndolo a la puerta—. Tranquilo, que te informaré de cualquier novedad, ¿de acuerdo?

—Está bien. —Camelia era consciente de la renuencia de Elliott a dejarla con Simon, pero él sabía que no podía imponer su presencia—. Señor Kent —dijo con educado movimiento de cabeza.

—Wicksted.

—Wickham.

—Naturalmente. —A Simon le sorprendía su absurdo deseo de fastidiarlo—. Le pido disculpas.

—Que tenga un buen día, señor. —Zareb acompañó a Elliott a la salida y cerró la puerta.

—Oscar, baja de ahí inmediatamente —ordenó Camelia, que extendió los brazos hacia el mono.

Oscar sonrió y sacudió la cabeza con insolencia.

—¿Siempre es tan efusivo? —preguntó Simon, alargando un brazo para soltar al tozudo mono de su pelo.

—Le ha caído usted bien —comentó Zareb asintiendo—. Y eso es bueno.

—Me siento halagado —repuso Simon con ironía. Al fin, logró sacarse al obstinado sinvergüenza del cuero cabelludo, que empezaba a dolerle, y dejarlo definitivamente en el suelo.

—¿Por qué no subimos a la sala de estar y tomamos un té, señor Kent? —sugirió Camelia.

—Ya está preparado —añadió Zareb, que intentaba persuadirlo—. Y hay galletas de jengibre. Me parece que están bastante buenas; las he hecho esta misma mañana.

Camelia miró a Zareb sorprendida, preguntándose qué diablos le había pasado de repente. No se había mostrado ni remotamente tan hospitalario con el pobre Elliott, y lo conocía desde hacía muchos años. ¿Acaso no percibía la hostilidad que emanaba de Simon?

Simon vaciló. Se había pasado la noche indignado, procurando asimilar el hecho de que se habían ido al traste varios años de trabajo, pero a la vez estaba hambriento; y eso que había ingerido un copioso desayuno a base de avena, salmón ahumado, salchichas y tostadas en la casa que sus padres tenían en la ciudad.

—¿Viene, señor Kent? —le instó Zareb, señalando las puertas abiertas de la sala de estar.

—Muy bien. —Simon siguió a Camelia esforzándose por no fijarse en el suave contoneo de sus caderas.

—Siéntese, por favor —le dijo Camelia señalando una silla desvencijada mientras ella se sentaba en un sofá igualmente desgastado.

—Sí, siéntese y tómese un té. —Sin molestarse en preguntarle cómo lo tomaba, Zareb puso tres cucharadas colmadas de azúcar en una taza, añadió un generoso chorro de leche y luego la llenó de té—. Y una galleta —comentó colocando un plato delante de Simon.

Simon aceptó el té y lanzó una mirada a las pastas oscuras que Zareb le ofrecía.

—Gracias —repuso, cogiendo educadamente una galleta.

—¿Le apetece un poco de pastel de pasas? —inquirió Zareb.

Camelia no lograba entender por qué su viejo amigo se esforzaba tanto por ser simpático con Simon. Desde su llegada a Londres no había hecho semejante despliegue de hospitalidad con nadie. Quizá creyese que Simon había cambiado de idea y estaba dispuesto a ayudarle.

Aunque, a juzgar por la cara de enfadado del señor Kent, a Camelia no le cabía ninguna duda de que no estaba ahí para brindarle su ayuda.

—El pastel de pasas está muy bueno con el té —le informó Zareb—. Voy a buscar un poco. —Salió de la habitación apresuradamente mientras las túnicas crujían en una explosión de intensos colores.

Hubo un tenso y momentáneo silencio.

—No esperaba verlo tan pronto —empezó Camelia con tiento.

—He tenido una noche movida; mi casa se ha incendiado.

Camelia se quedó boquiabierta.

—¡Oh, no! ¿Y se ha quemado todo?

Su sorpresa parecía auténtica, Simon advirtió. Pero no estaba seguro; algunas personas actuaban de maravilla cuando tenían que hacerlo, y algo le decía que lady Camelia entraba en esta categoría.

—Lamentablemente, sí.

—¿Qué provocó el fuego?

—Esperaba que usted pudiese arrojar un poco de luz sobre eso.

Camelia enarcó las cejas, asombrada.

—No creerá que yo he tenido nada que ver.

Simon permaneció callado.

—Le aseguro que mientras estuve en su laboratorio no hice nada que pudiese provocar un incendio. Claro que difícilmente hubiese podido hacerlo, porque usted no me quitó el ojo de encima en todo el rato.

—Pues no debí de vigilarla bastante, teniendo en cuenta que logró robar uno de mis dibujos.

Camelia estaba indignada.

—Yo no incendié su casa, señor Kent —insistió Camelia categóricamente—. ¿Por qué motivo iba a hacer algo semejante?

—Le dejé muy claro que no podía construir su bomba porque tenía muchos otros proyectos que requerían mi atención. Y hoy todos esos proyectos han sido reducidos a escombros, por lo que de pronto mi agenda está vacía. ¿No le parece una extraordinaria coincidencia?

¡Qué extraño!, pensó ella. En Suráfrica se habría culpado de un incidente como ése a los malos espíritus o a la maldición que ella y su padre habían supuestamente atraído a la excavación. O tal vez fuese parte del viento oscuro del que le había hablado Zareb.

Sintió un escalofrió en la espalda.

No creía en las maldiciones, se recordó a sí misma con firmeza. Cuanto ocurría tenía una explicación lógica y científica. Su padre le había enseñado eso desde que era pequeña y era un lema al que se había aferrado a lo largo de los años.

Incluso cuando había deseado con desespero un poco de suerte o el consuelo de algún buen espíritu que velase por ella.

—Lo que encuentro extraordinario, señor Kent, es que un hombre de su aparente inteligencia llegue a una conclusión tan irracional —contestó Camelia con frialdad—. Cuando ayer fui a verlo, lo hice con la esperanza de que estuviese dispuesto a suministrarme una bomba. Pero creo que también le dejé claro que respeto su trabajo, aunque es verdad que me decepcionó que no lo aparcase temporalmente para ayudarme. Como arqueóloga de cierto prestigio en el entorno académico y como empresaria de la que en este momento dependen un montón de hombres para su subsistencia, le aseguro que jamás arriesgaría mi reputación ni el bienestar de quienes dependen de mí para involucrarme en actividades ilegales. Estoy dispuesta a hacer muchas cosas para acelerar mi excavación, pero provocar incendios y destruir propiedades ajenas no está entre ellas.

Se puso de pie con solemnidad, con la espalda completamente recta y la barbilla levantada.

—Ahora que está todo aclarado, le ruego me disculpe, pero tengo una serie de asuntos urgentes que atender. Espero que sepa encontrar la salida.

—Muy bien, pero no se mueva —dijo Simon en voz baja y tensa.

Confundida por la repentina palidez de su rostro y su asustada mirada, Camelia se volvió.

—¡Oh, Rupert! —Soltó un suspiro, cogió a la serpiente de fiero aspecto del sofá y la dejó en la alfombra—. Sé un buen chico y quédate en el comedor. Prometo darte pronto de comer.

Rupert la miró apenado con sus ojos protuberantes y sin párpados, y se enroscó junto a sus pies en una brillante espiral de color naranja y negro.

Simon estaba estupefacto. Respiró hondo y procuró relajarse.

—¿También es suya?

—No la he comprado, si eso es a lo que se refiere. El año pasado me la encontré herida y cuando se curó por lo visto decidió que le gustaba vivir conmigo.

—Ya veo.

Inmensamente aliviado por no tener que reducir a una serpiente de un metro de largo, Simon dejó la taza y la galleta y observó al animal desde una distancia considerable.

—Siempre me han fascinado las serpientes. —Intentó hablar como si la súbita aparición del terrorífico reptil fuese de lo más normal—. Tienen una fuerza y una fluidez de movimientos increíble. ¿Es una serpiente coral?

—No, una tigre.

Simon asintió.

—Sí, debería haberlo sabido por las bandas. Entonces no es tan venenosa.

¡Menudo alivio! Porque, si no recordaba mal, cuando se ponían nerviosas las serpientes tigre podían atacar y pegar un mordisco fatal.

—Cuando era joven estuve un tiempo estudiando las serpientes —continuó—. ¿Qué le llevó a traérsela de viaje?

—Fue ella la que decidió venir. Se metió en uno de mis baúles mientras hacía las maletas. Cuando me di cuenta ya estábamos en el barco.

—De modo que es un polizón. —Si Simon se hubiese encontrado con una serpiente en la maleta, la habría cerrado y habría salido corriendo del camarote, sin importarle llevar la misma ropa durante todo el viaje—. ¿Y Oscar?

—Oscar no hubiese soportado mi ausencia y la de Zareb. Y como era imposible hacerle entender que volvería, no tuve más remedio que traerlo conmigo. También me traje a Harriet, mi turaco unicolor. Supongo que le parecerá ridículo. —Estaba ligeramente a la defensiva—. Por lo visto la mayor parte de la ciudad piensa eso.

—Hay familias de todos los tamaños y formas, lady Camelia. Empezando por la mía. —Siguió observando a Rupert, sin acercarse a la serpiente pero sin alejarse tampoco.

Camelia no dijo nada. Puede que al documentarse sobre Simon se hubiese equivocado con respecto a su edad, pero había logrado reunir unos cuantos datos de su infancia. Por lo visto era un huérfano escocés que había sido adoptado por Haydon y Genevieve Kent, marqueses de Redmond. Pese a que saltaba a la vista que las cosas le habían ido bien, recibiendo una educación excelente y convirtiéndose en un respetado conferenciante sobre un sinfín de temas, Camelia tenía la sensación de que no había salido indemne de su vida anterior; de que durante una parte de su infancia había estado solo y atemorizado.

Como ella muy bien sabía, era posible curar las heridas, pero las cicatrices permanecían para siempre.

—¿Por qué ha venido a verme? —preguntó en voz baja—. ¿De verdad pensaba que mi admiración por todo lo que ha conseguido era fingida? ¿Que soy el tipo de persona que para lograr mis objetivos destruiría egoístamente todo aquello que tanto ha luchado por crear?

Dicho así, sonaba horrible, pensó Simon. Pero si bien la noche antes había considerado esa opción, en el fondo sabía que no era posible. Tuviese los defectos que tuviese, estaba claro que a lady Camelia le gustaba descubrir y preservar, no destruir.

—No.

—Entonces ¿a qué ha venido?

Él siguió con los ojos clavados en Rupert, evitando mirarla. Lo cierto es que no sabía realmente por qué estaba ahí. Se había pasado la noche entera abrumado, presa de la ira y la desesperación. Sabía que podía volver a empezar. Como siempre, Genevieve y Haydon no habían dudado en mostrarle su apoyo. Ya se habían ofrecido a buscarle una nueva casa de alquiler, y Haydon iba a ingresarle dinero en su cuenta bancaria ese día para que pudiese comprar la maquinaria y el equipo preciso para continuar. Había sido un desagradable revés, pero no necesariamente insuperable. Ya no disponía de sus bocetos y dibujos, pero la información seguía grabada en su mente con relativa nitidez. Con mucho trabajo y muchas horas de dedicación podría recuperar lo que le habían arrebatado.

Entonces ¿qué hacía perdiendo el tiempo en casa de Camelia, dejando que un mono le revolviese el pelo y observando cómo se movía una maldita serpiente?

—Supongo que de algún modo intento comprender cómo una vida entera de trabajo puede haber quedado reducida a un amasijo de hierros y cenizas —comentó—. Esto no ha sido un simple accidente, lady Camelia. Quienquiera que incendiase mi laboratorio lo hizo con la intención de destruirlo junto con la casa entera.

—¿Qué le hace pensar eso?

—Cuando volví pude acercarme bastante a la casa para mirar por las ventanas de la cocina. Las mesas que yo había levantado estaban de nuevo volcadas y todo estaba esparcido por el suelo. La lavadora que había construido había sido destruida y su motor estaba volcado sobre un lateral. Debía de pesar unos doscientos veinticinco kilos; es imposible que las llamas lo tirasen al suelo.

—Pero había explosivos en su laboratorio, los que usó para fabricar los petardos —señaló Camelia—. A lo mejor hicieron explosión y el impacto hizo que el motor volcase.

—Esa es la razón por la que nunca guardo más explosivos de los que necesito para fabricar unos cuantos petardos. De joven ya viví unas cuantas experiencias que me enseñaron que el nitrato de potasio es peligroso. Incluso aunque hubiese explosionado mi arsenal de pólvora entero, lo único que se habría producido es una gran detonación y una humareda impresionante. Además, lo curioso es cómo se incendió la casa.

—¿A qué se refiere?

—Cuando llegué, las habitaciones del piso de arriba ardían, igual que mi laboratorio, que como sabe estaba en el sótano. Sin embargo, la planta baja y las escaleras no estaban en llamas, sólo había humo, que debía de haber ascendido por las escaleras de la cocina.

—Pero no tiene sentido —objetó Camelia—. ¿Cómo podían arder las habitaciones, si el incendio se había iniciado en la cocina y aún no había llegado a la escalera?

—Eso mismo pensé yo. La única explicación lógica es que alguien hurgara en mi laboratorio y lo incendiase, y luego decidiese quemar el piso de arriba... O a lo mejor eran dos personas y cada una se ocupó de incendiar un piso, pensando que probablemente el fuego se propagaría al resto de la casa.

—Suponiendo que el incendio haya sido provocado, ¿qué le hace pensar que yo he tenido algo que ver? Podría haber sido un inventor celoso que quisiese destruir todo lo que usted ha conseguido.

—Me halaga que crea que mi trabajo pueda haber atraído a tan devoto admirador. Pero, como ya le he dicho, nunca he ocultado mis ideas ni he llevado un gran control de mis patentes. La idea de que algún rival demente destroce mi laboratorio para ganar tiempo fabricando sus propios inventos me parece bastante improbable.

—Quizá no intentase comprometer su trabajo. Puede que le robase sólo un boceto y luego quemase su laboratorio para tener tiempo para concluir un prototipo, y registrar la patente de lo que le robó.

—En ese caso espero que consiga ajustar la tensión de la fregona; de lo contrario, que se prepare para recibir un montón de quejas.

Camelia lo miró exasperada.

—Yo no le veo la gracia.

—No creo que haya sido obra de un inventor obsesionado, lady Camelia. Mi intuición me dice que usted tiene algo que ver en todo esto. —La miró con seriedad—. ¿Qué querían ayer exactamente esos dos hombres de la callejuela?

Ella se encogió de hombros con indiferencia.

—Ya le dije que probablemente los hubiese contratado algún arqueólogo interesado en ahuyentarme de la excavación.

—Sé lo que me dijo, pero quiero saber la verdad.

Camelia sostuvo su mirada. Simon no le había dado esperanzas, se recordó a sí misma. Sin embargo, mientras nadaba en las profundidades de sus ojos azules grisáceos presintió que su negativa a ayudarle ya no era tan rotunda. Tal como le acababa de decir, todos sus proyectos habían desaparecido en cuestión de horas. Su agenda estaba completamente despejada. Después de todo, a lo mejor podía convencerlo de que le ayudase.

—Ya le he dicho la verdad —insistió—. No hay nada más.

Simon supo que mentía. Su rostro estaba inexpresivo, sus ojos verdes del color de la salvia brillaban con una seductora mezcla de determinación femenina y un ligero toque de fragilidad. Era como si se esforzase por evitar que él percibiese la leve esperanza que latía en su pecho, porque su orgullo y su independencia le impedían manifestar cualquier cosa que Simon pudiese interpretar como debilidad. Era una actuación realmente notable, que podría haber convencido a cualquier otro hombre. Pero Simon no era un hombre cualquiera.

Sus años de lucha por sobrevivir como mendigo y ladrón se habían encargado de que no lo fuera.

—He cambiado de opinión, lady Camelia —anunció de pronto—. Le construiré la bomba.

Camelia lo miró sorprendida. No esperaba que cambiase de idea tan rápido.

—¿Por qué? —preguntó con cautela.

Él se encogió de hombros.

—Tardaré años en volver a construir los inventos en los que estaba trabajando. Ahora que me ha recordado los retos que me planteaba el motor de vapor, me imagino que solucionarlos supone un desafío para mí; y éste es tan buen momento para empezar como cualquier otro.

—¿Y vendrá a África conmigo para asegurarse de que la máquina funciona?

—Por supuesto. Incluso me ocuparé de preparar a varios de sus trabajadores para que sean capaces de manejarla cuando yo me haya ido. Siento una gran curiosidad por ver su excavación y averiguar qué tiene que sea tan importante para que esos dos hombres la hayan atacado y amenazado de muerte.

Su tono era ligeramente jocoso y Camelia tuvo claro que se estaba burlando de ella.

—Me ocuparé de comprar los billetes para viajar a Ciudad del Cabo en el próximo barco que salga.

—Eso me parece un poco prematuro. Primero necesito tiempo para construir la máquina.

—Pero eso puede hacerlo en Suráfrica —objetó Camelia—. Puede llevarse todo lo que necesite y montarla allí.

—Por desgracia, no es tan sencillo. Quiero modificar el diseño, lo que significa que algunas piezas funcionarán y otras no. Y necesito estar en Londres; aquí hay un montón de fabricantes de confianza que pueden suministrarme piezas a medida. Necesitaré tiempo.

—¿Cuánto?

—Yo diría que podría crear una bomba eficaz en unas ocho semanas.

A Camelia se le cayó el alma a los pies.

—¡Eso es demasiado tiempo!

—Las reliquias que busca llevan probablemente miles de años enterradas; no creo que les pase nada por seguir ahí abajo unos cuantos meses más.

—Pero tengo que pensar en mis trabajadores —señaló Camelia—. En la actualidad, lo único que pueden hacer es intentar sacar el agua con cubos. Al margen de lo poco que consigan tengo que pagarles por su trabajo y, lamentablemente, mis fondos no son ilimitados. Pagarles dos meses más para que no logren prácticamente nada supone para mí un gran esfuerzo económico.

—Pues envíeles una carta dándoles la orden de que se vayan dos meses a casa —sugirió Simon— y vuelvan cuando lleguemos nosotros con la bomba.

—Esa gente procede de tribus que viven a muchos kilómetros de distancia, en algunos casos a cientos de kilómetros —le explicó Camelia—. Viajan a pie durante semanas o incluso meses para encontrar trabajo y, cuando lo encuentran, pactan quedarse un determinado periodo de tiempo tras el cual están ansiosos por regresar a casa con sus familias. No puedo pedirles que se vayan a casa y luego vuelvan. ¿No podría intentar construir la bomba más deprisa?

—Si trabajo día y noche, y mis proveedores cumplen los plazos, quizá podría tenerla lista en seis semanas.

Camelia lo miró implorante.

—¿Y cree que si trabajase aún más duro lograría acabarla en cuatro?

—Lo veo difícil.

—Pero ¿lo intentará?

Simon suspiró.

—Sí, lo intentaré.

—¡Magnífico! ¿Cuándo empezamos?

—Mañana me pondré a buscar una casa donde pueda montar mi nuevo laboratorio.

—¿Y por qué no se instala aquí? —le ofreció Camelia—. Podría ocupar la sala de estar o el comedor, o incluso los dos sitios, si quisiera. No los utilizamos mucho; raras veces tengo invitados y la verdad es que Zareb y yo preferimos comer abajo en la cocina.

—Es muy generoso por su parte, pero no creo que quiera que sus vecinos cuchicheen porque tiene usted a un extraño deambulando por su casa las veinticuatro horas del día.

—No me preocupa demasiado lo que la gente elija decir sobre mí. A nadie le gusta que viva aquí con mis animales, de modo que dudo que su presencia empeore mucho las cosas.

Simon no sabía si tomarse como un insulto el hecho de que lo hubieran comparado con un mono, un pájaro y una serpiente, o preocuparse de lo aparentemente ajena que era Camelia a lo hirientes que podían ser los rumores de la sociedad londinense.

—Ya encontraré otros sitio donde establecer mi laboratorio —le aseguró él—, pero gracias. En cuanto me haya instalado, tendremos que volver a reunirnos. Necesitaré hablar con usted de muchas cosas durante el proceso de diseño de la bomba. Tal como usted misma ha señalado, el duro entorno africano presenta desafíos únicos.

—Puede recurrir a mí a cualquier hora del día o de la noche. Estoy ansiosa por ayudarle de la forma que sea para que podamos volver a casa lo antes posible.

—Estupendo entonces, que tenga un buen día, lady Camelia. —Avanzó hasta las puertas de la sala de estar, manteniéndose a distancia de Rupert y luego se detuvo—. Sólo una cosa más: hemos olvidado hablar del tema de mi remuneración.

—¡Claro! Le pido disculpas. —Camelia frunció las cejas, fingiendo pensar durante unos instantes—. Si no me equivoco, ayer quedamos en que le daría el cinco por ciento de mis beneficios de los dos próximos años.

—Creo que cuando cejó en su extraordinario empeño por contratarme me había ofrecido el diez por ciento de los próximos cinco años.

Camelia lo miró con frialdad, molesta de que se hubiese acordado.

—Muy bien.

—Pero, por desgracia, eso fue ayer. Desde entonces mis circunstancias han cambiado considerablemente y me veo obligado a fijar mi remuneración en un veinte por ciento de los beneficios que obtenga durante dos años.

—¡No puedo pagarle tanto!

—En realidad, es una ganga. Si es cierto que está a punto de realizar un gran descubrimiento, ganará una fortuna y un veinte por ciento será una cantidad insignificante. Pero si resulta que el terreno no contiene las riquezas que usted prevé o no se pueden desenterrar con éxito en los dos próximos años, habrá obtenido mis servicios y experiencia a cambio de nada; no le pediré el porcentaje de unos cuantos cientos de libras. Entretanto, dedicaré todo mi tiempo y energía a la fabricación de la bomba, y pagaré a los proveedores y el material que necesite. Yo diría que es evidente que el negocio es mucho más arriesgado para mí que para usted.

—Tiene razón, Tisha. —Zareb estaba de pie en la puerta, sujetando algo envuelto con un trapo y con Oscar sentado en uno de sus anchos hombros—. Deberías aceptar.

—Muy bien, pues —concedió Camelia sucintamente. Era un precio exorbitante, pero no estaba en posición de regatear—. Acepto sus condiciones, señor Kent. ¿Quiere que lo pongamos por escrito?

—Me basta con su palabra, lady Camelia. Zareb es testigo.

—Por mí de acuerdo —dijo éste con una sonrisa.

—Vendré a visitarla dentro de unos días, lady Camelia, para que podamos repasar los detalles de mis bocetos. Que tenga una buen día. —Simon se despidió con una leve inclinación de cabeza.

—Tenga, señor Kent. Le he envuelto un trozo de pastel de pasas para que se lo lleve.

—Gracias, Zareb. —Simon pensó que el viejo criado era extraordinariamente atento.

—Ha sido un placer. Lo acompañaré a la puerta.

Camelia observó a Simon mientras seguía a Zareb y a Oscar escaleras abajo hasta la puerta principal. Luego cogió a Rupert del suelo y se sentó en el sofá con la serpiente enroscada en su regazo.

—Cuatro semanas más, Rupert —musitó mientras le acariciaba la escamosa cabeza naranja—. Me dedicaré a recaudar más fondos con los que seguir pagando a los trabajadores y después, al fin, podremos irnos a casa.

Rupert la miró fijamente, disfrutando en silencio de sus suaves caricias.

—Pasarán rápido —le prometió Camelia, pero el comentario iba más dirigido a sí misma que a Rupert—. Ya lo verás. Y ahora, ¿qué tal si bajamos y vemos si puedes comer algo? —Colocó al animal alrededor de sus hombros y se levantó del sofá. Cuatro semanas más viviendo en Londres.

Le parecía una eternidad.

—Ya sale —informó Bert mientras Simon se subía en su carruaje—. Venga, Stanley, andando.

Stanley apareció por detrás de un árbol con un pastel de carne grasiento y picante, que le goteaba por la mano.

—No me he acabado el pastel.

—¡Maldita sea, Stanley! Te he dicho que no lo robaras. ¿Quieres que la vieja que lo ha hecho empiece a dar alaridos o qué?

—Tengo hambre —declaró Stanley con ingenuidad.

—Siempre tienes hambre, pedazo de inútil —le espetó Bert—. Acabas de tragarte un plato de puré de patatas, y desde entonces no has parado de soltar eructos. ¿No puedes dejar de engullir un momento?

—Claro, Bert. —Stanley lo miró avergonzado—. ¿Quieres un poco? Está buenísimo.

Bert echó un vistazo al desmigajado pastel que Stanley tenía en su enorme mano. Como estaba enfadado, estuvo a punto de decir que no y obligar a Stanley a que lo tirase al suelo; al fin y al cabo, ¿cómo iba a aprender el pobre zoquete a distinguir entre lo que estaba bien y lo que no, si no se lo enseñaba él? A veces era peor que un jodido bebé, la verdad fuera dicha. Sin embargo y pese a que Stanley lo había espachurrado entero, el pastel olía bastante bien. Debía de tener buen aspecto, y estar jugoso y calentito cuando lo había robado; y eso que le había dejado más claro que el agua que no lo hiciese.

—¡Dame eso! —susurró Bert—. Un día te trincará la policía, ¿y qué pasará entonces? —dijo mientras se introducía en la boca las migajas del pastel de carne.

Stanley lo miró confuso.

—Que me meterán en el trullo, ¿verdad, Bert?

—Eso es: te encerrarán en el trullo durante Dios sabe cuánto tiempo, ¿y crees que ahí dentro te darán de comer pasteles de salchichas y puré de patatas?

Stanley frunció las cejas, pensativo.

—Tal vez sí. A mucha gente le gustan.

—En el trullo no dan de comer lo que a la gente le gusta —le aclaró Bert, que puso los ojos en blanco—. Te dan papillas compactas como el cemento y sopas agrias sin carne, y el pan está tan seco que al morderlo te rompes los dientes. Te morirías de hambre en menos de una semana, en serio, y yo no podría ayudarte porque también me estaría muriendo, ¿lo entiendes?

Stanley sonrió.

—Sí, Bert, lo entiendo.

Bert lo miró desesperado y convencido de que no había entendido nada. ¿Cómo iba a hacerlo? El pobre cabeza hueca era demasiado idiota para entender cómo funcionaba el mundo. Bert no sabía si había nacido así o si le dieron un puñetazo y perdió la sensatez para siempre. Supuso que daba igual.

Llevaban casi cinco años codo con codo, y durante ese tiempo Bert había hecho todo lo posible para que Stanley tuviese un techo bajo el que dormir la mayoría de las noches y comida que llevarse a la boca la mayoría de los días; lo que no era nada fácil, teniendo en cuenta lo mucho que comía. Era como alimentar a un jodido caballo. Bastaba que Bert tuviese un poco de pasta en el bolsillo para que el estómago de Stanley empezase a rugir. A este paso trabajarían hasta el día del juicio final y seguirían sin nada más que los andrajos que llevaban puestos y una fría salchicha en las manos.

Bert se hartó de paciencia.

—Cuando te diga que no hagas algo, tienes que obedecerme, ¿vale? O sea, que cuando te diga que no robes un pastel, no lo hagas, aunque tu barriga te diga que sí, ¿de acuerdo? —advirtió relamiéndose los dedos.

—De acuerdo, Bert —contestó Stanley deseoso de complacerlo—. No estás enfadado conmigo, ¿verdad?

Bert suspiró.

—No, no estoy enfadado. Sólo quiero que prestes atención a lo que te digo.

Stanley asintió.

—¿Y ahora qué hacemos, Bert? ¿Seguimos ese carruaje?

—Me temo que ya es demasiado tarde. Mientras perdía el tiempo explicándote que tienes que hacerme caso, el jodido carruaje ha desaparecido; y ahora hemos perdido a ese tipo de vista.

—A lo mejor se ha ido a casa —sugirió Stanley.

—¡Oh, sí! ¡Es una gran idea! El único problema es que su casa ha sido reducida a cenizas, de modo que ya no puede ir allí ¿no te parece?

—A esa casa no —aclaró Stanley—, pero sí a la de su padre. El carruaje lleva un elegante escudo, así que lo más probable es que sea de su padre. Deberíamos ir a esa casa a menos que creas que tenemos que quedarnos aquí y observar a esa señora. Lo que tú prefieras, Bert. El inteligente eres tú.

—Es verdad, lo soy. —Bert frunció las cejas, pensativo—. Iremos hacia Bond Street y entraremos en alguna de esas elegantes tiendas para preguntar si saben dónde vive lord Redmond —decidió—. Diremos que tenemos que entregarle un mensaje, pero que nos hemos hecho un lío con las calles. Cuando averigüemos la calle, preguntaremos en un número al azar y así nos contestarán: «No, vive en el número tal», y entonces sabremos adónde ir.

—Es un plan curioso, Bert —comentó Stanley con entusiasmo y sorpresa.

—Lo sé —repuso Bert satisfecho—. Venga, Stanley, vamos. El viejo petardo dijo que nos daría un extra si le dábamos un informe completo la próxima vez que lo veamos. Creo que si continuamos trabajando así durante un tiempo, pronto tendremos suficiente dinero para comprar un piso más grande y puede que también una cama para ti solo.

—¿De verdad? —Stanley no daba crédito—. ¿Con una almohada de plumas?

—Ya veremos —contestó Bert intentando no darle demasiadas esperanzas—. Si impedimos que esa señora vaya a África, ¿quién sabe cuánto podría pagarnos ese viejo chocho? Mientras ella esté aquí habrá que vigilarla, ¿y quién mejor que nosotros para no quitarle el ojo de encima?

—A mí me gusta vigilarla —declaró Stanley alegremente—. La señora pelea con fuerza.

—Pues gracias a ella viviremos mejor —prometió Bert mirando hacia la casa de Camelia con los ojos entornados—; eso siempre y cuando la tengamos controlada.

Capítulo 4

—Entonces pongo la moneda aquí, muevo la mano en el aire, digo la palabra mágica y... ¡la moneda ha desaparecido! —Simon movió los dedos para enseñarle a su embelesado público que no tenía el chelín escondido.

Byron arqueó las cejas confuso.

—Has olvidado decir la palabra mágica.

—En serio, Byron, ¿qué más da si la dice o no? —preguntó Frances, que puso en blanco sus enormes ojos de color zafiro. A sus catorce años empezaba a dejar atrás los últimos vestigios de la infancia y estaba ansiosa por demostrar que ya no era una niña pequeña—. En realidad no es magia, es sólo un truco.

—Pero es un truco muy hábil —declaró una leal Melinda, que no quería que Simon pensase que no valoraban sus gentiles intentos por entretenerlos. Melinda tenía diecisiete años y los mismos elegantes pómulos y brillante cabello cobrizo que lucía su madre. Tenía el porte esbelto y ligeramente coqueto de una adolescente que no tardaría en convertirse en una mujer exquisita—, ¿no te parece, Eunice?

—No veo qué tiene de estupendo meterse una moneda por la manga —comentó Eunice mientras trataba de amasar una harinosa masa de pan—. Preferiría que me ayudarais a preparar las albóndigas de carne, cebolla y beicon —añadió mientras se escondía un mechón de pelo níveo debajo de su sombrero blanco nuevo—. Los señores volverán pronto y todos protestaréis porque tenéis hambre.

—A tu edad me pasaba el día estafando a los ricos y jamás vi un solo penique —se jactó Oliver, cogiendo una cuchara de plata empañada con una mano acartonada mientras la frotaba enérgicamente con un paño ennegrecido—. Claro que tampoco me quedaba esperando a ver si se daban cuenta de que sus bolsillos pesaban menos; por aquel entonces corría como los conejos, así que como mucho lo que notaban era una sacudida de aire en el culo. ¡Eso sí que era magia! —Se rió a carcajadas.

—¿Por qué no les enseñas a los niños cómo convertir una moneda en tres? —sugirió Doreen con su rostro alargado y apergaminado aún más serio mientras pasaba con fuerza el rodillo por unos delgados filetes de ternera—. Al menos eso les serviría de algo.

—¿Te refieres a esto? —Simon puso la mano derecha encima de la mesa de la cocina, con la otra mano se dio unos golpes sobre los nudillos, luego levantó las dos manos y aparecieron tres brillantes chelines.

—¡Genial! —exclamó Byron—. Ahora que aparezcan seis.

—Me temo que tres es mi límite de hoy —confesó Simon—. Tal vez otro día.

—¿Sólo seis? —se mofó Oliver—. Cuando tenía un buen día yo conseguía una docena o más. ¡Eso sí que es magia!

—No, es un robo —observó Doreen con ironía.

—Pero no deja de ser arte y el pequeño Byron parece que tiene talento para ello. —Oliver entornó los ojos y miró al chico con ternura—. ¿Qué tal si después de cenar me pongo el abrigo y jugamos a robar en el jardín? ¿Qué me dices Frances? ¿Y tú, Melinda? La última vez Melinda me birló la tabaquera con tanta sutileza que ni me enteré.

—Sí, y el señor se quedó helado cuando Melinda fue después a darle un abrazo y le quitó su mejor reloj de oro del bolsillo sin que se diese cuenta —recordó Eunice con seriedad.

—Dijo que no entendía por qué todos sus hijos tenían que aprender a ser carteristas para ir por el mundo —añadió Doreen, mientras tiraba los filetes en una sartén.

—Que sepan hacerlo no significa que tengan que usarlo —dijo Oliver filosófico—. Simon es un buen chico, pero si no hubiese sabido robar cuando tuvo que hacerlo, el pobre se habría muerto de hambre; es la pura verdad.

Byron miró a su hermano mayor con admiración.

—¿Es cierto que pasaste hambre, Simon?

—No —le aseguró él—. Oliver es un exagerado.

Byron tenía sólo once años; apenas dos años más de los que tenía Simon cuando Genevieve lo rescató de una apestosa celda de la cárcel de Inveraray. Pero su hermano pequeño había vivido su corta vida en una burbuja de comodidad, privilegios y amor incondicional. Pese a que Genevieve había hecho lo posible por ayudar a sus tres hijos pequeños a comprender que había gente mucho menos afortunada que luchaba a diario por su supervivencia, a sus once años Byron no entendía realmente lo que eso quería decir.

Y Simon tampoco quiso explicárselo.

—Ahora que ya habéis acabado de hacer magia, me gustaría que exprimierais esas naranjas para la crema de naranja. —Con un brusco ademán y la mano llena de harina Eunice señaló el bol de naranjas que había en la encimera que quedaba a sus espaldas—. Hoy hay un postre especial en honor de Simon; sé que es uno de tus favoritos. Melinda, ayúdame a pelar estas patatas para hervir, y tú, Frances, puedes ir cortando esas cebollas de ahí.

—¿Y yo qué hago? —preguntó Byron.

—Tú ven conmigo y saca brillo con el paño a esta tetera de plata —propuso Oliver—. Frota con fuerza hasta que veas tu rostro en ella como en un espejo.

Simon se levantó de la mesa, se quitó la chaqueta y se arremangó las mangas de la camisa.

—Deberías haber visto el exprimidor que te había hecho, Eunice; creo que te habría encantado —dijo mientras cogía un cuchillo y empezaba a partir las naranjas por la mitad—. Se metía media naranja en el aparato y el zumo se obtenía al instante sin tener que hacer fuerza o retorcer la muñeca. Las pepitas quedaban separadas del líquido, se extraía el recipiente y se servía el zumo donde se quisiese.

Eunice lo miró asombrada.

—¿Había un recipiente?

—Uno pequeño con una pequeña boquilla en un lado para que servir fuese más fácil.

—¿Y dónde iban a parar las pepitas? —inquirió Doreen.

—Se quedaban en el colador de la parte superior del recipiente.

Doreen frunció las cejas.

—¿Para siempre?

—No, después había que tirarlas y limpiar el colador.

—¡Es una idea magnífica! —exclamó Oliver, que notaba que a las dos mujeres les resultaba difícil visualizar el invento—. No os imagináis la cantidad de veces que he deseado que existiese una máquina como ésa para no tener que rescatar las pepitas con una cuchara.

—Seguro que era un gran invento, Simon —concluyó Eunice no muy convencida mientras introducía la masa de pan en un bol, y la cubría con un trapo limpio.

—Te haré otro exprimidor, Eunice —prometió Simon, que se disponía a exprimir las naranjas en un sencillo exprimidor de cristal—. Así entenderás por qué es mucho mejor que este cacharro.

—Ese cacharro lo llevo usando desde hace más de veinte años —le informó Eunice—. Y a ti también te funcionaría bien, si te acordaras de rodar las naranjas con fuerza sobre la mesa antes de cortarlas; así el zumo sale más dulce.

Simon cogió la siguiente naranja y la frotó con suavidad contra la mesa.

—Me había olvidado de hacerlo. ¿Y si invento algo que las haga rodar?

—¿Tienes alguna idea para limpiar la plata? —le preguntó Oliver—. Ése sí que es un trabajo que me gustaría que fuese más sencillo.

—Intenté crear una máquina en la que se introducía el objeto de plata y se cubría con pasta de amoníaco. A continuación se giraba una manivela que accionaba unos cepillos redondos para quitar la pasta y sacar brillo a la plata.

—Suena fenomenal —intervino Melinda—. De esta forma a Oliver nunca más le quedarían las manos sucias y negras.

—El problema era que arrancaba casi todo el baño de plata —reconoció Simon—. Me cargué más de dos docenas de tenedores y cucharas antes de darme finalmente por vencido.

Oliver se rió entre dientes.

—No te alteres, chico, pero ¡si no hay baño de plata, ya no hace falta sacarle brillo!

—Hay cosas que es mejor hacer a mano —reflexionó Doreen.

—No te preocupes —le consoló Eunice, asintiendo—, yo estoy muy orgullosa del aparato que me diste para hacer puré de patatas; hace un puré finísimo.

—¿Y qué me decís del batidor de huevos que me regaló la pasada Navidad? —recordó Doreen—. Deja los huevos tan ligeros y esponjosos que da la impresión de que se van a evaporar.

—Estoy convencido de que si le propusieses la idea a algún fabricante, no tardarías en hacerte millonario —especuló Oliver.

—Simon no quiere ser millonario —comentó Genevieve con orgullo al entrar en la cocina—. Lo que quiere es inventar.

Simon alzó la vista y sonrió. Aunque su madre rozaba la cincuentena, aún conservaba la extraordinaria belleza que le había asombrado desde el primer momento en que la vio. Él era un niño harapiento y escuálido de apenas nueve años que llevaba desde los cinco o seis trampeando únicamente gracias a su ingenio y sus todavía más rápidas manos. Cuando lo metieron en la cárcel creyó que su vida había terminado. Era fuerte para su edad, pero tras la detención y la docena de latigazos que le dieron por haber robado, se sintió insignificante, débil y a punto de morir.

Entonces Genevieve apareció en su celda con su brillante pelo cobrizo y esos impresionantes ojos de color marrón chocolate. Se arrodilló junto a él y le acarició con suavidad las mejillas y la frente con el rostro lleno de rabia e inquietud.

Y por primera vez en su vida pensó que, después de todo, quizá Dios no se había olvidado de él.

—Pero seguro que ganará una fortuna igualmente, mami —le dijo Byron seriamente—. Porque si se da golpes en la mano le salen monedas.

—¡Eso sí que me gustaría aprenderlo a mí! —bromeó Haydon reuniéndose con su mujer.

El marqués de Redmond examinó con satisfacción la concurrida y ajetreada cocina. Antes de conocer a Genevieve no había pisado nunca la cocina, ni siquiera de pequeño. Y ahora era uno de sus lugares predilectos.

—Eunice y Doreen, no sé lo que están ustedes preparando, pero huele de maravilla —dijo agradecido mientras levantaba la tapa de la olla que había en el fuego.

—Hoy hay albóndigas con cebollas al jerez, salmón al horno con salsa de alcaparras, patatas con guisantes, espinacas a la crema, y de postre pudín de dátiles con salsa espesa de caramelo y crema de naranja —le explicó Eunice—. Me parece que con eso tendrán todos el estómago lleno hasta mañana.

—Yo estoy ayudando a hacer las patatas —le informó Melinda a su padre.

—Y yo, cortando cebollas —anunció Frances.

—Entonces seguro que la cena estará incluso más deliciosa que habitualmente. ¿Y tú qué haces, Byron?

—Sacar brillo a esta tetera —respondió el niño con seriedad—. ¡A ver si puedes verte en ella!

Haydon cogió la grasienta tetera con las manos.

—¡Desde luego que me veo! —exclamó mientras acariciaba con suavidad el pelo de su hijo—. Bueno, Simon, supongo que te gustará saber que a partir de mañana tendrás un nuevo laboratorio donde seguir trabajando en tus inventos.

Simon lo miró ansioso.

—¿Habéis conseguido alquilar la casa que vimos ayer?

Genevieve sonrió.

—Así es.

—El propietario ha titubeado un poco al enterarse de que era para ti —le contó Haydon—; por lo visto la ciudad entera sabe que tu casa ha ardido en llamas.

Simon ya sabía que el incendio le dificultaría encontrar una casa, razón por la cual le había pedido a Haydon que tramitase el alquiler por él.

—¿Has tenido que ofrecerle más dinero?

—Un poco.

—Lo siento, Haydon. Sea la cantidad que sea, te lo devolveré en cuanto pueda.

—No quiero que te preocupes por el dinero, Simon. Lo que Genevieve y yo queremos es que tengas un sitio donde estés cómodo y puedas concentrarte plenamente en tu trabajo. Sé que perder el laboratorio ha supuesto un serio revés para ti, pero espero que puedas recuperarte pronto.

—Jack me ha dicho que está deseando que fabriques una turbina de vapor más perfeccionada para que la pueda probar en uno de sus barcos —comentó Genevieve—. Está intentando hacer los itinerarios más deprisa y con el motor adecuado su empresa naviera podrá expandir su mercado y cubrir otras rutas que hacen sus competidores.

—Pues el motor de Jack tendrá que esperar un poco —informó Simon—, porque primero tengo que acabar otro proyecto que llevo entre manos.

—¿Te refieres a la lavadora esa de la que me has hablado antes? —preguntó Eunice con curiosidad.

—No, eso también tendrá que esperar. Ha venido a verme lady Camelia Marshall para pedirme que le construya una bomba de vapor.

Oliver arqueó las cejas.

—¿Una bomba para llenar la bañera?

—No, lady Camelia es arqueóloga y necesita una bomba para sacar el agua de la excavación que dirige.

—¿No es la hija de lord Stamford? —inquirió Genevieve.

—¿Has oído hablar de ella?

—Sí, lleva poco tiempo en Londres, pero ya ha llamado bastante la atención.

—Me lo puedo imaginar —replicó Simon con ironía.

—¿Y eso por qué? —quiso saber Eunice, preguntándose si se trataría de algo reprobable.

—Porque es una mujer guapa, inteligente y soltera que va por ahí sola intentando recaudar fondos para su excavación de Suráfrica.

Oliver enarcó sus espesas cejas, perplejo.

—¿Eso es todo?

Doreen soltó una risotada de desdén.

—Eso no es nada comparado con lo que han hecho las mujeres de esta familia. Así que, chicas, no quiero que vosotras también os metáis en líos —añadió con una mirada de advertencia a Melinda y a Frances—. Ya hemos tenido bastante con vuestra madre, Annabelle, Grace y Charlotte —dijo, refiriéndose a sus hermanas mayores.

—Lady Camelia no es conocida únicamente por ir sola a los sitios —observó Genevieve—. Capta la atención porque viaja con un criado africano que va vestido con túnicas muy llamativas y un mono como mascota.

Oliver, que encontraba el asunto divertido, dio unas palmadas sobre su rodilla

—¡A eso se le llama tener valor!

Byron miró a su padre con suspicacia.

—Me dijiste que no podía tener un mono porque la ley lo prohibía.

Haydon le lanzó una mirada de socorro a su mujer.

—Es probable que lady Camelia haya obtenido algún permiso especial —improvisó enseguida Genevieve—, porque el mono estará aquí temporalmente. Seguro que cuando regrese a Suráfrica se lo llevará consigo.

—Seguro que sí —afirmó Simon—, junto con su pájaro y su serpiente.

—¿Puedo tener una serpiente? —le preguntó excitado Byron a su padre.

Haydon se encogió de hombros.

—Pregúntaselo a tu madre.

—No creo que una serpiente sea una gran mascota —objetó Genevieve, que miró a su marido con las cejas fruncidas—. No se puede jugar con ella, y tampoco es cariñosa ni se la puede achuchar.

—Sí que se puede jugar con ella —insistió Byron con obstinación—. Podría construir una enorme torre de cubos de construcción y dejar que la horrible serpiente luchase por salir del castillo. También podría llevarla alrededor del cuello o dejarla en el suelo y jugar al escondite con ella.

—Ya, y luego me la encontraría enroscada en mi cama y yo me moriría del susto —musitó Doreen—. Sería mejor que te comprasen un gato bonito y tranquilo, así se comería los ratones.

—Las serpientes también comen ratones —señaló Byron.

—Me niego a tener una serpiente deslizándose por mi cocina en busca de ratones —le espetó Eunice.

—Vale, muy bien —concedió el muchacho enfadado—. ¿Y qué me decís de un lagarto? Los lagartos no se deslizan.

Oliver se rascó la cabeza.

—No es mala idea.

—¿Dónde has conocido a lady Camelia, Simon? —preguntó Genevieve, procurando cambiar de tema.

—Vino a verme el otro día porque había leído mis artículos sobre los motores de vapor —contestó Simon—. Me dijo que me pagaría si le construía una bomba y yo accedí. Oliver, ¿te importaría llevarme en coche a la casa nueva mañana a primera hora? Me gustaría tener el laboratorio montado lo antes posible.

—Doreen y yo no podremos salir hasta que hayamos recogido el desayuno y dejado la casa arreglada —objetó Eunice—. Si eso te parece demasiado tarde, Ollie, tendrás que volver a buscarnos.

—A las diez como muy tarde estaremos listas y con las maletas hechas —añadió Doreen.

Simon las miró confuso.

—¿Qué maletas?

—¡Ja! No pretenderás limpiar y organizar la casa tú solo, ¿verdad?

—Sois muy amables —se apresuró a decirles Simon—, pero no hace falta que os instaléis allí, en serio. Estoy convencido de que estaréis mucho más cómodos aquí, y Haydon y Genevieve os necesitarán mañana por la noche.

—En realidad, Haydon y yo habíamos pensado volver a Escocia con los niños mañana —le aclaró Genevieve—. Nos hemos quedado unos cuantos días más porque queríamos buscarte una casa. Y dado que Lizzie y Beaton regresarán mañana de visitar a sus respectivas familias —añadió, refiriéndose al ama de llaves y al mayordomo que vivían en la residencia londinense—, Oliver, Eunice y Doreen se han ofrecido muy amablemente a quedarse en Londres contigo para ayudarte a organizar tu nueva casa. —Sonrió con ternura al anciano trío—. Aunque les echemos de menos, tenemos suficiente personal en casa para que las cosas funcionen relativamente bien hasta que ellos vengan.

—Me aseguraré de que comes suficiente, muchacho —soltó Eunice—. Estás en los huesos. Ya es hora de alimentarte con unos deliciosos *haggis** y un buen pudín de tofe.

—Y yo quiero verte dormir en una cama de verdad con sábanas limpias —intervino Doreen— en lugar de quedarte dormido en una silla o encima de la mesa como me he enterado que haces. Además, me ocuparé de que tu ropa esté limpia y planchada; parece que te haya sacudido un vendaval.

—Y yo me aseguraré de que no incendias la casa —concluyó Oliver con sinceridad—. Y cuando se haga de noche, apagaré las lámparas y esconderé las cerillas, ¿me has entendido?

Simon miró a Haydon con impotencia.

—A mí no me mires, ha sido idea de Genevieve.

—Será sólo hasta que estés instalado, Simon —le dijo Genevieve con cariño.

Desde que Simon había llegado a su casa de madrugada varios días antes, Genevieve había estado tremendamente preocupada por él. Pese a que había insistido en que la causa del incendio había sido una vela desatendida y había prometido ser más cauto en el futuro, a Genevieve le daba miedo que volviese a producirse un accidente. Tal vez la próxima vez no tuviese tanta suerte. Sabía que Simon se abstraía de lo que le rodeaba cuando trabajaba, olvidándose a menudo de comer, dormir o incluso de salir a la calle para respirar un poco de aire fresco. Lo encontraba pálido, pálido y un poco nervioso, que era como solía estar cuando trabajaba en alguno de sus inventos. Por mucho que le asegurase que lo prefería así, no le gustaba el hecho de que quisiese vivir solo; Haydon y ella se habían ofrecido a pagarle un criado un montón de veces, al menos para poder estar seguros de que había comida en su casa y alguien con quien pudiese hablar ocasionalmente. Pero Simon siempre se negaba e insistía en que no podía trabajar con gente alrededor.

—Eunice, Oliver y Doreen aún no están del todo listos para regresar a Escocia y, de todas formas, tampoco hay mucho que hacer en casa —continuó Genevieve, intentando que pareciese que hacía esto en beneficio del trío—. Así que encuentro bien que se queden contigo un tiempo y te ayuden a organizar tu casa.

—Te lo pasarás bien con nosotros, muchacho —le aseguró Doreen.

—Te prepararé tus platos favoritos —prometió Eunice, colocando una torta recién hecha ante él.

—Y yo evitaré que incendies la casa entera —bromeó Oliver, que le guiñó un ojo.

Simon suspiró.

—¿Os quedaréis sólo hasta que esté todo organizado?

—Por supuesto, chico.

—En cuanto la cocina esté como a mí me gusta y haya conseguido que engordes un poco, me marcharé en el primer tren que salga hacia Inverness —le tranquilizó Eunice.

—Yo también me iré en cuanto te haya lavado y planchado la ropa, y la casa esté limpia —prometió Doreen.

—Muy bien —concedió Simon mientras cogía un trozo de torta y pegaba un mordisco.

—Como mucho serán dos meses.

Simon se atragantó.

—¿Dos meses?

—No te alteres, chico —le calmó Oliver, dándole una fuerte palmada en la espalda—. Te prometo que en un par de días ni siquiera notarás nuestra presencia.

Si alguien más le decía cuánto la admiraba por su dedicación al trabajo, lo estrangularía.

No obstante, Camelia sonrió e hizo todo lo posible por mantenerse serena y comportarse como una dama o al menos por poner la cara que ella creía pondría una dama. De vez en cuando lanzaba una mirada hacia las mujeres que llenaban el sofocante salón de baile en busca de alguna pista acerca de cómo se suponía que debía proceder en este evento tan tremendamente tedioso. Todas las chicas que daban vueltas con elegancia por el salón tenían la misma expresión insustancial; eran como preciosas muñecas de porcelana con los labios pintados dibujando pequeños y tensos arcos. El resto de mujeres solteras, que estaban de pie y en grupos alrededor de la pista de baile, se abanicaban y pestañeaban a los nerviosos jóvenes lo suficientemente valientes como para intentar entablar una conversación con ellas.

Algunas de las chicas daban la impresión de que querían salir de ahí corriendo, y con razón, pensó Camelia. Bastaba mirar el triste surtido de pretendientes de piernas larguiruchas y rostros granulosos que las rodeaban para entenderlo. Un par de torpes bailes, una nauseabunda copa de ponche tibio y un plato de pollo viscoso, y al instante sus madres decidirían que hacían buena pareja.

Se centró de nuevo en la monótona voz de lord Bagley, eternamente agradecida de haber dejado atrás los dieciocho años, cuando algunos amigos de su padre habían tratado de convencerlo de que tenía que encontrarle un marido a Camelia.

Por suerte, su querido padre no consideró que su única hija tuviese que contraer matrimonio nada más alcanzar la mayoría de edad; y dado que Camelia le aseguró que no tenían ningún interés en casarse y que lo que quería era trabajar con él, el tema se zanjó rápidamente.

—...y luego las cargamos en un barco y las enviamos al Museo Británico, donde desde entonces han sido la esencia de su colección de antigüedades griegas —concluyó lord Bagley, pasándose triunfalmente un grueso y enguantado nudillo por el bigote gris amarillento—. En aquella época le dije a tu padre que viniese conmigo, pero siempre fue muy tozudo. Decía que creía que en África había riquezas extraordinarias por descubrir y que él las encontraría. —Se rió entre dientes y sacudió la cabeza como si hubiese algo sumamente gracioso en la devoción que lord Stamford sentía hacia su trabajo en África.

—Y tenía razón. —Camelia aborrecía el desprecio con que lord Bagley hablaba de la labor de su padre.

—Sí, siempre y cuando se refiriese a los diamantes y el oro —convino lord Bagley—. Pero tu padre no se refería a los minerales. La última vez que hablé con él, unos seis meses antes de su muerte, no paró de quejarse de las grandes compañías mineras.

—Decía que destruían la tierra —intervino lord Duffield, un hombre delgado y de aspecto hosco de unos sesenta años, que llevaba el ralo pelo cano peinado sobre su cuero cabelludo lleno de manchas—. Aseguraba que, si no se impedía, acabarían destruyendo África.

—En eso también tenía razón —insistió Camelia—. Dígame, lord Duffield, ¿ha visto alguna vez de primera mano la devastación que produce en la tierra el proceso de extracción de diamantes?

—La industria minera es un negocio sucio —contestó él con indiferencia, recolocándose distraídamente unos cuantos mechones de pelo sueltos—. Me temo que eso es inevitable.

—Me imagino, querida, que convendrá en que gracias a los diamantes África ha sido incluida en el mapa —intervino lord Gilby mientras se acariciaba su exageradamente recortada y estropajosa barba gris.

—África estaba en el mapa millones de años antes de que esa detestable piedra preciosa fuese descubierta junto a las orillas del río Orange hace apenas dieciocho años —repuso Camelia en el mismo tono.

—Sí, pero ¿qué era? —Lord Pendrick frunció el entrecejo de su rostro rollizo y sonrojado por el alcohol—. Una árida y miserable extensión de tierra erosionada y llena de rocas habitada por unos bárbaros desnudos e ignorantes, unas bestias salvajes, y por esos ridículos boers holandeses. A nadie le importó África hasta que se descubrieron los diamantes; era indómita, incivilizada y estaba prácticamente deshabitada.

Lord Duffield asintió vehementemente.

—Estoy completamente de acuerdo.

—Y ahora, gracias a la industria minera se están construyendo vías férreas e instalando telégrafos, se están haciendo ciudades y formando gobiernos. Tengo entendido de que incluso ha llegado la electricidad a Kimberley, donde está el yacimiento más grande.

—Intentan que el lugar se vuelva más o menos civilizado y lo conseguirán siempre y cuando logren que esos salvajes se muevan y trabajen un poco. —Lord Gilby se rió, dejando claro que ése era un reto casi imposible.

—Es difícil que los nativos trabajen; no han recibido la pertinente ética laboral cristiana —reflexionó una pía lady Bagley mientras las abundantes arrugas de su cara prácticamente se tragaban sus diminutos ojos—. Estoy segura de que preferirían pasarse el día entero sentados al sol sin hacer nada.

Camelia apretó los puños dispuesta a decirle al ignorante grupo de arrogantes lo que pensaba de su asquerosa intolerancia. Notó que Elliott se acercaba un poco más a ella, no llegaba a tocarla, pero aun así Camelia sintió su reconfortante presencia; supo que intentaba ayudarle a mantener la calma. A Elliott siempre se le había dado mucho mejor jugar a este juego que a ella o a su padre, y era consciente de ello. Camelia inspiró todo lo hondo que su corsé dolorosamente apretado le permitió y se esforzó por controlar su ira. Si atacaba con dureza a los allí presentes, no conseguiría nada. Lo único que haría sería insultarles y enemistarse con los miembros de la Sociedad Arqueológica Británica, y por tanto perdería cualquier posibilidad de obtener su apoyo.

Si no lograba recaudar más contribuciones, le resultaría imposible hacer realidad el preciado sueño de su padre.

—Suráfrica es un país precioso que en la actualidad vive cambios tremendamente intensos —intervino Elliott con una sonrisa mientras conducía la conversación a un terreno menos conflictivo—. Durante los quince años que estuve trabajando al lado de lord Stamford aprendí a valorar todas sus riquezas, por sencillas que algunas puedan parecer. Lord Stamford estaba convencido de que África encerraba la llave de la historia de la humanidad, y creo que tenía razón.

—La tenía —insistió Camelia—. Demostrarlo será sólo cuestión de tiempo. En la excavación ya hemos desenterrado cientos de reliquias fascinantes cuya antigüedad estimo en miles de años. Y estoy segura de que en los próximos meses encontraremos piezas todavía más importantes.

—¿En serio? —Lord Bagley la miró con curiosidad por encima del borde de su copa de brandy—. ¿Y qué es exactamente eso que está usted a punto de descubrir, lady Camelia?

Camelia abrió la boca para responder, pero se detuvo. Pese a su rostro impasible, los ojos de lord Bagley la miraban con una repentina intensidad que le provocó un escalofrío.

«Aléjese de África si no quiere ver cómo la palma el resto de sus magníficos trabajadores.»

¿Habría sido lord Bagley quien había contratado a esos dos rufianes para amedrentarla?, se preguntó. Desde luego era factible. Lord Bagley era una reconocida arqueólogo con una extensa y notable carrera, pero no era la clase de hombre que dedicaría años de su vida a excavar la tierra sin ninguna garantía de encontrar algo. Su filosofía siempre se había limitado a llevarse lo que ya estaba ahí, incluso aunque eso significase levantar un templo maravillosamente ubicado o arrancar una escultura espléndida para poderla introducir en una caja y enviarla en barco al Museo Británico. Habían pasado muchos años desde el último hallazgo de lord Bagley, reflexionó Camelia. Y a pesar del manifiesto escepticismo respecto al trabajo de su padre, siempre se había mostrado sumamente ansioso por hablar con él de su excavación africana cuando viajaba a Londres.

¿Habría conseguido su padre persuadir a lord Bagley de la extraordinaria importancia de la excavación antes de morir?

—Estoy convencida de que encontraremos más reliquias que revelen lo rica y antigua que es la historia de los africanos —replicó Camelia sin dar detalles y sosteniendo la mirada de lord Bagley—. Quizás haya incluso pruebas que apoyen la teoría del señor Darwin en lo que concierne a la evolución de las especies.

—Pues a mí esta idea de que todos procedemos del mono me parece repugnante y absurda. —Lady Bagley agitó enérgicamente su abanico de plumas de avestruz frente a su delantera cubierta de diamantes mientras concluía—. Todo el mundo sabe que Dios creó al hombre.

—Yo entiendo que el señor Darwin deja abierta la posibilidad de que Dios creara primero al mono y luego lo vigilara en su evolución hasta convertirse en hombre —declaró lord Duffield—. Porque eso duró miles de años.

—¡Es absurdo! —se opuso lady Bagley—. Si lo que Dios quería era que el hombre poblase la Tierra, ¿por qué iba crear primero al mono para luego convertirlo en un ser humano? Dios es omnipotente, algo que demostró al crear a Adán y Eva.

—Hay muchas cosas acerca del origen de nuestra existencia que, simplemente, no entendemos, lady Bagley —señaló Elliott con diplomacia—. Como arqueólogos, nuestra misión es hacernos preguntas y no dejar de buscar para intentar que algunas piezas del puzzle encajen.

—Si tal como asegura el señor Darwin es cierto que la humanidad comenzó en África, mi pregunta es: ¿qué demonios han estado haciendo esos negros estos últimos miles de años? —inquirió lord Gilby.

Lord Bagley asintió mostrando su conformidad.

—¿Por qué no han construido grandes edificios ni espléndidas tumbas, o su arte no es espectacular como el que nos dejaron los antiguos egipcios, los griegos y los romanos? ¿Qué han hecho durante todos estos años?

—Los africanos no tienen necesidad de engrandecerse con la construcción de enormes pirámides y templos —le explicó Camelia procurando ser paciente—. Sus creencias espirituales están ligadas a la tierra y los animales de un modo inextricable; ellos creen que cuando una persona fallece, su espíritu permanece en la tierra que les rodea. No les hacen falta los rituales de enterramiento ni las tumbas. La construcción de viviendas permanentes carece de sentido en una sociedad nómada; la tierra y el clima pueden ser rigurosos y obligar a las tribus a desplazarse cuando aumenta la necesidad de encontrar comida.

—A lo mejor han sido demasiado vagos para construir algo importante —dijo lord Duffield con sarcasmo.

—No son inteligentes —afirmó lord Bagley—, y, en realidad, tampoco es culpa suya. Hay estudios científicos que demuestran que es debido al tamaño de sus cerebros.

—Y dígame, lord Bagley, ¿de qué tamaño cree usted que es su cerebro? —preguntó Camelia mordaz—. Se lo pregunto porque no veo que haya construido nada especialmente notable en toda su vida.

—Camelia... —intervino Elliott en tono de advertencia.

—Para que lo sepa, lady Camelia, soy uno de los principales colaboradores de la colección de antigüedades griegas y romanas del Museo Británico —soltó un ofendido lord Bagley—. Soy el responsable de la instalación de un templo griego entero en el interior del museo, que es ampliamente considerado una de las piezas más importantes de la colección. Mi trabajo en el campo de la arqueología es, como los socios aquí presentes no dudarán en convenir, de suma relevancia.

—Lo que usted hizo en Italia y en Grecia fue arrancar obras de arte y templos magníficos, y llevárselos antes de que nadie intentase detenerlo —replicó Camelia—. ¿Acaso no es eso destrozar lo que otros habían hecho?

Atónito, Elliott se acercó todavía más a ella.

—Lo que lady Camelia trata de decir es...

—Sé lo que lady Camelia intenta decir —le aseguró lord Bagley, con el rostro pétreo, surcado de arrugas y rojo de indignación—. Y debo decir que sus comentarios no sólo me parecen equivocados, sino extremadamente ofensivos.

Camelia abrió la boca para replicar que los comentarios de lord Bagley sobre los africanos le parecían igualmente ofensivos, pero Elliott le apretó la mano, suplicándole que se contuviese.

—¡Que no se diga que lady Camelia no comparte la pasión de su padre por crear debate! —exclamó riéndose con entusiasmo—. A lord Stamford nunca le importó en especial qué bando defendía siempre y cuando desafiase mi punto de vista. Y, por lo que veo, su hija es igual que él, ¿verdad, lady Camelia?

Su cara era una cuidadosamente estudiada máscara de alegría. Camelia notó que detrás de la aparente diversión de sus ojos de color marrón oscuro, Elliott le estaba suplicando que dejase de insultar al anfitrión y le siguiese el juego con la justificación que acababa de dar.

Ella le devolvió la mirada con serenidad, negándose a pedir disculpas por sus comentarios. Aborrecía el soberbio grupito de arrogantes damas y caballeros que le rodeaba y lo completamente convencidos que estaban de su propia superioridad. Tenía ganas de insultarles, de decirles a las claras lo que pensaba de su asquerosa ignorancia e intolerancia.

Sin perder la sonrisa, Elliott la miró arqueando las cejas, expectante.

«Discúlpate», le ordenó en silencio. «Ahora.»

Se sintió totalmente impotente al percatarse de que necesitaba la ayuda de esta gente. Sin su capital o su apoyo, aunque se lo diesen de mala gana, no podía continuar su trabajo. Era así de sencillo.

Y así de exasperante.

—Soy como mi padre —musitó Camelia, procurando fingir cierto arrepentimiento— y a veces me dejo llevar por el acaloramiento y supongo que me extralimito. —Contempló a los presentes con indiferencia.

Hubo en breve y tenso silencio.

—Tranquila, querida, no es necesario que se disculpe —le aseguró lord Bagley.

«Bien, porque no me estoy disculpando», pensó mirando a Lord Bagley inocentemente.

—Está claro que las mujeres se comportan de otra manera en Suráfrica —añadió lady Balgey como si quisiese hallarle alguna explicación al ultrajante comportamiento de Camelia—. Supongo que será debido a que es un país todavía joven; no me imagino viviendo en un lugar tan cálido y salvaje.

«No duraría ni un día allí. El sol la marchitaría o sería devorada por una fiera salvaje», dijo Camelia para sus adentros mientras sonreía, disfrutando perversamente del pensamiento.

Malinterpretando la naturaleza de la sonrisa de Camelia, lady Bagley hizo lo propio.

—Si nos disculpan, le he prometido a lady Camelia enseñarle los jardines —anunció Elliott, ansioso por llevarse a Camelia de ahí ahora que había cierta calma—. Tengo entendido que son sencillamente magníficos.

—¡Oh, desde luego que lo son! —exclamó lady Bagley con entusiasmo—. Dicen que nuestro jardín de rosas es uno de los más bonitos de Londres.

—En ese caso, estoy deseando que lady Camelia lo vea. —Elliott le ofreció un brazo, que ella aceptó—. Con su permiso. —Inclinó la cabeza levemente y alejó a Camelia rápidamente del lugar.

—El joven Wickham se va a llevar una sorpresa, si se piensa que logrará domarla —comentó lord Bagley cuando se fueron.

—No pasa nada porque la chica se muestre un poco temperamental —repuso lord Duffield comprensivo—, aunque sus argumentos son ridículos.

—Una cosa es ser temperamental, pero lady Camelia se ha convertido en una completa salvaje —se impacientó lady Bagley, que se abanicó enérgicamente—. Su padre nunca debió consentir que se fuese a vivir a África con él tras el fallecimiento de su madre. Debería haberla dejado en Inglaterra, al cargo de algunos familiares, y después haberle buscado un marido nada más cumplir la mayoría de edad. No es normal que una mujer joven y soltera trabaje en una excavación en medio de África rodeada de animales peligrosos y nativos desnudos.

—No seguirá ahí mucho más tiempo —le aseguró su marido—. Afirma que está a punto de descubrir algo importante, pero todo el mundo sabe que lo único importante que puede encontrarse en África son oro y diamantes. A menos que encuentre minerales, y rápido, se verá obligada a abandonar el disparatado sueño de su padre.

—¿Cómo ha conseguido aguantar tanto tiempo? —inquirió lord Pendrick.

—Stamford le dejó una herencia modesta, además de bastantes deudas —explicó lord Gilby—. Algunos miembros de la sociedad le han perdonado generosamente sus préstamos; otros incluso le han estado dando dinero estos últimos meses, por respeto a la memoria de su padre. Pero, por desgracia, me temo que su espíritu caritativo va en descenso.

—Es bien sabido que lady Camelia ha tenido problemas en la excavación, aunque no le guste reconocerlo. —lord Duffield se acarició el extremo de la barba mientras añadía—: Varios de sus trabajadores han muerto en accidentes laborales y muchos han huido. Por lo que sé, a consecuencia de las lluvias el terreno se ha inundado de agua y no logra sacarla. Los nativos creen que ha caído una maldición sobre el lugar.

—Los nativos siempre han creído en las maldiciones —se mofó lord Bagley con impaciencia—, forma parte de su ignorancia. Si yo hubiese dejado de excavar cada vez que alguien me hablaba de alguna estúpida maldición, jamás habría descubierto nada.

—Tienes razón, querido —convino su mujer—. Pero supongo que estarás de acuerdo conmigo en que en el caso de una mujer es distinto. Lady Camelia debería abandonar la excavación inmediatamente.

—Seguro que Wickham está rezando para que ella entre pronto en razón y venda el terreno —señaló lord Pendrick.

—Por lo visto la De Beers Company le ha hecho una oferta, aunque no sé para qué demonios quieren ese terreno —dijo lord Duffield cabeceando—, porque no han encontrado ni una sola chispa.

—Están intentando consolidar sus posesiones en los alrededores de Kimberley —especuló lord Gilby—. Mientras la zona sea suya nadie más podrá hacer nada ahí.

—Tal vez el terreno ahora no valga nada, pero ¡quién sabe dentro de treinta o cuarenta años! —añadió lord Pendrick—. Me imagino que la De Beers Company piensa que, aunque no se hayan encontrado diamantes, el lugar podrá destinarse algún día a la agricultura o la construcción de casas.

Lord Bagley se echó a reír.

—¡Eso sí que es una inversión a largo plazo! Desde luego yo no metería dinero en algo que tenga tan pocas posibilidades de dar beneficios. Yo preferiría sacar alguna rentabilidad antes de ser demasiado viejo para disfrutarla.

—Espero que lady Camelia recupere pronto la sensatez, antes de que se arruine del todo —deseó lady Bagley.

—No tardará en dar su brazo a torcer, querida. Haya o no caído una maldición sobre el terreno, si no puede pagar a sus trabajadores, tendrá que vender. —Lord Bagley hizo una pausa para tomar un sorbo de coñac antes de añadir enigmáticamente—: Tan sencillo como eso.

—No deberías haberle hablado así a lord Bagley, Camelia —la reprendió Elliott mientras la conducía por una senda de gravilla de color crema—. Le has ofendido.

—Lo merecía —replicó Camelia acaloradamente—. Todos ellos lo merecían. Me repugnan los comentarios que hacen sobre los africanos. ¿En serio creías que me quedaría callada escuchando lo que decían?

—Sé que te cuesta, Camelia, pero tienes que aprender que a veces es mejor callar —advirtió Elliott—. Por mucho que los desafíes no cambiarán de opinión; sólo conseguirás insultarles y que se muestren reacios a ayudarte. Y dado que necesitas su ayuda, deberías vigilar tu comportamiento.

—Su ayuda no me importa tanto como para tener que escuchar cómo denigran a una raza entera de gente que en un solo día trabaja más que la mayoría de los que están en ese salón en un año entero.

Elliott suspiró.

—¿Has apalabrado ya alguna contribución esta noche?

—Lord Cadwell me ha comentado que estaría dispuesto a darme un poco de dinero. Fue un buen amigo de mi padre hace muchos años.

—¿Te ha dicho cuánto?

—No, pero estoy segura de que será una cantidad generosa. Me ha parecido que estaba muy interesado mientras le hablaba de los últimos huesos que hemos encontrado y, por supuesto, está ansioso por saber más cosas de las pinturas rupestres.

—¿Alguien más?

—De momento, no.

Él la miró con severa resignación.

—La noche no ha terminado aún, Elliott.

—No, Camelia, aún no ha terminado, pero supongo que te habrás dado cuenta de que por parte de la Sociedad Arqueológica hay una acusada negativa a continuar apoyando el trabajo de tu padre.

—Lo que están es un poco renuentes a darle el dinero a una mujer —matizó Camelia—. Tengo que convencerles de que es irrelevante el hecho de que yo sea mujer, lo que importa es la excavación en sí.

—Es más que eso, Camelia, y lo sabes. Incluso a tu padre le costó persuadir a la gente de que invirtiera en su labor. A pesar de su entusiasmo y dedicación nunca descubrió nada de gran significación.

—Esta vez es diferente. Lo de Pumulani será importante.

—Eso es imposible saberlo con certeza, Camelia. Antes de su muerte tu padre y yo trabajamos juntos en Pumulani durante quince años, y tú llevas seis meses trabajando allí sin descanso. Todo lo que hemos encontrado son algunos huesos y collares, unas cuantas herramientas primitivas y las pinturas rupestres, que, si bien son interesantes, difícilmente constituyen un gran hallazgo arqueológico. —Y viendo que Camelia estaba a punto de protestar, añadió enseguida—: Al menos en opinión de la Sociedad Arqueológica.

—Hay más cosas ahí, Elliott —insistió Camelia—. Sé que te desanimaste cuando mi padre murió y que por eso decidiste montar un negocio de exportación. Y no te culpo.

—No me fui de África únicamente porque estuviese desanimado, Camelia —objetó Elliott—. Tú sabes mejor que nadie que me encantaba vivir y trabajar en Pumulani, al margen de lo mucho o lo poco que desenterrábamos. Me fui a África por elección propia, en contra de la voluntad de toda mi familia, porque amaba la arqueología y porque creía en tu padre, y quería aprender de él. Los años que pasé allí fueron increíbles. Por desgracia, tras el fallecimiento de mi padre he tenido que asumir otras responsabilidades; responsabilidades que, simplemente, no puedo afrontar sin una fuente de ingresos constante. Nuestras vidas han cambiado, Camelia. —Le rodeó los hombros con un brazo mientras paseaban—. Y, aunque sea difícil, debemos aceptar esos cambios y seguir adelante.

—Creo realmente que en Pumulani hay algo vital esperando a ser descubierto, Elliott —le dijo Camelia con seriedad—. Si aguanto un poco más, lo encontraré.

—Lo mejor que podrías encontrar son diamantes —señaló—. Así la De Beers Company te ofrecería incluso más dinero por el terreno del que te ha ofrecido. Resulta que está intentando adquirir los máximos terrenos posibles alrededor del yacimiento de Kimberley para proteger sus intereses. —Hizo un breve alto antes de añadir en voz baja—: Deberías plantearte seriamente su oferta.

—Jamás venderé el terreno ni a la De Beers Company ni a ninguna otra compañía minera —afirmó Camelia—. Ese lugar es una valiosa conexión arqueológica con el pasado, y debe ser protegido y conservado. No consentiré que nadie empiece a excavarlo y dinamitarlo hasta convertirlo en un enorme y horrible pozo, como los espantosos agujeros que han hecho en Kimberley.

—Pero ¿y si no hay nada más en ese terreno? —repuso Elliott—. Sé que tu padre estaba convencido de que allí hay una enorme cámara mortuoria, pero no hay ninguna prueba que evidencie que realmente exista esa cámara y, aunque así sea, es probable que sólo contenga unos cuantos huesos descompuestos y conchas rotas. No vale la pena arruinarse la vida por un hallazgo como ése, Camelia. —Se acercó a ella y su voz se volvió un susurro—: No vale la pena que desperdicies la oportunidad de tener un verdadero hogar, con un marido y unos hijos, aquí, en Inglaterra.

—Inglaterra no es mi hogar —objetó Camelia. Habían llegado a una bonita glorieta del jardín, y Camelia notó que tenía una espesa pared verde a sus espaldas—, es África.

—Pero Inglaterra también podría serlo —insistió Elliott persuasivo y en voz baja—. Sé que no te sientes cómoda aquí, pero acabaría gustándote. Y te prometo que, si me dejaras, haría cuanto estuviese en mis manos para hacerte feliz. —Colocó las manos sobre sus hombros y la atrajo hacia sí—. Desde que nos conocemos, no te había visto nunca tan triste, Camelia, y me duele verte así. Lo único que quiero es que seas feliz, como lo eras cuando te traía un libro nuevo de Ciudad del Cabo o un estilete especial que veías por primera vez.

Camelia le dedicó una melancólica sonrisa.

—No es tan sencillo, Elliott. No soy la niña despreocupada de antes, que podía pasarse horas distraída con un libro o un estilete nuevos, aunque me los regalases tú. Soy una arqueóloga a cargo de una excavación inundada en medio de Suráfrica, con docenas de trabajadores que dependen de mí para su subsistencia y un montón de deudas que trato de que no se coman cuanto poseo.

—Entonces deja que te ayude a salir de este embrollo —le suplicó Elliott—. Sé que cuando tomas una decisión detestas abandonar antes de llegar al final; siempre has sido así y te admiro por ello, pero me duele ver lo que sufres para perseguir el sueño de tu padre.

—También es mi sueño, Elliott —le recordó Camelia—. Mi padre y yo compartíamos el mismo sueño.

—Tu padre era hombre, aunque odies oír esto, su caso era distinto. No te puedes pasar la vida viviendo en tiendas de campaña inmundas y llenas de polvo en medio de la nada, rodeada de docenas de nativos, y escarbando la tierra en busca de huesos y herramientas de piedra. Tu sitio está aquí, en Londres, en una magnífica casa, educando a tus hijos y siendo una buena anfitriona para la flor y nata de la sociedad británica.

—Me temo que a la flor y nata británica no le gustaría ser mi invitada —replicó ella—. Lo único que les serviría es una copiosa cena a base de antílope asado y pudín de plátano, me pondría a defender que el hombre viene del mono y, mientras, Oscar, Harriet y Rupert se dedicarían a saltar, volar y escurrirse por encima y debajo de la mesa del comedor. ¡Dudo que nadie quisiese volver a mi casa después de eso! —exclamó riéndose.

—Pues cometerían una estupidez. —Elliott alargó el brazo y apartó un rizo rebelde de su mejilla.

Camelia lo miró confusa. Él dejó los dedos sobre su mejilla, el tacto era suave, pero poseía una determinación masculina que jamás había detectado en él. En ese instante supo que algo había entre ellos, sosegadamente, pero con absoluta certeza.

Sin dejar de mirarla a los ojos, Elliott empezó a inclinar la cabeza hacia la suya.

—Tú me perteneces, Camelia. —Sus labios se rozaban cuando él concluyó con voz ronca—: Siempre has sido mía.

Camelia se quedó helada, no podía respirar y su corazón latía con fuerza como una pájaro atrapado que aletea contra la firmemente encorsetada jaula de sus costillas. Elliott apretó los labios contra su boca, calientes, decididos y secos. Tenía las manos sobre sus hombros, la sujetaba con ternura pero con determinación. A ella le pareció un beso casto, incluso cuando él aumentó ligeramente la presión de los labios en un intento por obtener algún tipo de reacción.

Le atravesó un remolino de emociones. Elliott era un viejo y querido amigo, que había formado parte de su vida desde que tenía trece años. Desde que llegó a África, guapo y con sólo veintiún años, Camelia lo había adorado. Lleno de energía, inteligencia y determinación, Elliott le pareció admirablemente independiente y valiente; un hijo de un vizconde, que había tenido la desfachatez de contrariar los deseos de su padre y que había dejado Inglaterra para dedicarse a lo que amaba: la arqueología. Durante años había ardido en su totalmente inexperto corazón una intensa llama de deseo inocente y admiración. Incluso en algún momento dado había fantaseado con la idea de casarse con él. Pero Camelia ya no era una niña pequeña. Era una mujer, y sus sentimientos hacia Elliott hacía tiempo que se habían convertido en una afectuosa y agradable amistad. Elliott era parte de su familia. Sentía un gran cariño por él, pero no era suya. No era de nadie.

¿En serio creía que dejaría África, se casaría con él y viviría en Inglaterra?

El beso más enérgico e intenso.

De repente, el aire de la noche se había vuelto denso y cálido, tan sofocante como el del salón de baile. Londres era así. Elliott la encerraría en una casa oscura, polvorienta y atiborrada de terciopelo para que criase a los niños, dirigiese al servicio y tomase decisiones sobre temas ridículos e insoportables como la tapicería, los menús y el vestuario. Jamás le dejaría volver a África, a excepción, tal vez, de una corta visita cada varios años, pero cuando tuviesen hijos probablemente acabaría incluso con eso. No lo aguantaría, pensó, sintiendo que le faltaba oxígeno. No sabía nada de niños, de moda ni de cómo se recibía, aunque se conocía bastante para saber que se marchitaría y moriría si la obligaban a quedarse en Inglaterra y desempeñar el rol de esposa. Puso las manos sobre el pecho de Elliott para intentar apartarlo, pero éste malinterpretó el gesto y la atrajo más hacía su cuerpo mientras abría la boca para darle un beso más profundo.

—Lamento la interrupción —dijo alguien en voz baja y levemente burlona—. No me había dado cuenta de que estaban ocupados.

Sobresaltada, Camelia se apartó de Elliott tambaleándose hacia atrás y vio a Simon, que la contemplaba con aparente regodeo.

—Señor Kent —logró decir sin aliento, procurando en todo momento no dar la imagen de la mujer que acaba de recibir un beso romántico.

Simon la observó, reparó en el vestido escarlata que le envolvía y dejaba al descubierto la incitante piel marfileña de sus hombros. Por la columna de su cuello y sobre su pálido escote caían mechones rebeldes de su cabello dorado por el sol, y se preguntó si Camelia lograba alguna vez sujetarse bien el pelo con horquillas o si había algo especial en esos sedosos mechones que, simplemente, se negaban a obedecer. Su boca era una abochornada línea de color coral, los labios estaban rosados pero no hinchados, dando a entender que lo que sea que hubiese sucedido entre ella y Wickham no había durado mucho rato.

Aunque no entendía el porqué, sintió pensar que los había interrumpido; al fin y al cabo, Lady Camelia era una mujer adulta y, sin duda, estaba en su derecho de tomar sus propias decisiones acerca de a quién besaba y a quién no. Sin embargo, la esperanza que le había impulsado a correr a verla al baile de la Sociedad Arqueológica se había desvanecido, dejándolo desilusionado y un tanto irritado.

—¿Qué demonios hace aquí, Kent? —inquirió Elliott, molesto porque su momento a solas con Camelia se había ido al traste.

—Tengo que enseñarle unos dibujos, lady Camelia —anunció Simon sin dejar de mirarla—. Supuse que querría verlos lo antes posible.

Camelia también lo miró, paralizada. Un poco sorprendida por no haberlo notado hasta ahora, cayó en la cuenta de que Simon era más alto que Elliott. Llevaba un arrugado abrigo de día, chaleco y camisa, y pese a que se había puesto una corbata alrededor del cuello, ésta estaba medio suelta y torcida, como si se la hubiese puesto a toda prisa en el último momento para completar su desarreglado atuendo. Las ondas despeinadas de su pelo cobrizo se rizaban ligeramente al chocar con sus hombros, que a Camelia le parecieron mucho más anchos que antes, y si bien le dio la impresión de que el corte y la tela de sus pantalones eran buenos, hacía mucho tiempo que habían perdido el efecto del planchado que pudieran haber experimentado. Sus manos fuertes y alargadas estaban sin guantes y generosamente manchadas de tinta, lo que indicaba que se había pasado horas trabajando en el montón de papeles que sujetaba, parte de la cual había penetrado en los puños blancos de su camisa. La tranquilidad y una gran confianza en sí mismo emanaban de él mientras estaba ahí de pie, mirándola fijamente, lo que, teniendo en cuenta su inapropiado y desaliñado atuendo, no dejaba de ser curioso. Estaba claro que a Simon Kent no le preocupaba mucho lo que los demás pensasen de él.

—No puede irrumpir aquí sólo porque quiere ver a lady Camelia —protestó Elliott de manera sucinta—; para esta fiesta se precisa invitación.

—¡Oh! Seguro que la tenía en alguna parte —repuso Simon, encogiéndose de hombros—. La debí de perder en el incendio. Supongo que se habrá enterado de que mi casa ardió en llamas hace unos cuantos días.

—Pero no lleva la ropa adecuada —señaló Elliott, que en ese momento nada podía importarle menos que los problemas de Kent—. Los invitados tienen que ir vestidos de etiqueta.

—Lo lamento, Wickhip, pero me temo que no tengo tiempo para quedarme a bailar —replicó Simon con amabilidad—.

Sólo necesito hablar un momento con lady Camelia y luego dejaré que retomen lo que sea que estuviesen haciendo.

—No estábamos haciendo nada —se apresuró a asegurarle Camelia, abochornada pero profundamente agradecida de que Simon hubiese llegado en el instante oportuno—. ¿Qué es lo que quería consultarme?

La luz de la luna caía sobre ella como un velo plateado, que volvía su piel dorada por el sol en la más pálida de las sedas. Sus ojos eran como dos chispeantes lagos verdes y aunque se esforzaba por fingir calma, Simon pudo percibir que el deseo hervía en las profundidades de color verdeceledón.

«¿Qué demonios haces con un gallito idiota y presumido como Wickham con el fuego que arde en tu interior?», se preguntó.

Notó que estaba avergonzada, algo comprensible teniendo en cuenta que los había sorprendido en tan inoportuno momento; lo que no podía entender era qué hacía en brazos de Wickham. Aunque soso y sin ser nada del otro mundo, supuso que el vizconde era bastante guapo; el tipo de belleza masculina estandarizada que había visto inmortalizada en cuadros y esculturas en un sinfín de ocasiones. Indudablemente, Simon comprendía que la mayoría de las mujeres encontrasen atractivo a lord Wickham, con su pelo de color arena, sus elegantes rasgos marcados y su ropa impecablemente planchada y absolutamente a la moda. Sólo que Camelia no era como la mayoría de las mujeres. Era una mujer de una curiosidad y determinación únicas, que había dedicado su vida a observar el mundo que le rodeaba y es probable que a analizar y valorar hasta los detalles más infinitesimales.

¿Realmente no veía que debajo de su atuendo rigurosamente hecho a medida y sus botas esmeradamente lustradas lord Wickham era un idiota arrogante y engreído?

—He hecho unos bocetos para su bomba, lady Camelia. —Prescindiendo de Wickham, Simon se acercó a un banco de piedra sobre el que colocó una serie de arrugados papeles—. Tengo más o menos pensado cómo habrá que adaptarla, pero necesito saber más cosas sobre la densidad del suelo que se mezcla con el agua, la cantidad y tamaño de las rocas que podemos encontrar y la disponibilidad de combustible para la bomba...

—Kent, me veo obligado a protestar —le interrumpió Elliott—. Lady Camelia está aquí para disfrutar de un evento social y no para tener una especie de reunión de negocios con usted. Es totalmente inapropiado.

—Disculpe, Wickhip...

—Wickham —le corrigió Elliott con frialdad.

—Como prefiera —concedió Simon—. Lady Camelia y yo somos socios en un proyecto arqueológico y sé que para ella el tiempo es de suma importancia. Además, me aseguró que podía hablar con ella de cualquier asunto o problema que surgiese a cualquier hora del día o de la noche.

—Dudo que se refiriese a que la abordase en una fiesta privada y la arrinconase en un jardín —replicó Elliott.

—A mí me ha parecido que ya estaba arrinconada.

—Le dije al señor Kent que podía venir a verme cuando quisiese —se apresuró a intervenir Camelia al ver la crispada mandíbula de Elliott.

Éste se volvió y la miró con incredulidad.

—Una cosa es que te vaya a ver a casa, Camelia, pero que te venga a buscar a una fiesta para hablar de negocios es completamente inadecuado.

—Sí, tiene razón —convino Simon, recogiendo con descuido sus arrugados bocetos—. Lo mejor será que me marche.

—¿Por qué es inadecuado, Elliott? —preguntó Camelia, repentinamente molesta por la insistencia de su amigo.

—En primer lugar, el señor Kent no tiene invitación...

—En realidad, creo que la tenía, es más, estoy casi seguro de ello —se defendió Simon, rascándose la cabeza—. Me temo que soy un poco desastroso con esa clase de cosas. No sólo con las invitaciones, ya me entiende, sino con las citas y la correspondencia en general. Lady Camelia puede atestiguarlo.

—No veo qué importancia tiene que haya sido o no invitado, Elliott —continuó Camelia—, dado que no ha venido aquí a disfrutar de la fiesta, sino a hablar conmigo de un asunto de negocios.

—Pero ¡es que eso no está bien, Camelia! —insistió Elliott—. No está bien visto hablar de negocios en un acto social.

—¿Y a qué he venido yo, Elliott? —le recordó Camelia—. A mí no me parece que esté mal, sobre todo cuando a los hombres les encanta discutir temas de negocios prácticamente en todos los actos sociales a los que asisten. ¿O lo dices porque soy mujer y consideras que no tengo el mismo derecho?

—Yo no he dicho eso —objetó Elliott, dándose cuenta de que le había hecho enfadar.

—No —concedió Simon, que asintió con la cabeza—, lo que ha dicho concretamente es que usted no debería hablar de negocios —le aclaró a Camelia con seriedad—. Seguro que piensa que otras mujeres sí pueden hacer lo que les plazca, ¿me equivoco, Wickhop?

—Me llamo Wickham —repitió Elliott con los dientes apretados.

—Como veo que te parece tan indecoroso que hable aquí de trabajo, quizá lo mejor será que me vaya. —Camelia se volvió hacia Simon—. ¿Por qué no viene a mi casa, señor Kent? Allí podremos seguir hablando sin correr el riesgo de ofender a nadie.

—Me parece una idea excelente —declaró Simon con entusiasmo—. La seguiré en mi carruaje. Bueno, Wickhop, ahora ya no ofenderemos a nadie.

—No hablarás en serio, Camelia. —Elliott la miró como si pensase que se había vuelto loca—. Es casi media noche.

—Gracias por su interés, Wickhop, pero no estoy cansado lo más mínimo —le aseguró Simon alegremente.

—No me refería a eso —le espetó Elliott—. Camelia, no deberías recibir en casa al señor Kent en plena noche.

—No viene como invitado, Elliott; viene a hablar de negocios.

—Aun así, es impropio.

—Lo siento, Elliott, pero si me pasara la vida intentando observar las aparentemente infinitas normas británicas de lo que es apropiado para las mujeres y lo que no, estoy segura de que nunca haría nada.

—En ese caso, te acompañaré.

—Eres muy amable, pero ni se me ocurriría obligarte a abandonar el baile; deberías aprovechar el tiempo. Hablaré contigo dentro de unos días para informarte de cómo están las cosas.

—De verdad, Camelia, insisto...

—Y yo insisto en que te quedes, Elliott —repuso Camelia con énfasis—. Aprovecharás mejor el tiempo si consigues que alguien quiera invertir en tu nuevo negocio. A lo mejor hasta acabas concediendo un par de bailes; la música es maravillosa.

Estoy convencida de que hay un montón de jovencitas a las que les encantaría tener la oportunidad de bailar contigo —concluyó, dedicándole una dulce sonrisa.

Elliott la miró resignado. No podía acompañarla a la fuerza.

—¿Nos vamos, lady Camelia? —Simon le ofreció galante su brazo.

Al fin aliviada, Camelia puso una mano sobre la tremendamente arrugada manga de su camisa.

El calor le atravesó la mano y recorrió su brazo, haciéndole hundir los dedos en el brazo de Simon.

—¿Va todo bien? —le preguntó él con las cejas fruncidas.

De pronto se le ocurrió que tal vez no fuese lo más acertado que Camelia abandonase el baile con él; a fin de cuentas, estaba totalmente seguro de que no había sido invitado. Pese a que no acostumbraba a importarle lo que la gente pensara de él o de su forma de vestir, le repugnaba la idea de que los invitados de lord Bagley pudieran hacer comentarios despreciativos de Camelia por su culpa.

—Si lo prefiere, puedo salir por mi cuenta —sugirió— y encontrarme con usted junto a su carruaje.

—No será necesario —le aseguró Camelia, consciente de que él intentaba protegerla de las miradas curiosas que, sin duda, atraerían en el interior del salón de baile. Si la veían marcharse con el probablemente no invitado e inadecuadamente vestido Simon Kent, darían que hablar durante días. Le dedicó una decidida sonrisa antes de concluir—: He entrado por la puerta principal y no veo razón alguna por la que no podamos salir por la misma puerta.

Simon esbozó una sonrisa. Estaba claro que a Camelia no le asustaban los escándalos. De hecho, por lo que había constatado hasta el momento, nada parecía asustarle. Se le pasó por la cabeza si todavía llevaría ese peligroso puñal entre las abundantes capas de su asombrosamente sencillo vestido de noche.

—Como desee, lady Camelia. Buenas noches, Wickhip —añadió con una leve inclinación de cabeza dirigida a Elliott—. Espero que tenga una placentera noche.

Con acusada impotencia Elliott observó cómo Camelia volvía sobre sus pasos por la senda marfileña del brazo de su inventor cabeza hueca y ridículamente desaliñado.

Era un hombre paciente, se recordó a sí mismo con optimismo.

Toda gran recompensa requería su tiempo.

Capítulo 5

Algo iba mal.

En algunas ocasiones era un engorro tener el poder de percibir las cosas mientras que otros ignoraban las fuerzas que se movían a su alrededor. Era una carga que soportaba con estoica resignación, igual que lo había hecho su madre y anteriormente la madre de su madre.

Durante generaciones en su familia se había dado por sentado que ese poder era exclusivo de las mujeres; hasta donde cualquiera de sus miembros podía recordar, sólo en las mujeres había recaído lo que su madre le había asegurado que era sencillamente un don. Pero el día en que, al fin, ésta admitió que el poder no residía en ninguna de sus trece hermanas, sino que únicamente hervía en su hijo, Zareb sintió que se le helaba el corazón. Las mujeres estaban acostumbradas al dolor, el desengaño y la alegría, le había dicho su madre, lo que las hacía más aptas para soportar el considerable peso que suponía sentir las cosas antes de que sucediesen. Para aguantarlo debería ser más fuerte que el león más poderoso y más sabio que el chamán más anciano. Por aquel entonces Zareb era un niño, un orgulloso descendiente del gran Waitimu, uno de los guerreros más importantes que la tribu había tenido. La arrogancia juvenil le permitió no albergar duda alguna de que tenía la fuerza y la sabiduría suficientes para soportar su don sin problemas.

Pero se había equivocado.

—Iré a abrir la casa y a encender las lámparas, Tisha —le anunció a Camelia mientras se apresuraba a bajar del asiento del cochero del carruaje.

—Eso es una tontería, Zareb; podemos entrar todos juntos —protestó Camelia—. No me importa que la casa esté a oscuras.

—El señor Kent es nuestro invitado y no debería entrar en una casa en penumbra. —Zareb intentó que pareciese que lo único que intentaba era observar el código de conducta británico—. Tardaré un momento.

—Razón por la cual es absurdo que nosotros dos nos quedemos aquí dentro esperando en lugar de entrar juntos en casa —objetó Camelia—. Estoy segura de que al señor Kent no le da miedo la oscuridad.

—Por mí no hay problema siempre y cuando la serpiente no se me acerque —bromeó Simon, que apareció junto a Zareb—. No me apetece demasiado la idea de encontrármela de pronto en mi cabeza. —Se dispuso a abrir la puerta de Camelia.

Pero Zareb le puso su curtida mano sobre el brazo, obligándole a detenerse.

Simon frunció las cejas.

—¿Ocurre algo, Zareb?

El calor penetró la mano de Zareb al entrar en contacto con la manga de la camisa del inventor blanco. La dejó ahí unos instantes para asegurarse.

Quizá sus sentidos se equivocasen, pensó, confundido por el calor que latía en su interior. El inventor blanco lo miró con curiosidad, con sus ojos azules desmesuradamente abiertos, aunque no parecía molesto por el hecho de que Zareb se hubiese tomado la libertad de tocarlo, como se habría mostrado lord Wickham. Estaba todo bien, decidió Zareb, procurando mitigar la inquietud que momentos antes se había apoderado de él. Había oscuridad, pero también luz.

Deseó que la luz fuese bastante fuerte para contrarrestar lo que se avecinaba.

—Yo lo haré —declaró con modesta dignidad al tiempo que agarraba la manilla de la puerta del carruaje. Y luego, tal vez porque quería dejarle claro al inventor blanco que sólo a él le correspondía velar por Camelia, añadió con solemnidad—: Es mi deber.

Abrió la puerta y le ofreció la mano a Camelia, ayudándola a bajar del vehículo. La sostuvo unos segundos más de lo necesario, sus dedos largos y de color café rodeaban protectores la pequeña y enguantada palma de la mano de Tisha.

—¿Va todo bien, Zareb? —Camelia lo miró extrañada.

—No es nada —la tranquilizó con la esperanza de que así fuese—. Entremos.

Deseó seguir sujetando su mano hasta que llegasen a la casa, como había hecho cuando ella era pequeña, pero comprendía que ya no procedía. Se la soltó a regañadientes, pensando que se agarraría del brazo del inventor blanco, pero no fue así.

Y, en cierto modo, eso le hizo sentir un poco mejor.

—¡Qué raro! —musitó Camelia mientras subían las escaleras que conducían a la puerta principal—. La puerta está entreabierta.

Zareb se colocó delante de ella, impidiéndole el paso.

—Espera.

Escudriñó rápidamente las ventanas de la fachada delantera en busca de cualquier indicio de luz o movimiento detrás de las cortinas echadas. No vio nada y, sin embargo, la puerta estaba abierta un dedo.

Zareb estaba convencido de que la había cerrado con llave.

—No parece que la hayan forzado —comentó Simon al examinar la cerradura y el marco de la puerta—. A lo mejor no la cerró bien y el viento la ha abierto.

—La puerta estaba cerrada —repuso Zareb con tranquilidad—. Y no hace viento.

A Camelia se le encogió el corazón. Había dejado a Oscar, a Rupert y a Harriet solos en casa. Rodeó a Zareb y entró en casa corriendo.

—¡Tisha, espera! —chilló Zareb, que corrió tras ella—. ¡No sabemos lo que nos podemos encontrar!

—¡Oscar! —Camelia avanzaba a tientas por el vestíbulo, tratando de ver a través de las sombras—. Oscar, ¿dónde estás?

—Espera un poco, Tisha —le instó Zareb, que manoseaba torpemente la mecha de la lámpara—. Estate quieta hasta que haya un poco de luz. —Su voz era extrañamente firme; el mismo tono que a veces había usado cuando ella era pequeña y hacía algo peligroso o de manera impulsiva.

Camelia aguardó ansiosa mientras Zareb conseguía con paciencia encender una mecha. Un delgado velo de luz naranja bañó la habitación, que aumentó cuando introdujo la mecha en la lámpara y giró la llave.

—¡Dios mío! —exclamó Camelia. Entró lentamente en el despacho de su padre.

El escritorio y las sillas estaban volcados, y su gastada tapicería de cuero había sido brutalmente acuchillada, por lo que parte del seco y polvoriento relleno de cerdas grises de caballo había caído sobre la descolorida alfombra. Asimismo habían tirado al suelo la librería y una pequeña mesa auxiliar, que después habían sido golpeadas con un hacha hasta reducirlas a astillas. Todos los óleos de su padre, los extraordinarios bocetos de antiguas edificaciones y los mapas habían sido arrancados de las paredes y separados de sus marcos. Irreemplazables aparatos, máscaras y esculturas reunidas durante sus múltiples viajes, que ahora yacían hechos añicos en el suelo. Y sus adorados libros, que Camelia había conservado apilados por toda la habitación tal como él los había dejado en su última visita a Londres, habían sido desgajados y esparcidos por todo el despacho.

Se quedó inmóvil unos instantes, contemplando los destrozos y repentinamente sobrecogida y desesperada.

Y después se volvió con brusquedad y se dirigió hacia el oscuro comedor.

Zareb la siguió de cerca con la lámpara en la mano. La luz cobriza iluminó la mesa del comedor y las sillas despedazadas, así como la alacena volcada. Un mar blanquiazul de platos de porcelana, tazas y copas de cristal hechos añicos cubrían la alfombra. Camelia reparó en las diversas plumas grises que había esparcidas por la habitación.

—¡Harriet! —En su voz había pánico—. ¡Rupert! ¿Dónde estáis?

—Dudo que estén aquí abajo. —Simon se esforzaba por controlar la ira que hervía en su interior mientras inspeccionaba los destrozos causados en el comedor. Le tendió la mano a Camelia—. Vamos, Camelia —le dijo con suavidad y manifiesta calma—, seguramente estarán arriba.

Aturdida, asintió y le cogió de la mano. Sus fuertes dedos rodearon los suyos, calientes, firmes y reconfortantes.

—Seguro que sí —repitió ella, que intentaba aminorar los violentos latidos de su corazón—. Probablemente se hayan asustado y hayan subido arriba a esconderse.

Dejó a sus espaldas el destrozado comedor y siguió a Zareb escaleras arriba sin soltar la mano de Simon.

—Ya puedes salir, Oscar —advirtió Zareb—. Ya ha pasado todo, pequeño.

—Estoy aquí, Oscar —añadió Camelia nerviosa—. No hay nada que temer.

El miedo se apoderó de Simon a medida que subían lentamente las escaleras. No se oía ningún ruido de los pisos superiores, donde estaban la sala de estar y los dormitorios, pero la luz de la lámpara que llevaba Zareb revelaba que no habían tenido más suerte que la planta baja. Quienquiera que fuese el autor de todo esto, lo había hecho a conciencia. Debía de haber sabido que Camelia salía esa noche y se había tomado su tiempo para ir de habitación en habitación rompiendo, acuchillando y destrozando. Simon se preguntó si habrían encontrado lo que sea que buscasen.

En ese momento, lo único que realmente le importaba era que Camelia recuperase a sus queridos animales.

—¡Oscar! —chilló Camelia tratando de que no se le quebrase la voz mientras inspeccionaba su arruinada sala de estar. Sobre la alfombra detectó más plumas grises de Harriet—. ¡Harriet! —Soltó súbitamente la mano de Simon y subió corriendo al último piso.

—¡Tisha, espera! —Zareb fue tras ella con la máxima rapidez que le permitían sus voluminosas túnicas—. ¡No subas sin mí!

Ignorándolo, Camelia corrió por el pasillo y abrió la puerta de su habitación. Se encontró una silenciosa oscuridad.

—¿Oscar? —susurró con un hilo de voz.

Una pequeña y oscura silueta chilló aliviada y se abalanzó sobre ella, chocando con sus piernas. Camelia soltó un grito mientras cogía a Oscar del suelo y lo abrazaba contra su pecho.

—¿Estás bien, Oscar? —Se apresuró a palparle para ver si estaba herido—. ¿Te han hecho daño?

Contento, Oscar emitió unos cuantos sonidos y se acurrucó contra ella mientras con sus pequeños brazos le rodeaba el cuello con fuerza.

—Hemos encontrado a Harriet —declaró Zareb, que apareció en la puerta con el pájaro de Camelia sobre su hombro—. Ha perdido muchas plumas, pero, por lo demás, no está herida. Aunque no creo que le guste mirarse en el espejo hasta que le vuelvan a crecer.

Camelia alargó un brazo y Harriet no dudó en abandonar a Zareb para volar hacia ella.

—¡Oh, Harriet! ¡Sigues siendo una preciosidad! —dijo Camelia con ternura, acariciando el suave pecho gris del pájaro—. Esconderemos todos los espejos hasta que te hayan vuelto a crecer las plumas —declaró, poniéndose a Harriet sobre el hombro—. Ahora sólo falta Rupert.

Simon enarcó las cejas.

—¿Es mi imaginación o está debajo de ese montón de ropa que se mueve?

Camelia miró en dirección a las prendas de ropa que se habían caído de su armario volcado y que avanzaban a paso lento.

—¡Rupert! —gritó feliz, agachándose para desenterrar al animal cubierto de satén y seda—. ¡Qué buena idea has tenido escondiéndote entre mi ropa!

Rupert la miró con sus ojos protuberantes y vidriosos, y luego le sacó la delgada lengua.

Camelia cogió al reptil del suelo y lo besó con cariño en la fría y suave cabeza.

Simon la miró, atónito. La expresión de tremenda angustia de su rostro había desaparecido, dando paso a un alivio absoluto. Estas extrañas criaturas africanas lo eran todo para ella, reflexionó, inexplicablemente conmovido por la constatación. Una horrible serpiente naranja y negra, un mono travieso y desobediente y un exótico pájaro aparentemente neurótico. Esos animales, y Zareb, eran la única familia de Camelia.

Tragó saliva, sintiendo un gran alivio al comprobar que quienquiera que hubiese irrumpido y destrozado la casa no había logrado hacer daño a ninguno de sus animales.

—Tenemos que salir de aquí, Tisha —le instó Zareb de repente mientras gesticulaba hacia la puerta—. Ya tenemos a los animales, podemos irnos.

El acuciante tono de voz de Zareb era casi imperceptible. Tan imperceptible que a cualquiera podría haberle pasado desapercibido, pero Camelia conocía y quería a Zareb desde hacía demasiados años para no darse cuenta. Confusa, se volvió, y supo que su amigo intentaba protegerla de algo.

Entonces miró hacia la cama.

—Acércame la lámpara, Zareb —pidió en voz baja.

—Deberíamos revisar el resto de las habitaciones, Tisha —insistió Zareb para alejarla del lugar—. Aquí no hay nada...

—Acércame la lámpara —repitió ella mientras avanzaba despacio hacia su cama. Y a continuación, consciente de que lo único que él quería era protegerla, añadió con suavidad—: Por favor.

A regañadientes, Zareb se aproximó a Camelia con la lámpara en la mano.

Un ardiente resplandor iluminó el puñal que había clavado en su almohadón.

Era el arma favorita de su padre, pensó Camelia, un grueso puñal fabricado por un miembro de la tribu San, también llamados Bushmen por los blancos de Suráfrica. Era un bello ejemplo de excepcional artesanía, con su grueso mango de hierro repujado, soldado a una cuchilla tremendamente afilada de pulidísimo acero. No era una antigüedad, pero era una magnífica obra de artesanía de gran equilibrio; un arma impresionante para aquel que quisiese utilizarla como tal. Se le ocurrió que era imposible que quienquiera que la hubiese descolgado de su gancho, encima de la chimenea del despacho de su padre, para clavar una nota en su almohadón, supiese que un chamán había transmitido al puñal poderes oscuros.

Lo miró con fijeza, tratando de controlar el miedo que sentía. No creía en las maldiciones sobrenaturales, se recordó tajante. Aun así, tenía frío, como si a su alrededor soplase de pronto un viento helado.

—¡Menudo puñal! —observó Oliver alegremente desde la puerta—. Ese pobre cojín no ha podido ni rechistar.

Simon suspiró.

—Lady Camelia, permítame que le presente a Oliver, que supuestamente me esperaba fuera, en mi carruaje. Oliver, estos son lady Camelia y Zareb.

—Encantado de conocerlos. —Oliver los saludó con un movimiento de su nívea cabeza—. Y no me regañes por haber venido a ver qué sucede aquí. ¡Por el amor de San Columbano! —continuó diciéndole a Simon con seriedad—. Si lo único que veo es una luz que se va moviendo por toda la casa como un fantasma, cuando habéis tenido tiempo suficiente para que se prendiera la casa entera... con luz, me refiero —corrigió rápidamente mientras le lanzaba una mirada tranquilizadora a Camelia—. Me imagino que se habrá enterado de que el chico incendió su casa la otra noche, aunque ha sido la primera vez que un experimento se le ha ido de las manos; no quiero que piense que acostumbra a hacer esta clase de cosas. Claro que en cierta ocasión estuvo a punto de quemar la casa de miss Amelia con una bomba de humo —comentó, rascándose la cabeza—, pero no fue intencionado. De joven se pasaba el día haciendo volar la tapa de algo o introduciendo demasiadas mechas en una botella para luego hacerlas arder. Nos decía que sólo intentaba buscar un sistema de iluminación mejor. —Soltó una carcajada y concluyó con contundencia—: ¡Estábamos convencidos de que cualquier día nos despertaríamos entre llamas!

—Oliver, yo no tengo la culpa del incendio de la otra noche —intervino Simon, deseoso de poner fin a las confesiones del anciano. No creía que fuese precisamente un buen momento para obsequiar a Camelia con historias de travesuras infantiles—. No se lo he contado a Haydon y Genevieve porque no quiero preocuparles, pero alguien quemó mi laboratorio a propósito. Es más, yo diría que fueron las mismas personas que esta noche han destrozado la casa de lady Camelia.

—Pues no es obra de unos ladrones profesionales, eso te lo aseguro —reflexionó Oliver mientras miraba tranquilamente la habitación—. Yo mismo fui un ladrón —les explicó orgulloso a Camelia y a Zareb— y jamás dejé una casa tan desordenada. ¿Para qué morder la mano que te da de comer? —Frunció las cejas y terminó furioso—: Esto lo han hecho unos vulgares aficionados, y si alguna vez les echo el guante, ¡los moleré a palos!

De algún modo, a Camelia le tranquilizó la indignación del menudo y anciano escocés.

—Gracias, Oliver. —No sabía muy bien qué pensar de él, con su tupido cabello blanco y por la forma en que se jactaba de haber sido un ladrón. Simon le había comentado que era su cochero, pero Camelia supo con certeza que, en realidad, era mucho más que eso—. Es usted muy amable.

Oliver le sonrió y después levantó las cejas.

—¿Se ha dado cuenta de que lleva un animal alrededor del cuello?

—Es Rupert —le aclaró Simon—. La serpiente de lady Camelia.

—¿Y la tiene como una mascota? —Oliver miró a Rupert con recelo—. ¿No debería estar encerrada?

—Me temo que a Rupert no le haría mucha gracia que lo encerrase —contestó Camelia—. Está muy acostumbrado a moverse con libertad.

—La nota, Tisha. —Zareb señaló el papel atravesado con el puñal—. ¿Qué dice la nota?

Camelia arrancó lentamente el arma del cojín y a continuación acercó la nota a la lámpara que estaba sosteniendo Zareb. Esforzándose para que no le temblara la voz, leyó en voz alta:

—«Que mueran aquellos que alteran la paz de Pumulani.»

—¿Qué es Poo Moo Lanee? —inquirió Oliver.

—Es el nombre africano de la zona surafricana donde está mi excavación arqueológica —respondió Camelia—. En las lenguas nguni significa «descanso» o «lugar de descanso». Hace aproximadamente cien años fue ocupada por una familia de boers holandeses, que construyeron una granja. Mi padre le compró las tierras al nieto del propietario original y empezó a excavarlas hace veinte años. Murió hace seis meses y desde entonces yo he continuado su labor.

—Pues me da la impresión de que alguien quiere que se largue de ahí.

—Mi padre creía que bajo esas tierras se esconde un hallazgo arqueológico de suma importancia —prosiguió Camelia—. Durante estos años hemos encontrado numerosas reliquias que indican que en el pasado vivió allí una próspera comunidad, teoría que apoyan una serie de extraordinarias pinturas rupestres. En mi opinión, debe de haber algunos arqueólogos que quieren ahuyentarme y obligarme a abandonar la excavación. Supongo que pensarán que, si me rindo, podrán comprar el terreno por una porción de su valor y excavar ellos mismos.

Oliver frunció las cejas.

—¿Me está diciendo que ésta no es la primera vez que la amedrentan?

—No.

—¿Qué más han hecho? —quiso saber Simon.

—Unas cuantas cosas —confesó Camelia quitándole importancia al asunto—, pero eso da igual. Quieren asustarme y no lo conseguirán. Ese terreno es mío y seguiré excavando hasta que dé con lo que mi padre buscaba.

—¿Y qué buscaba?

—Pruebas de una civilización antigua.

Oliver se rascó la mandíbula pensativo.

—Demasiado alboroto para un puñado de huesos rotos.

—Sí, es cierto. —Simon miró a Camelia fijamente.

—Es normal que piensen eso, porque no han dedicado sus vidas a la arqueología —admitió ella—. Pero es de suma importancia para aquellos que viven toda su vida con la esperanza de realizar un solo descubrimiento de significación histórica.

—Debemos irnos de aquí, Tisha —advirtió Zareb con expresión adusta—. Ahora.

—No podemos irnos, Zareb —replicó Camelia—. El señor Kent todavía no ha podido terminar la bomba.

—No me refiero a volver a África esta misma noche —precisó Zareb—, sino a que en esta casa ya no estarás a salvo. Debemos irnos.

Camelia cabeceó.

—Ésta es la casa de mi padre y no pienso dejar que un par de miserables me intimiden. Ordenaremos todo y nos quedaremos.

—¡Eso es una chica valiente! —Oliver miró a Simon con aprobación—. Las ovejas mojadas no se encogen, se sacuden el agua.

—A las ovejas se las mata, Oliver —musitó Simon.

—Bueno, a veces sí —concedió Oliver con reserva—. Sólo intentaba ser positivo.

—Y se lo agradezco, Oliver —le aseguró Camelia—. Ésta no es la primera vez que alguien trata de apartarme de mi camino y supongo que tampoco será la última; pero no se saldrán con la suya.

—Lo que yo digo, ¡una chica valiente! —Oliver le sonrió—. No importa la fiereza del perro al que haya que enfrentarse, lo que importa es luchar.

—Lady Camelia no es un perro —objetó Zareb—. La han amenazado con el puñal de su padre; un arma a la que un gran chamán dotó con poderes oscuros. No puede permanecer aquí más tiempo. Debemos abandonar esta casa hoy mismo.

—¿Ha dicho con poderes oscuros? —Oliver arqueó las cejas y se rascó la cabeza—. Eso ya es harina de otro costal.

—Pero no podemos irnos esta noche —protestó Camelia—. No tenemos adónde ir.

—Podrían venir a casa —ofreció Oliver amablemente.

Simon no daba crédito.

—No creo que sea una buena idea...

—¿Por qué no? Hay espacio de sobras para todos ellos, aunque no será fácil que Eunice se avenga a tener una serpiente deslizándose por la casa. No le hacen mucha gracia los reptiles.

—Rupert puede quedarse en la habitación de lady Camelia —se apresuró a sugerir Zareb—. No creo que le importe.

—Pero a Oscar y a Harriet no puedo dejarlos todo el día encerrados en una habitación —objetó Camelia—. Necesitan espacio para moverse; será mejor que nos quedemos aquí.

—Bueno, no creo que Eunice y Doreen tengan ningún problema con eso siempre y cuando se comporten, y no alboroten demasiado —comentó Oliver.

—Yo me ocuparé de que se porten bien —aseguró Zareb antes de que Camelia pudiese decir nada—; les daré de comer y limpiaré lo que manchen. Eunice y Doreen ni siquiera notarán su presencia.

—Muy bien, pues ya está todo solucionado —concluyó Oliver contento.

—Sigo pensando que no es una buena idea —insistió Simon una vez más.

—No tema por la reputación de la chica —le dijo Oliver a Zareb, prescindiendo de Simon—. Eunice y Doreen están más que acostumbradas a vigilar a las señoritas de casa; llevan años haciéndolo.

—El único honor que cuenta es el que arde en el interior del corazón —declaró Zareb con solemnidad—. El honor de lady Camelia está a salvo vaya adonde vaya.

—Por supuesto, eso no hacía falta ni mencionarlo —coincidió Oliver—. Pero me refería a que seremos tantos que siempre habrá alguien para asegurarse de que lady Camelia está bien. Le diré una cosa: si los desgraciados que han entrado aquí esta noche intentan irrumpir en mi casa, les daré una patada en su maldito culo...

—Gracias, Oliver, estoy seguro de que lady Camelia agradece tus ganas de ayudar —le interrumpió Simon—. Sin embargo, no acabo de ver claro que ésta sea la mejor solución...

—Pero ¡si tú tendrás espacio más que suficiente para dedicarte a todos tus inventos! —exclamó Oliver—. Y no creo que lady Camelia se lleve mucho equipaje.

—Solamente un poco de ropa —concretó Zareb—. Y yo no necesito una habitación, puedo dormir en cualquier parte.

—¿Lo ves? Todo arreglado. —Oliver le dedicó una sonrisa a Camelia—. Joven, vaya a coger lo que necesite que Zareb y yo lo bajaremos al carruaje.

Camelia miró a Simon indecisa.

En realidad, ésta última agresión le había conmocionado. Cuanto había en la casa de su padre había sido brutalmente destrozado y ella no había podido hacer nada para impedirlo, aunque lo más importante era que sus animales no estaban heridos, pensó. Pero ¿qué pasaría la próxima vez que Zareb y ella saliesen, y Oscar, Harriet y Rupert se quedaran solos en casa? Si quienquiera que intentaba intimidarla acababa por hacerle daño a alguno de ellos, jamás se lo perdonaría a sí misma.

—¿Estás de acuerdo con esto, Simon? —Odiaba el hecho de que él se viese obligado a aceptar su presencia y la de sus animales. Pero la visión del puñal de su padre clavado en el cojín le inquietaba más de lo que quería reconocer—. Será por poco tiempo.

Simon suspiró. Oliver y Zareb tenían razón. Camelia no estaría a salvo en esa casa. Él no creía en los hechizos maléficos, pero estaba claro que alguien se había propuesto intimidarla para que abandonase la excavación.

Quizá la próxima vez no se limitasen a destrozar muebles.

—Me encantará teneros a ti, a Zareb, a Oscar y a Harriet —dijo al fin.

Camelia asintió y luego frunció el entrecejo.

—¿Y qué pasa con Rupert?

Simon miró con recelo la serpiente que Camelia llevaba alrededor del cuello.

—Rupert también puede venir —concedió a regañadientes— si me prometes encerrarlo en tu habitación. No quiero que Eunice grite horrorizada cada vez que tropiece con él. —Evitó mencionar que a él tampoco le gustaba especialmente la idea de toparse con esa horrible criatura en plena madrugada.

—No creo que le importe mucho quedarse en mi cuarto —dijo Camelia acariciando con ternura a la serpiente—. Pero ¿estás seguro de que no te molestará que Oscar y Harriet se paseen por ahí?

—¡Pues claro que no, jovencita! —exclamó Oliver sin dudarlo—. Darán un poco de vida a la casa.

Camelia miró a Simon.

—¿Simon?

Sus penetrantes ojos no estaban iluminados más que por la débil luz dorada de la lámpara de Zareb, pero Simon pudo ver el miedo en ellos. Camelia era fuerte y decidida; sin embargo, era evidente que este último incidente le había afectado profundamente. El terror se había apoderado de ella mientras buscaba a sus animales por la casa. Le había dicho a Simon que no creía en las maldiciones; y es posible que fuese verdad.

Pero aun así no había duda de que ver el puñal de su padre clavado en un cojín había disipado parte de su valor.

—Estoy convencido de que Harriet y Oscar no supondrán ningún problema en absoluto —mintió.

—¿Lo ve, jovencita? —Oliver sonrió—. ¿Y ahora qué le parece si recoge sus cosas y nos marchamos?

—Oliver y yo comprobaremos que todas las puertas y ventanas están cerradas mientras Zareb y tú hacéis las maletas. Cuando hayáis terminado, avisadnos. —Simon se volvió y salió de la habitación.

—Será mejor que les expliques a Eunice y a Doreen lo del mono y la serpiente —susurró Oliver al bajar las escaleras—, porque no creo que vayan a dar saltos de alegría.

—Dado que la idea ha sido básicamente tuya, Oliver —repuso Simon con tranquilidad—, dejaré que seas tú quien se lo diga.

—Vamos, chico, te conozco lo suficiente como para saber que no habrías dejado a esa chica en la estacada rodeada de puñales clavados en cojines y hechizos malignos. Lo único que yo he hecho es ayudarte a tomar la decisión de invitarle a casa.

—No es una mascota, Oliver.

—Tienes razón, es una chica muy valiente, y bastante guapa también. Me recuerda a la señora cuando era joven —concedió Oliver riéndose entre dientes—. Cuando se conozcan congeniarán enseguida.

—No se conocerán. Voy a trabajar día y noche para tener lista la bomba dentro de unas cuantas semanas y así poder acompañar a lady Camelia a África lo antes posible.

—¿Has dicho África? Nunca me habría imaginado que iría a África; me pregunto si hará tanto calor como dicen.

—Y no vendrás, Oliver.

—Supongo que el viaje será largo, incluso en uno de los barcos más rápidos que tenga Jack —comentó Oliver sin hacer caso a Simon—. Tendremos que decirle a Eunice que prepare un montón de galletas.

—Oliver...

—¡Menudo desastre han hecho aquí! —Oliver miró con solemnidad las reliquias hechas añicos del despacho—. Pero incluso en un nido caído puedes encontrar un huevo —añadió alegremente.

—Creo que quien ha destrozado la casa lo ha hecho a conciencia —opinó Simon recorriendo el suelo con la mirada.

—Por suerte a ella no le han hecho daño, ¿verdad?

—Verdad.

—Pues ahí tienes el huevo entero. —Sonrió, se fue al comedor a revisar las ventanas y dejó a Simon contemplando los escombros que le rodeaban.

Capítulo 6

A Camelia se le encogió el corazón cuando, al fin, el carruaje se detuvo.

Igual que la mayoría de las casas londinenses, la nueva casa de Simon era estrecha y alta, en un intento por aprovechar al máximo el escaso terreno disponible que había. Cuando era pequeña creía que todas las viviendas se construían así, excepto la destartalada finca familiar. Su madre nunca tuvo mucho interés en esa casa ruinosa y llena de corrientes de aire, con sus paredes desmoronadas y su tejado de incesantes goteras. Lady Stamford siempre había preferido las luces y el bullicio de Londres a ser secuestrada durante semanas en medio del campo, como solía decir. Dado que el padre de Camelia estaba constantemente de viaje en alguna de sus expediciones, su madre elegía quedarse en la ciudad, donde ocupaba el tiempo yendo de compras, al teatro o viéndose con sus amigas.

A Camelia le encantaban las raras ocasiones en que su padre regresaba a casa e insistía en que se fueran al campo a pasar varias semanas. Disfrutaba tumbándose sobre la hierba de un prado y contemplando el cielo mientras el sol le calentaba la piel, y el suave susurro del viento se colaba entre los árboles. Incluso la casa le gustaba, con ese olor a viejo y a musgo que impregnaba todas las habitaciones, las descoloridas tapicerías y desvencijados muebles que habían sido testigos de las vidas de varias generaciones. Todos los rincones estaban atestados de reliquias que su padre había coleccionado durante sus viajes; algunas eran antiguas y bastante valiosas, otras, en cambio, eran simplemente objetos corrientes y ordinarios que le habían parecido bonitos o interesantes. Extasiada, Camelia escuchaba cómo le contaba una historia maravillosa para cada pieza: cómo había estado a punto de morir para conseguirla o a qué personaje tremendamente miserable o pintoresco se lo había comprado. Durante el relato la animaba a acariciar con los dedos la reliquia para que sintiese su calor, su esencia, sus secretos.

Lo mejor de todo era cuando su padre aparecía en casa con una nueva arma. A su padre le encantaban las armas, no por el daño que podían causar, sino porque le fascinaba el hecho de que prácticamente en todas las civilizaciones los artesanos trabajaban para hacerlas tan hermosas como fatales. Le daba a Camelia afilados puñales, pesadas lanzas y espadas, y escudos de labrada ornamentación, y le pedía que los cogiese y comprobase cuánto pesaban. Algunas veces, si lograba convencerlo, le dejaba sacarlas al jardín y manejarlas. Entonces su padre se colocaba cerca de ella mientras le enseñaba a coger bien una espada, a tirar una lanza o un puñal, con su enorme y bronceada mano rodeando firmemente la suya, pequeña y suave, y su ronca voz resonando con oculta satisfacción al tiempo que hacía las demostraciones.

Cierto día su madre los sorprendió cuando Camelia se disponía a lanzar un puñal contra un árbol. La cuchilla se le escurrió y le hizo un profundo corte en la palma de la mano, produciéndole un brillante río de sangre que se deslizó por su brazo. Al borde de la histeria, lady Stamford agarró a Camelia y la condujo rápidamente a casa mientras acusaba a su marido furiosa de haber estado a punto de matar a su única hija. En vida de su madre, a Camelia se le prohibió volver a tocar un arma.

Sentada, se removió incómoda dentro de su vestido de noche de arrugada seda y crinolina, repentinamente consciente de la tirantez de la funda que le sujetaba el puñal en la pantorrilla.

—Vamos, Tisha —dijo Zareb, abriendo la puerta del carruaje y ofreciéndole su mano.

—Gracias, Zareb.

Al coger su mano se sintió un poco mejor. Aunque intentaba que no trasluciera, le había conmocionado profundamente ver su casa destrozada, y los libros y los objetos más valiosos de su padre hechos añicos. Sólo eran cosas, se recordó para serenarse, pero el hecho de que algunas de ellas fueran reliquias excepcionales le entristeció.

Lo que más le irritaba era que alguien hubiese conseguido sacarla del único lugar de todo Londres en el que al menos se sentía como en casa.

—¿Por qué no llevas la jaula de Harriet? Yo llevaré a Oscar y a Rupert.

—Quizá deberíamos dejarlos aquí un momento —sugirió Zareb—, hasta que el señor Kent advierta a Eunice y a Doreen de su existencia.

—Después de lo mal que lo ha pasado, dudo mucho que Oscar quiera quedarse en el carruaje sin mí —objetó Camelia mientras Oscar se abrazaba a ella con fuerza—. Y me temo que, si se enfada, Harriet y Rupert se asustarán. Es mejor que entremos todos juntos.

—Como quieras. —Zareb cogió a Harriet, a la que habían encerrado en una jaula durante el trayecto.

Simon esperó a que Camelia y Zareb se reunieran con él en el sendero de entrada a su casa recién alquilada. Hacían una extraña pareja: ella con su vestido de noche de color escarlata y él con sus espectaculares y vistosas túnicas, acompañados de un mono, un pájaro y un cesto con una serpiente. Sin embargo, emanaba de ellos una extraordinaria dignidad mientras se acercaban a Simon y a Oliver.

—Oiga, joven, ¿por qué no deja que lleve yo la cesta? —se ofreció Oliver, que se apresuró hacia Camelia mientras Simon abría la puerta—. Ya tiene bastante con ese mono agarrado a su cuello.

—Gracias, Oliver —dijo ella con una sonrisa—. Es usted muy amable.

—¡Ya estamos en casa! —anunció Simon abriendo la puerta.

—¡Menudas horas de llegar! —Seguida de Doreen, Eunice cruzó corriendo la puerta que conducía a la cocina—. Ya estábamos a punto de avisar a la policía... ¡por San Columbano! ¡Esa chica lleva una bestia peluda alrededor del cuello!

—Es Oscar —repuso Oliver alegremente—. Y estos son lady Camelia, Zareb, y en esa jaula está Harriet.

—Supongo que encantada de conocerlos. —Doreen miró a Oscar con cautela—. ¿Muerde?

—Sólo manzanas —le aseguró Zareb—. A las personas, no.

—Lady Camelia y Zareb han tenido un percance en su casa esta noche —explicó Simon— y se quedarán un tiempo con nosotros hasta que vuelvan a Suráfrica.

Eunice los miró sorprendida.

—¿Qué tipo de percance?

—Unos desgraciados han entrado en casa de lady Camelia estando ella fuera y la han destrozado —contestó Oliver—.

Han clavado un puñal en un almohadón con una nota que decía cosas horribles... Como coja a esos malditos cobardes, ¡les daré una paliza que jamás olvidarán!

Eunice miró a Camelia con compasión.

—Tranquila, joven, aquí estará a salvo.

—Estos ladrones de hoy en día ya no tienen dignidad —continuó Oliver enfadado—. Todo lo arreglan con pistolas y burdas amenazas, ¡que me expliquen dónde está el honor en eso!

—Lo que ha ocurrido en casa de lady Camelia no es obra de unos vulgares ladrones —señaló Simon—. Su intención era amedrentarla.

—Eso todavía es peor. ¡Serán miserables! —Doreen golpeó su huesudo puño contra la palma de la otra mano mientras proseguía indignada—. ¡Como se les ocurra aparecer por aquí les propinaré un sartenazo en la cabeza y les meteré una escoba por el culo antes de que puedan darse cuenta!

—Espero que las autoridades los encuentren antes de que averigüen que lady Camelia está aquí —declaró Simon—. Ahora me acercaré a comisaría para poner una denuncia.

Camelia lo miró asustada.

—La policía no tiene que enterarse de esto.

—¿Por qué demonios no?

—Si las autoridades investigan, saldrá en los periódicos, lo que significa que los miembros de la Sociedad Arqueológica se harán eco de ello. Los pocos socios que han accedido, a regañadientes, a darme su apoyo financiero se preocuparán y para protegerme me retirarán su apoyo. —Cabeceó con rotundidad—. No quiero que nadie sepa que han irrumpido en mi casa ni que me han amenazado.

—Si no damos el parte a la policía será imposible encontrar a los responsables de esto —advirtió Simon.

—De cualquier forma, a mí me da la impresión de que tampoco sería fácil —intervino Oliver—, a menos que se dediquen a irrumpir en otras casas destrozando cuanto encuentren a su paso.

—Al margen de lo que haga o deje de hacer la policía, los autores de los hechos serán encontrados a su debido tiempo —observó Zareb.

—Bueno, pues si la chica no quiere que se entere la poli, todos callados —decidió Doreen—. No alborotes la colmena si no quieres que te piquen las abejas.

Camelia sonrió.

—Gracias por comprenderlo, Doreen. Espero que no molestemos demasiado. —Igual que Oliver, estaba claro que esas dos mujeres eran para Simon mucho más que unas simples criadas, y eso le gustaba.

Tal vez así entenderían mejor su relación con Zareb.

—No molestan en absoluto —se apresuró a asegurarle Eunice—. La casa es grande para nosostros cuatro; hay espacio de sobras.

—¿Por qué no llevas este cesto mientras Zareb y yo vamos al carruaje a buscar el resto de las cosas? —le sugirió Oliver a Eunice—. Así Doreen y tú podréis acompañar a lady Camelia a su habitación, y ayudarle a instalarse.

—He pensado que estará más cómoda en el cuarto empapelado en verde —comentó Eunice mientras cogía el cesto—. No es nada del otro mundo, pero está limpio y, si lo desea, puedo traerle... ¡Dios mío! —chilló al ver a Rupert asomado a la superficie—. ¡Socorro!

Lanzó el cesto por los aires y se abalanzó contra Oliver, aplastándole la cara con sus grandes pechos. Camelia y Simon corrieron a rescatar el cesto, en cuyo interior había ahora un reacio pasajero. De pronto, la serpiente salió disparada del cesto y Simon cogió el cesto mientras Camelia se lanzaba sobre Rupert.

En ese momento Oscar decidió que se había cansado de estar con Camelia y, gritando como un loco, saltó sobre la cabeza de Doreen. Camelia perdió el equilibrio y cayó encima de Simon. Ambos fueron a parar al suelo y el cesto se fue rodando mientras Doreen chillaba, tratando de deshacerse del mono.

—¡Te cogí! —exclamó Zareb triunfalmente al recuperar a Rupert.

—¡Socorro! —gritaba Doreen, que se tambaleaba por el vestíbulo—. ¡Sacadme esta bestia salvaje de encima!

—¡Oscar, baja de ahí! —ordenó Zareb.

Oscar saltó contento de la inestable cabeza de Doreen al firme hombro de Zareb.

—No puedo respirar. —La voz de Oliver estaba amortiguada por los voluminosos pechos de Eunice.

—¡Oh, Ollie! —exclamó mientras le soltaba—. ¡Pensé que me moría!

Simon miró a Camelia, echada encima de él y con las piernas enroscadas en las suyas.

—¿Estás bien?

Camelia estaba perpleja. De repente había tomado plena conciencia de que Simon era muy alto, observación que no dejaba de ser extraña, teniendo en cuenta que estaban los dos tendidos sobre el suelo. Pero de alguna manera Simon había suavizado la caída protegiéndola por completo con su cuerpo, con todo su pecho y sus hombros, y sus largas, delgadas y musculosas piernas. Ella se estremeció y se fundió en los tibios contornos de su cuerpo, encajando en su silueta de granito. Era maravilloso estar echada sobre él. Su corazón latió con fuerza y sus sentidos se encendieron mientras analizaba cada uno de los rasgos de Simon. Olía a un aromático jabón y a algo más, un delicioso y misterioso olor masculino que le hizo desear apoyar la mejilla en su hombro para embriagarse con su aroma. Su pecho subía y bajaba debajo de ella, su respiración era profunda y constante, y si se quedaba inmóvil, podía sentir los latidos del corazón de Simon contra los suyos.

Camelia notó el calor por todo su cuerpo, en sus pechos, su estómago y entre sus piernas; una sensación confusa y embriagadora que le hizo sentirse extrañamente débil y excitada mientras se perdía en la ahumada, penetrante e insondable mirada de Simon.

—Creo que la chica se ha hecho daño —dijo Oliver frunciendo sus blancas cejas—. No se mueve.

Camelia suspiró y con un ruido sordo se apartó de Simon rodando por el suelo.

—Estoy bien.

—Deja que te ayude, Tisha —se ofreció Zareb—. Estás sonrojada, ¿seguro que te encuentras bien?

—Me he quedado sin aliento, eso es todo. —Aturdida, se apresuró a alisar las arrugas de su vestido.

—Supongo que no pretenderéis que esa cosa escurridiza se quede en esta casa —comentó Eunice, que miraba a Rupert con desaprobación.

—Siento mucho que Rupert la haya asustado, Eunice —se disculpó rápidamente Camelia—. Debería haber llevado yo el cesto, pero le aseguro que no había ningún peligro. El veneno de Rupert no es nocivo para las personas.

—Sea o no peligrosa, me niego a que vaya suelta por casa dándome sustos de muerte.

—No te los dará —quiso tranquilizarla Simon—. Rupert permanecerá encerrado en la habitación de lady Camelia; ni siquiera sabrás que está aquí, ¿verdad, Camelia?

—Sí. —En realidad, Camelia había tenido la esperanza de que Rupert se familiarizase gradualmente con los miembros de la casa y acabara no importándoles que paseara a sus anchas durante su estancia en ella.

—¿Y qué me dices del mono flacucho? —inquirió Doreen mientras se frotaba el cuero cabelludo, que le escocía—. ¿Se quedará también en la habitación de la chica?

—Por desgracia, Oscar necesita un poco más de espacio —explicó Simon al notar la angustia que sentía Camelia nada más pensar en encerrar a Oscar—. Pero estoy seguro de que en cuanto se haya acostumbrado a su nuevo entorno ni siquiera notaréis su presencia.

—Difícil lo veo —murmuró Doreen, mirando indignada a Oscar.

El mono le enseñó la dentadura dedicándole una amplia y burlona sonrisa.

—¡Bicho descarado!

—Por lo menos el pájaro se quedará en la jaula —intervino Oliver en un intento por decir algo positivo—. Además, es bastante bonito.

—La verdad es que Harriet sólo utiliza la jaula para viajar y dormir —aclaró Camelia—. Durante el día necesita volar y estirar un poco las alas.

—Cosa para la que, sin duda, encontrará espacio suficiente en la habitación de lady Camelia —añadió Simon al percatarse de que a Eunice y a Doreen no les gustaba especialmente la idea de que la casa se convirtiera en un auténtico zoo.

—Bueno, ahora que todo se ha solucionado, ¿qué tal si le enseñamos a lady Camelia su habitación? —propuso Oliver—. La chica ha tenido una noche dura y seguro que estará deseosa de acostarse.

—¡Claro que sí, pobrecita! —Eunice chascó la lengua, de pronto recuperada del susto—. Usted suba por aquí, que Doreen y yo la acomodaremos lo mejor que podamos; Oliver se ocupará de su amigo, el señor Zareb.

«Señor Zareb.» Nada más oír esas dos palabras, Camelia perdonó al instante a Eunice por no gustarle Rupert. Desde su llegada a Londres, casi todas las personas con las que Camelia había tropezado habían tratado a Zareb con diversos grados de recelo y condescendencia. Si bien el racismo también estaba extendido en Suráfrica, el padre de Camelia siempre se había asegurado de que en su excavación todo el mundo fuese tratado con igualdad y respeto, al margen del color de su piel. Naturalmente, durante casi toda su vida Zareb había sufrido el desdén de los blancos en lugares como Ciudad del Cabo y Kimberley, pero en África él formaba parte de una población de millones de personas, por lo que no atraía constantemente una atención indeseada. En Inglaterra, Zareb no podía evitar destacar, y nadie dudaba en dar por sentado que era una especie de criado de categoría inferior. Únicamente por su color, la mayoría de los ingleses se sentían al instante superiores a él. Pero Eunice se había referido a Zareb como al amigo de Camelia y había sido muy educada al concederle el título de «señor»; sólo por eso, Camelia haría cuanto estuviese en su mano para mantener a sus animales fuera del alcance de la vista de Eunice, al menos hasta que ésta entendiese que eran absolutamente inofensivos.

—Yo me quedaré esta noche con los animales, Tisha —declaró Zareb, que quería facilitarle las cosas a Eunice y a Doreen mientras acomodaban a Camelia en su cuarto—. No te preocupes.

—Para usted también tenemos una estupenda habitación —le anunció Oliver a Zareb mientras cogía la jaula de Harriet—. Si me sigue, lo acompañaré.

Zareb le dedicó una inclinación de cabeza a su nuevo amigo.

—Gracias, Oliver.

Simon observó cómo la curiosa comitiva subía las escaleras con Oscar sentado, cual pequeño rey peludo, en el trono de la cabeza de Zareb.

Después Simon se volvió y se dirigió a su estudio, sintiéndose extrañamente desconcertado y desesperado por echar un trago.

Algo había cambiado.

En realidad, se había quedado corto, pensó Simon apenado mientras miraba fijamente el líquido ámbar de su vaso. Desde que había conocido a Camelia un incendio había quemado su casa, destrozando cuanto tenía y, lo que era peor, todos los inventos en los que estaba trabajando; luego, sin saber cómo, lo habían engatusado para que dejase que Oliver, Eunice y Doreen se fuesen a vivir con él, erradicando por completo el silencio y la tranquilidad que, sin duda, necesitaba para trabajar. Y justo cuando creía que su casa y su vida no podían ser más ruidosas ni estar más atestadas de gente, Oliver había decidido invitar a Camelia y a Zareb con su séquito de animales salvajes; lo de séquito era una exageración, admitió, pero no del todo, teniendo en cuenta la propensión al conflicto que presentaban un mono, un pájaro y una serpiente.

Tomó un sorbo de brandy y contempló los arrugados bocetos que tenía esparcidos por la mesa, intentando concentrarse en la bomba de vapor que pretendía diseñar. El reto estaba en lograr que el vapor se expandiese de forma gradual con la ayuda de una serie de cámaras. Quizás aumentando el número de cámaras y haciéndolas más pequeñas...

—Perdona, pensé que no había nadie más despierto.

Alzó la vista y vio a Camelia de pie en la puerta de su estudio. Llevaba un camisón de seda de color marfil, cuyo cuello estaba adornado con una tira de exquisito encaje. Se había envuelto de cualquier manera los hombros con la colcha de la cama, pero este improvisado chal no hacía sino acentuar la delicadeza de su silueta. Su melena dorada colgaba suelta sobre sus hombros y por su espalda, un resplandor de oro a la luz de color albaricoque de la lámpara. Simon la miró fijamente, fascinado. Sus ojos descendieron lentamente desde el elegante pómulo de su mejilla por el contorno sutil de su cuello y el encantador hoyo latiente de la base de su garganta, y siguieron descendiendo hasta las sensuales colinas de sus pechos. Se descubrió a sí mismo recordando cómo se había sentido al tenerla tumbada sobre él hacía sólo unas horas; puro ardor femenino y suavidad, sus delgadas piernas enroscadas en las suyas, su cuerpo, que se movía y presionaba contra el suyo mientras lo miraba fijamente con esos magníficos ojos verdes del color de la salvia.

El deseo se apoderó de él, con intensidad y ardor, absolutamente arrollador.

—¿Está todo en orden? —preguntó Simon, que al levantarse de golpe de la mesa volcó su vaso.

«Contrólate», dijo para sí buscando torpemente un pañuelo al tiempo que el brandy empapaba sus bocetos. Al no encontrarlo, decidió coger los dibujos y sacudirlos, por lo que el líquido salpicó toda la superficie de la mesa.

«¡Por el amor de Dios! ¿Se puede saber qué te pasa?»

—¿Te gusta tu habitación? —añadió apurado mientras los papeles que llevaba en la mano seguían goteando.

Camelia lo miró vacilante, extrañada por su aparente aturdimiento.

—Sí, me gusta, gracias.

Se fijó en que aún llevaba la misma camisa de hilo arrugada y los mismos pantalones oscuros, pero se había quitado la chaqueta y la corbata, y se había desabotonado el cuello insinuando su musculoso pecho. Su pelo cobrizo estaba despeinado y una sombra canosa oscurecía su mandíbula, haciendo que su aspecto fuese incluso más desaliñado que habitualmente. En ese momento volvió a recordarle a un guerrero escocés, con su imponente silueta y sus anchos hombros, y sus penetrantes ojos extraordinariamente azules; aunque era ridículo y lo sabía. Simon Kent era un reservado intelectual y científico que se pasaba la vida encerrado en un laboratorio, tratando de perfeccionar nuevas maneras de lavar la ropa, fregar el suelo y transformar el vapor en energía. Difícilmente sería el tipo de hombre que se lanzaría con valentía a la batalla esgrimiendo una pesada espada.

Más bien lo que haría sería lanzarle al enemigo unos inofensivos petardos con la esperanza de que su color y estruendo lo ahuyentase.

—¿Tienes hambre? —Como su mesa era ahora un completo desastre, empezó a colocar torpemente los bocetos empapados en el suelo para que se secasen—. Si quieres, podemos bajar a la cocina y cenar algo.

—No, gracias. Eunice y Doreen han sido muy amables y antes me han subido una bandeja a mi habitación. Me han dicho que también le llevarían una a Zareb, lo que ha sido todo un detalle por su parte. Zareb no está acostumbrado a que lo traten con tanta cortesía lejos de su hogar, especialmente aquí, en Londres.

—Para bien o para mal, Eunice, Oliver y Doreen siempre han tratado a todo el mundo igual. No les impresionan los títulos ni el dinero, ni siquiera el color de la piel de la gente. Lo único que les importa es el interior.

—Zareb también es así —afirmó Camelia, sentándose en la silla que había frente a la mesa de Simon—. Creo que está contento de haber encontrado, al fin, a personas que ven el mundo como él. Me temo que empezaba a pensar que todos los ingleses eran unos arrogantes y unos estúpidos.

Simon sonrió.

—En realidad, somos escoceses, pero yo no me atrevería a condenar a toda la población inglesa basándome sólo en la experiencia de Zareb. Tal vez no haya dado con la gente adecuada.

—Tal vez. —Camelia subió los pies y los escondió debajo de las piernas. No había podido dormirse en la agradable cama que Doreen y Eunice le habían preparado. Pese a su determinación de ser fuerte, ver la casa de su padre y sus valiosas posesiones destrozadas le había afectado profundamente. Lo peor de todo era que habían usado su puñal para clavar esa repugnante nota en un cojín; aunque ella no creía en las maldiciones, se recordó con firmeza.

Aun así, le inquietaba la obstinación mostrada por Zareb al insistir en que debían marcharse.

—¿Cómo conociste a Oliver, Eunice y Doreen? —preguntó, cubriéndose todo el cuerpo con la colcha.

—Mi madre se los llevó a casa cuando salieron de la cárcel —explicó Simon—; aunque nunca los trató como a unos criados. En aquella época tenía que cuidar de varios niños que había rescatado de la cárcel y necesitaba ayuda desesperadamente, así que Eunice, Oliver y Doreen pasaron a formar parte de la familia y desde entonces han estado en casa.

—¿Cuántos niños acogió lady Redmond?

—Contándome a mí, somos seis —respondió Simon con resignación mientras se sentaba de nuevo frente a su mesa—. Con la minuciosa investigación que has hecho sobre mi pasado, supongo que ya sabrás que es así como pasé a formar parte de la familia Kent.

—Mi interés en tu pasado estaba puramente centrado en tus logros como científico e inventor —repuso Camelia—. Alguien me había comentado que lord y lady Redmond te habían adoptado, pero lo cierto es que no le presté atención. Lo único que me importaba era que eras un brillante científico que yo pensaba que podría ayudarme a sacar agua de mi excavación.

La miró durante un buen rato y ella le devolvió la mirada con naturalidad y sincera tranquilidad.

Decía la verdad, pensó, maravillado ante algo tan sencillo como sorprendente.

Hasta donde podía recordar, Simon se había sentido avergonzado de su pasado, aunque no tanto como su hermano Jack. Jack se había visto obligado a sobrevivir en las calles de Inveraray hasta que tuvo casi quince años. Durante todo ese tiempo la violencia y la maldad levantaron un muro a su alrededor, que sólo el cariño y el amor de su mujer, Amelia, consiguieron, finalmente, derrumbar. Pero hasta que Genevieve encontró a Simon acurrucado en el suelo de una celda a los nueve años de edad, también tuvo que arreglárselas solo. No guardaba ningún recuerdo de su padre biológico y los que tenía de su madre eran vagos. Durante muchos años se formó en la mente una inocente imagen infantil de ella: una mujer guapa, de pelo castaño y de grandes ojos grises, que lo abrazaba con fuerza por las noches y le acariciaba la cara con suavidad.

Después de que Genevieve se lo llevara a casa y en cuanto, por fin, pudo empezar a dormir sabiendo que estaría a salvo hasta la mañana siguiente, sus recuerdos dieron un giro de ciento ochenta grados. La mujer que invadía sus sueños nocturnos era sucia y malhablada, su aliento apestaba a ginebra y sus mugrientos puños le pegaban hasta dejarlo encogido en el suelo. Entonces se despertaba sobresaltado, con el corazón latiéndole, la boca seca y temblando sin parar.

Y a continuación bajaba de su nueva y cómoda cama, y se acurrucaba en el suelo suplicándole a Dios que por la mañana sus sábanas empapadas de orina estuviesen secas para que Genevieve no se enterase de su terrible secreto y lo echase de casa.

—¿Estás bien? —Camelia lo miró preocupada, preguntándose qué sombras habrían de pronto oscurecido su mirada.

—Sí —afirmó enseguida—, estoy bien.

Evitando su mirada, empezó a secar el brandy derramado en la mesa con la manga de la camisa. Sabía que Camelia lo estaba mirando y se preguntó si ella habría percibido su estado de ánimo. No quería que Camelia supiese de la existencia de ese chico vagabundo, acobardado y ladrón. Por algún motivo que no alcanzaba a comprender, quería que ella pensase que era mejor de lo que en realidad era; quería que lo viese como un hombre fuerte, seguro de sí mismo y capaz de resolver problemas. Un científico brillante, tal como ella había dicho exageradamente. Bueno, quizá no fuese brillante, rectificó, pero al menos era bastante educado e inteligente. Un hombre capaz de ayudarle cuando lo necesitaba, fuese ahuyentando a los dos ladrones que habían intentado agredirla u ofreciéndole cobijo cuando ya no estaba a salvo en su propia casa. Un hombre que controlaba perfectamente tanto sus emociones como su vida. Lo que no era tan peculiar, dijo para sus adentros; al fin y al cabo, ella dependía de su ayuda. Y si bien siempre se había prestado a ayudar a su familia, no recordaba una sola ocasión en que una mujer hubiese recurrido a él para pedirle ayuda.

Claro que tampoco había conocido a muchas mujeres.

—¿Podrías servirme una copa de brandy? —preguntó de pronto Camelia.

—Naturalmente —contestó Simon, volviendo a la realidad—. Disculpa que no te haya ofrecido una copa hasta ahora. Si lo prefieres, también hay jerez.

—La verdad es que el jerez no me gusta mucho. Lo encuentro demasiado dulce... Supongo que te parecerá bastante inusual que una mujer prefiera el brandy al jerez.

—Yo diría que echar un trago de brandy no es nada comparado con el hecho de que viajas con un mono en el carruaje y una serpiente en la maleta —replicó él en tono burlón mientras le daba el vaso.

Camelia tomó un sorbo y suspiró.

—Supongo que en Londres la gente piensa que soy algo excéntrica.

—¿Te importa lo que piensen de ti?

Ella se encogió de hombros.

—No mucho.

—Bien, porque precisamente en ese caso no dejarás que la opinión de los demás te influya a la hora de decidir por dónde quieres conducir tu vida. No hay muchas mujeres tan valientes.

—Elliott considera que es un disparate. Cree que soy una ingenua y que, en realidad, no entiendo cómo funciona el mundo que me rodea; por eso está tan ansioso por protegerme.

—¿Es eso lo que intentaba hacer cuando os sorprendí en el jardín? —inquirió Simon con ironía—. ¿Protegerte?

—En cierto modo, sí. —Camelia clavó los ojos en el fondo de su copa, avergonzada por el hecho de que Simon la hubiese visto en tan ridícula situación—. Elliott quiere casarse conmigo —añadió incómoda.

¡Así que ése era el objetivo de Wickham! Simon supuso que debería sentirse aliviado porque, por lo menos, las intenciones de ese estúpido eran honorables. Pero, aunque ignoraba el motivo, la idea de que Wickham se casase con Camelia le parecía una completa equivocación. Wickham trataría de enjaularla y Camelia era un ser demasiado maravilloso para que ese necio y arrogante le cortase las alas.

—¿Y tú qué quieres, Camelia?

—Yo quiero volver a África a seguir excavando.

—Algo me dice que a Elliott no acaba de gustarle esa idea.

—Yo creo que está algo confuso —reconoció Camelia—. Elliott vino a Suráfrica justo después de licenciarse en Oxford, porque quería trabajar con mi padre. En aquel entonces sólo tenía veintiún años y estaba lleno de la vitalidad y el idealismo de la juventud. Mi padre lo protegió y le enseñó todo lo que sabía de la profesión. Pero a medida que fueron pasando los años, creo que a Elliott le decepcionó bastante que mi padre no le hubiese proporcionado ni un solo hallazgo importante.

—En otras palabras, que se había pensado que el campo de la arqueología sería más lucrativo de lo que resultó ser.

—Elliott valora mucho más el reconocimiento de sus logros que el dinero —matizó Camelia, deseosa de defenderlo—. Hace dos años, cuando su padre murió, heredó su título y las pertenencias que éste tenía aquí, en Inglaterra, que no son pocas. Pero Elliott quiere que lo conozcan por sus propias conquistas, y con razón; por eso se ha volcado en montar un negocio en la ciudad.

—Y quiere que abandones la excavación y te instales en Londres con él.

—Le preocupa mi bienestar —explicó Camelia—. Teme que esté malgastando mi tiempo y mi dinero en una excavación que tal vez esté agotada, pero eso no significa que no me apoye. Elliott y yo somos grandes amigos desde que yo era pequeña. Vino a África en contra de la voluntad de su familia, porque admiraba a mi padre y su labor, y con el paso del tiempo su relación fue muy estrecha, la verdad es que eran como padre e hijo. Aparte de Zareb, Elliott es lo más cercano que tengo a una familia. Siempre hará lo posible por ayudarme, por eso quiere casarse conmigo. —Tomó un sorbo de brandy y soltó un suspiro—. Elliott me tiene un gran cariño, pero hasta cierto punto también se siente responsable de mí, sobre todo ahora que mi padre ha fallecido. Supongo que piensa que mi padre quería que él cuidase de mí y por eso está dispuesto a casarse conmigo, aunque sabe que sería una esposa horrible.

¿En serio era tan ingenua que no entendía por qué Wickham quería casarse con ella?, se preguntó Simon. Al observarla allí sentada en una silla, hecha un ovillo mientras bebía brandy, decidió que a lo mejor sí lo era. Camelia era una mujer inteligente e independiente de veintiocho años, pero Simon tuvo la sensación de que su experiencia con los hombres era escasa. No le daba la impresión de que fuese consciente de su extraordinaria belleza, así como de la natural y espontánea sensualidad que emanaba constantemente de ella. Hasta cierto punto es probable que Wickham valorase la perspicacia de Camelia y su devoción por el trabajo de su padre, por mucho que le hubiese desilusionado que ella no accediese a abandonar la excavación en cuanto él decidió que había sido un fracaso. Camelia era tan exquisita y magnífica como cualquiera de las reliquias que Elliott hubiese podido desear descubrir, pensó Simon. Posiblemente él la consideraba el premio final a todos esos años que había pasado en tierras africanas.

Por lo menos a Wickham no le faltaba inteligencia para entender lo especial que era Camelia, si bien no acabase de comprender que estaba destinada a mucho más que a ser la mujer de un atildado vizconde.

—Cuando se entere de lo que ha pasado esta noche en tu casa, no le hará ninguna gracia —comentó Simon—. Porque me imagino que no le has contado lo de tu encuentro en la callejuela con esos dos ladrones, ¿verdad?

Ella sacudió la cabeza.

—Creo que es mejor que no sepa algunas cosas; tiene tendencia a alterarse, y eso no sirve de gran ayuda.

—En cuanto se dé cuenta de que no estás en tu casa, no tardará mucho en venir aquí a buscarte. Dudo que le parezca buena idea que estés instalada aquí conmigo.

—Cuando se lo explique, lo entenderá.

—¿Qué tiene que entender? ¿Que alguien ha amenazado conmatarte si vuelves a la excavación? ¿No crees que hará todo lo posible para convencerte de que no regreses allí?

—Nadie me sacará de Pumulani —afirmó Camelia con énfasis—. El sueño de mi padre era excavar ese terreno como es debido, documentar minuciosamente sus reliquias y trasladarlas a un museo para su conservación. Me prometí a mí misma llevar a término su sueño y no pararé hasta que lo haya hecho.

Sus ojos del color de la salvia brillaban con una mezcla de obstinación y determinación. Simon se percató de que cuando se enfadaba se oscurecían un poco, adquiriendo la variación de verdes de un bosque.

—Lo de Pumulani no lo haces realmente por ti, ¿verdad, Camelia? —observó Simon con tranquilidad—. Lo haces para asegurar el legado de tu padre.

—Su legado ya está asegurado. —Hablaba con orgullo, pero se había puesto ligeramente a la defensiva dándole a entender que era muy consciente de que la cúpula arqueológica no compartía su convicción—. Era un gran hombre y un destacado arqueólogo, que escogió ir en contra de los convencionalismos imperantes en su campo y trabajar en un continente donde, por falta de visión o de valor, ninguno de sus colegas quiso hacerlo. Durante los años que pasó en Suráfrica encontró un sinfín de importantes reliquias, pinturas rupestres y tumbas, que ponían de relieve lo extremadamente inteligentes, capaces y hábiles que eran las tribus que habían habitado esas tierras desde tiempos inmemoriales. No excavó la tierra con la esperanza de obtener fama o veneración, aunque, sin duda, habría agradecido el respeto y el apoyo de sus colegas. Tampoco consagró su vida al continente africano porque pretendiese hacerse rico. Mi padre era un explorador; para él, el propio viaje era una recompensa. Y yo quiero seguir su viaje.

—¿Durante cuánto tiempo?

—Durante el resto de mi vida.

—No creo que la bomba dure tanto —bromeó Simon. Y añadió con expresión más seria—: Tenía entendido que estabas a punto de realizar un importante descubrimiento en Pumulani.

—Y así es, pero sea lo que sea lo que descubra tardaré años en desenterrarlo, y cuando haya terminado buscaré otro lugar de África donde excavar. Llevo la arqueología en la sangre, Simon, igual que mi padre. Mi primera excavación la viví con diez años. Desde el instante en que tuve un cubo en una mano y un pequeño pico en la otra supe que era lo único a lo que me quería dedicar.

—Deduzco entonces que tu madre compartía la pasión de tu padre por explorar África.

Camelia suspiró.

—Por desgracia, mi madre no conocía nada de África. Le parecía un lugar cálido, sucio e incivilizado que le robaba a su marido durante varios meses seguidos cada vez. Mi madre era hija de un vizconde y la educaron para ser una buena dama inglesa apropiadamente frágil. Creo que en algunas ocasiones no podía evitar decepcionarse conmigo, porque se daba cuenta de que me parecía mucho más a mi padre que a ella.

—Si tanto detestaba África, ¿por qué te dejó ir allí?

—No lo hizo. Murió cuando yo tenía diez años, y mi padre regresó a Londres sin saber muy bien qué hacer conmigo. Le supliqué que me llevase a África con él, y accedió.

—Pues debió de costarte mucho el cambio. Dejar tu casa y cuanto te rodeaba para irte a un país desconocido.

—La pérdida de mi madre fue una tragedia, pero irme a vivir con mi padre fue fácil. En realidad, me daba igual adónde me llevase siempre y cuando estuviésemos juntos.

Pensativo, Simon permaneció unos instantes en silencio.

—¿Y cuándo apareció Zareb en tu vida?

—Zareb y mi padre eran amigos mucho antes de que yo fuese a África. El día que llegamos en barco a Ciudad del Cabo, Zareb estaba allí para recibirnos. Alargó el brazo, me acarició la mejilla y susurró unas cuantas palabras que no entendí. Entonces se agachó, me miró directamente a los ojos y me dijo que siempre me protegería. —Se echó a reír—. Debo reconocer que por aquel entonces me daba un poco de miedo, con esas extraordinarias túnicas, su piel tibia y oscura y esa intensa manera de mirarme. En Inglaterra no había conocido a nadie como él. Pero Zareb cumplió su palabra. Permaneció a mi lado y cuidó de mí con más celo que mis propios padres o ninguna de las institutrices que había tenido. Solía decirme que yo era un regalo de los espíritus y que por eso debía cuidarme tanto. Creo que fue su modo de hacerme sentir parte de África. En ese momento lo único que yo quería era estar a toda costa con mi padre.

Allí sentada, envuelta en la colcha con desenfado y con la enmarañada melena de color miel que caía sobre sus hombros, Simon pudo imaginarse perfectamente a la niña asustada pero decidida que debía de haber sido antaño. Su padre amaba África y ella quería a su padre, y quería estar con él, sobre todo tras la muerte de su madre. Ahora que lord Stamford también había fallecido, Camelia estaba resuelta a continuar su trabajo. Y no sólo porque quisiera asegurar su legado, como Simon había pensado, aunque, sin duda, eso era un factor que había que tener en cuenta.

Camelia necesitaba seguir excavando en Pumulani, porque eso le hacía sentirse más cerca del hombre al que tanto había idolatrado.

—Si tienes la intención de estar el resto de tu vida excavando en África, ¿qué pasará con Wickham?

—En realidad, Elliott no quiere casarse conmigo —afirmó Camelia—. Siente la obligación de cuidar de mí por la estrecha relación que nos une desde hace un montón de años y porque quería a mi padre. Lo que de verdad quiere es casarse con la percepción de lo que cree que yo podría llegar ser, si consiguiese hacerme entrar en razón y que fuese más parecida a las demás mujeres.

—¿Estás segura de lo que dices?

—Sí, lo que ocurre es que aún no se ha dado cuenta. Pero creo que lo entenderá mejor ahora que ha visto lo mal que he encajado en esta ciudad. Estaba bastante enfadado conmigo por la manera en que le he hablado a lord Bagley esta noche. Y, honestamente, no creo que fuese una buena esposa para ningún hombre —continuó con irreverencia, sin que tampoco pareciese muy molesta por ello—. No sé cómo se lleva una casa, ni hacer de anfitriona ni educar niños, y soy absolutamente incapaz de morderme la lengua cuando alguien dice o hace algo que considero insultante u ofensivo. No puedo estar encerrada en una casa más de un par de meses; necesito estar al aire libre, trabajando. Y, luego, por supuesto, están Zareb y mis animales, que siempre van conmigo. —Al concluir sus ojos se iluminaron, alegres—. ¡Dudo que muchos hombres considerasen atractivo mi equipaje!

Tenía toda la razón, admitió Simon. La mayoría de los hombres pensarían que una mujer tenaz, que se pasaba el día desenterrando huesos en África mientras paseaba por ahí con sus animales exóticos, no era una candidata a esposa especialmente atractiva. Pero eso era lo que hacía que fuese tan fascinante. Camelia vivía su vida a sus anchas, con sus propios objetivos y principios. No le interesaba lo más mínimo lo que los demás pensasen de ella, excepto en lo que concernía a sus logros en el campo de la arqueología. Y estaba entregada en cuerpo y alma a honrar el trabajo de su difunto padre, persiguiendo su sueño hasta el final al margen de los sacrificios y riesgos que ello implicase.

Simon tomó otro sorbo de brandy, conmovido y hechizado por ella. ¿Por qué demonios Wickham era incapaz de quererla tal y como era en lugar de intentar que se convirtiese en algo que jamás sería?

—Bueno, será mejor que te deje trabajar —dijo Camelia levantándose de la silla—; al fin y al cabo, cuanto antes acabes la bomba antes podremos irnos a Suráfrica.

Simon se puso de pie. Camelia tenía razón; debería volver al trabajo. Sin embargo, ya no le apetecía la idea de seguir enclaustrado en su estudio, leyendo detenidamente sus apuntes y dibujos hasta el amanecer.

—Lo echas mucho de menos, ¿verdad? —le preguntó mientras caminaba con ella hacia la puerta.

—Estoy ansiosa por reanudar la excavación.

—No me refería a la excavación; hablaba de Suráfrica.

Ella asintió.

—Sí.

—¿Cómo es todo aquello?

—Es... el paraíso —se limitó a contestar—. Es un lugar de contrastes brutales, pero magníficos. El cabo está rodeado por la franja de océano más azul, transparente y tibia que jamás te hayas podido imaginar; cuando el sol se pone es como si miles de estrellas se hubiesen caído del cielo y bailasen sobre las olas. Alrededor de Ciudad del Cabo hay árboles y plantas de toda la gama de verdes imaginables, que dan la fruta más dulce que nunca hayas probado. Y al caminar algo suave te acaricia la mejilla y desordena tu pelo, es tan suave que al principio casi ni se nota hasta que, finalmente, caes en la cuenta de que es la limpia brisa del océano, que roza tu piel. Y luego, si viajas al interior, la tierra se vuelve más cálida, seca e inhóspita, pero todavía es más maravillosa. La tierra te rodea como un mar infinito verde y dorado, salpicado de fuertes arbustos y matorrales a los que no les importa estar meses sin oler la lluvia. Hay montañas antiguas y enormes que se prolongan hasta el cielo e intentan tocar el sol cada mañana para luego transformarse en serrados e imponentes picos negros cuando por las noches el cielo se oscurece y la luna se eleva en lo alto. Y cuando estás a solas debajo de esa brillante luna nacarada y escuchas los latidos de tu corazón y tu respiración mientras la tierra se va quedando dormida, no hay ningún lugar del planeta en el que pudieras encontrar mayor belleza.

La colcha que envolvía sus hombros había resbalado ligeramente, como si Camelia visualizase la cálida caricia de esa brisa africana en su piel. Durante unos instantes se produjo un silencio perfecto entre ellos mientras ella lo miraba seria tratando de transmitirle lo que uno sentía debajo de la luna de África.

Aturdido, Simon la miró fijamente. Nunca había estado debajo de la luna africana, pero estaba convencido de que era comparable a la extraordinaria belleza de Camelia, de pie frente a él. Lo había hechizado, decidió, pese a que su mente de absoluto científico sabía que eso era imposible. Pero debía ser así, porque de algún modo lo había hechizado hasta el punto que ya no recordaba con exactitud quién era. La maraña de recuerdos del pasado y las necesidades futuras lógicas e inexorables de pronto se habían desvanecido, existiendo sólo ese momento, con Camelia de pie delante de él, enfundada en su sencillo camisón y cubierta con una descolorida colcha, y sus ojos brillando al recordar un mundo que amaba y añoraba desde lo más profundo de su ser.

Ella lo atraía hacia sí, lo notaba con la misma certeza con la que podía sentir cuanto acababa de describirle: la sedosa brisa que le rozaba la piel, la fragancia de flores exóticas flotando a su alrededor y la imponente quietud de la noche africana. Se inclinó hacia Camelia, acortando el espacio que había entre ellos, creyendo que estaba a punto de perder la razón y, curiosamente, sin importarle.

Un beso nada más, se dijo para sus adentros con fervor sin dejar de mirarla a los ojos mientras apoyaba los labios sobre su boca. Ella se quedó completamente inmóvil, no abrió la boca pero tampoco se apartó de él. El aire de su nariz acarició su áspera mejilla, cálido y suave como la brisa del océano de la que hablaba, y el aroma del sol y de los prados inundó sus sentidos hasta que ya no supo si era de día o de noche, si estaba en Londres o en África. Entonces Camelia suspiró, abriendo levemente la boca, invitación que a Simon le pareció desgarradoramente tímida, cándida y maravillosa. Camelia no era suya; lo supo con certeza mientras le pasaba la lengua por sus aterciopelados y dulces labios con sabor a brandy, despacio, con suavidad, jurándose a sí mismo que pararía enseguida.

Un beso nada más. Sólo uno y tendría bastante. Después dejaría que se marchara, que cruzase el océano hasta África, donde podría vivir con la libertad que tan desesperadamente ansiaba, entre sus misteriosas reliquias y animales salvajes, y mares llenos de estrellas bailarinas.

Camelia se quedó helada, plenamente consciente de la tibia lengua de Simon, de la suave aspereza de su piel contra su mejilla, de la intensa promesa del cuerpo marmóreo que estaba frente a ella. La pasión la recorrió por dentro, ardiente y urgente, completamente distinto al pánico que había sentido cuando Elliott le había besado hacía unas horas. En este momento estaba tensa, y se sentía extraña y derretida como si su cuerpo se hubiese despertado de repente de un profundo sueño y ahora ardiese de pasión. Permaneció inmóvil, sus músculos tensos ante lo que se avecinaba, su cuerpo entero presa de un desconocido e inquietante deseo. Esto era desear a un hombre, pensó aturdida, asustada y paralizada por las intensas sensaciones que experimentaba.

Y entonces, con la misma rapidez con la que había comenzado, Simon empezó a alejarse de ella, interrumpiendo el ardiente contacto de sus labios y dejándola sola y perdida.

Camelia emitió un gemido gutural, alargó los brazos y atrajo a Simon hacia ella una vez más, besándole con fuerza en la boca. Entreabrió los labios y deslizó la lengua titubeante en el oscuro y dulce misterio con sabor a brandy de su boca. La colcha que llevaba sobre los hombros se le cayó al suelo; ahora sólo le cubría el delgado velo del camisón. Se pegó más a su cuerpo caliente, desesperada por sentir su ardor y la dureza marmórea de su cuerpo contra el suyo mientras, inexperta, enroscaba su lengua a la de Simon con el único anhelo de estar cada vez más y más cerca de él hasta que entre ellos no hubiese nada salvo este maravilloso y extraordinario deseo.

Una honda pasión floreció en el interior de Camelia, tierna, dolorosa y atemorizante, que abrió la puerta a un frágil anhelo que en algunas ocasiones había sentido, aunque sin acabar de entenderlo. Pero mientras rodeaba con fuerza los anchos hombros de Simon lo único que importaba era que no dejase de abrazarla, de tocarla o de besarla. Algo había cambiado en su interior y pese a que no lo comprendía, sabía con absoluta certeza que no quería que acabase.

Simon la abrazó con más fuerza, los últimos vestigios de cordura que le quedaban protestaban en vano recordándole que aquello no estaba bien, que no debería tocarla, que no tenía derecho a acariciarla con sus manos y su boca de esta manera. Pero su cuerpo ardía del deseo más apremiante que jamás había conocido, y no podía reunir la sensatez suficiente para analizar correctamente por qué motivo exactamente no debía probar con su lengua la rosa tibieza de la deliciosa boca de Camelia o deslizar las manos por las suaves curvas de sus hombros, su cintura y sus caderas. Ella soltó un gemido y se pegó a él hasta que sus sensuales muslos rozaron la dureza de Simon.

Él también gimió y puso las manos debajo de sus nalgas mientras presionaba su cuerpo contra el de ella, con la mente embriagada con el aroma a limón de Camelia, la intensa y ardiente humedad de su boca y la increíble sensación que suponía notar su esbelta silueta moviéndose ansiosa contra él. Simon no era un hombre dado a la pasión, sin embargo, en ese momento su deseo era tal que creía que no podría soportarlo. Nada importaba salvo que Camelia lo deseaba, podía sentirlo en su desesperado tacto y en el dulce ardor de su beso, y podía oírlo en los hechizantes gemidos que salían de su garganta.

Y él también la deseaba con una intensidad ilógica, desconcertante, y total y absolutamente irrefrenable.

De modo que la devoró con su boca mientras la cogía en brazos, acunándola posesivo. Cerró la puerta del estudio de una patada y a continuación la tumbó en el pequeño sofá que había contra la pared. Separó los labios de su boca y empezó a regalarle una lluvia de hambrientos besos por la mejilla bronceada, la elegante curva de su mandíbula y la cavidad de la base de su garganta, que latía salvajemente. Su camisón traslúcido se escurrió hacia abajo mientras él seguía descendiendo hasta que sus labios llegaron a la pálida seda de sus bellos pechos. Colocó la lengua sobre un pezón coralino, cerró la boca sobre él y chupó con fuerza un buen rato hasta que éste despertó y se endureció. Lo soltó para darle la misma atención al otro pecho, que lamió, chupó y besó mientras las manos recorrían nerviosas las curvas y llanos del precioso cuerpo de Camelia.

Camelia cerró los ojos y enredó los dedos en los desordenados rizos cobrizos del cabello de Simon, presionándolo contra su pecho, que él acariciaba con la boca. El camisón, que estaba ahora a la altura de la cintura, caía en cascada hasta el suelo dejando su piel desnuda en contacto con el tibio aire nocturno. En algún lugar recóndito de su mente era vagamente consciente de que no estaba bien que Simon la besara y la tocara así, pero no lograba comprender el motivo; al fin y al cabo, ya no era una niña tímida a la que unos padres protectores reservasen pura a la espera de un interesante contrato matrimonial.

Era una mujer adulta e independiente de veintiocho años, que había dejado atrás hacía tiempo cualquier idea infantil de un matrimonio romántico. Desde los diez años África había sido su hogar y en la vida a la que su padre la había habituado no había cabida para un marido que pretendiese que su existencia girase únicamente alrededor de sus necesidades. Esta situación le había proporcionado una gran libertad, pero también momentos de absoluta soledad, sobre todo desde el fallecimiento de su padre.

Desechó el pensamiento y se concentró en las sensaciones que le producía tener el rostro de Simon enterrado en el valle que había entre sus pechos, y el reguero de besos que le daba por el liso vientre y que le empujaba el camisón cada vez más abajo. Siguió descendiendo, la aspereza de la mandíbula de Simon rascó ligeramente su ardiente piel, vertió el aliento tibio y reconfortante en el hoyo de su ombligo, en su pronunciada cadera y el marfileño terciopelo de su muslo. Su camisón continuó cayendo gradualmente hasta que el aliento de Simon tanteó el sedoso y anhelante triángulo escondido entre sus piernas.

Se quedó inmóvil, repentinamente vacilante, pero antes de que pudiese protestar le besó allí, con suavidad y atrevimiento mientras le acariciaba con las manos en un incesante descenso. Entonces introdujo en ella la punta de la lengua, y un placer puro y auténtico recorrió su cuerpo entero.

Gritó atemorizada y se puso rígida, pensando que debería apartarlo, pero Simon se anticipó a su súbito recato y le agarró de las muñecas, sujetándolas suavemente junto a su cuerpo mientras seguía lamiendo la oscura y ardiente piscina que acababa de descubrir. Lamió hacia arriba y hacia abajo, moviendo la lengua entre los lisos labios rosas de la vulva, saboreándola y probándola hasta que sus huesos empezaron a derretirse y su carne ardió. El placer le inundó, misterioso, impactante e intenso, llevándose consigo cualquier pensamiento recatado o de control. Si quería, podía decirle que parase, seguro que sí, aunque, en cierto modo, el asombroso descubrimiento de que, en realidad, no quería que lo hiciese erradicó los últimos vestigios de sus escasas reticencias.

Camelia suspiró y se hundió en el sofá, sintiendo el calor de África en su piel, pese a que la noche era fría, y el aire de sus llanuras, pese a que estaba en una pequeña casa londinense. Ahora el placer latía en su interior, pero venía de la mano de una especie de inquietud que no alcanzaba a comprender. Comenzó a agitarse y moverse debajo de la tierna embestida de Simon, excitada y, sin embargo, levemente insatisfecha mientras su cuerpo empezaba a estirarse en busca de algo más. Abrió más los muslos, invitándole a saborearla en profundidad, sin importarle ya si él la consideraba frívola o casquivana. Simon gimió y la chupó con mayor intensidad, reclamando conocer los secretos más íntimos de su cuerpo, y después introdujo un dedo en ella y empujó, al principio despacio y luego más deprisa, llenándola y vaciándola mientras con la boca y la lengua dibujaba círculos sobre su vulva.

Camelia jadeó, sus pechos subían y bajaban mientras, con desesperación, trataba de llenar sus pulmones de aire, pero por alguna razón no había aire suficiente y su cuerpo se tensó al esforzarse por llenar el horrible vacío que crecía ahora en su interior. Este deseo era nuevo para ella, pero ignoraba qué era lo que quería. Simon siguió embistiéndola con las manos y los dedos, devorándola mientras sus dedos entraban y salían de ella, impulsándola a continuar persiguiendo lo que sea que él intentaba darle. Ella se removió y se arqueó, se sentía ardiente, derretida y extraña, y su respiración aún era jadeante, como súplicas en medio del quedo aire nocturno.

«Por favor, por favor, por favor», suplicó en silencio, sin saber por qué suplicaba; lo único que sabía que era que no quería que Simon se detuviese, se alejase de ella ni la abandonase cuando tanto lo necesitaba. El placer que le proporcionaban las deliciosas embestidas de Simon era cada vez mayor y más hondo; su boca y sus manos le acariciaban ardientes y la saboreaban mientras la hacían suya. Se estaba entregando a él, se estaba entregando a la misteriosa pasión que él le mostraba, y si estaba cometiendo un error, ya era demasiado tarde. El placer seguía creciendo, traspasaba su ser y creyó que no podría soportarlo, pero sí pudo, cada vez más, hasta que finalmente no podía respirar, moverse ni pensar. Y, de repente, se quedó helada y su cuerpo entero disfrutó de una deliciosa explosión de placer y felicidad. Soltó un grito ronco y desesperado, y Simon la sujetó con fuerza mientras se sucedían los rápidos espasmos del orgasmo, que la liberaron de cualquier tensión conocida hasta que no hubo nada excepto Simon y ella, y la arrolladora pasión que los unía.

Simon se abrazó unos segundos a Camelia, embriagándose con su suave ardor y aroma mientras el corazón le latía con tal violencia que estaba convencido que se le romperían las costillas. Y entonces se levantó y se quitó rápidamente las gastadas botas, la camisa y los pantalones llenos de arrugas y se quedó desnudo frente a ella, su piel bronceada a la luz de la lámpara. Fascinada, Camelia lo miró fijamente con sus ojos de color verdeceledón, pero Simon no detectó en ellos ni una pizca de sorpresa o miedo. No, Camelia había pasado la mayor parte de su vida en la selva africana, donde sin duda habría visto a cientos de hombres desnudos o semidesnudos, que vivían sus vidas orgullosamente indiferentes a los dictámenes de la castidad victoriana. Su mirada resuelta sólo sirvió para que aumentara el deseo que ya hervía en Simon; cualquier duda o reparo que hubiese podido albergar acerca del deseo de poseerla se había desintegrado al comprobar la intensidad de la pasión sincera y pura de Camelia. Ella lo deseaba tanto como él a ella.

Más allá de eso, no había nada.

De modo que se echó encima de ella, cubriéndola con el ardor de su cuerpo marmóreo, y pese a la excitación experimentada en cada uno de sus sentidos, se esforzó para no penetrarla enseguida. Camelia suspiró y lo rodeó con los brazos, recibiéndolo y envolviéndolo en su suavidad y su tibieza mientras la humedad de color miel que había entre sus muslos le rozaba como una tentadora promesa. Apretó la mandíbula, procurando controlarse y recuperar al menos suficiente cordura para poder entrar en ella lentamente.

Era la mujer más maravillosa que había conocido, no sólo por su belleza, sino por la profunda e inquebrantable determinación que hervía en ella. Camelia tenía algo salvaje que le parecía exquisito; era un espíritu exótico, desconcertante y magnífico. Era perfectamente consciente de que su hogar no estaba en Londres, pero de pronto la idea de que volviese a su amada África y se alejase de él le resultaba insoportable. Ella no le pertenecía y al darse cuenta de ello sintió un gran vacío. La penetró, despacio, con cuidado, abrazándola con fuerza mientras la miraba con fijeza a los ojos, perdido en las brillantes profundidades de esos impresionantes ojos verdes del color de la salvia.

«Quédate conmigo», suplicó para sus adentros, consciente de que eso jamás sucedería, de que Camelia jamás querría vivir atada a nadie ni encarcelada. «Conmigo estarás a salvo», juró con fervor, embistiéndola con más fuerza, pensando que quizá pudiese hacerle entender así lo que nunca podría expresar con palabras. Pero ella no buscaba seguridad, se lo había dejado muy claro al negarse a abandonar la excavación del terreno que tanto amaba pese al serio peligro que ello conllevaba. Camelia suspiró y empezó a agitarse debajo de él al notar que Simon estaba distraído. Entonces se quedó inmóvil. Estaba perdiendo la razón, ahora se daba cuenta, él, que durante tantos años se había regido por la preponderancia de la razón sobre la pasión. Se estaba entregando a ella y no podía evitarlo; Camelia ya había conquistado su cuerpo, su corazón y su alma.

Reculó levemente en un intento por recuperar un poco su voluntad, un poco de control que por lo menos le permitiese templar sus emociones dentro de lo posible. Y entonces ella le abrazó con fuerza, levantó las caderas, disipando las pocas dudas que aún tenía, y lo atrajo hacia sí con exquisito ardor. Simon gimió de placer y desesperación, y se hundió en ella tanto como pudo mientras le daba un profundo beso que la ató a él, aunque fuese por unos segundos.

Camelia se quedó petrificada, sobresaltada por la repentina y aguda punzada que le dio.

—Tranquila, mi amor —susurró Simon, que procuró no moverse en absoluto—. Abrázame fuerte y el dolor pasará enseguida.

Esperaba desesperadamente que así fuese. Teniendo en cuenta que hasta el momento su experiencia con vírgenes era nula, no estaba del todo seguro.

Camelia enterró el rostro en su cuello, relajándose al calor del cuerpo protector de Simon, relajándose con los tiernos besos que éste depositaba ahora sobre su frente, mejillas y boca, y su suave movimiento mientras lentamente empezaba a agitarse dentro de ella. Se centró en el caliente mármol de su espalda, que recorrió con los dedos descubriendo la masculina estructura de sus hombros, costillas y columna para a continuación deslizar las palmas de las manos hasta acariciarle las musculosas colinas de sus nalgas. El deseo se despertó en ella de nuevo, primero despacio y luego más deprisa, disipando su miedo mientras su cuerpo se estremecía, se tensaba y se erguía para poseerlo. Simon le dio un profundo beso sin detener sus embestidas suaves y lentas, que la llenaban y la vaciaban. Colocó una mano en la unión de sus cuerpos y le prodigó caricias allí, excitándola hasta que volvió a arder de deseo. Camelia empezó a moverse con él, al mismo ritmo que él, y después lo abrazó con más fuerza y se movió más deprisa, atrayéndolo más hacia sí con cada ardiente embestida.

Simon estaba perdiendo la razón. Tenía que ser así, porque en ese momento no podía pensar en nada excepto en la insoportable tortura de su deseo. Quería permanecer así para siempre, unido a ella, atado a ella, perdido en ella. Ahora era consciente de que le había entregado parte de su ser a Camelia, aunque no estaba seguro de si ella se lo había robado o él se lo había dado voluntariamente. Lo único que sabía era que no importaba nada salvo ese momento, el maravilloso abrazo de Camelia, el aroma de las praderas soleadas y de frutas exóticas que le rodeaba, la llamada de África y el canto del corazón de Camelia. Supo que ella no le pertenecía, y sintió que se desgarraba por dentro. La embistió una y otra vez, intentando atarla a él, intentando hacerle entender que sí le pertenecía, por ilógico o imposible que eso fuera. Pensó que necesitaba más tiempo, que debía ir más despacio. Necesitaba que el fuego que ardía entre ambos durase para que ella pudiese entenderlo. Pero no quedaba tiempo, Camelia se movía a su ritmo, susurrando pequeñas y frenéticas súplicas mientras le incitaba a que fuera más y más rápido. Simon luchó por dominar su deseo, pero era como intentar impedir que una ola rompiese contra una orilla rocosa. De repente, Camelia se incorporó y le besó con fervor mientras su sedoso y ardiente cuerpo lo apresaba con firmeza. Él soltó un gemido, un grito de éxtasis y desesperación, y la penetró con fuerza. La sujetó y le dio un intenso beso mientras se entregaba a ella, se sentía a punto de morir, pero por algún motivo le daba exactamente igual.

Camelia estaba tumbada debajo de Simon y notaba los fuertes latidos de su corazón contra el suyo propio. Cerró los ojos y se imaginó que los rayos del sol africano caían sobre ellos, unos rayos calientes, limpios y suaves. Ya no tenía el frío habitual que había sentido desde que llegase a Londres. Suspiró y atrajo a Simon hacia sí, escuchando sus jadeos.

No estaba preparada para lo que acababa de suceder entre ambos.

Hacía tiempo que había decidido que nunca se casaría y por lo tanto su concepto de intimidad entre un hombre y una mujer se había quedado simplemente en eso: un mero concepto. Había conocido los pormenores del acto años antes cuando su padre y ella tropezaron con dos leones, que estaban apareándose. Pese el bochorno sentido, su padre respondió a sus preguntas con su característica sinceridad pragmática; al fin y al cabo, era un hombre culto y de ciencia, que no veía ninguna utilidad en que su hija siguiese ignorando un tema que, teóricamente, algún día necesitaría conocer. Después de aquello Camelia se interesó sobremanera en las burlas de las nativas que de vez en cuando acompañaban a sus maridos a Pumulani. Gracias a ellas supo que el acto en sí no era desagradable, algo que ya se había imaginado al presenciar el apareamiento de los dos leones, pero que su objetivo era principalmente la procreación. Y dado que Camelia no se veía a sí misma casada y con hijos, desechó el tema.

Ahora se había dado cuenta de que había muchas cosas que no sabía.

Cuando su cuerpo fue enfriándose gradualmente, empezó el miedo. ¿Y si había empezado a gestarse un niño en su vientre? No había sitio en su vida para los hijos. Necesitaba ser libre para excavar su terreno, para trabajar durante largos y calurosos días prácticamente en medio de la nada. Un hijo le haría engordar y cuando hubiese nacido, la necesitaría y absorbería todo su tiempo. No podía permitirlo; debía mantener su libertad para ser fiel a la promesa que le había hecho a su padre, una promesa que sabía que tardaría meses e incluso años en cumplir.

Apartó a Simon y bajó del sofá de un salto, recogiendo su camisón del suelo.

—Tengo que irme —anunció mientras se ponía rápidamente por la cabeza el camisón de cuello de encaje. Recuperó la colcha y se la puso sobre los hombros en un intento por levantar el muro que ahora necesitaba que hubiese entre ellos.

Simon la miró confundido, sin saber qué decir. ¿Qué demonios iba a decirle? ¿Que lo sentía? ¿Que lamentaba haberla tocado? ¿Que a pesar de que lo que acababa de suceder entre ellos era lo más maravilloso que le había pasado nunca, se arrepentía de ello?

Decir algo semejante no haría sino quitarle importancia a lo ocurrido y entristecerla a ella; y se negaba a hacer eso.

—Camelia... —susurró mientras se ponía de pie.

—Lo siento —le interrumpió ella, retrocediendo para evitar el aturdimiento que le producía su preciosa silueta desnuda. ¡Dios! Pero ¿qué había hecho? Posiblemente acababa de estropear su relación con el único hombre que se había ofrecido a ayudarle en su excavación. Bueno, lo cierto es que no se había ofrecido, pero ahora eso era lo de menos. Necesitaba su ayuda con urgencia y si ahora él se desdecía y la echaba de su casa, se agotaría el dinero y jamás encontraría la tumba—. No era mi intención que pasase esto, pero ha pasado, y me temo que ya no podemos dar marcha atrás, aunque estoy convencida de que si pudiésemos hacerlo, los dos lo haríamos sin dudarlo —le espetó disculpándose.

Simon la miró con incredulidad. Ahora sí que se había quedado sin habla.

—Lo mejor que podemos hacer, dadas las circunstancias, es reconocer que esto ha sido un error, un momento... digamos, que de locura total y absoluta —continuó Camelia ansiosa por disminuir el daño que le había hecho—. Supongo que no suelen ocurrirte este tipo de cosas, pero Zareb dice que de vez en cuando las estrellas se alinean de tal forma que la gente hace cosas que, de lo contrario, jamás haría, y aunque no creo demasiado en los mitos y las supersticiones, quizá deberíamos convenir en que en este caso concreto eso es, probablemente, lo que ha ocurrido; que las estrellas se han alineado de alguna forma extraña provocando que hayamos actuado como lo hemos hecho. Pero te aseguro que no volverá a ocurrir, te doy mi palabra.

Camelia deseaba con todas sus fuerzas que él dijese algo, casi tanto como deseaba que se pusiese los pantalones.

—No te preocupes por mí —añadió nerviosa, esforzándose por no apartar los ojos de su rostro—. Te garantizo que en adelante no tendré ningún problema en absoluto para controlarme debidamente en lo referente a tu persona. —Lo miró con seriedad, preguntándose si habría logrado convencerlo.

Simon estaba completamente perdido, pensó, estaba atónito y, por qué no decirlo, también un poco ofendido. Sabía que Camelia podía reaccionar de diversas maneras, pero lo que desde luego no se había imaginado era que saltaría del sofá y pronunciaría un discurso sobre Zareb, las estrellas y el autocontrol, como si creyese que le había obligado a hacer algo en contra de su maldita voluntad.

—Me asombra tu aparente determinación, Camelia —musitó con frialdad mientras recogía sus pantalones del suelo—. Pero supongo que eso es lo que siempre te ha diferenciado del resto de las mujeres, tu extraordinaria determinación.

—Entonces ¿no me echarás de tu casa?

Él la miró sorprendido.

Camelia sujetaba los bordes de la descolorida colcha con tanta fuerza que sus nudillos se habían vuelto blancos. Entonces Simon comprendió. Lo que a Camelia le aterraba era que después de lo ocurrido entre ellos, él decidiese echarla de su casa. Supuso que no tenía ningún otro sitio adónde ir en Londres (excepto a casa de Wickham, naturalmente) y le gustó constatar que Camelia prefería estar con él, aunque eso implicase que las estrellas tuviesen que realinearse.

—¡Pues claro que no! —contestó con rotundidad—. ¿Qué te ha hecho pensar eso?

Ella lo miró insegura.

—¿Y construirás la bomba de vapor y vendrás a África conmigo para enseñarles a mis hombres cómo funciona?

Simon se puso los pantalones y se los abrochó. Ahora que estaba al menos parcialmente vestido se sentía un poco menos vulnerable.

—Sí.

El alivio inundó a Camelia, que se relajó y dejó de apretar la colcha con tanta fuerza.

—De acuerdo, pues, muy bien —dijo—. En ese caso, te dejo para que puedas seguir trabajando. —Abrió la puerta y añadió—: Buenas noches.

Simon la observó mientras salía silenciosamente del estudio y cerraba la puerta tras ella.

Y luego se acercó a su mesa y se sirvió una generosa copa completamente convencido de que esa noche no podría reanudar el trabajo.

Capítulo 7

—¿Dónde está el fuego, chico? —inquirió Oliver malhumorado al abrir la puerta.

Elliott lo miró confuso.

—¿Qué fuego?

—El que le hace a usted aporrear la puerta como si estuviésemos todos a punto de quedar reducidos a cenizas como no salgamos de aquí corriendo —replicó Oliver con sequedad.

—Vengo a ver al señor Kent —le informó Elliott, que decidió ignorar el sarcasmo del anciano—. Dígale que lord Wickham desea hablar con él.

—No quiere que se le interrumpa —objetó Oliver como si tal cosa—. Está trabajando en uno de sus inventos y cuando está concentrado no le gusta que lo molesten.

—Se trata de un asunto muy importante —insistió Elliott.

Oliver le lanzó una recelosa mirada.

—Tendrá que ser más concreto.

—Se trata del paradero de lady Camelia Marshall —argumentó Elliott, perplejo por el hecho de estar justificando su presencia ante un criado. Éste aún era más insolente que Zareb. Por lo menos el africano hacía algún esfuerzo para fingir cierta deferencia delante de él—. Seguro que si le dice esto, querrá hablar conmigo.

Oliver se rascó la cabeza pensativo.

—Si quiere saber el paradero de lady Camelia, ¿por qué no habla directamente con ella? Yo creo que eso es más sencillo que tener que molestar al señor Kent.

—Porque no sé dónde está —explicó Elliott con paciencia—. Y ahora, si es tan amable de anunciarle al señor Kent que estoy aquí...

—¡Vuelve aquí, bestia insolente —chilló una voz furiosa desde el piso de arriba— o me haré un sombrero con tu asquerosa piel!

Oscar bajó las escaleras dando saltos con unas braguitas de franela rojas ondeando alegremente tras él. Vio a Elliott en la puerta principal y soltó un grito, que él no supo con seguridad si era de alegría o irritación. El mono huidizo se abalanzó sobre él y se encaramó a su hombro, colocando las braguitas sobre su cabeza cual vistosa bandera escarlata.

—¡Te trituraré y haré unos *haggis* contigo! —advirtió Eunice furiosa y resoplando mientras bajaba las escaleras—. Pero antes te arrancaré ese roñoso pelo y lo usaré para limpiarme los zapatos, ¡bestia... San Columbano! —Presa de la vergüenza su arrugado rostro se volvió casi tan rojo como sus braguitas cuando vio que éstas estaban sobre la cabeza de Elliott.

—Disculpe, señora. —Con la mayor dignidad posible, Elliott se sacó las braguitas de la cabeza—. Creo que esto es suyo.

—No son mías —protestó Eunice mientras se apresuraba a introducir la deformada bandera roja en el bolsillo de su delantal—. Me disponía a lavar la ropa de una señora que vive en esta misma calle cuando esa mala bestia ha entrado y me las ha robado —explicó Eunice mirando indignada a Oscar.

—¿Qué señora? —inquirió Oliver arqueando las cejas.

—¿Está lady Camelia aquí? —quiso saber Elliot, que intentaba ahora deshacerse del mono, agarrado firmemente a su hombro.

—Una *señora* —dijo Eunice, lanzándole a Oliver una mirada de advertencia—. No la conoces, Ollie.

—No sabía que le hacías la colada a otras personas, Eunice —repuso Oliver, todavía confundido—. ¡No será porque aquí falte trabajo con la chica y todos sus animales salvajes correteando por la casa!

—¿Está aquí lady Camelia Marshall? —repitió Elliott mientras seguía peleándose con Oscar, que por lo visto había decidido que en ese momento su hombro era más seguro que cualquier otro lugar.

—¡Elliott! —Camelia apareció por la puerta que conducía a la cocina con Harriet encima del hombro—. No esperaba verte aquí.

Elliott la miró fijamente, desconcertado por su sencillo vestido de día y por el hecho de que había salido de lo que dedujo que era la cocina con su ridículo pájaro sobre el hombro.

—He ido a verte a casa, pero las cortinas estaban echadas y Zareb no me abría la puerta —explicó—. La primera vez me imaginé que habías salido, pero hoy he tropezado con tu cartero y me ha dicho que no ha podido entregarte el correo en toda la semana. Naturalmente, me he empezado a preocupar pensando que te había ocurrido algo. Y como la última vez que te vi la semana pasada te fuiste del baile de la Sociedad Arqueológica con Kent, he pensado que tal vez él supiese alguna cosa; por eso he venido aquí. —Al fin, logró sacarse a Oscar del hombro y dejar bruscamente al mono travieso en el suelo—. ¿Debo inferir entonces que te has instalado aquí,

Camelia? —Lo preguntó con suavidad, pero estaba claro que la posibilidad no le hacía ninguna gracia.

—Será por poco tiempo —le aseguró ella—. He tenido ciertos problemas en casa de mi padre y Simon, el señor Kent, fue tan amable de invitarnos a todos; así que aquí estamos.

Elliott arqueó las cejas.

—¿Qué clase de problemas?

—Detalles sin importancia que me dificultaban bastante la estancia en casa —contestó Camelia quitándole gravedad al asunto. No quería que Elliott se enterase de que habían entrado en su casa y la habían amenazado. Si Elliott sabía que ella corría cualquier tipo de peligro, insistiría en cuidar de ella, y eso era lo que no quería—. Nada preocupante.

—El tejado tenía unas goteras tremendas —intervino Oliver, tratando de echarle una mano a Camelia—. Aquello parecía un colador gigante, ¡hasta las patatas se podrían haber lavado ahí debajo!

Elliott lo miró con recelo.

—No ha llovido en las últimas dos semanas.

—¡Exacto! Lo que significa que está a punto de caer una buena —repuso Oliver sin titubear—. No podíamos dejar a la chica sola en esas condiciones.

—Camelia, ¿qué ocurre realmente?

—Ya te he dicho que hay ciertos problemas en casa —insistió Camelia—. Cuando se hayan solucionado, Zareb y yo volveremos...

—¡*Socorro*! —Se oyó gritar una voz procedente de la cocina—. ¡*Me está persiguiendo*!

—¡Dios mío, están atacando a alguien! —Elliott se quitó el sombrero y corrió hacia la puerta de la cocina.

—Tisha, ¿has visto a Rupert? —preguntó Zareb desde el rellano de arriba.

Camelia se mordió el labio.

—Creo que está en la cocina con Doreen. Lord Wickham va ahora a ver qué pasa.

—Buenas tardes, lord Wickham —saludó Zareb con simpatía—. Si encuentra a Rupert, ¿sería tan amable de subírmelo?

Elliott se detuvo en seco.

—¿Se refiere a la serpiente?

—¡*Socorro*! —Doreen apareció como un rayo por la puerta de la cocina, con el pelo blanco despeinado por debajo de su gorro de hilo y una pesada sartén negra en la mano—. ¡Casi me muerde, de verdad! —protestó furiosa—. Si vuelvo a verlo en los hornillos, ¡le aplastaré la cabeza con la sartén y lo freiré para cenar!

—¡Oh, Doreen, cuánto lo siento! —se disculpó Camelia—. Juraría que esta vez he cerrado la puerta de mi habitación.

—Y así ha sido, Tisha —le aseguró Zareb—. Yo mismo lo he comprobado.

Oscar se subió al pasamanos de la escalera y se rió.

—Oscar, lo que has hecho está muy mal —le reprendió Camelia—. Sabes que a Doreen y a Eunice no les gusta que Rupert se deslice por la casa; se ponen nerviosas.

—No pienso entrar en esa cocina hasta que alguien saque de ahí a ese escurridizo bicho y lo encierre como es debido —declaró Doreen inflexible—. ¡Ya estoy harta de encontrármelo metido en los armarios y las ollas! ¡Me da unos sustos de muerte!

—A Rupert le gusta la cocina porque es el lugar de la casa donde hace más calor —explicó Camelia en tono de disculpa—. Me temo que no está acostumbrado a la fría humedad de Londres; le gusta mucho más el calor de África.

—El calor del más allá es lo que le enseñaré como no deje de asustarme —advirtió Doreen con dureza—. Y ahora le agradecería, señor, que sacara a esa bestia de mi cocina —dijo mirando a Elliott expectante.

Elliott retrocedió unos cuantos pasos.

—Seguro que Zareb será más persuasivo que yo para la lograr que salga.

—¿Qué demonios sucede aquí? —gritó Simon malhumorado mientras abría las puertas del comedor—. Es imposible trabajar con tanto alboroto... ¡Ah, hola, Wickhop! ¿Qué le trae por aquí?

—Es Wickham —le recordó Elliott tenso—. Y he venido para preguntarle si sabía el paradero de lady Camelia.

—Ahí la tiene —repuso Simon inclinando la cabeza hacia ella—. ¿Puedo hacer algo más por usted?

—Elliott se ha preocupado al ver que Zareb y yo no estábamos en casa —se apresuró a aclarar Camelia, esforzándose por aparentar que entre ella y Simon había una relación absolutamente normal.

Durante la semana transcurrida desde su extraordinaria noche de pasión, Camelia había hecho lo posible por esquivar a Simon. Lo que había sido bastante sencillo, teniendo en cuenta que éste se había pasado día y noche encerrado en el comedor, donde había establecido su nuevo laboratorio. Eunice y Doreen le habían llevado bandejas con comida y bebida cada cierto tiempo, y en algunas ocasiones había podido oír a Oliver decirle con dureza que ya era suficiente y que tenía que acostarse. Aunque Camelia dudaba que Simon hubiese seguido el consejo de Oliver, porque las puertas del comedor habían permanecido cerradas las veinticuatro horas del día y había escuchado a Simon martilleando, golpeando y hablando en voz alta; de modo que, si había dormido, no debía de haberlo hecho más de un par de horas seguidas y seguramente encima de la mesa o en el suelo.

Al reparar en su desaliñado aspecto Camelia se preocupó. Tenía cercos oscuros debajo de los ojos y la piel pálida y arrugada a causa de haber pasado demasiados días sin ver la luz del sol, sin que le diera el aire fresco y sin hacer ningún ejercicio físico. El cabello sedoso en el que, con tanta pasión, había enredado sus dedos era ahora una maraña cobriza y una barba castaña rojiza de una semana oscurecía la elegante línea de su mandíbula, proporcionándole un aspecto ligeramente peligroso, casi salvaje.

—Y le hemos explicado que me he instalado aquí unos cuantos días hasta que me hayan arreglado el tejado de la casa —terminó en un tono fingidamente alegre.

Simon frunció las cejas, confundido.

—¿El tejado?

—Sí, hombre, el que tiene tantas goteras que parece un colador —intervino enseguida Oliver—. Le he dicho al señor Wickham que se avecina una gran tormenta y que por eso lady Camelia está con nosotros.

—Ya veo.

—¿Qué tal si hablamos un momento a solas, Camelia? —sugirió Elliott, molesto por el hecho de que, al parecer, todos lo considerasen un completo idiota—. Me gustaría discutir un par de cosas contigo.

—¿De qué se trata? —Pese a que Camelia agradecía el deseo de Elliott de hablar a solas con ella, el recuerdo del beso que le había dado en el jardín le hacía mantener una actitud de reserva. No tenía precisamente ganas de volver a hablar de matrimonio.

—Es sobre tu excavación, Camelia —concretó Elliott—. Es importante que hablamos de esto en otra parte.

Camelia miró a Zareb expectante.

—El viento oscuro continúa, Tisha —declaró Zareb con expresión grave—. No podemos luchar contra algo que no vemos.

Camelia asintió, intentando reprimir el miedo que sintió en su interior.

—Subamos a la sala de estar, Elliott. Allí podremos hablar.

—Les traeré un poco de té —se ofreció Doreen.

—La acompaño, Doreen. —Las llamativas túnicas de Zareb crujieron sonoramente mientras bajaba las escaleras—. Sacaré a Rupert de su escondite para que no vuelva a asustarla.

—Naturalmente, señor Zareb —repuso Doreen con una sonrisa—. Es usted muy amable.

—Quizá podrías llevarte también a Harriet, Zareb —propuso Camelia mientras le daba el pájaro.

—¿Quieres que te acompañe, Camelia? —inquirió Simon.

La miró fijamente. Un súbito temor había ensombrecido su mirada cuando Zareb había mencionado el viento oscuro. Simon notó que a Camelia le daba miedo lo que Wickham pudiera decirle. Por rara que se hubiese vuelto su relación durante esa última semana, quería que ella supiese que, si lo necesitaba, seguía estando ahí para apoyarle.

Camelia miró a Simon sorprendida. Su penetrante mirada azul diluyó las máscaras de protección que tanto se había afanado en construirse durante toda la semana. Una oleada de ardor recorrió su cuerpo, calentando su sangre y provocándole escalofríos en la piel al recordar su tacto.

—No, gracias —logró contestar—. Estoy bien.

Por supuesto, era una absoluta mentira; no estaba nada bien. Le aturdía el efecto que Simon causaba en ella, aunque sólo la mirase; y tenía miedo de lo que sea que Elliott fuese a decirle. Pero no quería que Simon lo supiese. Necesitaba que pensase lo que los demás pensaban: que era una mujer fuerte, capaz y de una inquebrantable determinación. Si manifestaba el más mínimo atisbo de debilidad, tal vez reconsiderase el pacto que habían hecho y se negase a hacer la bomba. Y sin la bomba la excavación seguiría llena de agua.

Así que a menos que sacase pronto el agua de ahí y encontrase la tumba de cuya existencia su padre estaba absolutamente convencido, los últimos inversores con los que aún contaba le retirarían su apoyo, dejándola con un montón de deudas y un trozo de tierra yerma, que no podría permitirse seguir excavando por su cuenta.

Entonces, para no arruinarse del todo, se vería obligada a vender el terreno.

—De acuerdo. —Simon se volvió de golpe, entró en el comedor y cerró las puertas.

—Por aquí, joven —dijo Oliver señalando las escaleras—. Los acompañaré a la sala de estar mientras Doreen y Eunice preparan el té.

Sacando pecho para lo que sea que Elliott estuviese a punto de decirle, Camelia siguió a Oliver escaleras arriba y entró en la sala de estar modestamente decorada. Se sentó en el raído sofá de terciopelo verde esmeralda y entrelazó las manos nerviosa. Elliott anduvo de un lado a otro de la habitación hasta que Oliver se marchó. Al fin, él y Camelia estaban solos.

—¿Por qué estás aquí en realidad, Camelia? —le preguntó—. Y, por favor, no vuelvas a contarme esa estupidez de las goteras. Pensaba que con la estrecha amistad que nos une desde hace tantos años tendrías al menos suficiente confianza en mí para decirme la verdad.

Parecía dolido y Camelia se sintió culpable, insignificante y avergonzada. Elliott tenía razón, dijo para sí. Había sido el protegido de su padre, su socio y gran amigo casi desde que Camelia era una niña, tiempo durante el cual había demostrado su lealtad y cariño tanto hacia ella como hacia lord Stamford en un sinfín de ocasiones. Elliott haría cualquier cosa por ella; incluso se casaría con ella para protegerla.

No merecía que Camelia le mintiese.

—Lo lamento, Elliott —se disculpó—. Tienes razón. Lo cierto es que he venido aquí porque alguien irrumpió en mi casa la semana pasada y la destrozó entera, rompiendo la mayoría de antigüedades y objetos valiosos que mi padre coleccionaba. Fue en la noche del baile de la Sociedad Arqueológica. Simon entró conmigo en casa y cuando vio lo que había ocurrido, insistió muy amablemente en que me instalase aquí.

—¡Dios mío! —Elliott la miraba con preocupación—. ¿Ya ha investigado la policía? ¿Tienen a algún sospechoso?

—No he acudido a la policía.

Elliott la miró atónito.

—Y ¿por qué demonios no lo has hecho?

—Por desgracia, no ha sido un simple robo. Yo diría que no se llevaron nada. Creo que quien entró en casa lo hizo con la intención de asustarme, no para robar nada.

—¿Qué te hace pensar que alguien quería asustarte?

—Hicieron todo añicos, Elliott. Es como si hubiesen querido romper absolutamente todo cuanto me importa.

—Tal vez hayan sido unos jóvenes borrachos, que pensaron que sería divertido destrozar una casa —aventuró Elliott.

Camelia permaneció callada.

—¿Hay algo más, Camelia?

Ella confesó a regañadientes:

—Dejaron una nota.

—¿Qué clase de nota?

—Una nota en la que me advertían que no continuase excavando.

Elliott frunció la boca.

—Pero ¿qué ponía exactamente?

Camelia se encogió de hombros.

—No lo recuerdo.

Él se arrodilló frente a ella y le cogió de las manos, obligándole a mirarlo a los ojos.

—Dímelo, Camelia.

Suspirando, dijo:

—Ponía algo sobre que mueran aquellos que alteran la paz de Pumulani.

—¿Que mueran...? —preguntó indignado—. ¿Estás segura de que aparecía la palabra muerte?

—Quizá fuese otra cosa —concedió Camelia, preocupada por haber hablado demasiado—; no me acuerdo bien.

—Hay que avisar a la policía ahora mismo —decidió mientras se ponía de pie—. No me puedo creer que hayas dejado pasar una semana; y no me puedo creer que el estúpido de Kent no te haya insistido en que des parte a la policía. Si hubiese estado yo contigo esa noche... ¡maldita sea! ¡Me habría asegurado de que las autoridades se presentasen en tu casa y empezasen a buscar a los desgraciados que hicieron esto!

—No quiero que la policía lo sepa —protestó Camelia—. Si se lleva a cabo una investigación, los periódicos se harán eco y todos los miembros de la Sociedad Arqueológica Británica se enterarán. Y entonces los pocos socios que han accedido a regañadientes a darme su apoyo financiero se preocuparán por mí, y retirarán el dinero con la intención de protegerme. Además, cuestionarán la viabilidad de la excavación en sí y echarán por tierra la posibilidad de que pueda ayudarme cualquier otra persona.

—Son científicos, Camelia —replicó Elliott—. El rumor de una maldición no les amedrentará.

—Eso no lo sabemos con seguridad, Elliott. Yo no creo que todos los arqueólogos sean tan escépticos como dicen, por mucho que aseguren que no creen en las maldiciones. Tú y yo sabemos que a lo largo de la historia son muchos los hombres que en distintas partes del mundo han muerto en extrañas circunstancias mientras desenterraban tumbas sagradas y tesoros. En mi opinión, a todos nos preocupa en un momento dado estar desenterrando algo que sería mejor dejar donde está.

—No me puedo creer que esas palabras salgan de tus labios, Camelia.

—Lo sé. —Paseó los dedos por el desgastado terciopelo del brazo del sofá y esbozó una forzada sonrisa—. No me está sentando muy bien la estancia en Londres. A veces me siento perdida, aquí... como si no supiese quién soy.

—Te has ido de tu casa tras sufrir un brutal contratiempo, abandonando todos tus recuerdos para instalarte en casa de un completo desconocido —comentó mientras se sentaba a su lado—. Podrías haber venido conmigo, Camelia —le reprendió con suavidad, cogiendo una de sus manos entre las suyas—. Me sorprende que no me pidieras que te fuese a buscar de inmediato. Pero ahora estoy aquí y esperaré mientras recoges tus cosas; puedes incluso traerte a Zareb y tus animales. —Y concluyó con cierta resignación—: Supongo que tendré que acabarme acostumbrando a ellos.

Camelia lo miró desconcertada.

—Yo no he dicho que quisiese ir a tu casa, Elliott —aclaró—. Es Londres lo que se me hace extraño, no esta casa. La verdad es que aquí todo el mundo es muy simpático con nosotros, siempre y cuando Rupert no asuste a Doreen más de una vez al día y se le pongan los pelos de punta. También debo reconocer que Oscar atormenta bastante a la querida Eunice, pero creo que en su fuero interno se gustan. Eunice siempre amenaza con convertirlo en un trapo para sacar brillo, pero a la hora de comer es la primera que le prepara un plato lleno de cosas deliciosas. Me preocupa un poco que al volver a África tenga antojos de tortas y pudín de tofe espeso.

Elliott no daba crédito.

—No hablarás en serio, Camelia. ¡No puedes quedarte aquí!

—¿Por qué no?

—En primer lugar debes pensar en tu reputación... por mucho que sea un tema que prefieras ignorar —insistió al ver que Camelia estaba a punto de protestar—. Todo el mundo opina, y supongo que tú también te habrás dado cuenta, que Kent está un poco loco; basta con fijarse en cómo va vestido y en lo solo que está siempre. ¡Por Dios! No se afeita ni se peina. Parece haber salido de un manicomio.

—Se pasa día y noche trabajando en la construcción de mi bomba de vapor, Elliott —señaló Camelia, que salió en defensa de Simon—. Creo que su capacidad para concentrarse en sus inventos y abstraerse de todo lo demás no demuestra sino su extraordinaria dedicación y disciplina.

—Lo que demuestra es su obsesión anormal por las cosas —replicó Elliott—. No hay que olvidar el hecho de que tuvo un pasado muy oscuro. ¡Por Dios! Pero ¡si lady Redmond lo encontró en una cochambrosa celda de una cárcel de Escocia! ¡Lo encarcelaron por robar!

—No era más que un niño, Elliott.

—Tenía casi quince años, Camelia, era prácticamente un hombre; especialmente tratándose de un ladronzuelo que se había pasado la vida en la calle. Todo el mundo sabe que tiene un pronto violento y peligroso; por lo visto estando en prisión pegó a un carcelero con tanta fuerza que el pobre hombre jamás pudo volver a andar bien.

—El que pegó a un carcelero fue mi hermano Jack —dijo alguien recalcando las palabras con voz grave e indiferente—. Yo me limité a vomitar encima de sus botas.

Camelia levantó la vista y vio a Simon de pie en la puerta, apoyado con naturalidad en el marco. Tenía los brazos, sucios de grasa, cruzados delante del pecho y las manchas de tinta de sus dedos habían ensuciado las tremendas arrugas de su camisa. Su semblante era relajado, como si no le importara lo más mínimo haberlos sorprendido en su sala de estar cuchicheando acerca de los sórdidos detalles de su pasado. Pero sus ojos azules habían adquirido el color plomizo del cielo justo antes de una tormenta veraniega. Había ira en ellos, aunque Camelia detectó también vulnerabilidad.

La misma vulnerabilidad aguda que había observado en su mirada la noche que fue a verlo a su estudio.

—Te ruego que nos perdones, Simon —se apresuró a disculparse Camelia—. No deberíamos estar hablando de tu pasado.

Simon se encogió de hombros.

—Me da igual que habléis o no de mi pasado. —Era mentira, pero se negaba a que Wickham creyese que había conseguido ofenderlo—. Como lo veo tan interesado, Wickhip, me parece que debería cuando menos aclararle unos cuantos puntos a tener en cuenta. En primer lugar, lady Redmond me sacó de la cárcel cuando tenía nueve años, no quince. Me encarcelaron por colarme en una casa de campo y devorar un cesto de manzanas y una botella de alcohol; puede que fuese whisky, pero como por aquel entonces no estaba muy versado en bebidas alcohólicas, no estoy seguro. Sí recuerdo que las manzanas estaban podridas y tenían un sabor horrible, pero llevaba más de tres días sin comer y no me importó demasiado. El alcohol me dejó completamente ido, razón por la cual seguía ahí cuando los propietarios regresaron a su casa. Me metieron en la cárcel de Inveraray, donde no tardé en vomitar todo encima de las botas del carcelero, con lo que no me gané precisamente su simpatía. Recibí doce latigazos y me condenaron a treinta días de cárcel seguidos de cinco años en un reformatorio. Lady Redmond vino a la cárcel al cabo de unas tres semanas y sobornó al alcaide para que me soltase, prometiendo responder por mí durante todo el tiempo que durase la condena. ¿Hay algo más que quiera saber?

Camelia lo miró fijamente, incapaz de articular palabra. En ese instante comprendió con absoluta claridad hasta qué punto a Simon le atormentaba todavía su pasado, aunque no sabía con certeza si era porque las desagradables heridas de ese pasado jamás se habían curado o porque el mundo que le rodeaba no le permitía olvidar.

—Discúlpeme, señor Kent —dijo Elliott, rompiendo el tenso silencio—. Como sabe, lo único que me preocupa es lady Camelia y su reputación.

Simon ladeó levemente la cabeza.

—Naturalmente.

—Y yo le he asegurado a Elliott que no necesito que me proteja —añadió Camelia en un intento por disipar la tensión que se respiraba en la habitación.

—Me parece que no acabas de entender lo poderoso que es el chismorreo en Londres —insistió Elliott—. Pero Kent seguro que lo entiende, ¿verdad?

—Procuro no prestar atención a eso, Wickhip —declaró Simon, que fingió una indiferencia absoluta—. Tengo muchas otras cosas en qué pensar.

—En ese caso déjeme que alabe su habilidad para desoírlos; por desgracia, lady Camelia es una mujer y no puede permitirse el lujo de ignorar lo que se dice de ella.

—Tonterías, Elliott —protestó ella—. Sabes muy bien que nunca me ha importado lo que le gente pueda decir de mí.

—Eso era en Suráfrica; aquí las cosas son diferentes.

—Pero es que no tengo intención de quedarme aquí. En cuanto Simon termine de construir la bomba zarparemos hacia casa.

—Da igual; los próximos dos meses que pases aquí, deberías esforzarte para evitar que hablen mal de ti y hagan cometarios.

—En realidad, nos iremos a Suráfrica dentro de muy pocos días —anunció Simon.

Camelia lo miró sorprendida.

—¿En serio?

Él asintió.

La mirada de Camelia se iluminó de pura felicidad. Simon la miró totalmente fascinado. Había estado esa última semana trabajando como un loco, sin dormir más de una o dos horas seguidas y parando sólo los minutos necesarios para comer y beber lo que Oliver, Eunice y Doreen amablemente le habían traído a intervalos que intuía regulares. Y todo porque estaba decidido a construirle a Camelia su bomba de vapor. Se había dicho a sí mismo que cuanto antes regresase ella a África y reanudase su excavación, antes podría él volver a Inglaterra y continuar con su maldita vida. Pero ahora, al verla ahí de pie, con esa alegría que le contagiaba como si fuese una gigantesca y reconfortante ola, se dio cuenta de que, por más que le hubiese gustado creerlo, su principal motivación no había sido apartar a Camelia de su vida. Lo que quería era que dejase de añorar tanto África.

Y la única forma de conseguirlo era hacer la bomba y llevarla a su hogar.

—¿Está diciendo que ha logrado construir una bomba de vapor en tan sólo un par de semanas? —preguntó Elliott con incredulidad.

—No está del todo acabada —reconoció Simon, encogiéndose de hombros—, pero el viaje en barco a África durará más de tres semanas y luego tardaremos días en llegar a Pumulani en tren y en carro; acabaré de montar y ajustar la bomba durante el viaje.

—¡Qué maravilla! —Camelia se levantó de un brinco para ir a abrazar a Simon, pero se detuvo en seco—. Es realmente maravilloso —repitió mientras lo miraba con fijeza—. Gracias por trabajar tan duro.

—¡Vaya, qué buenas noticias! —Elliott hizo lo posible por mostrar entusiasmo al tiempo que se levantaba lentamente del sofá.

Simon se relamió con la situación. Sabía que Wickham estaba desesperado por retener a Camelia en Londres; al fin y al cabo, era donde él estaba intentando establecer su nuevo negocio y su nueva vida. Y quería a Camelia a su lado, revoloteando tranquila y sumisamente a su lado. Sería un poco difícil cortejarla y convencerle de que se casara con él, si ella estaba excavando felizmente la tierra a varios miles de kilómetros.

—Camelia, quizá deberías reconsiderar la idea de instalarte en mi casa al menos hasta que puedas regresar a Ciudad del Cabo —sugirió Elliott—. Están mi madre y mis tres hermanas, y tendrás una dama de compañía como Dios manda. Creo que el entorno será mucho mejor que el que el señor Kent con tanta amabilidad te ha ofrecido aquí. No creo que quieras seguir abusando de su confianza.

—Camelia no ha abusado de mi confianza en ningún momento —le aseguró Simon, que procuró que la expresión de su rostro fuera creíble—. De hecho, ni siquiera he notado su presencia. Sin embargo, si prefiere trasladarse a su casa, depende, naturalmente, de ella.

Camelia lo miró sorprendida. El rostro de Simon era de absoluta indiferencia, como si no le importase un ápice que se quedase en su casa o no. Pero una sombra cubría el azul claro de sus ojos, enmascarando cualquier emoción que hirviese en su interior.

Lo observó unos instantes, la palidez de su cara, las ojeras negras que tenía debajo de los ojos, la desaliñada maraña cobriza de su cabello originalmente largo. Este hombre había llegado a la extenuación porque le había construido la bomba que ella con tanta desesperación necesitaba. Era su socio en la excavación, y por lo tanto tenía un interés económico en ayudarle para que regresase a África a completar su misión. También estaba el hecho de que hasta que le entregase la bomba y enseñase a sus hombres a manejarla, Simon no podría continuar con sus otros inventos. Sin embargo, algo le decía a Camelia que no era ésa la razón por la que se había encerrado en el comedor a trabajar afanosamente durante la última semana.

—Es mejor que me quede aquí, Elliott —repuso Camelia de pronto.

Elliott no daba crédito.

—¿Por qué?

—Porque así estaré disponible por si Simon me necesita.

—¿Para qué?

—Para preguntarme alguna cosa —contestó Camelia lanzando una mirada a Simon—. Ya sabes, sobre la bomba.

—¡Ah..., sí, la bomba! —Simon asintió—. Siempre surgen dudas acerca de la bomba, Wickhip; me temo que es inevitable.

—Muy bien, pues, como no hay forma de convencerte de que vengas a casa conmigo, Camelia, no te entretendré más. Pero antes de irme, te daré una cosa. —Introdujo la mano en el bolsillo de su abrigo y extrajo un sobre sucio y manoseado—. Por lo visto el cartero lleva varios días intentando entregártelo. Al ver que era de Trafford he pensado que era importante y le he persuadido de que me lo dé a mí, asegurándole que te lo entregaría enseguida.

Camelia alargó el brazo y cogió el sobre de Elliott con disgusto. No había olvidado ni mucho menos la advertencia de Zareb.

«No podemos luchar contra algo que no vemos.»

Con el corazón latiéndole, abrió el sobre y echó un rápido vistazo a la carta que contenía.

Simon vio que Camelia se ponía pálida.

—¿Qué ocurre, Camelia?

—Ha habido otro accidente en la excavación —musitó—. Una explosión.

—¿Qué quiere decir una explosión? —inquirió Elliott—. Nunca hemos usado explosivos.

—Pues, al parecer, alguien lo ha hecho. Sucedió de noche, mientras la mayoría de los trabajadores dormía. Uno de los hombres que hacía guardia murió. Los demás están convencidos de que la explosión tiene que ver con la maldición. Unos diez hombres abandonaron la excavación esa misma noche y el señor Trafford asegura que cada día se va alguno; creen que estoy demasiado lejos para seguirlos protegiendo de la maldición.

Simon frunció el ceño.

—¿Qué maldición?

—Los nativos creen que ha caído una maldición sobre Pumulani —explicó Camelia a regañadientes—. Eso quiere decir que cada vez que pasa algo, sea debido al mal tiempo o a un derrumbamiento, culpan de ello a las fuerzas malignas, cuando en realidad en una excavación arqueológica es normal que ocurran esas cosas.

—A mí no me parece normal que una explosión mate a un hombre —comentó Simon—. ¿Ha habido más accidentes?

—En una excavación siempre hay accidentes. Lamentablemente, forma parte del trabajo.

—Y supongo que los nativos no piensan lo mismo.

—Me temo que es un poco más complicado que eso —intervino Elliott—. Hay quien cree que en el terreno donde lord

Stamford decidió excavar están las antiguas tumbas de una tribu que se asentó allí hace cientos o quizás incluso miles de años —dijo—. Hará unos sesenta años se instaló en la zona una familia de boers, que cultivó la tierra durante apenas dos generaciones. Tuvieron problemas; la tierra era árida la mayor parte del año, lo que hacía prácticamente imposible cosechar, y el ganado enfermaba y moría en los campos. Los nativos decidieron que era debido a una maldición. Y cuando el padre de Camelia se presentó allí y les propuso a los boers comprar el terreno, la familia no dudó en vender.

—¿Y por qué lord Stamford estaba tan interesado en ese terreno? —inquirió Simon.

—Mi padre había estado trabajando en una excavación en la que descubrió una serie de extraordinarias pinturas rupestres —explicó Camelia—. Pinturas que retrataban una sociedad tribal muy activa que, obviamente, estuvo muchos años en la zona. Al hablar con los ancianos de una tribu cercana se enteró de que esa antigua tribu practicaba complejos rituales de enterramiento, y de que se creía que los reyes de la misma habían sido enterrados en un lugar determinado; el lugar en cuestión era la granja de esa familia de boers.

—¿Te refieres a que ahí hay una tumba?

—No como las que hay en Egipto o en China —matizó Camelia—. Los africanos no suelen construir grandes estructuras donde enterrar a sus muertos; pero los ancianos hablaron de una «Tumba de los Reyes», dando a entender que había un montón de reyes enterrados en el mismo sitio junto con los objetos que necesitaban para el más allá.

—¿Qué clase de objetos?

—Normalmente son objetos muy sencillos. Debería haber joyas hechas con cáscaras, piedras, conchas de tortuga, piedras agujereadas y en algunas ocasiones cáscaras de huevo de avestruz convertidas en recipientes.

—Pero eso no son reliquias valiosas.

—Lo son desde un punto de vista arqueológico —defendió Camelia—. Nos ayudan a entender las vidas y creencias de esas antiguas tribus.

—Y me imagino que también serán valiosas para los nativos de la zona, que tal vez no comprendan tu deseo de desenterrarlas.

—Yo sólo quiero desenterrarlas para que puedan ser estudiadas y conservadas en lugar de que los elementos las destruyan.

—Estoy de acuerdo, pero es posible que haya algunos nativos que consideren que es mejor dejar esos objetos donde están. ¿Y si fueran ellos los autores de la explosión?

—No, imposible.

—Porque siempre hablas de que hay algún arqueólogo rival que intenta ahuyentarte de la excavación para poder desenterrar él esos huesos y huevos de avestruz.

—A mí me parece mucho más probable.

—¿Por qué?

—En primer lugar, los nativos ni siquiera sabrían cómo contactar con un par de ladrones que viven al otro lado del océano, en Londres, para que destrozaran mi casa y me intimidaran. Y en segundo lugar, jamás utilizarían explosivos, porque lo que quieren es conservar las tumbas y no correr el riesgo de que sean destruidas.

—Razonable argumentación —convino Simon—. ¿Y usted qué opina de todo esto, Wickham?

—Para mí lo de menos es el autor de los hechos —declaró Elliott con rotundidad—. Los nativos creen que ahí hay una tumba enterrada por los dioses y que son los propios dioses quienes los están castigando por intentar desenterrarla. Yo no creo en las maldiciones, pero me preocupa la seguridad de Camelia, sobre todo después del ataque que ha sufrido en su casa y de que la hayan amenazado.

—Elliott considera que debería abandonar la excavación y vender el terreno al precio que me ofrezcan —añadió Camelia—, cosa que no haré, jamás.

—¿Y a quién cree que debería venderle Camelia el terreno? —le preguntó Simon a Elliott—. Si este misterioso rival se presenta ante ella diciendo que quiere comprarlo, estoy convencido de que se aferrará aún más a él y continuará excavando.

—De eso puedes estar seguro —se apresuro a afirmar Camelia, que le lanzó a Elliott una suplicante mirada.

No quería que Simon supiese que la De Beers Company le había hecho una oferta para comprar Pumulani. Si Simon se enteraba de que la compañía de diamantes estaba interesada en su terreno, aunque no se había encontrado un solo diamante en él, tal vez se pusiese de parte de Elliott y dijese que lo mejor era vender y seguir con su vida. Entonces se ahorraría el arduo trabajo de terminar la bomba y realizar el pesado viaje a África, que desde el principio se negó a hacer.

—A lo mejor hay otras posibilidades —apuntó Elliott sin precisar, respetando el deseo de Camelia de no revelar ningún tipo de información sobre la oferta de la De Beers Company—. Por desgracia, Camelia ha preferido no tenerlas en cuenta, y eso a pesar de que cada día que pasa es más difícil seguir excavando. Yo dediqué muchos años de mi vida a excavar en Pumulani y doy fe de que no hay ninguna prueba tangible de que la tumba exista, aparte de los delirios de unos cuantos ancianos de la tribu kaffir, que probablemente nos desprecien y, de todas formas, nos hayan mentido.

—Nosotros no mentiríamos para ver cómo excavan la tierra, lord Wickham. —Zareb apareció en la sala de estar llevando una gran bandeja de plata con el té y Oscar sentado majestuosamente en su hombro—. Los africanos respetamos mucho a la tierra para hacer algo así.

—No me refería a usted, Zareb —corrigió Elliott—. Me refería a los nativos que convencieron a lord Stamford de que excavase allí.

—Lord Stamford tomó la decisión solo —replicó Zareb—. El señor no era un hombre que se dejase convencer de nada en lo que él mismo no creyese realmente.

—Las grandes convicciones empiezan en uno mismo —observó Oliver, que entró con un plato lleno de tortas y queso. Harriet se había posado elegantemente sobre su hombro, mirando a su alrededor como una reina que desaprueba ligeramente lo que ve.

—Y la carne se cocina mejor a fuego lento —añadió Eunice, que iba detrás de Oliver con unas galletas de jengibre.

—Conseguir un sueño a veces requiere tiempo. —Doreen fue la última en entrar, llevando un plato con trozos de pastel—. Si lady Camelia no ha encontrado lo que sea que su padre buscaba, a lo mejor es que la carne aún no está a punto.

—Bueno, ahora que Simon ya casi ha acabado de construir la bomba para extraer el agua de la excavación y que falta poco para volver a casa, estoy segura de que avanzaremos a pasos agigantados —declaró Camelia esperanzada.

La expresión de Zareb era cautelosa.

—¿Nos vamos a casa, Tisha?

Camelia le sonrió. Sabía que Zareb estaba tan ansioso como ella por volver a África.

—Nos iremos dentro de una semana, Zareb.

—¿Ha dicho una semana? —Oliver frunció las cejas, pensativo—. El tiempo justo para comprarme unos pantalones y un par de botas nuevas.

—Tú no vas a venir, Oliver —le espetó Simon.

—Vamos, chico, no pensarás que la señora dejará que vayas solo a la selva africana sin nadie que cuide de ti —objetó Oliver—. No has salido de Gran Bretaña en toda tu vida.

—Tú tampoco —repuso Simon.

—Por eso será una gran aventura para ambos —concluyó Oliver alegremente mientras frotaba sus agarrotadas manos—. Además, el sol me irá muy bien para el dolor de huesos.

—Más bien te freirá como un bistec de ternera —predijo Eunice.

—Y te pondrás más rojo que una langosta —añadió Doreen.

—No sufran por Oliver —las tranquilizó Zareb—. Le daré unas cuantas túnicas y un buen sombrero, y estará completamente protegido.

—¿Qué? ¿Lo veis? El señor Zareb me equipará como es debido y seguro que a ti también, chico, así no se te quemará esa piel lechosa que tienes.

—Estaré bien, Oliver. —A Simon no le gustaba que calificasen su piel de «lechosa» delante de Camelia—. Y repito, tú no vendrás.

—Estaba pensando que deberíamos ir en uno de los barcos de Jack —continuó Oliver sin prestarle atención—. Seguro que tiene uno que va hasta África.

—A lo mejor hasta va con vosotros —sugirió Eunice—. A mí me tranquilizaría saber que cruzáis el océano con nuestro Jack dirigiendo la expedición.

—¿Se refiere a tu hermano Jack? —inquirió Camelia.

Elliott abrió los ojos desmesuradamente.

—¿El que le dio una paliza al carcelero?

—Sí, y es el propietario de una gran flota de barcos —contestó Oliver orgulloso—. Supongo que habrá oído hablar de la North Star Shipping.

Camelia lo miró con incredulidad.

—¿La pequeña empresa naviera que hace un par de años absorbió la Great Atlantic Steamship Company?

—Ésa misma. —Oliver estaba encantado de ver a Camelia sorprendida—. Nuestro Jack es el dueño y es el mejor marinero que encontrará en el océano Atlántico, o en cualquier otro. Si nos lleva a África, llegaremos todos sanos y salvos.

—Avisaré al jefe de oficina para decirle que nos gustaría viajar en uno de sus barcos —decidió Simon—. No sé exactamente dónde está Jack ahora, tampoco es necesario que gobierne él mismo el barco; estoy convencido de que cualquiera de sus tripulaciones es buena.

—Pero Jack gobernaría el barco con suavidad —señaló Eunice—, lo que os iría bien a los dos, que nunca habéis estado más de una hora en el agua.

—Lo superaré, Eunice.

—Yo también —añadió Oliver.

—¡Oh, sí, claro! Como aquella vez que os fuisteis los dos a dar una vuelta en barco por el lago con Charlotte y Annabelle, y media hora después las chicas tuvieron que traeros de vuelta. Estaban mareados como una cuba, y Ollie me suplicó que le envenenase para acabar con su tormento.

—Comí algo que me sentó mal —explicó Oliver en tono defensivo.

—Si insinúas que mi comida te sentó mal, a partir de ahora te harás tú la cena —advirtió Eunice.

—Lo que te sentó mal fue el lago —insistió Doreen—. Con tanto meneo y tantas sacudidas me extraña que llegaseis a tierra firme sin vomitar.

—Por si acaso os daré un poco de mi remedio especial para el mareo —dijo Eunice—. Si os lo tomáis en cuanto empecéis a encontraros mal, impedirá que echéis las entrañas.

—Me parece magnífico, Eunice —afirmó Camelia—. El viaje a África será largo y aunque yo nunca he tenido problemas, el océano a veces puede ser muy bravo.

—Muy bien, pues todo aclarado —concluyó Oliver con una sonrisa—. Marchando cuatro billetes a África en el primer barco de Jack que zarpe.

—Serán cinco.

Camelia miró a Elliott sorprendida.

—No estarás pensando en venir con nosotros, Elliott. ¿No crees que es mucho más importante que te quedes en Londres para ocuparte de tu negocio?

—Para mí no hay nada más importante que tu seguridad, Camelia —contestó él con seriedad—. Has tomado la decisión de continuar excavando, y yo iré a ayudarte. Mi negocio puede esperar hasta que regrese.

Simon miró a Elliott con curiosidad. Al parecer, Wickham era bastante astuto para darse cuenta de que cuando Camelia se pusiese a desenterrar fragmentos de huesos en su excavación prácticamente se olvidaría de él. Y estaba claro que eso no le hacía ninguna gracia. Aun así, a Simon no dejaba de asombrarle que Elliott tuviese la capacidad y la disposición de abandonar su incipiente negocio de importación de un día para otro e irse a pasar varios meses a África. Daba la impresión de que su lealtad a Camelia era mucho más profunda que su preocupación por sus asuntos de negocios. Quizás Elliott abrigaba la tenue esperanza de que, después de todo, la Tumba de los Reyes existiese, y quería estar al lado de Camelia en caso de que lograse encontrarla. Simon intuía que a Elliott no le gustaría nada que otra persona descubriese lo que él no había conseguido desenterrar tras muchos años de trabajo.

Sea por la razón que fuere, el hecho de que Elliott viajase con ellos avivó el recelo de Simon y le produjo cierta irritación.

—De acuerdo, entonces, cinco billetes. —Oliver miró a Oscar, que había bajado del hombro de Zareb y ahora devoraba las galletas de jengibre—. Se me ocurre que tal vez no deberíamos decirle nada a Jack de los animales. No sé si le gustará la idea de que deambulen por su barco.

—No tendrá por qué preocuparse —le aseguró Camelia—. Me aseguraré de que Oscar, Rupert y Harriet se queden en mi camarote durante la mayor parte del viaje.

—Decídselo cuando ya hayáis embarcado —sugirió Eunice—. Jack es muy especial en lo referente a sus barcos y puede que no le apetezca tener a un mono comiendo de su plato o a una serpiente husmeando en sus cazuelas.

—No se altere, jovencita —dijo Oliver al notar que a Camelia le disgustaba que sus animales no fueran bienvenidos—. Jack ha dado la vuelta al mundo un montón de veces y ha visto cosas que ni siquiera podemos imaginarnos. Dudo que le molesten un pequeño mono, una serpiente escuálida y un pájaro que ha perdido varias de sus plumas.

—Bien, todo arreglado. Iré a escribirle una carta al señor Trafford para avisarle de que vamos para allá. Si sale en el correo de hoy, el señor Trafford sabrá que llegamos al menos con unos cuantos días de antelación. Le encantará saber que, por fin, tenemos una bomba para sacar el agua de la excavación. La maldición no podrá asustar a una máquina.

Oliver arqueó las cejas.

—¿Qué maldición?

—Nada importante, Oliver, no hay de qué preocuparse.

Oliver miró expectante a Zareb.

—No se altere, Oliver —dijo Zareb en un torpe intento por utilizar una de las expresiones de éste—. Le prepararé un poderoso amuleto para protegerlo de cualquier espíritu maligno.

Oliver no parecía convencido.

—¿Por qué no le hace también otro al chico? —propuso mientras señalaba a Simon.

—No será necesario, Zareb. No creo en las maldiciones. —Simon hizo una mueca de dolor cuando Harriet aterrizó de pronto en su hombro batiendo sus alas grises.

Zareb lo observó unos instantes, analizando el hecho de que Harriet hubiese elegido ese momento concreto para volar hasta él.

—Es posible que no necesite un amuleto —concedió—, pero le haré uno de todas formas; ya lo llevaré yo.

—Ya puestos, ¿podría hacerme uno a mí también? —preguntó Doreen—. Así evitaría que esa peligrosa serpiente se me acercase.

—Rupert no es peligroso, Doreen —protestó Camelia—. Le cae bien.

—Vale, entonces hágame un amuleto para no caerle tan bien. O eso o lo frío en la sartén.

—Le haré un amuleto para que Rupert no se le acerque, Doreen —ofreció Zareb—. Pero le advierto que es posible que le cueste llevarlo debido a su olor.

Doreen se encogió de hombros.

—Pues lo colgaré encima de la puerta de la cocina.

—Lamento tener que interrumpirles —se disculpó Camelia—, pero debo escribir la carta para el señor Trafford.

—Y yo será mejor que empiece a preparar las medicinas que necesitaréis —decidió Eunice—. Creo que os irá bien tener a mano un jarabe de violetas para purgar vuestras barrigas de vez en cuando. No quiero ni imaginarme lo que comeréis allí.

—Preferiría que nos dieses algo para mantener la comida en el estómago en lugar de devolverla —apuntó Oliver.

—Os prepararé las dos cosas —resolvió Eunice—. Sólo por si acaso.

—Yo también tengo numerosos asuntos que atender antes de partir —anunció Elliott.

—Será un placer acompañarlo a la puerta, señor —repuso Oliver amablemente, abriendo el desfile.

Simon observó cómo la pequeña comitiva abandonaba la sala de estar y se dirigía ruidosamente hacia las escaleras.

Después se sentó en el sofá y miró fijamente a Oscar, que engullía felizmente las olvidadas galletas de jengibre.

—¡Para ya de comer o le diré a Eunice que fuiste tú el que tiró sus enaguas buenas por la ventana! —ordenó Simon alargando el brazo mientras Oscar cogía con avidez la última galleta.

Oscar protestó con insolencia.

—No te gustará convertirte en un trapo para sacar brillo —le advirtió Simon—. El abrillantador que usa Eunice huele realmente mal.

Oscar se detuvo, pensativo y luego, a regañadientes, le dio la codiciada galleta a Simon.

—Chico listo —dijo Simon a punto de morder la galleta.

Sobre su hombro, Harriet graznó con fuerza en señal de protesta.

—Te cedo las tortas, Harriet. —Simon cogió una y se la ofreció al pájaro—. También son muy buenas.

Harriet agarró la torta con el pico y, enfadada, la tiró al suelo sin dudarlo.

—De acuerdo —concedió él—. Pero solamente te daré la mitad. —Partió la galleta en dos trozos y le dio uno a Harriet.

Se reclinó de nuevo, mordió su media galleta y suspiró. Tras treinta y cinco años sin aventurarse más allá de Inverness o Londres estaba a punto de cruzar el océano y adentrarse en las zonas más recónditas de África para encontrar una tumba sobre la que, al parecer, había caído una maldición.

En ese momento sólo se le ocurría rezar por dos cosas. La primera, porque la bomba que acababa de construir funcionase.

La segunda, porque sobreviviese al maldito viaje.

SEGUNDA PARTE

El viento oscuro

Capítulo 8

Camelia se agarró a la gruesa barandilla de hierro e inspiró profundamente, dejando que la rociada fría y negra del océano le arrancara la suciedad y la agitación londinense.

Llevaban sólo tres días de las tres semanas que duraría el viaje, pero ya se sentía mejor de lo que se había sentido en meses. El aire del océano era fresco y puro, no como el de Londres, denso debido al hedor de los humeantes fuegos, los perfumes fuertes, el estiércol almacenado y las alcantarillas. Ignoraba cómo había logrado aguantar tanto tiempo sin que sus pulmones enfermaran de forma terrible. Aunque no habían llegado aún a la costa de Marruecos, ya podía sentir la llamada de África a través de los oscuros kilómetros de olas salpicadas de estrellas.

«Ven a casa, Camelia», le susurraba cada vez que las aguas bravas y agitadas golpeaban el casco del barco. «Ven a casa.» Cerró los ojos y se inclinó más hacia delante, sintiéndose libre, sin miedo y cautelosamente esperanzada.

Por fin regresaba a casa.

Unos tres meses antes, al partir de Ciudad del Cabo en dirección a Inglaterra, Zareb estaba preocupado por la posibilidad de que tal vez nunca volviesen. Le había advertido a Camelia de que Londres era un lugar indómito y peligroso, donde el espíritu podía perderse para siempre. Camelia había desechado sus miedos considerándolos propios de un africano de edad temeroso de un mundo que desconocía; un mundo donde, tal como ya le había avisado a Zareb, quizá tuviese que hacer frente incluso a más prejuicios de los que había tenido que soportar en su tierra natal. ¿Cómo no iba a tener miedo de viajar a un sitio como ése un hombre bueno, honorable e inteligente como Zareb, nacido en el seno de una de las tribus más poderosas del Cabo?

Pero se había equivocado. Camelia no había perdido su espíritu en Londres; ni mucho menos. Los fastuosos bailes y fiestas a los que había acudido palidecían al lado del terrible anhelo que sentía por la serena belleza del cielo nocturno africano. Los altos y churriguerescos edificios y las estrechas y atestadas calles le habían hecho sentirse atrapada, como si le faltase oxígeno. Y esos días interminables redactando cartas para suplicarle a algún inversor potencial que la recibiese, o esas aburridas conferencias y fiestas a las que había asistido con la esperanza de obtener una promesa económica o de una bomba le habían dejado vacía y frustrada, con la sensación de que no estaba consiguiendo nada en absoluto. Su padre tenía razón, pensó mientras se asomaba todavía más al mar.

Cuando removía la tierra era realmente feliz.

—Preferiría que no te asomaras tanto al agua —dijo una voz grave—. No tengo muchas ganas de darme un chapuzón a estas horas.

Camelia se volvió y vio a Jack, el hermano de Simon, que la observaba desde las sombras. Estaba apoyado con indiferencia en un mástil, con los brazos cruzados delante del pecho; su relajada postura le recordó muchísimo a la que a menudo adquiría Simon. Aunque cualquier semejanza acababa ahí.

Jack Kent debía de ser un par o tres centímetros más alto que Simon y su bello rostro tenía arrugas y estaba curtido debido a los años que se había pasado de pie en una cubierta, de cara al viento y al sol, mientras gobernaba sus barcos por el océano. Su pelo, del color de la madera bien encerada, tenía unos cuantos mechones dorados aclarados por el sol y sus ojos eran de un gris acerado que a Camelia le recordaron la reluciente hoja de un puñal. Tenía treinta y ocho años, sólo tres más que Simon, pero había visto tanto mundo que parecía mucho más maduro. Posó su mirada en la delgada cicatriz blanca que serpenteaba por el anguloso contorno de su mejilla izquierda y recordó que Simon le había comentado que Jack tenía casi quince años cuando, al fin, lady Redmond lo rescató de la celda de una cárcel en Inveraray.

Intuyó que esos años de soledad y lucha por la supervivencia habían sido extremadamente duros.

—Me encanta sentir el océano, y su aroma —repuso Camelia, retrocediendo un poco—. Hace que me sienta libre.

—Lo entiendo perfectamente —le aseguró Jack—. Sin embargo, creo que Simon se enfadaría bastante conmigo si dejara que te cayeras por la borda.

—¿Dónde está?

—En la sala de máquinas. Está intentando construir un motor de vapor más eficiente que los actuales para incrementar la propulsión de mis barcos. Dice que se le ha ocurrido una idea en la que empezará a trabajar en cuanto vuelva de África.

—Eso significa que ya se encuentra mejor.

—Sí, supongo que sí. Por lo visto ya se le ha pasado el mareo.

—O eso o que el medicamento de Eunice le ha hecho echarlo todo —intervino Oliver, que acompañado de Zareb se reunió con ellos en la cubierta—. Pobre muchacho; por un momento pensé que le pediría a Jack que virase y lo llevase de vuelta a Londres. Tenía miedo de pasarse todo el viaje mareado como una cuba.

—No se habría encontrado tan mal si me hubiese dejado practicar mi ceremonia de curación —insistió Zareb—. Pero, por desgracia, no logré convencerle.

—No debería haber salido de su camarote —comentó Camelia—. Si está débil, no debería intentar trabajar todavía.

—¡Ay, preciosa! —exclamó Oliver—. El chico es feliz cuando está lleno de grasa de arriba abajo y rodeado de metal.

Jack asintió.

—Recuerdo que la primera vez que fuimos a la finca de Haydon, Simon estaba fascinado con todos los relojes que había allí. De modo que los desarmó uno por uno y los intentó montar otra vez para ver si sabía cómo funcionaban. Pero, por alguna razón, al acabar de montarlos siempre sobraban unas cuantas piezas.

—Durante casi un año entero hubo relojes sonando en casa a cualquier hora del día y de la noche —continuó Oliver riéndose—. Finalmente, el señor los cogió todos y los envió a un famoso relojero de Inverness, ¡que estuvo otro año entero tratando de que volviesen a funcionar como Dios manda!

Camelia sonrió. No le costaba nada imaginarse a Simon de pequeño, dedicándose a desmontar cuanto sus manos tocaban.

—¿Consiguió averiguar cómo se fabrica un reloj?

—Al final, Haydon contrató al relojero para que viniese a la finca y le enseñase a Simon cómo funcionaban tanto los relojes de pared como los de bolsillo —contestó Jack—. Al cabo de una semana el hombre dijo que Simon tenía un talento increíble y que debería plantearse ser relojero.

—Pero, para entonces, al chico ya habían dejado de interesarle los relojes —añadió Oliver, cabeceando—. Había decidido construir otras máquinas a partir del mecanismo de los relojes; máquinas más grandes.

—¿Como cuál? —inquirió Camelia.

—Un día, Eunice y Doreen les pidieron a Simon y a su hermano Jaime que lavaran los platos de la cena, y a Simon se le metió en la cabeza la idea de que lo mejor era que fuese una máquina la que los lavara —explicó Oliver—. Así que amontonó platos y vasos en un viejo barreño de madera con agua jabonosa, y fijó un gran dispositivo que había construido encima del cubo. Cuando Eunice y Doreen regresaron a la cocina un poco después, se encontraron a Jaime moviendo una manivela que hacía que el barreño se sacudiera con bastante fuerza mientras Simon le instaba a que la girase más deprisa para que los platos se lavasen antes.

—Estaba tremendamente decepcionado cuando Eunice empezó a sacar de la máquina trozos de platos rotos y la cristalería hecha añicos —prosiguió Jack con ironía—. Después de aquello no tuvo más remedio que revisar su invento.

Camelia sonrió.

—Pero nunca dejó de inventar cosas.

—No podía; lo llevaba en la sangre de la misma manera que Jack lleva el mar en la sangre —repuso Oliver—. El señor y Genevieve contrataron los mejores tutores y todos coincidieron en que el chico poseía una inteligencia fuera de lo común, incluso aquel que se despidió del empleo después de que Simon hiciese volar accidentalmente su escritorio por los aires. —Se dio unas palmadas en la rodilla divertido—. Le chamuscó las cejas al pobre hombre; su hermana Annabelle tuvo que dibujárselas con un corcho quemado antes de salir a la calle. Cuando por fin Simon se marchó a la universidad a todos nos dio miedo que la incendiase sin querer.

—¿Y lo hizo? —inquirió Zareb.

—Sólo quemé un laboratorio de ciencias. —Simon apareció en la cubierta con Oscar cómodamente sentado en su hombro—. De todas formas, había que reformarlo.

La suave luz de la luna le iluminó mientras se acercaba. Llevaba una sencilla camisa blanca, pantalones oscuros y un holgado abrigo hecho a medida. Le pareció más delgado en la oscura noche y, durante los últimos días de indisposición, su piel se había vuelto aún más pálida. Camelia se sintió un tanto culpable; antes de embarcar en el *Independence* había estado trabajando día y noche en la bomba, y se había agotado. No podía dejar de pensar que el débil estado de Simon había contribuido a que enfermase en cuanto el enorme barco de vapor de Jack zarpó de Londres. Se encontraría mejor al llegar a África, decidió mientras observaba cómo Oscar buscaba cariñosamente piojos en su enredado pelo cobrizo. Cuando estuviera de nuevo en tierra firme, y el cálido sol africano y el viento le acariciaran la piel, se repondría enseguida.

—Jack y Oliver nos estaban contando algunas de tus travesuras de niño —explicó Camelia con una sonrisa—. Por lo visto ya por aquel entonces intentabas mejorar las cosas.

—Siempre he sentido curiosidad por saber cómo funcionan las cosas —replicó Simon, intentando apartar las fisgonas pezuñas de Oscar de su pelo—. Si entiendes cómo funciona algo, puedes concentrarte en tratar de mejorarlo.

—Aunque hay cosas que no necesitan mejorarse —observó Oliver.

—¿Como qué?

—Como este cielo. —Oliver miró hacia lo alto—. Todas esas estrellas llevan ahí miles de años y seguirán miles de años más. No hay nada que mejorar, sólo hay que disfrutarlo.

Simon levantó la vista y frunció las cejas.

—Para estudiar las estrellas necesitamos máquinas y las máquinas siempre pueden perfeccionarse. Algún día inventaré un telescopio mejor, que permita observar los planetas con más claridad.

—¿Para qué quieres ver los planetas? ¿No tienes suficiente con todas las estrellas que hay? —preguntó Oliver con impaciencia.

—Me gustaría ver qué hay más allá de las estrellas.

—¿Por qué?

—Porque me intriga lo que pueda haber ahí arriba. Quiero conocer lo que no puedo ver fácilmente.

—¿Y nunca has pensado que puede haber cosas que no tienes por qué ver?

Simon se encogió de hombros.

—Si hay algo que no tengo que ver, supongo que no podré verlo.

—Después de ver los planetas, querrás ver a Dios y Él mismo te dirá: «Jovencito, ya está bien, no seas indiscreto».

—Cuando Dios me diga eso, miraré hacia otra parte, Oliver —repuso Simon tranquilo—. Aún quedan muchas cosas por descubrir.

—Buenas noches a todos. —Elliott subió de la cubierta inferior—. Camelia, ¿no crees que es un poco tarde para que estés aquí fuera? El aire es frío.

—Estoy bien, Elliott —le aseguró Camelia—. Sólo estábamos disfrutando de este maravilloso cielo nocturno.

—¿Qué tal va nuestro rumbo, capitán Kent? —quiso saber Elliot, que no se molestó en mirar al cielo—. ¿Navegamos según el calendario previsto?

—Estos últimos días hemos navegado a buen ritmo —contestó Jack—, pero se avecina mal tiempo y es probable que mañana y pasado haya que aminorar la marcha. Espero que después podamos volver a navegar más deprisa.

—¿Has dicho mal tiempo? —se mofó Oliver—. ¡Pero si el cielo está completamente despejado!

—Hay nubarrones al sureste.

—¿No te estarás refiriendo a ese punto oscuro de ahí? —le espetó Oliver—. Pero ¡si eso no es más que una pequeña nube que ha perdido a su madre?

—Pues su madre está justo detrás —replicó Jack, divertido con la analogía de Oliver—. Y su padre también.

—El capitán tiene razón. —Zareb miró a lo lejos con los ojos entornados—. Se avecina tormenta. Lo presiento.

—Tal vez deberíamos navegar más deprisa —sugirió Camelia— e intentar esquivarla antes de que se desate.

—Lamentablemente, con el rumbo que llevamos lo único que conseguiríamos es acercarnos a ella aún más rápido —le explicó Jack—. No se preocupe, el *Independence* ya ha hecho frente a un montón de tormentas.

—Quizá tu barco esté acostumbrado a ellas, pero el estómago de tu hermano no es tan fuerte —declaró Oliver, señalando a Simon con un movimiento de cabeza—. Si se pasa tres días más con la cabeza metida en un cubo, cuando llegue a Ciudad del Cabo se habrá convertido en un pellejo.

—Sí, no se ha encontrado muy bien desde que zarpamos, ¿verdad, Kent? —preguntó Elliott con cierto tono de superioridad—. Supongo que no está acostumbrado a viajar en barco.

—Estoy bien. —De hecho, Simon estaba hecho un trapo, pero no tenía por qué compartir eso con Wickham. Le irritaba que, al parecer, a nadie más le hubiese afectado el infernal vaivén del barco, mientras él había estado padeciendo miserablemente en la estrecha cama de su camarote.

—Eso espero, porque en Pumulani necesitará todas sus fuerzas.

—No se preocupe por mí, Wickhip —comentó Simon—. He tenido unos cuantos días para acostumbrarme al balanceo del barco y estoy disfrutando bastante del viaje. Si me disculpan, debo volver al trabajo. Los veré a todos por la mañana. Buenas noches.

Se volvió y se dirigió a su camarote silbando alegremente.

Odiaba el maldito océano.

Ése era su único pensamiento mientras, tumbado en su cama, se asía con desesperación a los bordes del colchón. Gracias a Dios, sus náuseas se habían suavizado, pero la tormenta anunciada por Jack había hecho que el mar se enfureciese. Como resultado de ello, el *Independence* había empezado a balancearse incluso más que antes y aproximadamente cada minuto las entrañas de Simon bajaban con violencia desde su garganta hasta las rodillas y viceversa.

¿Cómo podía la gente soportar un vaivén tan brusco y angustioso?, se preguntó furioso. ¿Y cómo era físicamente posible que un enorme barco de vapor de hierro pudiese ser movido con tanta violencia como si fuese un simple y maldito corcho?

«Si consigo sobrevivir a este estúpido viaje, no volveré a subirme a un barco en toda mi vida.» Vio con impotencia cómo su jofaina de metal y su jarra se deslizaban por el palanganero y aterrizaban ruidosamente en el suelo. «No, hasta que construya uno que no se balancee como si fuera de juguete.»

Tragó con dificultad y cerró los ojos, lo que sólo sirvió para empeorar las cosas. Los abrió de nuevo y miró el escritorio fijamente, intentando fijar la vista en el montón de libros y dibujos que había dejado encima. Tal vez debería levantarse e intentar trabajar. Quizá eso le ayudaría a no pensar en el movimiento. Sus libros empezaron a deslizarse lentamente de un extremo de la mesa a otro. Clavó la vista en ellos mientras se desplazaban de un lado a otro, incapaz de decidir si era peor mirarlos y ser consciente del tremendo vaivén del barco o simplemente cerrar los ojos y notar el movimiento. Al final, los libros se cayeron del escritorio, seguidos de su pluma y su tintero.

Sin duda, era peor la primera opción.

Cerró los ojos y procuró anular cualquier sensación. Se planteó subir a la cubierta, pensando que tal vez el aire fresco y la rociada del océano le reanimarían un poco. Además, si acababa devolviendo, era mucho más fácil apoyarse en la barandilla y vomitar sobre las miserables aguas que tanto le estaban haciendo padecer. Pero la idea de salir de la oscilante cama, arrastrarse por el inestable pasillo y subir por el balanceante tramo de escaleras requería un esfuerzo físico muy superior al que podía realizar. De modo que se limitó a permanecer tumbado, agarrándose con fuerza al colchón mientras sopesaba las consecuencias de ingerir otra dosis del asqueroso elixir estomacal de Eunice. Si el océano no acababa con él, el elixir de Eunice seguro que lo haría.

Y en ese momento esa posibilidad resultaba enormemente tentadora.

Pero de pronto alguien llamó a la puerta interrumpiendo su desdicha.

—¡Señor Kent! Soy Zareb, ¡por favor, venga enseguida!

Sin saber cómo, Simon logró levantarse de la cama, tambalearse hasta la puerta y abrirla.

Zareb estaba en el pasillo con el pánico reflejado en la mirada.

—Se está muriendo, señor Kent —susurró Zareb con voz temblorosa—. Ha llegado el viento oscuro y no puedo ahuyentarlo.

Presa del miedo, Simon olvidó su propio malestar.

—¿Qué quiere decir que se está muriendo?

—El viento oscuro —repitió Zareb, convencido de que Simon sabría de qué hablaba—. Al fin la ha encontrado. He intentado evitarlo, pero es demasiado fuerte. ¡Acompáñeme!

El africano de edad se volvió y voló por el pasillo; sus vistosas y coloridas túnicas ondeaban tras él como el plumaje de un pájaro exótico. Simon lo siguió corriendo.

Una espesa y acre nube de humo emergió del camarote de Camelia cuando Zareb abrió la puerta.

—¡*Fuego*! —gritó Simon, casi sin poder respirar mientras se precipitaba al camarote inundado de humo—. ¡*Camelia*!

—No, no es fuego —se apresuró a asegurarle Zareb, que entró tras él—. Estoy intentando ahuyentar los malos espíritus.

Simon parpadeó debido a la acre neblina. Camelia estaba echada en el suelo, acurrucada y tiritando, vestida sólo con un camisón y rodeada de unos protectores Oscar, Harriet y Rupert. Un velo gris espesaba el aire del camarote tenuemente iluminado, envolviéndolos a todos con su nauseabundo hedor dulce. A su alrededor había dibujado un círculo de arena y junto a su cabeza, brazos, piernas y pies había dispuestos media docena de recipientes humeantes, de cada uno de los cuales emanaba una sofocante niebla. Cuando entró Simon, Camelia intentó levantar la cabeza, pero no logró llegar a la palangana porque su cuerpo entero se retorcía con la arcada más feroz que había visto jamás.

Corrió junto a ella, se arrodilló para apartarle con suavidad el pelo de la cara y le sujetó la cabeza mientras vomitaba.

—Tranquila, Camelia. —Le habló con voz seria y grave procurando aparentar una calma que no sentía. Cuando por fin sus arcadas se suavizaron, la acunó en sus brazos, consternado por la espectral palidez de su piel.

—Me estoy muriendo —gimoteó Camelia con un hilo de voz apenas audible con el rugido del barco.

—No te estás muriendo —repuso Simon con firmeza—. Si yo puedo sobrevivir a este horror de viaje, Camelia, tú también puedes —le dijo mientras la cogía en brazos.

—Déjela donde está —protestó Zareb—. ¡Necesita protegerse de la maldición!

—Lo que necesita es estar tumbada en su cama —le espetó Simon, llevándola hasta la cama y echándola con cuidado sobre ella.

—Pero la cama está apoyada en el suelo y entonces no podré dibujar un círculo de protección alrededor de ella.

—El círculo de protección no sirve de nada, Zareb —argumentó Simon mientras tapaba a Camelia con las mantas—. ¡Mírela, está congelada!

—¿Dónde está el fuego, muchacho? —Oliver irrumpió en el camarote, sacudiendo sus delgados brazos y tosiendo—. ¡Por el amor de San Columbano! ¡Esto apesta!

—Estoy intentando ahuyentar los malos espíritus. —Zareb acercó a Camelia los recipientes de hierbas humeantes.

—Yo más bien diría que lo que hace es ahuyentar el poco oxígeno que queda —comentó Oliver con voz ronca.

—¡Camelia! —Elliott entró a toda prisa en el camarote y espantado miró fijamente a Camelia, que yacía débil y pálida en su cama—. ¡Dios mío, Zareb! —logró exclamar pese a la sofocante neblina—. Pero ¿qué le ha hecho?

—Han sido los espíritus malignos. —Con afligida expresión, colocó los humeantes recipientes de hierbas alrededor de la cama de Camelia—. La han seguido a través del océano y ahora se la quieren llevar.

—¿De qué demonios está hablando? —Horrorizado, Elliott vio cómo Camelia volvía la cabeza a un lado y vomitaba en la palangana que Simon sostenía. Estaba pálida—. ¡Jesús! ¿Qué le pasa?

—Es la maldición —insistió Zareb a punto de echarse a llorar—. El viento oscuro la ha encontrado.

—¿Se puede saber qué pasa aquí? —inquirió Jack, que apareció en la puerta vestido sólo con unos pantalones—. ¿Se ha quemado algo?

—¡Necesitamos un médico! —suplicó Elliott—. ¡Ahora!

—No hay ningún médico a bordo. —Jack se aproximó a la cama de Camelia.

—Esto es indignante. ¿Cómo demonios es posible que en un barco no haya un médico a bordo?

—¿Cuánto tiempo lleva así? —le preguntó Jack a Simon, ignorando a Elliott y fijándose en los pálidos labios de Camelia, que castañeteaban, y en su cérea piel.

—No lo sé; acabo de llegar y me la he encontrado así. —Simon alargó el brazo para coger una toalla del lavabo y le enjugó la boca con cuidado. Después le preguntó a su hermano con voz grave y tensa—: ¿Tú qué crees que le pasa?

—Lo más seguro seguro es que alguno de sus asquerosos y malditos animales le haya contagiado una horrible enfermedad. —Elliott miró furioso a Oscar, Harriet y Rupert—. A lo mejor le ha mordido esa maldita serpiente, ¡y eso que le advertí que no la dejara suelta!

Rupert se irguió y le enseñó a Elliott la lengua amenazadoramente.

—Los espíritus malignos no se manifiestan a través de los animales —objetó Zareb, que acercó a la cama de Camelia otro recipiente humeante—. Tienen suficiente poder para entrar en un cuerpo por sí mismos.

—Deme eso, Zareb. —Jack cogió el cuenco, abrió la ventanilla y lo arrojó al agitado océano—. Oliver, por favor, ¿podrías pasarme el resto de recipientes?

—¡No, capitán! —exclamó Zareb mientras sujetaba dos de ellos con firmeza—. ¡Debemos luchar contra el espíritu maligno desde el interior del camarote!

—Lo único maligno que hay en este camarote es el hedor y el humo que usted ha producido —repuso Jack mientras tiraba otro cuenco por la ventanilla—. Si yo apenas puedo respirar y no me encuentro mal, no quiero ni imaginarme el efecto que este aire venenoso está produciendo en lady Camelia —dijo al tiempo que arrojaba otro recipiente humeante al mar.

—Se está enfrentando a un poder oscuro que usted no comprende —protestó Zareb—. ¡La maldición que ha caído sobre Pumulani es muy poderosa!

—Puede que no sepa mucho de poderes oscuros, pero reconozco un caso grave de mareo nada más verlo —replicó

Jack, cogiendo otro recipiente que le había dado Oliver y lanzándolo a la tormenta—. ¡Y sé con toda seguridad que obligarle a respirar ese asqueroso humo cuando no para de vomitar no le ayudará en absoluto!

Simon lo miró confuso.

—¿Mareo?

—Imposible. —Zareb sacudió la cabeza enérgicamente—. Tisha nunca se marea.

—Para todo hay una primera vez —soltó Jack.

Oliver se rascó la cabeza, perplejo.

—¿Cómo puede ser que la chica esté mareada, si durante los tres primeros días de viaje se ha encontrado bien?

—En las últimas cuatro horas el mar se ha embravecido. ¿No has notado lo mucho que se mueve el barco?

—A mí no me ha parecido que se moviese más que antes —contestó Simon con pesar.

—Pensaba que era el trago de wkisky que me he tomado después de cenar —comentó Oliver.

—Yo que tú no bebería más, Oliver; de lo contrario, tendrás la sensación de que el barco se bambolea todavía más —advirtió Jack, que le pasó a Oliver la palangana—. ¿Te importaría aclararla e ir a pedirle a Will, el joven grumete, que me consiga dos cubos limpios, unas cuantas toallas, una jarra de agua para beber, una cuchara y un par más de mantas? Zareb, es preciso que esté toda la noche junto a lady Camelia y que la vigile bien. Probablemente seguirá encontrándose mal hasta que esté tan cansada que sólo pueda dormir. Procure que beba un poco de agua a sorbos de la cuchara, pero más o menos cada diez minutos, si no volverá a vomitar. Si empeora o le sube la fiebre, avíseme de inmediato, ¿de acuerdo?

Zareb asintió lentamente, esforzándose por centrar los ojos en el rostro de Jack mientras el camarote se inclinaba y se balanceaba.

Y entonces, de repente, se tapó la boca con la mano y huyó del dormitorio para no devolver delante de todos.

—Iré con él para comprobar que se encuentra bien —dijo Oliver, súbitamente ansioso por subir a la cubierta—. No creo que esta noche le sirva de mucha ayuda a la chica.

Jack suspiró y miró expectante a Elliott y a Simon.

—Yo cuidaré de ella —anunció Simon.

—No, lo haré *yo* —insistió Elliott—. Hace muchos años que conozco a Camelia; mi relación con ella es mucho más estrecha que la suya, Kent.

—Está bien —concedió Jack—. Lo dicho, Wickham, es importante que beba un poco de agua, pero despacio. En cuanto deje de vomitar, intente que beba un poco de té de jengibre. Mañana, si Camelia tiene fuerzas suficientes para incorporarse, podrá comer una galleta de soda troceada y si el estómago aguanta, entonces podrá tomar... ¿Me escucha, Wickham?

—Por supuesto que le escucho —afirmó Elliott, luchando por mirar a Jack mientras el camarote se bamboleaba de un lado a otro. Pegó bien los pies al suelo en un intento por buscar un poco de estabilidad—. Decía algo de unas galletas de soda y... —Alargó el brazo y se apoyó en la pared para no caerse.

—¿Está usted bien, Wickhip? —Simon frunció las cejas—. Está completamente pálido...

—Estoy bien —contestó Elliott, que tragó con dificultad—. Entonces, le tengo que dar galletas y té... —Hizo una pausa con cara de horror.

Después salió volando del camarote y apenas llegó al pasillo se puso a vomitar.

—¡Maldita sea! —Jack se volvió para mirar a su hermano—. ¿Tú te encuentras bien o también estás a punto de devolver?

—Puedo cuidar de ella perfectamente —aseguró Simon.

—De acuerdo. Lo más importante es que esté lo más abrigada y cómoda posible, e intenta que beba un poco de agua. El aire del camarote es ahora más fresco y menos denso, pero creo que habría que sacar esos animales de aquí para que esté más tranquila. Los llevaré a tu camarote. —Miró a Rupert con cautela—. Pensándolo bien, será mejor que cojas tú a la serpiente; yo cogeré a los otros dos.

Harriet voló hasta el hombro de Simon y graznó con fuerza al ver que Jack se aproximaba a ella. Entonces Jack se volvió a Oscar, que trepó por el cuerpo de Simon, plantándose encima de su cabeza. Rupert permaneció donde estaba, con el cuerpo erguido y arqueado listo para el ataque.

Cuando Oscar se agarró del cabello de Simon, éste hizo una mueca de dolor.

—Tal vez deberíamos dejar que se quedaran aquí.

Jack miró a su hermano extrañado.

—No sabía que te gustasen los animales.

—Y no me gustan —declaró Simon mientras procuraba que Harriet no hundiese sus patas en su hombro—, pero por alguna razón ellos no se han dado por aludidos.

—Aquí tiene lo que ha pedido, capitán. —Un chico soñoliento de unos doce años entró en el camarote con un montón de mantas, toallas, cubos y agua—. Creo que lord Wickham no se encuentra muy bien; lo acabo de ver intentando llegar a su camarote y estaba pálido... ¡Mierda, una serpiente!

—Así es, Will —constató Jack—. Es de lady Camelia. Deja las cosas encima de esa mesa.

—¿Muerde? —preguntó Will temeroso, sin avanzar.

—Yo no le he visto morder a nadie. —Como no había conseguido que Harriet se moviera de su hombro, Simon intentó ahora sacar al tozudo de Oscar de su cabeza—. Y aunque lo hiciera, sus mordiscos no son venenosos para los humanos.

—¿Por qué lady Camelia no la mete en una jaula? —inquirió Will, que se acercó lentamente a la mesa manteniéndose lo más alejado que pudo de Rupert.

—Porque no es partidaria de las jaulas.

—Admirable filosofía —observó Jack—. A mí tampoco me convencen. ¡Venga, Will! Subiremos a la cubierta para ver cómo va todo. Si la tormenta se desata, tendremos más cosas de qué preocuparnos que de unos cuantos pasajeros mareados.

—¿Qué quiere decir «si se desata»? —quiso saber Simon mientras cogía la jarra de agua, que estaba a punto de caerse—. ¿No estamos ya en plena tormenta?

—¿Llamas a esto una tormenta? Esto no es nada. Tú espera a que el barco empiece a ladearse como si fuese a volcar, ¡y entonces sí que te sentirás realmente vivo!

Simon abrazó contra su pecho la oscilante jarra de agua y gimió.

—¿Sabe Amelia lo excéntrico que eres en todo lo relativo al mar? —le preguntó, refiriéndose a la mujer de Jack.

—Amelia sabe todo sobre mí y por alguna razón que desconozco me quiere igualmente. —Jack le dedicó una sonrisa a su hermano, cuyo aspecto en ese momento era ridículo con un mono sobre su cabeza, un pájaro encima de su hombro y una serpiente, que se deslizaba por sus pies—. Lo que me lleva a pensar que hay una esperanza para todos los que nos hemos descarriado, Simon. —Lanzó una mirada a Camelia, que estaba silenciosamente tumbada en su cama—. Ya no tiene tantas arcadas, y eso es bueno. No le des agua todavía, sólo mantenla abrigada. Volveré dentro de un rato para ver cómo se encuentra. —Se marchó con Will y cerró la puerta al salir.

Simon se quedó en el centro del camarote, observando cómo los baúles de Camelia y la silla del pequeño escritorio se desplazaban por el suelo. Rupert se apartó de en medio culebreando mientras de un salto Oscar se refugiaba sobre el escritorio, que estaba sujeto al suelo. Harriet batió las alas y se agarró con más fuerza al hombro de Simon.

—Consideradlo una aventura —sugirió al tiempo que detenía la díscola silla—. Algo que podréis contarles a todos los demás monos, pájaros y serpientes cuando lleguéis a casa.

Oscar arqueó las cejas y cabeceó enérgicamente.

—Sí, supongo que tienes razón; no se lo creerían. Te aseguro que yo tampoco lo haría si alguien me lo contase. —Colocó la silla con decisión junto a la cama de Camelia y se sentó. Después puso agua fresca en la jofaina, mojó y escurrió una toalla, y empezó a humedecerle la cara con suavidad.

Estaba pálida, debajo de sus ojos se le habían formado ojeras moradas y sus labios eran una tensa raya, como si estuviese aún luchando contra las náuseas que le sacudían. Mientras le mojaba despacio la cara y la nuca le inundó una desconocida necesidad de protección. Dejó la toalla en la jofaina y puso una mano sobre la frente de Camelia para saber si tenía fiebre. Tenía la piel fría. Recordó que Jack le había aconsejado que estuviese abrigada y se levantó para coger las mantas que el joven Will había dejado bruscamente en el suelo del camarote.

Cuando regresó a su lado, Camelia lo estaba mirando.

—Me has dejado sola —susurró. Daba la impresión de que le costaba articular las palabras, como si hablar requiriese un gran esfuerzo.

—Ha sido sólo un momento. He ido a buscar unas mantas. —Las extendió sobre su cuerpo.

—Me estoy muriendo, Simon —dijo en voz baja—. Lo siento.

—No te estás muriendo, Camelia. Sé que lo que digo no te parecerá especialmente reconfortante, porque acabo de pasar por una experiencia similar a la tuya, pero no te vas a morir.

Ella arrugó la frente, tratando de comprender lo que Simon le decía.

—¿No me estoy muriendo?

—No.

—Pero Zareb ha dicho que ha llegado el viento oscuro.

—Tenía entendido que no creías en las maldiciones. —Habló en tono ligeramente burlón mientras se sentaba junto a ella y se disponía a recolocar las sábanas y las mantas más a su gusto.

—Y no creo en ellas. —Lo miró fijamente con los ojos nublados por la desesperación—. Pero tengo la sensación de que me voy a morir.

Simon alargó el brazo y le acarició con ternura la fría y sedosa mejilla.

—Está oscuro, Camelia, y sin duda sopla el viento ahí fuera. Y el viento ha agitado el océano, por eso el barco sube y baja como una pelota. Si tú estás mareada, tendrías que ver al pobre Wickham. —Se mofó con una sonrisa—. Debe de estar apoyado en la barandilla pensando en tirarse al mar y poner fin a su misera vida.

—¿Y Zareb?

—Por desgracia, también se encuentra mal. Me parece que Oliver está con él.

—La culpa es mía —declaró con tristeza.

—No creo que se te pueda responsabilizar del mal tiempo, Camelia.

—Estáis aquí por mi culpa.

—Estamos aquí porque así lo hemos querido —le corrigió Simon—, que es muy distinto.

Camelia cerró los ojos, demasiado cansada para seguir discutiendo.

Él permaneció un largo rato sentado a su lado, contemplando la lasitud de su pálido y bello rostro mientras el dormitorio se bamboleaba y sus baúles se movían de un lado a otro. Pensó en lo pequeña y frágil que se la veía ahí tumbada, imagen que tanto contrastaba con la mujer decidida y joven que había irrumpido en su laboratorio sin ser anunciada, y que le había insistido en que le construyese una bomba de agua. Había cruzado este mismo océano antes de aparecer en su vida. Ahora, por fin, regresaría a la tierra que tanto amaba. Ningún viento oscuro, maldición o amenaza de muerte lograría evitar que volviese a África, su hogar. Volvería a su excavación, sacaría el agua y reanudaría el trabajo, y descubriría la antigua tumba con la que su padre había soñado o moriría en el intento. Si algo sabía de Camelia era que nunca se rendía.

Luchaba con el corazón de un guerrero.

Ahora respiraba más profundamente y los pliegues de su frente se habían suavizado; al fin, las náuseas se habían mitigado. Simon pensó que tal vez fuese un buen momento para ir a buscar el té de jengibre que Jack le había mencionado. Cuando Camelia se despertara, debería animarla a beber un poco; también le traería unas cuantas galletas, por si después tenía hambre. Se levantó y la arropó con las mantas para que en su ausencia no pasase frío.

—No me dejes —musitó ella. Con las embestidas del océano contra el *Independence* su voz apenas era audible.

—No te dejo, sólo voy a buscarte un poco de té —le dijo mientras le apartaba de la frente un mechón de pelo dorado.

Camelia frunció las cejas y buscó su mano, que rodeó débilmente con los dedos.

—No me dejes —repitió, esta vez más despacio, como si estuviese empeñada en hacerse entender—. Por favor.

Simon miró con fijeza la palidez de sus largos dedos, que se agarraban con desesperación a los suyos. Tenía la mano pequeña y suave al tacto, como los aterciopelados pétalos de una flor. Recordó cómo esa mano le había acariciado, cómo le había tocado y presionado hasta que se creyó enloquecer. Esa noche había tenido la sensación de que se había entregado a ella, de que había perdido una parte profunda e íntima de su ser que ya nunca podría recuperar, por mucho que lo intentase. Y lo había intentado durante las semanas siguientes. Había hecho lo posible para esquivarla, para concentrarse en su trabajo, en los detalles de la organización del viaje y, en esos últimos días, en el inmenso desafío que suponía sobrevivir en este maldito y miserable barco.

Pero mientras sostenía su mano, se sintió nuevamente perdido. «No me dejes.» Se refería sólo a ese momento, porque estaba enferma, se sentía vulnerable y tenía miedo. Sin embargo, las palabras de algún modo se abrieron paso hasta los más recónditos rincones de su alma, y se sintió unido a ella de una forma incomprensible. Camelia le había robado una parte de su ser; ahora lo entendía. No lo había hecho intencionadamente, pero eso apenas importaba. Le había robado un trozo de su corazón y de su alma, trozos que ella se quedaría cuando, por fin, él abandonase África y regresase a casa.

Sabía que nunca le convencería de que volviese a Londres con él. Su lugar estaba en África, con sus montañas bañadas por el sol, sus animales salvajes y sus misteriosos fragmentos de huesos y cáscaras. No se podía comparar con una vida banal junto a un antiguo ladrón olvidadizo y despistado, en una casa llena de gente de una calle lluviosa y tiznada de Londres.

Y, a diferencia de Elliott, Camelia le importaba demasiado a Simon como para intentar que viviese una vida con la que jamás sería feliz.

—No te dejaré, Camelia —susurró, volviéndose a sentar en la silla.

Ella le apretó la mano con debilidad, luego suspiró y volvió la cabeza, y finalmente se quedó dormida.

Y Simon se quedó sentado, mirándola, con la mano unida a la suya, protegiéndola del viento oscuro mientras su corazón empezaba a desgarrarse.

Capítulo 9

—Se coge el estómago, se limpia la sangre y después se deja diez horas en agua fría con sal. Así las asaduras quedan bien saladas.

Zareb miró a Oliver confundido.

—¿Qué son las asaduras?

—Las entrañas de la oveja —explicó Oliver, sumergiendo una bolsa cruda del estómago del animal en un recipiente con agua—. El corazón, el hígado, los pulmones y la tráquea.

Zareb titubeó.

—¿La tráquea?

—Se pone más por la textura que le da que por el sabor. —Oliver agitó el estómago en el agua sanguinolenta con la misma naturalidad que si estuviera lavando un par de calcetines—. Me gustan los *haggis* bien fuertes, con un buen pellizco de pimienta negra y pimienta inglesa.

—¿Y las asaduras se ponen dentro de la bolsa y después se condimentan?

—Primero se hierven hasta que estén tiernas —continuó Oliver— y luego se cortan bien, en trozos no demasiado finos, porque esto no es un pudín. Después se mezclan con harina de avena tostada, una buena taza de sebo, unas cuantas cebollas troceadas y las especias, y se introduce todo en la bolsa del estómago, que se cose.

—¿Y la bolsa se come cruda? —Zareb parecía asqueado.

—No, se hierve —contestó Oliver—. Se hierve en agua durante tres horas a fuego lento. Después se sirve caliente con un montón de whisky y puré de patatas. —Extrajo el resplandeciente estómago del agua ensangrentada y lo introdujo en otro recipiente con agua salada—. Le aseguro que no hay nada comparado con un buen plato de *haggis*. ¡Le sentará de maravilla! Le saldrá pelo en el pecho.

Zareb abrió los ojos desmesuradamente.

—¿Le saldrá a Tisha pelo en el pecho?

—Es una forma de hablar —le aseguró Oliver, que se limpió las manos con un trapo—. No hay ninguna chica escocesa que tenga pelos en el pecho y eso que empiezan a comer *haggis* prácticamente en cuanto aprenden a coger una cuchara.

—No le haga caso, Zareb —advirtió Simon con la cabeza inclinada sobre la tabla que usaba a modo de mesa para hacer sus dibujos—. Es bastante improbable que Oliver haya podido verle realmente el pecho a todas las escocesas.

—¡Oye, cierra el pico! —le reprendió Oliver.

—Los khoikhoi, pastores y cosechadores nómadas que habitan gran parte de la antigua Provincia del Cabo, sólo comen carne de oveja cuando sacrifican animales para un ritual —comentó Zareb, nada convencido con el *haggis* de Oliver—, pero la mayoría usamos las vacas y las ovejas únicamente para obtener leche.

—¿Y qué clase de carne comen? —inquirió Oliver con interés.

—Lo que cazamos: cebras, rinocerontes, antílopes, búfalos... La carne de avestruz es muy buena y también comemos algunos insectos. Debería probarlos durante su estancia allí, son realmente sabrosos.

Oliver arqueó las cejas.

—¿Qué clase de insectos?

—Pues hay varios tipos: termitas, saltamontes y gusanos *mopane*. Hay muchos que son excelentes y muy digestivos.

—¡No sé si me atreveré a probarlos! —Oliver se rió entre dientes y arrojó el agua ensangrentada del recipiente por la borda.

—Cuando lleguemos al campamento de Pumulani, le prepararé algunos —insistió Zareb—. Le gustarán, ya lo verá.

—¿Qué es lo que verá? —preguntó Camelia, que apareció en la cubierta seguida de Oscar.

—Zareb está intentando convencer a Oliver de que coma insectos cuando esté en África —le explicó Simon, levantándose de su improvisado asiento de madera al verla acercarse.

Habían pasado dos semanas desde aquella terrible noche en que Camelia empezara a sentirse mal y su recuperación había sido lenta. Simon la había cuidado durante casi cuatro días, que Zareb, Oliver y Elliott habían pasado gimiendo con impotencia en el interior de sus respectivos camarotes. Durante ese tiempo Simon no se había movido de su lado, tratando de animarla para que bebiese agua a sorbos, comiese galletas y pan, y sujetando la palangana cuando su cuerpo rechazaba lo poco que había ingerido.

Jack le había asegurado que era absolutamente normal que la indisposición durase tantos días, pero aun así Simon se había preocupado. Cada vez que había ido a ver a Zareb para llevarle un poco de agua y algunas galletas, éste había insistido en que la maldición era la causante de la enfermedad y en que necesitaba poner más recipientes humeantes en el camarote de Camelia para protegerla. Simon le había asegurado que el lamentable estado de todos ellos no era debido a la maldición, pero no hubo forma de persuadir a Zareb, que le ordenó embadurnar a Camelia con *buchu*, una aromática planta africana, para protegerla y se enfadó muchísimo cuando Simon le dio un no por respuesta.

A los cuatro días lo peor ya había pasado, pero la indisposición dejó huellas en ella. Mientras que los hombres, aparentemente, recobraron las fuerzas en pocos días, Camelia estaba muy débil, envuelta en un cansancio del que no acababa de recuperarse. Las ojeras moradas que tenía debajo de los ojos se negaban a diluirse y su piel había perdido su maravilloso lustre dorado. Todo el rato tenía frío y acabó llevando un chal sobre los hombros incluso cuando brillaba el sol y hacía calor. La ropa bailaba sobre su esbelta silueta y aunque todavía hablaba de la excavación y de lo que tenía planeado para cuando, al fin, llegasen, a Simon le preocupaba que en su estado actual tuviese dificultades para aguantar las exigencias físicas de su trabajo.

—¿Qué tal te encuentras, Tisha? —le preguntó Zareb con las cejas fruncidas.

—Estoy bien, Zareb —contestó Camelia—. Hoy me encuentro mucho mejor.

—Voy a preparar un plato especial para que engorde un poco y le crezca el pelo en el pecho. Bueno, es una forma de hablar. —Oliver le lanzó a Simon una mirada de advertencia.

—¿Qué es?

—Un buen *haggis* picante —le contestó con orgullo—. Acabo de poner el estómago en remojo y esta noche estará relleno, cocinado y listo para comer.

Camelia contempló cautelosa el estómago amarillo del recipiente.

—Creo que no lo he probado nunca.

—Está hecho a base de tráquea y pulmones —advirtió Zareb mirándola con complicidad— mezclados con grasa animal.

—Suena peor de lo que es en realidad —intervino Simon, preguntándose si al ver el estómago de oveja Camelia se marearía—. Pero, si no te apetece, no tienes por qué comerlo.

Oliver miró a Simon perplejo.

—¿Y por qué no iba a querer comerlo? A cualquier mujer que esté acostumbrada a comer insectos y gusanos no puede darle miedo una pequeña bolsa de un buen *haggis* escocés.

—La verdad es que yo nunca he comido ni insectos ni gusanos —confesó Camelia—. Y aunque no dudo de que el *haggis* que cocina es una delicia, Oliver, ahora mismo no tengo mucha hambre.

—Espere a verlo servido en un plato con una buena ración de puré de patatas untado con mantequilla. Creerá que ha muerto e ido directa al cielo.

—Y si no lo estarás deseando —soltó Simon.

Camelia observó el reluciente estómago crudo y tragó saliva intentando reprimir las náuseas que empezaba a sentir.

—¿El estómago también se come o sólo el interior?

—No te preocupes, Camelia. Si no te gusta, Simon, Oliver y yo nos comeremos tu parte en un santiamén —la tranquilizó un Jack sonriente que acababa de aparecer en la cubierta—. Cuando éramos pequeños nos encantaban los *haggis* que preparaba Eunice.

—Sí, y eso que cuando llegaron a casa de la señora estaban en los huesos —comentó Oliver—. Apestaban y estaban muertos de hambre; podría habérselos llevado un soplo de viento. Entonces los alimentamos a base de *haggis*, patatas, guisos y pudines, ¡y ya ve lo fortachones que están!

—Hubiese lo que hubiese para comer, Simon siempre tenía más hambre —explicó Jack, que divertido le lanzó una mirada a su hermano pequeño—. Diez minutos después del desayuno ya quería comer y justo después de comer le preguntaba a Eunice cuánto faltaba para el té. Y cuando merendábamos pactaba con alguno de nosotros para que le diéramos una de nuestras galletas o bollos a cambio de otra cosa.

—Eunice y yo no podíamos creernos que un chico tan menudo pudiese comer tanto, así que llegamos a la conclusión de que se guardaba la comida envuelta en una servilleta para más tarde —añadió Oliver—. Es lo que hacían sus hermanas Annabelle, Grace y Charlotte cuando llegaron a casa; no acababan de creerse que al cabo de sólo unas cuantas horas volverían a ver comida encima de la mesa. Pero cada vez que lo comprobábamos, la servilleta de Simon estaba vacía. Entonces Doreen sospechó que escondía la comida por la casa, pero jamás encontró una mísera miga de pan. Así que no nos quedó más remedio que aceptar que el chico era un pozo sin fondo y que por mucho que lo intentáramos ¡nunca se saciaba! —Oliver se dio unas palmadas en la rodilla y se rió.

Camelia vio que Simon sonreía mientras Oliver y Jack contaban la historia. Iba vestido con su habitual camisa blanca arrugada y sus pantalones oscuros, arremangado con descuido hasta los codos y con el cuello desabrochado. Por alguna razón, su informal atuendo encajaba perfectamente en la soleada cubierta del barco, si bien no se ajustaba a los cánones de la vestimenta apropiada que había que llevar en público. La brisa marina jugueteaba con las ondas cobrizas de su cabello, que en el transcurso del viaje se había aclarado, y lucía un saludable bronceado. Parecía de lo más relajado ahí de pie, rodeado de sus dibujos, del mar, el sol y el aire fresco, mientras su hermano y su viejo amigo bromeaban sobre su juventud.

Los primeros días de viaje había estado preocupada por él, porque se encontraba tan mal que no se había atrevido a salir de su camarote. Pero no sólo se había repuesto totalmente de sus mareos, sino que además estaba más fuerte y tenía más energía que nunca. En Londres, Simon pasaba la mayor parte del tiempo encerrado, pensó Camelia, siempre oculto detrás de montañas de libros y papeles, y docenas de inventos. Cuando trabajaba en algo a menudo perdía la noción del tiempo, en ocasiones durante días, como le había ocurrido cuando ella se coló en su laboratorio. Seguro que hasta que Eunice, Doreen y Oliver se instalaron a vivir con él, más de una vez se había olvidado de comer. Sin embargo, ahora se le veía increíblemente fuerte, guapo y relajado.

—Te sienta bien tomar el aire —le dijo mientras se acercaba a él.

—Me sienta bien desde que el mar se ha calmado. —Simon apartó a un lado los dibujos y señaló la tabla de madera—. ¿Te apetece sentarte?

—Gracias. —Al sentarse, ella se ajustó el chal sobre los hombros y contempló la infinita extensión de mar espumoso—. Es bonito, ¿verdad?

Sin dejar de mirar a Camelia, Simon contestó:

—Sí.

—Creo que nos estamos acercando a la costa —observó Camelia, levantando la cara para recibir los agradables rayos del sol.

—¿Cómo lo sabes?

—Lo presiento. Sé que no suena muy científico, pero lo cierto es que no tengo otra explicación.

—Muchos descubrimientos científicos empiezan con un simple presentimiento —le aseguró Simon—. A veces la intuición es lo único en lo que podemos confiar. ¿Y qué sientes?

Ella cerró los ojos, embriagándose del sedante calor del sol, del aroma del océano y de la extraordinaria sensación que le producía el suave vaivén del barco, que la acercaba más y más a su hogar.

—Tengo más calor —contestó, disfrutando de los cálidos rayos del sol—, y el aire es más dulce, no sé, no es tan salado como en alta mar. Pero sobre todo lo que siento es que mi corazón late más despacio. En África me siento más calmada que en ninguna otra parte. Es como si cuando por fin estoy en casa, no pudiese pasarme nada malo. —Abrió los ojos y su mirada encontró la de Simon.

—Todavía sopla un viento oscuro, Tisha —intervino Zareb con solemnidad—. Créeme.

—Siempre sopla un viento oscuro. —Camelia se envolvió mejor con el chal y miró fijamente al horizonte—. Si sigue ahí cuando lleguemos a Pumulani, le haré frente, Zareb, como siempre he hecho.

—Tal vez en esta ocasión sea diferente, Camelia —dijo Elliott, haciendo acto de presencia.

A diferencia de Simon, Elliott se había propuesto vestir con elegancia en todo momento durante el viaje. Esa mañana había elegido unos impecables pantalones grises oscuros, un chaleco a rayas amarillas y de color crema y un magnífico abrigo marengo hecho a medida. Como era propio de todo caballero, también llevaba unos guantes blancos y un sombrero de fieltro.

—Con la cantidad de accidentes que se han producido en la excavación —continuó—, es posible que al llegar nos encontremos que todos los nativos se han marchado.

—Muchos hombres se han quedado porque querían y respetaban a mi padre, Elliott —señaló Camelia—. No se asustarán fácilmente.

—No, pero si sigue habiendo accidentes...

—Si se producen más accidentes y se marchan todos, seguiré excavando yo sola —insistió ella con obstinación—. Ya sabes que mi padre siempre decía que no se puede descubrir nada a menos que uno ponga el corazón en lo que hace, Elliott. Y mi corazón está en Pumulani.

—Un corazón valiente puede con lo que le echen —dijo Oliver reflexivo y con aprobación—. Puede que yo esté viejo, pero si me necesita, aún puedo coger una pala y excavar.

—Gracias, Oliver. —Camelia le sonrió cariñosamente—. Aunque no creo que lleguemos a ese extremo. No a todos los trabajadores les asusta la idea de una maldición.

—¿Por qué no le hace a cada trabajador uno de sus amuletos especiales? —le preguntó Oliver a Zareb—. Los que nos dio al chico a mí nos han ido de maravilla.

—A mí no me pareció que el mío funcionara cuando estaba enfermo —recalcó Simon.

Oliver frunció las cejas.

—No te has muerto, ¿verdad?

—No.

—Entonces, ¿de qué te quejas?

—Habría preferido no ponerme enfermo.

—Pues haberte quedado en casa —le dijo Jack divertido—. El que viaja en barco se marea, Simon, al menos hasta que se acostumbra.

—No todos los trabajadores pertenecen a los pueblos khoikhoi; son de muchas tribus distintas —le aclaró Zareb a Oliver—. Tienen sus propios métodos para luchar contra los malos espíritus y prefieren hacerse sus propios amuletos.

Oliver se rascó la cabeza.

—Sí, supongo que es lógico. En Escocia hay por lo menos doce formas distintas de combatir la brujería.

—¡Mirad! —Camelia corrió emocionada hasta la barandilla; su corazón latía con fuerza—. ¡Tierra!

—¿Está segura, joven? —Oliver aguzó la vista hacia el horizonte—. Yo no veo nada.

—Sí, estoy segura —insistió Camelia, señalando—. No se ve muy bien, pero donde termina el océano hay una delgada franja de tierra gris. ¡Estoy segura de que es tierra! —Se volvió y miró a Jack con expresión casi suplicante—. ¿Verdad que sí?

Jack sonrió.

—Así es. Estamos acercándonos a la costa. Según mis cálculos dentro de unas horas deberíamos atracar en Ciudad del Cabo, eso siempre y cuando el mar esté tranquilo y el viento estable.

Simon observó fascinado la alegre sonrisa que iluminó el rostro de Camelia. Con un nudo en la garganta, miró de nuevo hacia la apenas visible franja de tierra. El chal con el que se había envuelto durante las últimas dos semanas se deslizó por sus hombros al inclinarse hacia el viento en un intento por estar más cerca de la imperceptible costa esmeralda. Sintió la imperiosa necesidad de estar junto a ella, de abrazar su dulce silueta y notar el estremecimiento de su cuerpo contra el suyo, de sentir la presión de sus deliciosas curvas mientras permanecían los dos de pie contemplando cómo los rayos del sol cubrían las cálidas olas turquesas de África con miles de puntos centelleantes. De forma repentina e inesperada, el deseo se apoderó de él, calentando su sangre y tensando sus extremidades hasta que no pudo pensar en otra cosa salvo en el exquisito recuerdo de embestir a Camelia, embriagado con la fragancia que olía a verano y a flores silvestres mientras la abrazaba con fuerza y, poco a poco, la hacía suya.

Respiró hondo tratando de recuperar el control.

¿Qué demonios le ocurría?

—¿Unas horas? —Oliver miró a Jack exasperado—. ¿Y qué pasa con mi *haggis*?

—Tranquilo, Oliver. Cuando lleguemos a Ciudad del Cabo, iré a comprar los billetes para ir a Kimberley y el primer tren no saldrá por lo menos hasta mañana por la mañana —le dijo Camelia al constatar su decepción—. Habrá tiempo más que suficiente para acabar de preparar el *haggis* y comerlo.

—De acuerdo. —Visiblemente aliviado, dio unas suaves palmadas sobre el viscoso estómago en remojo y concluyó animado—: Porque sería un crimen desperdiciar unas deliciosas asaduras de oveja.

—¡Dios! ¿Por qué no me matas y acabamos con esto? —gimió Bert, asomado a la barandilla del *Sea Star*.

—Dice el capitán que te sentirás mejor dentro de un par de días, Bert —le dijo Stanley alegremente.

—Dentro de una hora estaré fiambre como un arenque —repuso Bert, agarrándose como podía a la barandilla—. ¡Joder! Preferiría que Dios me llevara consigo de una vez.

—No hables así, Bert. —Stanley pegó un mordisco de la enorme lengua adobada que tenía en la mano antes de añadir—: No creo que a Dios le guste.

—¿Y a quién coño le importa lo que le guste a Dios? —inquirió Bert malhumorado—. Si quiere que me muera, que lo haga ya de una vez. ¡Maldito inútil! ¿Me has entendido? —gruñó.

—Estás enfadado porque llevas mucho rato con dolor de barriga —contestó Stanley compasivamente.

—Me estoy muriendo —insistió Bert—. No llegaré a África. Tendrás que tirarme por la borda y los malditos peces me devorarán.

—Quizá si comieras algo, te encontrarías un poco mejor. ¿Quieres probar esta lengua en adobo? —le preguntó, poniéndole delante de la cara la tira gris de carne avinagrada.

—Aparta eso, ¡pedazo de inútil! —le espetó Bert, que golpeó a Stanley en la mano—. ¿Quieres matarme o qué?

—Lo siento, Bert. —Avergonzado, Stanley bajó los ojos y los clavó en sus gastadas botas—. No quería hacerte enfadar.

Bert notó una punzada de culpabilidad, lo que le hizo sentir aún más desdichado. Odiaba cuando Stanley se ponía así, con sus enormes hombros inclinados hacia delante y la barbilla entrecana gacha hacia el maldito pecho. Stanley no tenía la culpa de que Dios hubiese decidido darle al pobre mentecato un cerebro de bebé. Si, finalmente, la palmaba y se iba al cielo, tendría unas palabras con Dios al respecto. ¿Para qué quería tanto poder si no podía arreglarle el cerebro a Stanley para que el pobre mentecato pudiese al menos valerse por sí mismo?

—No te preocupes, Stanley —lo tranquilizó Bert—. Es que estoy un poco harto de estar mareado, eso es todo.

Stanley levantó la cabeza con cautela.

—¿No estás enfadado conmigo?

—No, no estoy enfadado contigo. —Suspiró—. Estoy cansado de encontrarme mal, nada más.

—Cuando lleguemos a África te encontrarás mejor. Lo que necesitas es pisar tierra firme.

—Pero queda por lo menos una semana para que lleguemos a África —observó Bert con pesar—. Y una vez hayamos llegado, tendremos que ir al sitio ése que el viejo chocho nos ha dicho que vayamos; a Poomoolanee. Seguramente estará en medio de la maldita jungla, donde las moscas serán del tamaño de los murciélagos y habrá animales salvajes escondidos detrás de los árboles. Si Dios quiere que siga con vida sólo para que algún tigre me devore, prefiero que me mate ahora y así acabar de una vez con esto.

Stanley se puso pálido.

—¿En serio son las moscas tan grandes como los murciélagos?

—No creo que todas —concedió Bert. No serviría de nada asustar a Stanley. Ya había sido bastante difícil convencer a su amigo de que se subiese al barco. ¡Qué injusto era que después de haberle suplicado, discutido y ordenado que embarcase, Stanley pareciese estar disfrutando del viaje mientras él sufría tantísimo! Debía de ser otra jodida broma de Dios, pensó con acritud. Toda su vida había sido así.

—Seguro que no será tan terrible; de lo contrario, lady Camelia no viajaría hasta allí —añadió—. Al fin y al cabo, es una mujer.

—Sí, supongo que tienes razón, Bert —afirmó Stanley, que pegó un gran mordisco a la lengua adobada—. Aunque a mí me da que no es como la mayoría de las mujeres.

—¿Y tú cómo lo sabes, si las únicas mujeres que has visto son las putas y las rameras del barrio obrero de Seven Dials?

—He conocido a más mujeres —insistió Stanley—. A veces voy a Mayfair y las veo pasear con sus parejas o subidas en sus elegantes carruajes. Parecen muñecas; da la impresión de que si las coges demasiado fuerte se van a romper. Pero ninguna es como lady Camelia; ésa los tiene bien puestos y, además, es muy lista.

—Si fuese lista, se habría quedado en Londres, que es lo que tendría que haber hecho en lugar de obligarnos a perseguirla por el maldito océano —comentó Bert con amargura—. Ahora estaríamos bien situados, viviendo en un bonito pisito de Cheapside, comiendo cada día un bistec y pudín de riñones con ginebra, y durmiendo en una cama con sábanas limpias por las noches.

—Todo llegará, Bert, ya lo verás. Aún falta un poco, pero llegará.

—Si aquel jodido capitán hubiese accedido a llevarnos en su barco, a estas alturas estaríamos a punto de llegar. Cuanto antes lleguemos antes liquidaremos el trabajo y podremos volver a casa.

—Tranquilo, Bert. El dandi ése dijo que si llegábamos unos cuantos días después que ella, no pasaba nada; que de ahí no se movería.

—Ese bribón debería habernos pagado lo que hemos hecho en lugar de hacernos viajar hasta la maldita África —repuso Bert malhumorado—. Hemos hecho todo lo que nos dijo que hiciéramos y aun así ella no se amilanó. ¿Cómo íbamos a saber que no se asustaría después de ver su casa destrozada?

—A eso me refería cuando he dicho que no es como el resto de las mujeres —dijo Stanley sonriendo—. Es muy valiente.

—Cuando lleguemos a la maldita excavación de Poomoo-lanee, se arrepentirá de no haberse quedado en Londres. —La expresión de Bert se ensombreció antes de que concluyera—: No le quedará mucho valor cuando hayamos acabado con ella, te lo prometo.

TERCERA PARTE

El resplandor de las llamas

Capítulo 10

Simon se apeó del tren con Oscar felizmente sentado en su hombro y miró a su alrededor con asombro.

—¿Cómo es posible que haya electricidad aquí, en medio de la nada —inquirió mientras señalaba el cableado que se extendía entre las farolas y las casas—, si ni siquiera había en Ciudad del Cabo?

—Kimberley ha crecido gracias a las minas de diamantes —le explicó Camelia, colocando la jaula de Harriet encima de sus baúles—. Hace quince años aquí no había más que tierra y toscas cabañas. Entonces, de la noche a la mañana, algunas personas empezaron a enriquecerse y quisieron que se construyesen casas en condiciones y tiendas con luz eléctrica.

—Ése ha sido uno de los aspectos positivos de las minas —señaló Elliott—. Ha convertido una tierra desolada y deshabitada en una ciudad moderna y productiva.

—Aquí vivía gente, Elliott.

—Unas cuantas familias de boers y un puñado de tribus nómadas medio muertas de hambre. Si no se llegan a descubrir los diamantes, nadie habría conocido ni se habría preocupado por esta parte de África, excepto tu padre, claro —se apresuró a añadir al ver el habitual destello de irritación en los ojos de Camelia.

—Y los nativos que vivían aquí.

Elliott soltó un suspiro. ¿Desde cuándo Camelia y él discutían por absolutamente todo?, se preguntó cansado. Al parecer, y pese a sus tremendos esfuerzos por mostrarle su apoyo, estaban casi todo el rato en desacuerdo. Ella siempre había tenido su propia opinión respecto a todo y nunca eludía el debate. Su naturaleza apasionada era parte de lo que al principio le había hecho a Elliott sentirse atraído por ella; sin embargo, después, le hubiese gustado que empezara a ver las cosas de otra manera.

Su vida habría sido infinitamente más fácil si Camelia se hubiese desencantado de Pumulani a la vez que él.

—Sea como sea, los diamantes harán que Suráfrica sea un país rico —insistió Elliott, consciente de que ella rebatiría ese punto.

—No, los que se enriquecerán serán los blancos que envían a otros hombres bajo tierra —le corrigió Zareb—. Los africanos que se arrastran en la oscuridad para encontrar los diamantes se quedarán con las migajas.

—Pero eso no es justo —observó Oliver, encargado de llevar el cesto en cuyo interior estaba Rupert—. ¿Por qué los nativos no delimitan un trozo de su tierra y buscan sus propios diamantes?

—Porque no les dejan —contestó Camelia—. Al principio, algunos nativos reclamaron sus derechos, hubo reclamaciones de los griquas, los coloreds del Cabo, una tribu mestiza seminómada, pero a los propietarios europeos eso no les hizo gracia y al cabo de unos años se aprobó una ley que prohibía a los nativos y hombres de color obtener licencias para excavar.

—O sea, que los nativos solamente pueden trabajar para los blancos sin la posibilidad de beneficiarse de lo que encuentren en su propia tierra. —Simon sacudió la cabeza asombrado por lo injusto del tema—. No me extraña que les parezca injusto.

—Cobran por su trabajo —objetó Elliott—. La mayoría proceden de tribus que se mueren de hambre y para ellos trabajar en las minas es un regalo del cielo, porque cuando vuelven con su gente tienen dinero para comprar rifles de caza, munición, arados y hacer una oferta a otra familia para concertar una boda. Las minas les han dado la oportunidad de ser independientes económicamente. Ahora tienen dinero para adquirir cosas, mientras que antes sólo podían intercambiar pieles de animales y unas cuantas armas primitivas.

—Las pieles de animales abrigan y nos protegen del sol, y las armas nos pueden salvar la vida —señaló Zareb con tranquilidad—. Son cosas útiles para quien las lleva. En cambio, las monedas carecen de valor hasta que se intercambian por otra cosa; y los africanos reciben muy pocas monedas.

—Debes de estar cansada, Camelia —comentó Elliott, cambiando de tema—. Tendríamos que ir al hotel y pedir unas cuantas habitaciones para pasar la noche.

Camelia cabeceó.

—No quiero pasar la noche aquí. Si nadie tiene inconveniente, me gustaría continuar hasta Pumulani.

Elliott la miró con incredulidad.

—Son más de las siete de la tarde y nos hemos pasado el día entero metidos en ese tren sofocante. Seguro que estarán todos exhaustos. Lo mejor sería dormir aquí y que mañana por la mañana fuéramos a la excavación.

Camelia se dio cuenta de que Elliott tenía razón, pero por algún motivo no podía soportar la idea de permanecer allí. Odiaba Kimberley. Tal vez a Simon y a Oliver les pareciese una ciudad razonablemente próspera, con luz eléctrica y un hotel decente (ambos rasgos bienvenidos después de estar casi tres semanas en un barco y doce horas dentro de un tren), pero Kimberley había sido construida con el sudor y la sangre de los nativos que trabajaban como esclavos en las minas. Para Camelia era otro eslabón de la larga cadena con que se había atado a los africanos. Además, como debido a la excesiva oferta, el mercado de diamantes había caído en picado arrastrando consigo a las fortunas recientes, en los últimos tiempos se habían suicidado varios inversores blancos. La desesperación y la avaricia habían vuelto el aire irrespirable.

No podría soportar estar ahí un segundo más de lo necesario.

Simon estudió a Camelia atentamente. La fatiga se reflejaba en su rostro, pero percibió su absoluta renuencia a pasar la noche en Kimberley. A pesar de que la idea de tomar un baño caliente y dormir en una cama de verdad le resultaba de lo más tentador, apoyaría a Camelia.

—¿A qué distancia estamos de Pumulani? —quiso saber.

Ella lo miró esperanzada.

—Sólo a unas dos horas.

—O menos —añadió Zareb—. Por la noche el aire es más fresco. Los caballos podrán ir más deprisa sin tener que parar tanto.

Elliott sacudió la cabeza.

—No me gusta la idea de viajar sin luz.

—Pero no oscurecerá por lo menos hasta dentro de una hora —observó Zareb.

—¿Y qué pasará después?

—Conozco el camino, lord Wickham —le aseguró Zareb con tranquilidad—. No necesito luz para llegar a Pumulani.

Las estrellas me guiarán. Si lady Camelia quiere que vayamos ahora, yo la llevaré. Usted puede ir con el señor Kent y con Oliver por la mañana.

Simon se encogió de hombros.

—A mí me apetece ir esta noche. ¿Y a ti, Oliver?

—No sé si será por lo cálido que es el aire africano —respondió Oliver alegremente, entrelazando sus deformadas manos—, pero yo estoy más despierto que nunca.

—De acuerdo, pues. Nosotros iremos con Camelia y usted, Wickham, puede venir mañana a lo largo del día, después de descansar, que seguro que lo necesitará, ¿le parece bien?

—Si todos quieren continuar el viaje, iré con ustedes. —Se negaba a dejar que pareciese que Kent tenía más aguante que él—. Además, necesitarán mi protección, a menos, por supuesto, que Kent sepa cómo disparar un rifle —añadió enarcando las cejas.

—Pues no, Wickham, no he disparado un rifle en toda mi vida —reconoció Simon sin problemas—. Pero estoy convencido de que, en caso de necesidad, sabría desenvolverme. Creo que sólo hay que apuntar hacia donde uno quiere y luego disparar el gatillo ¿no?

—Me temo que es un poco más complicado que eso...

—Yo te enseñaré —se ofreció Camelia.

Elliott hizo una mueca de disgusto. Incitar a Camelia a que pasase tiempo con Simon para enseñarle a disparar no había sido precisamente su intención.

Oliver frunció sus blancas cejas.

—¿Cómo es posible que una preciosa joven como usted sepa cómo disparar un rifle?

—En África es necesario saber manejar un arma —contestó Camelia—. Mi padre me enseñó a disparar a los quince años.

Oliver se rascó la cabeza, pensativo.

—¿Y de qué hay que protegerse?

—La zona que atravesaremos está plagada de animales salvajes —explicó Elliott— que siempre están hambrientos.

—¿Eso es todo? —se burló Oliver—. Entonces no hará falta que se preocupe por mí, joven. Puedo lanzar un puñal con la rapidez y la precisión de una bala.

—¿Y qué me dice de usted, Kent? ¿Sabe lanzar un puñal? Simon le rascó la cabeza a Oscar.

—Sabré hacerlo en caso de necesidad.

—Simon puede darle a un árbol desde una distancia de veinte pasos —comentó Oliver con orgullo—. Yo mismo le enseñé cuando no era más que un crío, ¡y se aficionó como las pulgas a los perros!

—Estupendo, será útil, si nos vemos amenazados por un árbol —replicó Elliott con frialdad.

—Muy bien, todo arreglado. —Ahora que la decisión estaba tomada, Camelia estaba ansiosa por proseguir el viaje—. Zareb, ¿te importaría ir a las caballerizas a buscar nuestro carro y nuestras armas, y cargar todas las cosas mientras yo me acerco a la tienda y compro algunas provisiones?

—Por supuesto que no, Tisha —dijo Zareb con una inclinación de cabeza—. Ahora mismo voy.

—Yo iré contigo, Camelia, así te ayudaré —se ofreció Simon.

—Y Rupert, Harriet y yo nos quedaremos aquí vigilando el equipaje hasta que Zareb traiga el carro. —Oliver se sentó lentamente en una enorme maleta frente a la pequeña montaña de baúles y el motor de vapor envuelto en lona que habían sido descargados sobre el andén del tren—. Si quieres, deja también a Oscar con nosotros.

Oscar sacudió la cabeza y se abrazó con fuerza al cuello de Simon.

—Creo que Oscar quiere estar conmigo —repuso Simon intentando que el mono le soltara—. ¿Qué hace usted, Wickham?

—Voy a ver si me compro un caballo —contestó Elliott—. El carro irá muy cargado y prefiero viajar por mi cuenta.

—Buena idea. —Camelia sabía que a Elliott no le gustaba viajar en carro. Además, con el espacio que ocuparían el equipaje, las provisiones y la preciada bomba de Simon, sería mejor que fuese a caballo—. Nos veremos aquí dentro de una hora para cargar el carro y salir hacia Pumulani.

Todo saldría bien.

En eso trataba de pensar mientras viajaba apoyada en el duro saco de trigo molido que usaba a modo de silla improvisada. El carro no tenía más que un banco para el conductor y un pasajero, que ocupaban Zareb y Oliver; Elliott se había comprado una preciosa montura negra en las caballerizas. Por desgracia, el animal tenía tanta energía como fuerza tenía el pobre Elliott, que se pasó gran parte del trayecto galopando de un lado a otro para intentar controlar al imparable caballo. Camelia dudaba que Elliott tuviese tiempo suficiente para llegar a una entente con el animal antes de que, al fin, él se cansase de Pumulani y decidiese regresar.

A pesar de su insistencia para acompañarla a África, Camelia sabía que, en realidad, Elliott no quería estar ahí. Había venido únicamente por ella. Y a ella le había conmovido sobremanera que él hubiese renunciado a las numerosas obligaciones que tenía en Londres para volver con ella a Pumulani. Durante años Elliott la había cuidado como un hermano mayor, haciéndole pequeños regalos, intentando hacerla sonreír, escuchándola cuando ella había necesitado hablar con alguien que no fuese su padre o Zareb. Camelia había crecido queriendo a Elliott por su carácter serio, paciente y pragmático, quizá porque era completamente opuesto al suyo. Cuando a la muerte de su padre, él le había anunciado que dejaba la arqueología para embarcarse en un negocio de exportación en Inglaterra, ella se había sentido decepcionada, aunque no la cogió del todo por sorpresa. Elliott era inteligente y ambicioso; tenía derecho a perseguir un objetivo en el que creyese que tenía mayores posibilidades de éxito. Fue al intentar convencerla con ahínco de que vendiera el terreno heredado de su padre y se marchase con él a Inglaterra cuando se dio cuenta de que apenas la comprendía. Su padre había soñado toda su vida con el descubrimiento de la Tumba de los Reyes.

Y Camelia estaba decidida a hacer ese sueño realidad, no sólo por el amor que sentía hacia su padre, sino por su amor por África y su gente. Conmemorando el pasado, Camelia tenía la esperanza de ayudar al mundo a entender la riqueza de la historia y la cultura africanas. Tal vez entonces su gente recuperaría parte de la dignidad que otros tanto se esforzaban por arruinar.

—Ahora lo siento.

Camelia miró a Simon confusa. Estaba en el fondo del carro apoyado en un enorme cesto de boniatos, con los pies tranquilamente colocados encima de un saco de arroz y los brazos cruzados sobre el pecho. Parecía de lo más cómodo, a pesar del traqueteo del carro y de que el cesto en el que se apoyaba se le estaba clavando en la espalda. Por lo visto Simon estaba dotado de una capacidad única para adaptarse al entorno, incluso cuando éste estaba lejos de ser hospitalario.

Camelia se preguntó si también habría gozado de esa habilidad en la cárcel o si la habría desarrollado a raíz de su estancia en prisión.

—¿El qué? —inquirió ella.

—Lo que intentaste describirme aquella noche que nos encontramos en mi estudio. —La miró con sus penetrantes ojos azules mientras añadía en voz baja y ligeramente burlona—: Te acuerdas de aquella noche, ¿verdad, Camelia?

Una oleada de excitación recorrió su cuerpo. Por supuesto que se acordaba de aquella noche. Recordaba cada detalle de la misma como si hubiese sucedido hacía un instante, y eso a pesar de las numerosas noches que se había pasado en vela tratando de extirpar el recuerdo de su mente. Había sido un momento de locura, dijo para sí, convencida de que si pensaba en esos términos, nunca más volvería a ocurrir. Pero, al parecer, su cuerpo no entendía la decisión de su mente, especialmente ahora que se había recuperado de sus mareos. Un dulce calor inundó su cuerpo mientras Simon seguía mirándola con fijeza, haciendo que su sangre se alborotara y el deseo se asomara a su piel en forma de cosquilleo.

—Sí, me acuerdo. —Se concentró en alisar las irremediables arrugas de su falda para intentar fingir cierta formalidad—. Intenté describirte cómo es Suráfrica.

—Exacto. —Las comisuras de sus labios se elevaron levemente. Simon encontraba una arrogante satisfacción en el efecto que el recuerdo obraba en ella—. Me hablaste de la sensación que produce la brisa contra la piel, de las impresionantes montañas negras y la brillante luna nacarada. Pensé que había sentido todo esto a través de tus palabras, pero me equivoqué. —Simon observó cómo el rubor coralino de sus mejillas y su cuello descendía hasta la piel pálida de sus clavículas antes de concluir con un susurro—: Lo cierto es que es uno de los lugares más paradisíacos de la Tierra.

Una bala cruzó el aire justo encima de su cabeza.

—¡*Al suelo*! —gritó Simon al tiempo que se lanzaba sobre ella.

Otro disparo sacudió la penumbra que les rodeaba, y luego otro más. Oscar chilló, bajó de un salto del hombro de Zareb y se escondió debajo de la lona que cubría la bomba de Simon.

—¡Simon, déjame moverme! —ordenó Camelia forcejeando—. ¡Necesito coger mi rifle!

—Pero ¿qué pasa aquí? —preguntó Oliver contrariado mientras sacaba el puñal que llevaba en la bota—. ¡En nombre de San Columbano! ¿Por qué nos disparan?

—¡Agáchense! —Elliott detuvo el caballo junto al carro y apuntó su rifle hacia la oscuridad.

—No dispare, lord Wickham. —Zareb no se había movido de su sitio—. Las balas no van dirigidas a nosotros.

—¿Cómo que no van dirigidas a nosotros? ¿A quién demonios van dirigidas entonces?

—A nosotros, no —repitió Zareb, insistente—. Pero si mata a alguien, entonces sí que nos dispararán.

—¡No creerá que voy a quedarme aquí sentado mientras me disparan...!

—Escuche. —Oliver frunció las cejas y aguzó el oído—. Los diparos han cesado.

Zareb asintió.

—Sí. Sólo querían advertirnos de que estaban aquí. Todo está en orden.

—Ya no hace falta que me protejas, Simon. —Camelia lo empujó, aturdida por la manera en que su cuerpo ansioso se había fundido con su musculosa silueta—. Zareb ha dicho que está todo en orden.

—Lo lamento, pero no acabo de entender cómo puede estar todo en orden cuando han estado a punto de matarnos —musitó Simon con frialdad y sin apartarse de Camelia—. ¿Cómo sabe Zareb que no se están acercando para tener mejor puntería?

—Porque lo sabe. Si Zareb dice que todo está bien, es que lo está.

—¿Cómo puedes estar tan segura?

—Porque Zareb siempre peca de un exceso de proteccionismo —contestó Camelia—. Si dice que estamos a salvo, yo le creo.

Simon la miró con escepticismo y continuó cubriéndola con su cuerpo.

—Soy Zareb, hijo de Waitimu —anunció Zareb con solemnidad poniéndose de pie—. Me dirijo a Pumulani con unos amigos. Venimos en son de paz.

Reinó un breve silencio sepulcral.

—¡Bienvenido a casa, Zareb! —exclamó de pronto una voz llena de entusiasmo—. ¡La espera ha sido larga!

Simon echó un vistazo por el lateral del carro y vio que dos nativos negros emergían de la oscuridad y ahora eran iluminados por la luz de la luna. Iban tapados sólo con pieles de leopardo y de antílope, y plumas soberbias de grulla y de avestruz ondeaban en sus hombros y cinturas. Sus pulseras de marfil contrastaban con sus negros y musculosos brazos, y gruesos collares de cuentas hechos de huesos y cáscaras relucían sobre sus pechos. Cada uno de ellos llevaba un imponente puñal enfundado en la pantorrilla y un enorme rifle cruzado sobre el pecho.

—Badrani, Senwe, me alegro de volveros a ver. —Zareb sonrió mientras bajaba del carro—. He traído a lady Camelia de vuelta, como os prometí. —Miró en dirección a Camelia, que seguía forcejeando para liberarse del abrazo protector de Simon—. Ya puede soltarla, señor Kent. No hay ningún peligro.

—Gracias por haber protegido Pumulani tan bien, Badrani y Senwe —dijo Camelia, que se puso de pie en el carro—. Me alegro de verlos.

—Bienvenida a casa, lady Camelia. —Badrani inclinó la cabeza respetuosamente. Era un guapo joven que debía de rozar la treintena, alto y fuerte, con una angulosa mandíbula que indicaba determinación—. Y usted también, lord Wickham —añadió al reconocer a Elliott.

—Estamos encantados de tenerla otra vez entre nosotros, lady Camelia. —Senwe era más joven y más bajo que Badrani, pero los musculosos contornos de su pecho y brazos dejaban entrever que no era menos fuerte—. Teníamos miedo de que no volviera.

—Nada hubiese podido evitar mi regreso a Pumulani —les aseguró Camelia—. Nos acompaña un poderoso profesor que puede ayudarnos a solucionar todos los problemas que hemos tenido. Les presento al señor Kent. —Señaló a Simon, que se puso de pie con Oscar agarrado a su hombro.

Badrani y Senwe lo miraron fijamente con los ojos muy abiertos.

—Es un placer conocerlos. —Simon se preguntó por qué parecían tan atónitos. Decidió que lo de «poderoso profesor» les había desconcertado.

—¡Su pelo es del color del fuego! —Badrani se volvió a Zareb asombrado—. ¿Tiene poderes especiales?

—Sí —afirmó Zareb con solemnidad—. Poderes buenos.

—No exactamente. —Simon no quería que los nativos pensasen que tenía poderes especiales sólo porque era pelirrojo.

La expresión de Senwe enseguida se ensombreció.

—¿No son buenos sus poderes? —preguntó apuntando a Simon con el rifle.

—No, quiero decir, sí, bueno, he venido a ayudarles, pero no tengo ningún poder especial —se apresuró a aclarar Simon. Nervioso, Oscar saltó de sus brazos para irse con Zareb—. Soy inventor.

Los dos nativos lo miraron estupefactos.

—El señor Kent ha venido para combatir la maldición —explicó Zareb—. Traerá otra vez la buena suerte a Pumulani.

—Lo intentaré —matizó Simon, deseoso de controlar sus expectativas.

—Si Zareb lo dice, así será. —Senwe seguía mirando con incredulidad el cabello de Simon.

—Y éste es Oliver —continuó Zareb—. Viene de un país lejano llamado Escocia y es un buen amigo.

—Encantado de conocerlos, jóvenes. —Al constatar, aliviado, que los nativos de extraño aspecto no iban a disparar a Simon, Oliver bajó el puñal—. ¿Han oído hablar de Escocia?

Senwe y Badrani sacudieron sus cabezas.

—Es un lugar maravilloso, aunque no hace tanto calor como aquí, en África. Les invito a venir a verlo cuando quieran.

—Gracias. —Badrani inclinó la cabeza con solemnidad para agradecer la invitación—. Los acompañaremos hasta Pumulani. Los hombres estarán encantados de que, al fin, lady Camelia haya vuelto. Tenían miedo de que el viento oscuro se la hubiese llevado para siempre.

—¿A cuánto estamos de Pumulani? —inquirió Simon.

—Está justo al pie de esa montaña. —Badrani señaló la puntiaguda cima hacia la que se habían dirigido desde que salieran de Kimberley—. Si se fija bien, verá el resplandor de las hogueras. Las llamas sirven para ahuyentar los espíritus malignos.

Camelia miró fijamente el suave fulgor naranja que había al pie de la montaña.

—Ya casi hemos llegado. —La excitación floreció en su interior y se sintió mejor de lo que se había sentido desde hacía meses.

Casi había llegado a casa.

—La conduciremos hasta ahí, lady Camelia —anunció Senwe—. Pero tenga cuidado; los espíritus están muy enfadados desde que se marchó. ¿Lleva el rifle encima?

—Sí. —Se agachó y cogió el arma, que estaba en un extremo del carro—. Pero a partir de ahora todo irá bien, Senwe. —Nada podía empañar la emoción que sentía al volver, finalmente, a la excavación—. Ya lo verá.

—Aun así, tenga cuidado —insistió Badrani—. Vayan todos con cuidado.

Camelia asintió, agradecida por su preocupación.

—Gracias, lo tendremos en cuenta.

Se sentó de nuevo en el saco y clavó los ojos en las espirales azafranadas que relucían en el pie de la montaña, sintiéndose cada vez más fuerte y llena a medida que se aproximaban lentamente a las refulgentes hogueras de Pumulani.

Capítulo 11

—¡Lady Camelia ha vuelto! —anunció Senwe contento al llegar al silencioso campamento.

Los gritos de alegría inundaron la noche tranquila. Entusiasmados, los nativos empezaron a salir de sus tiendas dispuestas alrededor del campamento, sonriendo y agitando sus brazos en señal de bienvenida. La mayoría iban vestidos con pieles de animales, plumas y cuentas, pero Simon se fijó en que algunos también llevaban pantalones gastados, un abrigo raído o un chaleco. Se agolparon alrededor del carro, chillando y cantando emocionados. Simon se puso de pie, le ofreció la mano a Camelia y le ayudó a apearse del carro.

Entonces los nativos soltaron un grito de sorpresa al que siguió el silencio.

—Éste es el señor Kent, un poderoso profesor que ha venido desde Inglaterra —declaró Camelia, señalando a Simon—. Nos ayudará a combatir las fuerzas que tanto nos han dificultado la excavación en Pumulani.

—¿Es necesario que uses la palabra poderoso? —susurró Simon, que dedicó una tensa sonrisa a los cautelosos nativos—. No sé si sirve de mucho.

—Es preciso que confíen en ti, y tu pelo les pone nerviosos.

—¡Su cabello es como el fuego! —exclamó uno de los hombres, señalando temeroso a Simon.

—¿Entiendes a qué me refiero? —Camelia sonrió y cogió a Simon de la mano en un intento por demostrar que era inofensivo—. Nunca habían visto algo parecido.

—¡Genial! De habérmelo dicho, habría hecho algo al respecto.

—¿Cómo qué?

—Me habría afeitado la cabeza.

—No creo que estar completamente calvo debajo del sol africano hubiese sido muy práctico. Además, el vello de los brazos, las piernas y el pecho seguiría siendo pelirrojo...

—Me halaga que te acuerdes.

—Y dudo que hubieses estado dispuesto a afeitarte el cuerpo entero —concluyó Camelia inquieta, reprimiendo el impulso de soltarle la mano—, porque cuando vuelve a crecer pica bastante.

—Tu preocupación es conmovedora.

—El cabello del señor Kent es sólo un indicio de su gran poder —anunció Zareb con solemnidad, de pie frente a la multitud—. En su interior arde un fuego abrasador y puro, que devolverá a los espíritus malignos de Pumulani al lugar donde pertenecen.

—¡Oh, por el amor de Dios! ¡No es más que pelo! —Cansado y molesto por la atención centrada alrededor de Simon, Elliott bajó de un salto de su anárquico caballo—. ¿Dónde demonios está Trafford?

—¡Estoy aquí, lord Wickham! —Un robusto hombretón emergió de una de las tiendas, abrochándose con torpeza los botones de su abrigo lleno de manchas mientras avanzaba entre la multitud de trabajadores.

—¡Bienvenida a casa, lady Camelia! —exclamó pasándose rápidamente los dedos por su rizado cabello entrecano. A juzgar por su curtida piel y su arrugado rostro, que indicaban una vida llena de aventuras y desafíos, Simon dedujo que tendría unos cuarenta y cinco años—. Me alegra que por fin haya vuelto. Los hombres la han echado mucho de menos, servidor incluido.

—Gracias, señor Trafford. —Camelia le dedicó una cálida sonrisa y bajó del carro—. Simon, éste es Lloyd Trafford, el capataz de la excavación. Señor Trafford, le presento a Simon Kent, el afamado inventor, y a su fiel socio y amigo, Oliver. El señor Kent nos ha construido una bomba de vapor que utilizaremos para poder extraer toda el agua de la excavación y Oliver ha venido a ayudarnos.

—Encantado de conocerlos a los dos —dijo Lloyd, dándoles la mano—. Esperábamos ansiosos su llegada.

—¿En serio? Bueno, en ese caso nos aseguraremos de no decepcionarlos. —Saltaba a la vista que Oliver estaba disfrutando enormemente con la atención que les dispensaban.

—Debe de estar cansada después de un viaje tan largo —continuó Lloyd—. Los acompañaré a sus tiendas; no son lujosas, pero están relativamente limpias. Si tienen hambre, en un momento les prepararán un poco de comida, aunque me temo que nuestra dieta se basa en carne de antílope y de cebra.

—Hemos traído cereales y hortalizas frescas —comentó Camelia—. Seguro que a los hombres les encantará complementar su dieta con eso.

—Entonces descarguemos el carro. —Lloyd les hizo un gesto a los nativos, que rápidamente empezaron a bajar los pesados sacos, cestos y cajas llenas de deliciosa comida y provisiones.

—Badrani y Senwe, ¿les importaría hacerme el favor de llevar a mi tienda la jaula de Harriet y ese cesto de ahí? —pidió Camelia—. Dentro está Rupert.

—¡*Tengan cuidado con eso*! —chilló Simon cuando varios hombres levantaron con torpeza la bomba envuelta en lona.

Boquiabiertos y petrificados, a los hombres estuvo a punto de caérseles la bomba al suelo.

—Chico, ¡no les grites así! —sugirió Oliver—. Entre que eres pelirrojo y todo lo demás, me parece que les has dado un susto de muerte.

—Disculpen. Por favor, tengan cuidado —suplicó Simon inquieto, intentando aparentar tranquilidad—. No es nada peligroso, pero les pido que lo trasladen con cuidado, eso es todo.

Los hombres lo miraron nerviosos y asintieron. Titubeando, agarraron mejor la bomba y empezaron a moverla con energía.

—Lleven la bomba a la tienda del señor Kent —ordenó Camelia.

—Pueden dejarla fuera —comentó Simon—. Dudo que esta noche haga nada salvo dormir.

—Aun así, la bomba estará más segura contigo —insistió Camelia—. ¿Por qué no vamos todos al comedor y bebemos algo, y de paso me cuenta qué tal están las cosas, señor Trafford? Estoy ansiosa por obtener un informe completo.

—Muy bien, lady Camelia —contestó Lloyd.

Condujo a la pequeña comitiva entre el laberinto de gruesas tiendas de lona hasta que, finalmente, llegaron al comedor. En su interior, protegidas de los elementos africanos, había una mesa de considerables dimensiones y sillas para trabajar y comer.

—Me temo que hemos avanzado muy poco desde que se fue a Inglaterra —informó Lloyd con seriedad mientras Senwe y Badrani servían una sencilla comida a base de carne de antílope desecada, galletas duras de trigo, plátanos cocidos al vapor y agua—. Hemos intentado sacar el agua a mano, pero, por desgracia, no es un método práctico para un terreno tan grande. Ha caído tanta agua durante la estación lluviosa que la verdad es que la excavación casi se ha convertido en un pequeño lago. Después se sucedieron los accidentes y los hombres empezaron a marcharse, lo que implicaba que había menos manos para una tarea que ya era difícil con el número de trabajadores que había antes.

—¿Cuántos hombres hay ahora? —inquirió Camelia.

—La última vez que hice el recuento había treinta y ocho, pero fue a la hora de cenar —contestó Lloyd—. Y cada mañana descubro que uno o dos hombres han cogido sus cosas y se han ido.

—¿Y cuántos hombres le harían falta? —preguntó Oliver.

—Cuando lord Stamford empezó a trabajar aquí teníamos más de doscientos —le explicó Lloyd—. Dadas las dimensiones del terreno, era suficiente para mantener un ritmo de excavación constante; pero treinta y ocho es un número realmente escaso.

Elliott arrugó la frente.

—Esos nativos habían firmado un contrato. ¿Cómo pudo dejar que se marcharan, Trafford?

—¿Y cómo iba a evitarlo, señor? —replicó Lloyd—. Esto es una excavación arqueológica, no una cárcel. Si los hombres deciden abandonar, pierden su derecho de remuneración; ésa es nuestra única arma. Por desgracia, con todos los accidentes que han ocurrido, los nativos creen que ha caído una maldición sobre la excavación. Para muchos el dinero ya no basta para retenerlos aquí. Incluso creen que las lluvias las enviaron los espíritus para inundar el terreno e impedir que excaváramos.

—Eso es absurdo —protestó Camelia—. Cada año llueve muchísimo durante la estación de las lluvias; seguro que se habrán dado cuenta.

—Eso no importa, Tisha —dijo Zareb con tranquilidad—. Un hombre asustado ve las cosas de otra manera. Para ellos la lluvia es parte de la maldición. No hay dinero suficiente capaz de convencer a aquellos que tienen realmente miedo de quedarse.

—Si de verdad pretendes continuar excavando, Camelia, no puedes permitirte perder más hombres. —La expresión de Elliott era severa—. Tendrás que idear un sistema mejor para controlar a los trabajadores.

—Mi padre nunca creyó en confinar a los nativos, Elliott, y yo tampoco —repuso Camelia con obstinación—. Los hombres que deciden trabajar para mí son empleados, no prisioneros.

Simon la miró confuso.

—¿Qué quiere decir confinar?

—Es un sistema que desarrollaron las compañías mineras hace varios años para hacer frente a los problemas de robos y deserciones —explicó Elliott—. Consiste únicamente en amurallar el recinto donde viven los nativos mientras duren sus contratos, que suelen ser de tres meses. Se construyen barracas en el recinto en las que duermen y comen, y se dispone un acceso de las viviendas a la mina. De este modo los nativos no pueden robar los diamantes que encuentren y huir con ellos, ni marcharse antes de que sus contratos finalicen.

Oliver frunció el ceño.

—¿Y si esconden los diamantes hasta que terminen sus contratos y luego se los llevan?

—Se les registra.

—De la forma más humillante que se pueda imaginar —añadió Camelia indignada.

Elliott suspiró.

—Sí, pero lamentablemente es necesario hacerlo.

—Es terrible privar a un hombre de su libertad, lo sé —comentó Oliver con seriedad—, pero es mucho peor quitarle su libertad cuando no ha hecho nada malo.

—Los hombres que están aquí le son leales a lady Camelia —insistió Zareb—. No hace falta encerrarlos como a animales y tratarlos como a esclavos.

—En cuanto vean la bomba de Simon en funcionamiento, se darán cuenta de que la lluvia no es consecuencia de ninguna maldición —agregó Camelia—. La bomba hará el trabajo de cincuenta hombres o más, lo que significa que podremos avanzar a buen ritmo pese al escaso número de trabajadores. —Miró a Simon esperanzada.

—Aún está por ver si la bomba funcionará bien. —Aunque agradecía la fe que ella tenía en sus capacidades, Simon no quería que Camelia tuviese demasiadas expectativas—. No puedo prometer nada hasta que la haya puesto en marcha y sepa qué tipo de ajustes necesita.

—Entonces, será mejor que nos vayamos a dormir —sugirió Camelia, que se levantó de la silla—. Empezaremos a trabajar a primera hora de la mañana.

Oliver reprimió un hondo suspiro y se desperezó.

—Dormiré un poco y mañana estaré fresco como una rosa y listo para trabajar.

—Me temo que su cama no será tan cómoda como a lo que está acostumbrado, Oliver. Espero que eso no le impida dormir.

—Puedo dormir en casi cualquier sitio, jovencita, igual que Simon —le aseguró Oliver—. Cuando se ha vivido en la calle y se ha estado en la cárcel, uno aprende a conformarse con lo que hay.

Los ojos de Badrani se abrieron desmesuradamente.

—¿Ha estado en la cárcel?

Oliver se encogió de hombros.

—Un par de veces.

—¿Qué delito cometió? —Senwe también miraba a Oliver con especial interés.

—Ratear.

Los dos hombres lo miraron atónitos.

—Robé —les aclaró Oliver—. Era uno de los mejores ladrones del condado de Argyll, y aún lo sería, si quisiera. Estas viejas manos pueden birlar un reloj en un periquete y apuesto a que no hay puerta en Londres que yo no pueda abrir.

—¿En serio? —Badrani estaba visiblemente impresionado. Abrió la lona de la tienda de campaña para que Oliver saliese y añadió—: ¿Cómo se abre una cerradura, señor Oliver?

—Bueno, pues hay distintos sistemas —contestó Oliver, encantado con su fascinado público—. En la mayoría de los casos lo único que se necesitan son un par de varillas de hierro y un poco de paciencia...

—Te acompañaré a tu tienda, Simon —se ofreció Camelia—. Está al otro lado del campamento.

—Ya le acompaño yo —se apresuró a intervenir Elliott.

Simon sonrió.

—Es usted muy amable, Wickham, pero no quisiera molestarlo después de un viaje tan largo, sobre todo después de los problemas que ha tenido con ese caballo que ha comprado.

—Que duermas bien, Elliott —le deseó Camelia—. Te veré por la mañana.

Elliott forzó una sonrisa, irritado por el hecho de que Kent hubiese encontrado la manera de estar a solas con Camelia y él no.

—De acuerdo, pues. Buenas noches.

Cuando Camelia salió de la tienda de campaña el aire era agradable y fresco. Estaba impregnado del aroma de la rica tierra africana y de las delicadas y jóvenes plantas, mezclado con el inconfundible olor de los animales salvajes que vivían justo pasado el perímetro del campamento. A pesar del poco halagüeño informe del señor Trafford sobre el número de hombres que habían desertado estaba más feliz que en los meses pasados. Había regreado a Pumulani y con ella estaban Simon y su bomba de vapor. Mientras caminaba junto a él notó que corría por sus venas un renovado optimismo, que le hizo sentirse emocionada y ansiosa por volver al trabajo.

De no ser porque era de madrugada y todos estaban exhaustos, le habría pedido a Simon que desenvolviera la bomba para ponerla en marcha de inmediato.

—Ésta es tu tienda —anunció mientras abría la pesada lona de la tienda de campaña, colocada en un extremo del campamento—. No es gran cosa, pero espero que te encuentres a gusto.

Camelia entró y su rostro se ensombreció al constatar lo estrecho que era el catre de madera, y ver la pequeña mesa sobre la que había una vieja jofaina metálica, una jarra y una lámpara de aceite, y la desvencijada silla. El motor de vapor ocupaba casi la mitad del espacio disponible, quedando sólo un paso estrecho por el que, para acceder a la cama, Simon prácticamente tendría que saltar por encima de las maletas.

—Quizá sería mejor que te quedaras con mi tienda. —De pronto le disgustó la idea de encerrar a Simon en tan diminuto y abarrotado espacio—. Es más grande y tú necesitarás más sitio que yo...

—No pasa nada, Camelia —le aseguró Simon—. Estaré muy cómodo. Ya sabes que puedo dormir casi en cualquier parte.

Ella asintió sin convicción. Ojalá les hubiese dicho a sus hombres que llevasen las cosas de Simon a su tienda para quedarse ella con la pequeña. Era como si se hubiese olvidado de lo espartanas que eran las instalaciones de Pumulani; tal vez fuese porque hasta entonces nunca le habían parecido incómodas o austeras.

—Bueno, pues si no necesitas nada más, buenas noches.

—Buenas noches, Camelia.

Ella avanzó hacia la abertura de la tienda y luego se detuvo.

—¿Ocurre algo? —inquirió Simon.

Camelia lo miró vacilante.

—Me gustaría hacerte una pregunta.

—Adelante.

Permaneció largo rato callada.

—¿Cómo es la cárcel? —preguntó al fin con un susurro de voz temblorosa.

Simon se puso tenso, aunque supuso que la curiosidad de Camelia era razonable. En su primer encuentro ella le había asegurado que lo único que le interesaba de él era su talento como científico e inventor. Pero habían pasado muchas cosas entre ellos desde aquel día. No sólo había conocido la pasión más intensa de toda su vida, sino que además desde entonces había florecido en él algo que iba mucho más allá del deseo que sentía por ella. Y era eso lo que le hacía mostrarse reacio a contestar su pregunta.

Por algún motivo que no alcanzaba a comprender; quería que Camelia tuviese la mejor imagen de él, la mejor imagen posible, habida cuenta de su sórdido pasado, sus preocupaciones de carácter obsesivo y su comportamiento excéntrico. Así que titubeó, como si no hubiese entendido del todo la pregunta, cuando lo cierto era que sabía perfectamente lo que Camelia había querido decir.

—Supongo que debió de ser terrible. —Camelia no quería que él pensase que vivía en una burbuja y que ignoraba las crueldades del sistema de prisiones—. No me refiero a las condiciones en las que vivías; lo que me gustaría es poder entender cómo lograste sobrevivir. No eras más que un niño y, sin embargo, tuviste que vivir varios años en las calles y en la cárcel y sólo hay que verte...

—¿Qué parte de mí estás mirando exactamente? —replicó en tono burlón en un intento por desviar el interés que ella sentía por su infancia.

—Todos sois disciplinados y brillantes...

—Yo no soy brillante, Camelia —objetó Simon—. Sólo veo las cosas de una forma distinta al resto de la gente.

—*Sí* que eres brillante —insistió ella—. Basta echar un vistazo a tus éxitos académicos y a los maravillosos artículos que has escrito para darse cuenta de ello.

—Hay muchos idiotas que se licencian en la universidad y escriben artículos. Te aseguro que las personas más inteligentes que he conocido jamás han pisado un colegio.

—Lo que te hace brillante es que ves posibilidades donde otros ven el fin —aclaró Camelia—. Tú no miras una cosa y piensas: «¡Esto es magnífico!», como hacemos la mayoría.

No, tú miras algo y dices: «Esto no es perfecto, ¿cómo puedo mejorarlo?» Y te da igual si se trata de una mopa que lleva un siglo en el mercado o del último motor para un barco de vapor; tienes la capacidad de desarrollar ideas para mejorarlo todo.

—Todo no —repuso con expresión indescifrable al tiempo que añadía—: A veces encuentro cosas que ya son perfectas.

—No hay nada perfecto.

Tú eres perfecta.

La observó allí, de pie frente a él, con el entrecejo fruncido intentando traspasar las máscaras de protección que él se había puesto tantos años atrás. Casi todo su cabello color champán, que se había soltado de las horquillas, caía sobre sus hombros en una maraña dorada y la luz de la lámpara había vuelto su piel de color albaricoque. Copiosas arrugas y suciedad cubrían la seda gris de su vestido de viaje, y una mancha veteaba la aterciopelada perfección de su mejilla.

Jamás le había parecido más bella.

Desde que había pisado suelo africano algo había cambiado en ella, algo que se había multiplicado por cien al llegar a Pumulani. Ahora parecía más fuerte, más fuerte y más segura, como un animal enjaulado que, finalmente, es devuelto a su hábitat. Le asombraba que Camelia pudiese florecer en un entorno tan duro y aislado, claro que era completamente distinta al resto de las mujeres que había conocido. Fue esta percepción la que empezó a derrumbar el muro que había construido a su alrededor desde el beso que le dio hacía ya tanto tiempo, en Londres. Eso, y sus magníficos y penetrantes ojos verdeceledón, el ligero aroma de limón que daba la impresión de que la seguía a donde quiera que fuese e incluso esa mancha oscura que tenía en su sedosa mejilla.

Respiró hondo con la absoluta sensación de que estaba entrando en un lugar al que le daba miedo acceder, pero por alguna razón ya no podía dar media vuelta.

—La cárcel fue como un infierno —confesó en voz baja.

Ella lo miró con seriedad; en su rostro no había lástima, cosa que a él le habría amilanado, sino aceptación y pena. Eso le reconfortaba, si es que tenía algo de reconfortante que a uno le pidiesen que mostrase unas heridas que habían permanecido largo tiempo ocultas. Nadie le había preguntado nunca directamente por su pasado; ni siquiera Genevieve y Haydon, quienes consideraban que sus hijos tenían que destapar las vendas de sus antiguas heridas sólo si así lo decidían. Pero mientras Camelia estaba ahí de pie, mirándolo con fijeza, Simon sintió que algo cambiaba en su interior. Ella estaba intentando entrar en él, y por alguna razón que apenas conseguía entender, quería comprender cómo había llegado a ser quien era.

Y por primera vez en su vida, aunque fuese sólo durante un instante, realmente deseó abrir la puerta del infierno del que tanto había luchado por escapar.

—En aquella época no tenía ni nueve años —prosiguió en voz baja—, pero ya estaba muy curtido. Y aun así la cárcel fue terrorífica, mucho peor que todo cuanto había conocido hasta entonces. Por primera vez en mi vida no tenía absolutamente ningún control sobre lo que podía pasarme. Y cuando me dijeron que permanecería allí cinco años, quise morirme.

Hizo una pausa.

—Lo siento, Simon —se disculpó Camelia con voz suave y teñida de arrepentimiento—. No era mi intención hacerte evocar tan dolorosos recuerdos. No tenía ningún derecho a hacerte esa pregunta.

—Tienes todo el derecho del mundo a preguntármelo, Camelia. —Se acercó a ella y le apartó un mechón suelto de la cara—. Y quiero que lo sepas.

Ella levantó la vista y lo miró, hipnotizada por el cálido tacto de sus dedos, la ardiente intensidad de sus ojos azules plateados y la lenta cadencia de su voz suave. Tuvo ganas de rodearlo con sus brazos y abrazarlo con fuerza, de hacer suyo de algún modo el dolor que él sentía únicamente porque ella le había preguntado. Sin embargo, una voz interior le dijo que no lo hiciera, que si lo abrazaba iniciaría algo que no podría parar, algo que sólo serviría para aturdirla cuando necesitaba con desesperación estar despejada y centrada. Por eso se quedó inmóvil, aceptando en silencio la suave caricia de sus dedos, que abrieron un lánguido sendero por la curva de su mandíbula.

—Entonces apareció lady Redmond y te sacó de la cárcel —dijo con un susurro, procurando ignorar el ardor que sentía allí por donde pasaban los dedos de Simon.

—Sí, ella me rescató. —Sus dedos seguían descendiendo por la delgada columna de su cuello y la sedosa cavidad de la base de su garganta—. Pero pasaron años hasta que me convencí de que nadie vendría de pronto para arrastrarme allí de nuevo o de que mis circunstancias no cambiarían repentinamente y volvería a dormir en la calle. Cuando pierdes el control sobre tu vida, haces lo posible por protegerte, porque sabes que te puede volver a suceder. No confías ni crees en nadie. Sobre tu vida planea una sombra, porque crees que ahí fuera no hay nada realmente bueno, bonito ni puro. —La rodeó con un brazo y la atrajo hacia sí mientras con la otra mano seguía acariciando la sedosa palidez de su garganta y su mejilla—. Pero entonces había algo que no sabía, Camelia.

—¿Qué? —preguntó ella con un hilo de voz y el corazón martilleando.

Él inclinó la cabeza hasta que sus labios prácticamente se rozaron.

—Que tú existías.

La besó para hacérselo comprender. Sólo un beso, dijo para sí desesperado, y pararía. Sólo un simple beso para apaciguar el fuego que ardía en él desde aquella noche que habían pasado en Londres. Cumpliría su palabra, prometió, aunque ella acabase de soltar un gemido y hubiese abierto la boca invitándolo a probar su dulce oscuridad. Simon deslizó la lengua en su interior, ansioso por redescubrir los secretos que Camelia ya había compartido con él la vez anterior.

No era más que un beso, se repitió Simon fervientemente mientras sus manos empezaban a recorrer las exuberantes curvas de sus pechos, cintura y nalgas. Sólo un beso, en realidad, pensó, atrayéndola hacia sí hasta que el suave triángulo secreto que había entre sus muslos presionó contra su insoportable dureza. Sólo un sencillo y apasionado beso, se repitió, incapaz de entender cómo sus dedos habían empezado a desabotonarle la chaqueta. Se la quitó y a continuación le desabrochó la blusa que llevaba debajo, todavía pensando que esto no era nada, que simplemente estaba liberando a Camelia de una ropa que tampoco necesitaba. La falda cayó al suelo en un charco de arrugada seda gris a la que enseguida le siguieron las diversas capas de sus enaguas marfileñas.

No dejaba de decirse que esto no era más que un beso, que podía parar en cualquier momento, si ella así lo deseaba.

La levantó en brazos y la tumbó sobre la estrecha cama, volviéndose a decir que le daría un beso más, sólo uno. Pero ahora ella le acariciaba con las manos, y le quitó la camisa y los pantalones dejando su piel expuesta al cálido aire nocturno de África y al ansioso ardor del tacto de Camelia, que empezó a explorar los contornos de su cuerpo. Los besos de Simon descendieron y decidió desabrochar los corchetes de su corsé, descubriendo centímetro a glorioso centímetro la belleza de sus senos de pezones coralinos y su vientre de color cremoso. Le bajó las braguitas por las piernas y le soltó las medias hasta dejarla al fin espléndidamente desnuda debajo de él.

Le regaló una lluvia de besos en la pálida seda de sus muslos y luego hundió la lengua en su hirviente vulva rosa. Camelia gimió y se removió sobre la cama, abriéndose a él, acariciándole el cabello y sujetándole la cabeza entre sus esbeltas piernas. Él la saboreó intensamente, lamiendo sus misteriosos y deliciosos jugos hasta que ella acabó jadeando y apretándole el cuerpo con las piernas. Simon le abrió más las piernas y deslizó un dedo en su interior, despacio, lánguido, buscando los más íntimos secretos de su cuerpo mientras seguía acariciándole con la lengua y la movía en círculos.

Camelia se retorció, aceptando el placer que él le daba y deseando más. Simon introdujo otro dedo y aceleró el ritmo, lamiendo y chupando con más fuerza y rapidez mientras metía y sacaba los dedos. Notaba cómo aumentaba el placer de Camelia como si fuese suyo, su cuerpo se tensaba y los jadeos se incrementaban. Eran una súplica desesperada que inundaba el silencio de la tienda en su ansiosa búsqueda por alcanzar lo que él intentaba darle.

Simon no paró de besarla, lamerla y llenarla; tenía la sensación de que el salvaje deseo que crecía en él al ver cómo ella reaccionaba a sus apasionadas caricias le haría enloquecer. De repente, el cuerpo de Camelia se puso rígido y soltó un grito, tan intenso fue su placer que él casi estuvo a punto de perder el poco control que aún le quedaba. Se tumbó sobre ella y la penetró mientras las contracciones de su orgasmo le apretaban el miembro una y otra vez.

Entonces empezó a embestirla, tratando de controlarse, y ella le abrazó y lo atrajo hacia sí para darle un profundo beso.

Quería ir despacio, quería que durase para de algún modo hacerle comprender lo que sea que había entre ellos, aunque ni él mismo lo entendía. Pero su cuerpo no le escuchó. Había esperado tanto tiempo para poder volver a vivir el milagro de estar dentro de Camelia que se dio cuenta de que no podía ir despacio, de la misma manera que no hubiese podido impedir que la noche se convirtiese en día. Así que gimió y la besó con fervor, acariciándola por donde podía mientras la embestía con fuerza.

La deseaba con una desesperación abrumadora, más de lo que había deseado nada en toda su vida. Y esa certeza resultaba angustiosa, porque en el fondo su mente era todavía bastante racional para saber que ella nunca le pertenecería. Camelia pertenecía a África, con toda su magnífica y áspera belleza, viviendo una vida completamente ajena a la suya; una vida en la que él jamás encajaría. Continuó embistiéndola con fuerza, abrazándola y besándola con pasión, y empujándola contra el chirriante catre. Y ella se movió al mismo ritmo que él, subiendo y bajando con cada intensa embestida, instándole a que fuese más deprisa.

De pronto, Simon empezó a adentrarse en un torbellino de luz y oscuridad. Gritó, era un grito de éxtasis y desesperación, porque sabía que cuando esto acabase ella volvería a apartarse de él. La abrazó y le dio un apasionado beso lleno de ansiedad y de posesividad; quería que ella entendiese que le pertenecía mucho más de lo que pertenecía a África. Pero estando ahí echados, mientras la cubría con su ardor, su fuerza y su deseo, empezó a notar que ella se alejaba de él igual que notaba que había aminorado el ritmo de los latidos de su corazón. Hundió la cabeza en el cuello de Camelia y permaneció inmóvil, negándose a salir de ella.

«Quédate conmigo», le suplicó en silencio consciente de que era una petición inútil. Le apartó con suavidad un mechón dorado de la frente y después le acarició las suaves curvas de su mejilla, nariz y barbilla intentando memorizar cada maravilloso detalle de su cuerpo. Acariciarla de esta manera era una pequeña tortura, pero lo hizo de todas formas, así, cuando finalmente tuviese que dejarla marchar, podría recordar lo que era estar sobre ella y rozar con los dedos su piel de satén.

Tumbada debajo de Simon, el corazón de Camelia latía con fuerza contra el sólido muro de su pecho. Le sacudían intensas emociones que le hacían sentirse frágil y temerosa. No había pretendido hacerlo, dijo para sí, pero sabía que era mentira. El recuerdo de las caricias de Simon llevaba semanas atormentándola; esos labios aterciopelados sobre su boca, esas manos ardientes sobre su piel. Había sido un error, naturalmente; era muy consciente de ello. Él no le pertenecía, igual que ella no le pertenecía a él. Su corazón y su vida estaban en África, el corazón y la vida de Simon estaban en Londres, donde podía pasarse sin problemas varias semanas seguidas encerrado en un laboratorio mal ventilado y atestado de cosas, sin nadie que lo molestara para cosas tan mundanas como comer, conversar o hacerle compañía. En su vida no había sitio para el matrimonio y los hijos, de igual modo que en la de Camelia no había sitio para tantos convencionalismos. Ahora lo entendía con dolorosa claridad.

Sin embargo, ella tampoco se movió.

—Será mejor que me vaya —dijo al fin con un susurro, más por decir algo que porque realmente quisiese irse.

Simon levantó la cabeza y la miró. Había lágrimas temblorosas en sus profundos ojos; su mirada estaba llena de dolor.

—No han sido las estrellas, Camelia —comentó él en voz baja y ronca—. Esta vez no.

Ella alzó la vista y lo miró, hipnotizada por la suave cadencia de su voz, la ternura de su tacto y la maravillosa sensación que le producía que su escultural cuerpo la presionara contra el delgado colchón.

—Entonces ¿qué es?

Simon le enjugó con la yema del dedo una brillante lágrima que rodaba por su mejilla.

—No estoy seguro.

Camelia cerró los ojos, incapaz de mirarlo. Sabía que le había entregado parte de su ser y no podía soportarlo.

—No puedo irme de África, Simon —susurró con esfuerzo—. No puedo.

Las lágrimas comenzaron a brotar más deprisa de sus ojos, resbalando por su bronceada piel y su sedoso cabello de color miel. Con el corazón encogido, Simon se dio cuenta de que a Camelia le había costado mucho hacerle esa confesión. Quería ser lo más honesta posible con él. Aunque apenas importaba que lo hubiese verbalizado; él ya sabía la profunda conexión que le unía a Camelia a este extraño y salvaje lugar.

Y si pensaba que podría debilitar esa conexión uniéndola más a él, se equivocaba.

—Nunca te pediría que te marcharas de aquí, Camelia —le dijo mientras le acariciaba el pelo con suavidad—. Pero también quiero que entiendas que yo no puedo quedarme. Tengo mi propio trabajo y mi familia, y la vida que me he organizado en Inglaterra y en Escocia. No puedo dejar todo eso para venirme a vivir a África, en medio de la nada. Estos son tu mundo y tu vida, no los míos.

Ella tragó saliva, estaba inmóvil.

—Lo entiendo.

Simon la miró, nada convencido.

—¿De verdad lo entiendes?

Camelia asintió.

—Tengo que irme —anunció con un hilo de voz.

—Quédate conmigo, Camelia —le suplicó con suavidad. No quería que se fuese. Ni ahora ni nunca—. Sólo un rato más.

Ella sacudió la cabeza. No podía estar con él ni un segundo más. Se le estaba desgarrando lentamente el corazón y no creía que pudiese soportarlo.

—Déjame marcharme, Simon. —Se movió para incorporarse, pero él se quedó quieto—. Por favor.

Simon no tuvo opción. Se apartó de ella, recogió sus pantalones y se los puso de espaldas a ella para dejar que se vistiera también.

Camelia se abrochó con torpeza los corchetes del corsé y las cintas de las enaguas, esforzándose por vestirse lo más deprisa posible. Cuando al fin terminó fue hasta la entrada de la tienda.

Simon se volvió para darle las buenas noches.

Pero Camelia ya se había ido, dejando a su paso el lento aleteo de la abertura de la tienda y el ligero aroma a limón y a pradera se quedó flotando en el fresco aire de la noche africana.

• • •

Esto no era lo que había previsto.

Zareb frunció las cejas al ver a Camelia salir apresuradamente de la tienda de campaña de Simon, con el pelo cayendo en cascada por sus espaldas y las manos sujetando la chaqueta sobre su blusa a medio abotonar. Aunque estaba demasiado oscuro para que pudiese verle la cara con claridad, emanaba de ella una indudable desesperación.

Esto no iba bien.

Zareb sabía que se estaba haciendo mayor, lo que le producía rabia y frustración. Era la única explicación para el hecho de que no hubiese intuido el daño que Kent le había causado a su querida Tisha. No pensó que sus poderes disminuirían con la edad, claro que tampoco los había entendido nunca del todo. Su madre le había advertido de que a lo largo de su vida irían aumentando o debilitándose en función de su propia evolución. Ésa era una de las razones por la que había decidido no contraer matrimonio. La miríada de exigencias que suponían una mujer y unos hijos habrían socavado su fuerza y nublado su visión. Y si bien era cierto que en algunas ocasiones era una maldición tener la capacidad de sentir las fuerzas que lo rodeaban, a veces le producían un placer indescriptible. Era como si estuviese más conectado con los poderes de los cielos y la tierra que los más grandes chamanes que le habían precedido.

Pero ¿de qué servía esta habilidad, si era incapaz de evitar el sufrimiento de la persona que más le importaba?, se preguntó indignado.

—Vete con ella —le ordenó a Oscar, que estaba sentado en su hombro mientras comía una galleta—. Te necesita.

Oscar bajó de un brinco y corrió hacia la tienda de Camelia.

Con cauto silencio, Zareb examinó la oscura silueta de Simon a través del velo de lona de su tienda. ¿Se había equivocado al pensar que este blanco extraño de pelo de color fuego y ropa arrugada les ayudaría a luchar contra el viento oscuro de Pumulani? E incluso aunque fuese Kent el encargado de combatir las fuerzas que lord Stamford había desatado involuntariamente cuando empezó a excavar en esta zona, ¿qué precio tendría que pagar Tisha por su presencia?

Zareb observó cómo en el interior de su tienda Simon sacaba el envoltorio de la bomba de vapor, cogía una herramienta y empezaba a hacer una serie de ajustes a la máquina. Al menos parecía decidido a proporcionarle a Camelia el instrumento para extraer el agua de la excavación.

Y eso estaba bien.

Cabeceó, confundido por el remolino de poderes buenos y malos que se agitaban a su alrededor. A veces no resultaba fácil comprender las fuerzas. Quizá, pensó con disgusto, su avanzada edad fuese también responsable de eso.

Se refugió de nuevo en la oscuridad de su tienda, cansado y confuso.

Y completamente ajeno al hecho de que no había sido el único que, agazapado en las sombras, había visto a Camelia perderse a medio vestir en la noche.

Capítulo 12

—Tengo buenas y malas noticias —informó Oliver seriamente.

Simon apretó la mandíbula y giró un poco más el tornillo que estaba ajustando, rompiéndolo en el proceso.

—¡Por el amor de Dios! —exclamó—. ¡Es el quinto maldito tornillo que rompo intentando montar esta maldita máquina! —Se incorporó y se dio un golpe en la cabeza con el borde de la bomba—. ¡Jesús!

Oliver arrugó la frente.

—Bueno, ya vale de blasfemias, jovencito, ¡o te lavaré la boca con el jabón de Eunice!

—No creo que sepa peor que la carne seca y fibrosa que hemos tomado en el desayuno —replicó Simon malhumorado mientras se frotaba la cabeza.

—Se llama *biltong* —le informó Zareb ofendido—. Es carne de antílope sazonada y secada al viento. Buenísima para estar fuerte.

—Me temo que todas mis fuerzas están concentradas en digerirla —musitó Simon—; me siento como si me hubiese comido una bota vieja. A ver, ¿cuáles son las buenas noticias?

A Oliver se le iluminó la mirada.

—La buena noticia es que he estado indagando y todo el mundo coincide en que la estación de las lluvias ha llegado a su fin. Hasta octubre el clima será totalmente seco.

—¡Magnífico! —celebró Simon silabeando—. Por lo menos no tendremos que preocuparnos de que caiga más agua en ese agujero enfangado. —Rebuscó impacientemente en su caja de herramientas para dar con otro tornillo—. ¿Y las malas noticias?

—Me temo que he tenido algún que otro problemilla para encontrar la leña que me pediste.

—¿Qué clase de problemillas?

—Bueno, es que no hay leña.

Simon levantó la vista con incredulidad.

—¿Qué quiere decir que no hay leña?

—Echa un vistazo a tu alrededor, chico. —Oliver hizo un gesto con sus delgados brazos—. Hay un poco de hierba y un montón de arbustos, pero no hay ni un solo árbol; a menos que cuentes como árboles esos pequeños brotes que no podrán talarse hasta dentro de unos cuantos años.

Oliver tenía razón, pensó Simon asombrado. Aparte de unos cuantos árboles jóvenes y unos pequeños arbustos no había árboles a la vista. Miró a Zareb confuso.

—¿Dónde están los árboles, Zareb?

—Antes había árboles, hace mucho tiempo —contestó—, pero las tribus que habitaban estas tierras los talaron para construir sus cabañas y hacer hogueras.

—Luego llegaron los Boers —añadió Senwe— y cortaron aún más árboles para poder cultivar la tierra.

—Después los exploradores —continuó Badrani— vinieron a los ríos Vaal y Orange en busca de diamantes, y talaron árboles para hacerse sus cabañas y sus hogueras.

Zareb asintió.

—Entonces apareció la industria maderera y taló los árboles que quedaban para poderlos llevar a las minas y venderlos a los excavadores.

—Luego llegaron las lluvias —intervino Senwe de nuevo— y...

—Lo he entendido; no hay árboles. —Simon se frotó las sienes, tratando de apaciguar el martilleo que llevaba toda la mañana sintiendo en la cabeza—. Entonces, ¿se puede saber con qué hicieron los hombres las hogueras de anoche?

—Con estiércol desecado.

Miró a Badrani con incredulidad.

—¿Con estiércol? ¿Con excrementos de animales?

Senwe asintió.

—Exacto.

—¿Y eso es lo que se supone que tengo que quemar para poner mi bomba en marcha?

—No le estamos diciendo lo que debe o no debe usar para su bomba —respondió Zareb—. Lo único que le hemos dicho es que no hay madera. Lo único que hay es excremento de buey desecado.

—¿Y qué tal prende el fuego en los excrementos de buey?

—Pues es lento y bastante humoso —reconoció Badrani.

—Y, por desgracia, si el estiércol no se ha secado bien a veces huele mal —añadió Senwe.

«¡Genial! —pensó Simon con amargura—. Realmente, el día no puede ir mejor.»

—Muy bien, pues. Oliver, Senwe y Badrani, necesito todo el estiércol posible para empezar a hacer una hoguera. Si es necesario, pidan ayuda a otros hombres para traerlo hasta aquí. Necesito hacer una buena hoguera para calentar bien la caldera. Probablemente la bomba tarde varios días en sacar el agua, así que necesitaremos mucho estiércol.

—Sí, señor Kent —dijo Senwe con una inclinación de cabeza.

—No te alteres, muchacho —lo tranquilizó Oliver, que percibió la desesperación de Simon—. Te traeremos el mejor estiércol que encontremos.

—No me altero —replicó Simon—. Es sólo que estoy deseando poner la bomba en marcha.

—De acuerdo, entonces deja de perder el tiempo hablando —lo regañó Oliver—. ¡A trabajar!

Simon observó al anciano escocés alejarse alegremente con sus nuevos amigos africanos. Excremento desecado. Sacudió la cabeza con incredulidad antes de enjugarse las gotas de sudor que resbalaban por su frente con la manga sucia y volverse a echar en el suelo para ponerse a trabajar de nuevo.

Después de que Camelia se fuese de su tienda de campaña no había podido conciliar el sueño, de modo que se pasó toda la noche intentando montar la bomba. Lamentablemente, la tarea estaba siendo mucho más complicada de lo que se había imaginado. Tras tres semanas de viaje con un aire húmedo y salado algunas de las piezas se habían oxidado y diversos dientes de la rueda estaban torcidos. Simon dedujo que habría sucedido en algún momento del trayecto hasta allí. Había tardado varias horas en reparar los daños y no sabía con seguridad si había enderezado los dientes lo suficiente para que su movimiento no se viese alterado.

Otra cosa más que añadir a su estado malhumorado de por sí.

—¿Va todo bien, Kent?

Simon alzó la vista con los ojos entornados a causa del sol y vio a Elliott de pie frente a él. Wickham iba vestido con un bonito traje hecho a medida, pantalones de color crema, una camisa asombrosamente almidonada, una corbata perfectamente anudada y un abrigo a cuadros grises y de color marfil. Un elegante sombrero de paja de alas anchas completaba su impecable atuendo. Parecía que estuviese a punto de asistir a algún picnic o fiesta al aire libre, dijo Simon para sí, en lugar de trabajar en una excavación inundada de barro en medio de Suráfrica.

—Buenas tardes, Wickham —lo saludó con amabilidad—. Espero que haya dormido bien esta noche.

—Así es. ¿Y usted?

—He dormido como un bebé —mintió Simon.

—¿Cómo va la bomba? —preguntó Elliott mientras observaba la máquina que Simon ensamblaba—. Lleva un montón de horas trabajando —comentó enarcando las cejas—, ¿va todo bien?

—Perfectamente. Dentro de unas horas estará lista para funcionar.

—Me alegra oír eso. Sé que Camelia está ansiosa por continuar excavando. Cuanto antes podamos extraer el agua antes podremos volver a excavar.

—Lo noto extrañamente ilusionado con la excavación, Wickham. Siempre he tenido la sensación de que no le hacía mucha gracia que Camelia siguiese trabajando aquí.

—Lo que no me hace gracia es que Camelia se arruine para perseguir el sueño de su padre —replicó Elliott—. Así que cuanto antes saquemos el agua y los nativos puedan continuar excavando, antes podrá Camelia darse cuenta de que aquí no hay nada más que desenterrar.

Simon lo miró con curiosidad.

—¿Por qué está tan seguro de que ahí abajo no hay nada?

—Pasé quince años de mi vida íntegramente dedicado a esta excavación. Camelia era aún una niña cuando vine a ayudar a su padre. Durante años estuve convencido de la existencia de la Tumba de los Reyes, sobre todo por la fe ciega que lord Stamford tenía en ella. Pero al ver que iba pasando el tiempo y no la encontrábamos, poco a poco empecé a dudar de que realmente existiera. Cuando lord Stamford murió, decidí que no iba a perder más tiempo en busca de lo que, sin duda, no es más que una leyenda de los kaffirs.

—La mayoría de las leyendas tienen un origen real —objetó Simon—. Por eso perduran.

—Está hablando de gente que tiene una historia para todo, incluso para explicar cómo el sol y la luna llegaron a gobernar el cielo. No son más que mitos infantiles.

Simon se encogió de hombros.

—No es ninguna locura pensar que una tribu reservase un lugar especial para enterrar a sus reyes.

—En ese caso, no habrá más que un montón de huesos descompuestos y unas cuantas conchas rotas. Por muy fascinante que eso le resulte a Camelia, no bastará para reunir el dinero necesario para seguir pagando a los nativos y continuar excavando. Lo que debería hacer es vender el terreno por lo que le ofrezcan y volver a casa.

—Camelia considera que ya está en casa.

—Este terreno perdido en medio de la nada no es en absoluto su hogar —protestó Elliott—. Es su locura, como lo era de su padre.

—Si tan convencido está de que la excavación carece de valor, ¿por qué ha vuelto a venir?

—Porque, lo sepa o no, Camelia me necesita. Soy el único que puede ayudarle a entender que aquí no hay nada más que desenterrar. Es preciso que lo comprenda antes de que dilapide la pequeña herencia de su padre y se quede sin nada.

—¿Y qué pretende que haga Camelia cuando haya tomado conciencia?

—Podrá hacer un montón de cosas —le aseguró Elliott—. Londres está lleno de comités de mujeres que se dedican a recaudar fondos para beneficencia, museos y arte. No creo que una mujer con la inteligencia y la determinación de Camelia tenga problemas para llenar el tiempo.

—Pero a ella no le gusta Londres, Wickham. Seguro que se habrá dado cuenta de eso.

—Tampoco conoce bien la ciudad —objetó Elliott—. Sólo ha ido allí para buscar una bomba y reunir el dinero que le permita continuar excavando, y no para entablar amistades y disfrutar de la ciudad. Cuando nos hayamos casado, aprenderá a disfrutar de ella. Y si se agobia en la ciudad, siempre puede instalarse en la casa que tengo en el campo.

—Veo que lo tiene todo planeado.

—Sí, así es —afirmó Elliott mirando a Simon fijamente.

Se sacudió una mota de polvo que tenía en la solapa de su impoluta chaqueta y se ajustó el sombrero.

—Le dejo trabajar, Kent. Cuanto antes consiga poner la bomba en funcionamiento antes conseguiremos que Camelia se dé cuenta de aquí no hay nada, y todos podremos dejar de perder el tiempo e irnos a casa.

Simon lo observó mientras se alejaba y luego cogió una llave inglesa y se dispuso a ajustar la presión de un tornillo. Realmente, Wickham no comprendía en absoluto a Camelia, pensó.

«No puedo irme de África», le había confesado ella la noche anterior. Y al ver sus ojos llenos de dolor, Simon supo con absoluta claridad que le decía la verdad. Tal vez Camelia se equivocase con relación a la Tumba de los Reyes, pero no era la tumba lo que la retenía allí. A pesar de que no lograba entenderlo, el calor, la belleza y la pureza de África corrían por sus venas. Le daban vida y energía, y le llenaban de determinación. Además, en el fondo de su corazón, Camelia se conocía bastante para saber que no podría ser feliz en ninguna otra parte.

Y si Elliott no entendía eso, es que era idiota.

Aunque más idiota era él por haberse enamorado de una mujer que jamás le acompañaría y abandonaría ese lugar, que amaba más que ninguna otra cosa.

CUARTA PARTE

Susurros de pasión

Capítulo 13

Sentada en el suelo, Camelia escudriñaba la enorme roca que había justo pasado el perímetro cercado de la excavación.

Era una roca impresionante, de unos dos metros de alto y más de cuatro en su punto más ancho. Miles de años de exposición al fuerte viento y la lluvia que arreciaban en Pumulani durante los meses de verano habían alisado su superficie al igual que habían estropeado y difuminado los dibujos realizados sobre la misma. En muchos aspectos se parecía a los cientos de ejemplos de pinturas rupestres africanas que su padre había descubierto y documentado a lo largo de los años.

Pero cuando lord Stamford tropezó con esta roca en concreto, se persuadió de que encerraba el secreto del emplazamiento de la Tumba de los Reyes.

—No tengo más nueces —le dijo a Oscar con firmeza, que había introducido su pequeña pata en el bolsillo de su arrugada chaqueta de hilo—. Te las has comido todas.

Oscar se sentó sobre las nalgas y señaló con reprobación a Harriet y a Rupert.

—Harriet se ha comido unas cuantas y yo habré tomado unas cinco —dijo Camelia mientras estudiaba los dibujos de la roca que había en el cuaderno de notas de su padre—. Y a Rupert no le gustan las nueces; así que el resto te lo has comido tú, Oscar. No me extrañaría que acabaras con dolor de barriga.

Oscar dio un brinco y empezó a girar en rápidos círculos para demostrarle lo bien que se encontraba.

—Bueno, vale, pero ya no comas más a menos que quieras que Zareb te meta en su tienda y se ponga a hacer hogueras a tu alrededor y a darte uno de sus asquerosos remedios.

—Mis remedios no son asquerosos —protestó Zareb, haciendo acto de presencia.

Ante la idea de tener que beber uno de los elixires de Zareb, Oscar corrió hasta Camelia y trepó a su hombro en busca de protección.

—¿Qué tal va la bomba? —preguntó Camelia, que levantó la vista del cuaderno de notas de su padre.

—Igual que todos estos días. Funciona durante unos minutos, a veces suficiente para extraer varios cubos de agua y luego no sé qué pasa que se para.

—¿Sabe Simon el motivo?

—No está seguro. El agua está muy fangosa y a la bomba le cuesta un sobreesfuerzo sacarla. Y aunque está convencido de que el motor de vapor es potente, tiene problemas con el combustible porque el estiércol no arde con mucha fuerza. Y eso le dificulta la producción de vapor, que a su vez afecta a la potencia del mecanismo de bombeo.

Camelia reanudó el estudio del diario de su padre, intentando no dejar traslucir su decepción.

—Ya veo.

Zareb tomó asiento en el suelo junto a ella, colocando las túnicas hasta que formaron un brillante lago de color escarlata y zafiro. La observó en silencio unos instantes, reparando en las arrugas de preocupación que le habían salido en el entrecejo y en el firme ángulo de su mandíbula. Había cambiado desde el primer viaje a Londres, pensó con orgullo y también con inquietud. Naturalmente, le había dado pena marcharse de África. La muerte de su padre le produjo una sensación de vacío y pérdida, además de la ansiedad que conlleva irse a otro lugar, lejos del hogar que uno ama. Pero Zareb detectó que el dolor que ahora anidaba en ella no era como el de entonces.

—¿Te ha hablado ya, Tisha? —le preguntó en voz baja.

Ella alzó la vista confusa.

—¿El qué?

—La roca. ¿Te ha susurrado ya su secreto?

Camelia soltó una carcajada.

—De ser así, no seguiría aquí sentada día tras día, como solía hacer mi padre, intentando averiguar el significado de estos dibujos.

—Pues empecemos por ahí. ¿Qué crees que representan?

Camelia examinó la roca unos instantes.

—Parece una escena de caza normal, con una manada de antílopes rodeada de unos guerreros. Pero las estrellas de encima indican que es de noche, lo que significa que la escena tiene una interpretación mítica. Luego está el león de cara a la manada, que puede significar una amenaza para los antílopes o los guerreros, o ambos. O puede que sea el propio león el que está en peligro, ya sea porque los antílopes vayan a atacarlo o porque los guerreros lo cacen. —Cabeceó con frustración—. Mi padre estaba convencido de que esta piedra era la llave para la localización exacta de la Tumba de los Reyes, pero nunca logró descifrar el mensaje. A veces me pregunto si estaremos excavando en el lugar adecuado.

—Eso depende de lo que estés buscando.

—Ya sabes qué busco, Zareb. Quiero encontrar la Tumba de los Reyes que mi padre se pasó la vida buscando.

—Tu padre buscó muchas otras cosas, Tisha. La Tumba de los Reyes fue sólo una de ellas.

—Pero era la más importante para él. Habría dado cualquier cosa por encontrarla antes de morir.

Zareb miró fijamente la roca y no dijo nada.

—Lo echo de menos —confesó Camelia con un hilo de voz mientras acariciaba las gastadas páginas del diario de su padre—. ¡Ojalá estuviese aquí para decirme lo que debo hacer!

—Tu padre nunca te dijo lo que debías hacer, Tisha. Era su forma de amarte y de darte libertad para que tú misma averiguaras lo que realmente querías.

—Quería ser arqueóloga como él y dedicar mi vida a desenterrar los secretos de África.

—Hay secretos que nunca podrán ser desenterrados. Si así está escrito, saldrán a la luz, de lo contrario permanecerán ocultos; no es algo que tú puedas decidir.

Ella lo miró confusa.

—¿Me estás diciendo que no encontraré la Tumba de los Reyes?

—Lo que digo es que será la propia Tumba la que decida si quiere o no ser descubierta. Lo único que tú puedes hacer es decidir hasta dónde estás dispuesta a llegar en esta búsqueda.

—Hasta el final. Igual que mi padre.

—Tu padre tenía otras cosas en la vida, Tisha. La Tumba de los Reyes era sólo una pequeña parte de ella.

—Hizo otros descubrimientos a lo largo de su carrera, pero ninguno fue relevante para el mundo arqueológico, básicamente porque todos estaban ubicados en África.

—No me refería al trabajo, Tisha, sino a su vida.

—El trabajo era su vida.

Zareb sacudió la cabeza.

—Cuando conocí a lord Stamford su vida estaba dividida entre su profesión y su alma. Los nativos lo llamaban Talib, que significa «el que busca».

—Tiene sentido; era arqueólogo.

—Los nativos no sabían qué era un arqueólogo. No podían entender que un hombre blanco excavara lo que sus antepasados habían dejado al morir. Lo llamaron Talib porque percibían su infelicidad; creían que había venido a África en busca de lo que añoraba.

—No añoraba nada, excepto el reconocimiento del mundo de la arquelogía.

—Estás viendo a tu padre a través de tus ojos; no puedes evitar hablar desde el reflejo de su amor. Antes de que tú vinieras a vivir con él, tu padre era un hombre distinto. Había un vacío terrible en su interior. Ni siquiera su amor por África pudo aliviar el dolor de ese vacío.

—Pero lo tenía todo —objetó Camelia—. Un título nobiliario, una profesión, una esposa, una hija...

—Una esposa y una hija que vivían a un océano de distancia.

—Supongo que nos echaba de menos —admitió Camelia—, pero su trabajo era muy importante para él. Le llenaba enormemente.

—Y sin embargo estuvo dispuesto a dejarlo por ti.

Ella lo miró atónita.

—Eso nunca me lo dijo.

Zareb clavó los ojos en la roca y permaneció en silencio.

¡Cuánto se parecía Camelia a lord Stamford! Su niña querida, cuya protección le habían confiado a Zareb hacía tantos años. Era obstinada, inteligente, decidida, tal vez incluso un poco egoísta, como son quienes están destinados a lograr grandes cosas; dueños de su tiempo, sus responsabilidades y sus corazones. Pero en su interior había desdicha y sus sombras habían crecido desde que Zareb la viera salir aquella noche apresuradamente de la tienda de campaña de Simon. También en el inventor blanco había germinado la infelicidad.

Entre los dos se había encendido un fuego y ni el tiempo ni el muro que ambos habían levantado entre ellos habían logrado apagar las llamas.

—Antes de que tu madre muriera —relató Zareb en voz baja— lord Stamford era consciente de que su trabajo no le permitía disfrutar de ti. Hubo una época en que estaba decidido a que dejaras de pagar ese precio. Pero entonces tu madre falleció y te trajo aquí, no para criarte en África, porque lo que pretendía era abandonar la excavación y volver contigo a Inglaterra.

Camelia frunció las cejas.

—Si lo que quería era abandonar la excavación, ¿por qué me trajo aquí? ¿Por qué no me dejó en Inglaterra hasta que se reuniese conmigo?

—Eras muy pequeña, Tisha, y acababas de perder a tu madre. Estabas sola y asustada, y tu padre pensó que necesitabas estar con él en esos momentos. Algunos opinaban que debía haberte metido en un colegio. Tu madre tenía una tía que insistía en quedarse contigo, y que le prometió a lord Stamford educarte para convertirte en una joven decente mientras él se dedicaba a su profesión. Pero tu padre no cedió. Te quería y quería ocuparse de ti, aunque eso implicase dejar de trabajar en África.

—Y ¿por qué no se fue a Inglaterra?

—Porque vio que África te gustaba, Tisha. Igual que le gustaba a él.

—Sí, supongo que era obvio —repuso Camelia—. Desde que puse un pie aquí me sentí como en casa.

—También tu padre se sintió como en casa a partir de entonces; cuando vio que eras feliz aquí. Pero su hogar no era África, Tisha, eras tú.

—Me imagino que yo también era parte de su hogar —concedió Camelia—. Pero mi padre pertenecía a este lugar. Nunca habría sido feliz en Inglaterra.

—Él eligió estar contigo, Tisha, fuese donde fuese. Tú eras su hogar.

Ella lo miró vacilante.

—¿Por qué me cuentas todo esto, Zareb?

—Porque algo ha cambiado en tu interior, Tisha. —Su expresión era grave—. Últimamente te veo triste, y eso me duele.

—Es que echo de menos a mi padre.

—Siempre lo echarás de menos, toda tu vida. Pero la tristeza de la que hablo no es la de una hija que añora a su padre.

Camelia desvió la vista, sintiéndose repentinamente vulnerable y desnuda.

—Mi vida está aquí, Zareb —insistió en voz baja—. Nada podrá cambiar eso.

—África es parte de tu vida, Tisha —replicó Zareb—. Una parte que te unía con fuerza a tu padre, y eso está bien. Pero no es toda tu vida. El futuro está por llegar; aún no está escrito. Ésa es la parte que puedes cambiar.

Se levantó, sacudió el polvo de sus túnicas y luego miró al cielo.

—El viento está cambiando de dirección —comentó al observar cómo un grupo de espesas nubes formaba un delicado velo alrededor de las picudas cimas de aquellas montañas.

—¿Significa eso que el viento oscuro dejará al final de soplar? —preguntó Camelia procurando sonar alegre—. Creo que nos vendría bien un poco de buena suerte.

Zareb contempló el cielo en silencio, intentando percibir las fuerzas que se movían a su alrededor. Supo que algo se aproximaba hacia ellos con la misma certeza con la que sentía los constantes latidos de su corazón.

Algo poderoso.

Cerró los ojos y aguzó los sentidos hasta que percibió con claridad el cegador brillo del sol, la cálida caricia del viento que agitaba sus túnicas y el olor acre y a humo de la hoguera a base de estiércol de Simon, que llegaba lentamente por el aire.

«Ten cuidado», le susurró el viento con voz tan suave que Zareb no estaba seguro de haberlo oído bien.

«Ten cuidado.»

Las gotas de sudor empezaron a resbalar por su frente mientras aguzaba el oído, tratando de entender el significado del mensaje.

«¿Que tenga cuidado con qué? ¿Con la excavación? ¿Con alguien? ¿Con un espíritu? ¿Con la Tumba?», se preguntó.

«Dime con qué», suplicó extendiendo los brazos hasta que sus túnicas formaron una gigante y vistosa bandera que ondeaba al viento. «Dime...»

—¿Qué ocurre? —le preguntó de pronto Camelia preocupada—. ¿Qué has oído?

El viento calló de golpe.

Zareb abrió los ojos y la miró con los ojos muy abiertos y llenos de miedo. Estaba claro que ella también había escuchado algo.

—Debemos vigilar nuestros movimientos, Tisha. —Su voz ocultó la ansiedad que crecía en su interior—. El viento oscuro sigue soplando.

—Pero ¿qué has oído, Zareb?

—Era una advertencia —contestó Zareb sin mentir—. Los espíritus siguen protegiendo el lugar. Debemos ser cautos para no disgustarlos.

Camelia clavó los ojos en la roca pintada, pensando en la advertencia de Zareb.

—Si de verdad la Tumba de los Reyes no quisiera ser descubierta, a estas alturas ya me habría echado de aquí.

—Algunos dirían que ha matado a varios hombres y ahuyentado a la mayoría de los trabajadores; que te ha enviado meses de sequía seguidos de meses de lluvias e inundaciones; que los pasadizos que se tardaron semanas en hacer se han derrumbado, que las máquinas han sido destruidas o no funcionan, y que no hay más dinero para continuar excavando. En Londres te agredieron, destrozaron la casa de tu padre y durante el viaje hasta aquí has estado tan enferma que pensé que no sobrevivirías. —Con expresión casi suplicante añadió—: ¿Te parece obstáculos suficientes para disuadirte, Tisha?

—Quizá sí —reconoció Camelia, con los ojos aún clavados en la roca. Alzó una mano para reseguir con los dedos la silueta del león—. O quizá son una serie de desafíos, pruebas que me revelan si realmente merezco descubrir la Tumba de los Reyes.

Zareb la miró en silencio. ¡Cómo iba a interpretarlo de otra manera! La sangre de lord Stamford fluía por sus venas y su padre jamás se había arredrado ante un desafío.

Aunque el desafío en cuestión fuera una niña de diez años sola y vulnerable que le había suplicado a su padre que no la enviase de vuelta a Inglaterra.

—¿Qué ha sido eso? —inquirió Camelia, dirigiendo la mirada hacia la excavación.

—Yo diría que eran aplausos —contestó Zareb.

Camelia se puso de pie y usó su mano a modo de visera para protegerse del sol.

—¿Ése no es Oliver bailando?

—Sí, con Senwe y Badrani —dijo Zareb sonriendo—. Deduzco que están contentos porque el señor Kent al fin ha logrado que la bomba funcione. Escucha, ¿oyes el ruido que hace?

Camelia inclinó la cabeza y escuchó las fuertes exhalaciones rítmicas de la bomba de Simon.

—¡Lo ha conseguido! —gritó eufórica—. ¡Sabía que lo lograría!

—¿Nos acercamos a verlo?

Camelia avanzó varios pasos y de repente se paró en seco.

—Ve tú, Zareb. Tengo mucho que hacer aquí.

—¿Estás segura, Tisha?

Se sentó de nuevo en el suelo, delante de la roca, y volvió a abrir el diario de su padre.

—Sí, ya me contarás luego qué tal funciona.

Zareb titubeó; por un lado deseaba quedarse a vigilarla, pero por el otro sabía que en ese momento ella necesitaba estar sola.

—Está bien. Tú quédate con Tisha —le ordenó a Oscar, que había bajado del hombro de Camelia para subirse al de Zareb—. Y ven corriendo a buscarme, si ves que me necesita.

Obediente, Oscar se sentó en otra piedra cercana.

Zareb se volvió y anduvo en dirección a la excavación, donde, al parecer, Oliver estaba enseñando a Badrani y a Senwe los pasos de algún baile escocés. Los dos khoikhoi se desternillaron de risa mientras, para divertimento del resto de nativos, imitaban los extraños y espasmódicos movimientos de Oliver.

Zareb decidió ir a comprobar qué tal iba la bomba, para ver con sus propios ojos que realmente funcionaba. Después volvería junto a Camelia y la acompañaría hasta el campamento. La advertencia del viento no había dejado lugar a dudas.

El peligro era inminente, estaba cada vez más cerca.

Capítulo 14

—De verdad, Oscar, mira la que estás organizando —lo regañó Camelia—. ¿Es necesario que comas las tortas de avena encima de mi mesa?

Oscar se introdujo el resto de tortas en la boca, con lo que un montón de migas cayeron sobre los libros y los papeles de Camelia.

—Además, ¿se puede saber de dónde narices las has sacado? —murmuró mientras levantaba el diario de su padre y sacudía las migas—. No recuerdo haber metido tortas de avena en mis maletas.

Oscar cogió una pluma que se le había caído a Harriet y se la puso sobre las cejas.

—Si te las ha dado Oliver, te agradecería que te las comieras en su tienda —le ordenó Camelia con firmeza—. Harriet, por favor, a ver si puedes picotear unas cuantas migas.

Le ofreció al pájaro un trozo de torta, tentándole a abandonar el respaldo de la silla de Camelia, y éste empezó a picotear con delicadeza los restos de comida de la mesa.

—A partir de ahora está prohibido comer en mi tienda de campaña; así no dejaréis todo perdido mientras intento trabajar.

Oscar la miró con pesar.

—Rupert nunca come aquí dentro —añadió Camelia lanzándole una mirada a la serpiente, que estaba enroscada en medio de la cama—. Sale a buscar una lagartija pequeña o algún ratón rollizo y luego vuelve y se enrosca para digerirla. Nunca desordena nada.

—No sabía que las serpientes fuesen tan pulcras —silabeó una voz en tono ligeramente burlón.

Boquiabierta, Camelia se volvió y vio a Simon de pie en la entrada de su tienda.

—Tendré que decírselo a Byron, mi hermano pequeño —comentó—. Así podrá añadirlo a la lista de atributos que está elaborando para mis padres sobre por qué las serpientes son unas mascotas excelentes —dijo arqueando las cejas—. ¿Puedo pasar, Camelia? ¿O estás decidida a seguir evitándome?

—Yo no te evito —contestó ella con ingenuidad, concentrada ahora en ordenar los libros y papeles de su mesa—. Es sólo que he estado muy ocupada.

—Eso me ha dicho Zareb. Pero aun así, pensé que podrías encontrar tiempo en tu apretada agenda para venir a ver lo bien que funciona la bomba. Durante más de una semana me he pasado día y noche peleándome con ella. En un momento dado hasta pensé que no lograría lidiar con el agua fangosa de la excavación.

En su voz había cansancio y Camelia dejó de ordenar la mesa, y lo miró.

Tenía ojeras y daba la impresión de que en la frente tenía más arrugas que antes. Su cabello era una salvaje maraña cobriza aclarada por el sol, que seguramente se había convertido en el súmmum para los trabajadores nativos, ya que ahora su color era más parecido al del fuego que la noche que llegaron. El sol africano había bronceado su piel, pero por la rojez de su nariz y mejillas Camelia supo que había estado demasiado rato bajo sus severos rayos. Tenía barba de varios días que oscurecía su mandíbula y sus mejillas estaban indudablemente chupadas, lo que indicaba que no había hecho pausas para comer o afeitarse. Llevaba su habitual conjunto de camisa blanca arrugada y arremangada, que dejaba a la vista un vendaje en su antebrazo izquierdo. Sus pantalones estaban tremendamente arrugados pero limpios, lo que quería decir que se había aseado y cambiado antes de ir a verla.

—Lo siento —se disculpó Camelia arrepentida—. Cuando me enteré de que al fin funcionaba la bomba y oí que todo el mundo aplaudía, estuve a punto de salir corriendo para ir a verlo. Me sentí tan aliviada, emocionada y feliz que yo también tuve ganas de aplaudir. Creo que de haber ido, incluso hubiese intentado bailar ese ridículo baile que Oliver les enseñó a Badrani y a Senwe.

Simon la miró con curiosidad.

—¿Y por qué no viniste?

Ella apartó la vista.

—Supongo que no sabía cómo hacerte frente.

—Pues de la misma manera que lo hiciste después de pasar nuestra primera noche juntos en mi estudio de Londres —repuso él—. No me dio la impresión de que tuvieses ninguna dificultad entonces.

—Fuiste tú quien me evitó en Londres —reprochó Camelia—. Te encerraste en el comedor durante una semana entera.

Él enarcó las cejas sorprendido.

—¿Es eso lo que crees que hice? ¿Evitarte?

—¿Acaso no es cierto?

—Estaba construyendo la bomba. Cuando trabajo en un invento me dedico a él por completo y me olvido de todo los demás, incluso de comer, dormir e interactuar con el resto de seres humanos. Mi familia no deja de decirme que no es normal —dijo sacudiendo con tristeza la cabeza—. Y supongo que tienen razón, pero para mí sí es normal. Como lo es para ti vivir en una tienda de campaña en plenas llanuras africanas excavando en busca de una mítica tumba antigua.

Camelia lo miró con incertidumbre.

—No podemos cambiar lo que ha ocurrido entre nosotros, Camelia. —Habló con voz grave y cargada de resignación—. Y aunque pudiese hacerlo, por muy descortés que te parezca, no lo haría. Lo único que podemos controlar es cómo reaccionamos a ello. Y al menos yo no pienso dejar que la... —Hizo una pausa tratando de dar con la palabra adecuada—... «fuerza» —dijo con torpeza— que surge entre nosotros cada vez que estamos juntos ponga en peligro tu trabajo. Te prometí que te construiría una bomba y que enseñaría a tus hombres a manejarla. Y tengo la intención de cumplir mi palabra, decidas o no evitarme durante el resto de mi estancia aquí. Eso es todo lo que quería decirte. —Abrió la tienda dispuesto a salir.

—Espera.

Simon se detuvo y la miró expectante.

—¿Qué te ha pasado en el brazo?

—Me corté con uno de los dientes de la bomba —contestó encogiéndose de hombros—. No es nada.

—¿Le has dicho a Zareb que le eche un vistazo?

—Zareb se ofreció muy amablemente a untarlo con estiércol y grasa de antílope, pero decliné su oferta.

—¿Y qué me dices de Oliver?

—Oliver decidió que había que sangrar la herida. Después de que le ordenase guardar su puñal, le preguntó a Zareb si sabía dónde podían encontrar unas cuantas sanguijue-las sedientas. Zareb se ofreció a buscar gusanos, asegurando que me chuparían la sangre tan bien como cualquier sangui-juela inglesa. Entonces fue cuando decidí vendarme el brazo yo solo.

—Déjame echarle un vistazo.

—No es más que un arañazo, Camelia.

—Aquí hasta un arañazo puede ser mortal, si no se cura adecuadamente. Siéntate y déjame examinar la herida.

Simon suspiró y se sentó a regañadientes en la silla.

—¿Te la habrás lavado al menos? —le preguntó mientras le sacaba con cuidado el vendaje.

—Sí.

—Pues jamás lo habría dicho. —Miró la herida al descu-bierto con la frente arrugada—. Esto está sucísimo.

—Tenía prisa.

—Hay que volverla a limpiar y me temo que tendré que darte unos cuantos puntos para cerrarla —decidió—; de lo contrario, se volverá a abrir y podría infectarse.

—No pienso dejar que Zareb ni Oliver se me acerquen: Oliver es capaz de hacerme un corte en el otro brazo mien-tras Zareb me cubre de gusanos. Prefiero correr el riesgo de que se me infecte.

—Yo te coseré.

Simon la miró con incredulidad.

—¿Sabes coser heridas?

—Sí. ¿Te sorpende?

—Supongo que no más que todas las otras cosas que he descubierto en ti —respondió, encogiéndose de hombros.

—Mi padre se empeñó en que aprendiese a curar heridas cuando tenía quince años. Era un poco aprensivo, como tú.

—Yo no soy aprensivo —protestó Simon ofendido.

—Verás, no creía en los métodos curativos de los nativos —rectificó Camelia mientras con una jarra de metal llenaba la jofaina de agua—. Así que un día, en nuestra casa de Ciudad del Cabo, hizo venir a un médico para que me enseñase a curar heridas, torceduras, quemaduras y demás. —Hundió una toalla en la palangana y cogió una pastilla de jabón—. Pensó que me resultaría útil saber algo de primeros auxilios cuando estuviésemos viviendo en una excavación. —Se acercó al gran baúl que había a los pies de su cama y se puso a buscar su botiquín.

—Veo que era tremendamente pragmático.

—Cuando quería, mi padre podía ser muy pragmático. —Abrió el botiquín y extrajo una aguja, hilo, unas cuantas gasas y un frasco de linimento—. Excepto en lo relativo a su trabajo. Ahí sí que no se dejaba intimidar por los obstáculos que se interponían en su camino; aunque todo el mundo le aconsejase que debía rendirse.

—A veces es más fácil no rendirse.

Ella lo miró sorprendida.

—¿Por qué dices eso?

—Porque rendirse le obliga a uno a volcar su tiempo y su energía en otra cosa. Si eso se hace con un proyecto relativamente pequeño, no cuesta mucho, pero si se trata de un objetivo que ha sido una obsesión durante toda una vida, admitir la derrota y seguir adelante es mucho más difícil.

—Mi padre no cometió un error al dedicar gran parte de su vida a la búsqueda de la Tumba de los Reyes. Me imagino que sabrás que algunos de los descubrimientos más importantes del mundo son el resultado de años y años de duro trabajo y una determinación inalterable.

—También hay un sinfín de casos de personas que se han pasado la vida buscando algo y no lo han encontrado.

—La Tumba de los Reyes existe, Simon. Estoy segura de ello.

—No te estoy diciendo lo contrario.

—Y no pararé hasta que la encuentre.

Él la miró fijamente.

—Lo sé.

Camelia desvió la vista, repentinamente incapaz de mirarlo a los ojos.

—Quizá sería mejor que te echaras en la cama mientras te curo —sugirió al tiempo que dejaba cuanto necesitaba en la pequeña mesa que había junto a la cama.

—En la silla estoy bien. Prometo no desmayarme.

—Lo decía por mí.

—Si vas a desmayarte, entonces eres tú quien debería usar la cama —le ofreció galantemente.

—Te aseguro que no me desmayaré —repuso Camelia, que trasladó a Rupert al mullido montón de ropa que había en su maleta—. Tardaré un rato en coserte la herida y me sería más cómodo hacerlo desde la silla mientras tú estás tumbado en la cama.

Simon suspiró.

—Muy bien. —Fue hasta el catre y se echó sobre él. La cama crujió en señal de protesta bajo su peso.

—Te has hecho un corte muy feo —comentó Camelia mientras le limpiaba la herida—. Habrá que irlo limpiando y cambiando el vendaje a menudo para que no supure.

Simon se incorporó sobre el otro codo para poder ver la herida.

—Pues a mí no me parece que sea tan grave, Camelia. No creo que haga falta coserlo. Cámbiame las vendas y ya está.

—Como acabes con fiebre, Zareb te meterá en la tienda de campaña y se pondrá a encender hogueras a tu alrededor —le advirtió Camelia con seriedad—. Y a la mínima que te despistes te cubrirá el brazo de gusanos.

—Supongo que si tengo que elegir entre tu afilada aguja y una horda de gusanos hambrientos, sin duda prefiero que me cosas la herida. —Se tumbó de nuevo y cerró los ojos, resignándose a su destino.

—No descartes los gusanos tan deprisa —replicó Camelia mientras enhebraba la aguja—. Se usan para curar desde hace siglos. Los soldados cuyas heridas eran infestadas de gusanos tenían más posibilidades de sobrevivir que los demás; esos bichos se comen el tejido muerto y ayudan a mantener las heridas limpias.

Simon frunció las cejas.

—¿Es ésta tu forma de distraer mi atención mientras me clavas una aguja?

—Pero si aún no he empezado.

—Ni lo harás como sigas hablando de gusanos.

—De acuerdo. Pensaba que, siendo científico, te parecería un tema interesante.

—Hay muchos temas que me interesan, pero hablar de gusanos que se comen tejidos muertos para que las heridas abiertas no supuren no es precisamente uno de ellos.

—¿Ves cómo eres *aprensivo*? —repuso Camelia triunfal.

—Lo único que he dicho es que intentemos hablar de algo más agradable mientras me coses —contestó Simon—. ¿Es eso mucho pedir?

—En absoluto. Ahora, por favor, échate antes de que apoyes demasiado peso en el brazo y vuelva a sangrar.

A regañadientes, Simon se tumbó de nuevo en la cama y cerró los ojos.

Camelia examinó el corte en silencio para decidir cuál era la mejor manera de coserlo. La herida era profunda pero bastante recta, lo que era bueno. Pensó que lo mejor sería hacer una serie de pequeños puntos, dejando entre ellos suficiente espacio para dejar paso a la sangre que pudiese seguir saliendo...

—¿A qué esperas? —inquirió Simon con irritación, incorporándose.

—Estoy pensando cómo coser el corte.

—No necesito que hagas ningún diseño especial; ¡ni que estuvieras tejiendo una colcha!

—No he tejido una colcha en mi vida, así que de diseños especiales nada de nada —dijo ella con socarronería—. Hay que cerrar bien el corte para que se cure bien. No querrás que te quede una cicatriz fea, ¿verdad?

—Te aseguro que me da igual cómo quede, pero me gustaría que acabaras antes de que me entierren.

—Si dejaras de incorporarte constantemente y de interrumpirme, ya habría terminado.

—No es necesario que lo cosas, en serio —insistió Simon—. La herida ya está limpia, véndala y me iré —dijo mientras empezaba a levantarse de la cama.

Camelia se puso de pie para impedírselo.

—Simon Kent, si no te echas ahora mismo, tendré que obligarte por la fuerza.

Él la miró divertido.

—Una amedrentadora amenaza viniendo de una mujer que apenas me llega al pecho. ¿Y cómo piensas obligarme exactamente?

—No me subestimes sólo porque sea una mujer —advirtió Camelia.

—Esto no tiene nada que ver con el hecho de que seas una mujer; es una constatación —le aseguró Simon—. Una cuestión de estatura.

—Pues no me parece un punto de vista muy científico —repuso ella—, al fin y al cabo, hasta se puede derribar un elefante con una bala diminuta.

—¿No pensarás dispararme?

—No, porque entonces tendría que curar dos heridas en lugar de una.

—¡Qué sensibilidad la tuya!

—Échate, Simon.

—De verdad, Camelia, tu oferta es tentadora, pero creo sinceramente que mi brazo tiene mucho mejor aspecto ahora que lo has limpiado. Véndalo en un momento y seguro que se curará de maravilla.

—No pienso vendarlo hasta que lo haya cosido.

—Muy bien, pues lo haré yo. —Empezó a levantarse.

—Lo siento mucho, Simon. —Le agarró del meñique de la mano derecha y tiró de él hacia atrás con fuerza.

—¡Dios mío...! —gritó, tambaleándose y cayendo en la cama.

Camelia le soltó el dedo y lo miró con naturalidad.

—¿Vas a dejar que te cosa?

Él la miró indignado.

—¿Dónde has aprendido este desagradable truquillo?

—Me lo enseñó Zareb —contestó ella mientras escurría la toalla—. Pensó que me iría bien saber unas cuantas tácticas de defensa, por si algún día me encontraba en una situación en la que pudiese necesitarlas.

—A juzgar por tu habilidad diría que has tenido ocasión de ponerla en práctica con anterioridad.

—No, en realidad es la primera vez que uso este truco. —Volvió a limpiarle la herida—. Hasta ahora sólo había ensayado con Zareb, y lógicamente no hacía fuerza de verdad. —Tiró la toalla en la jofaina y sonrió—. Le gustará saber que ha funcionado.

—Preferiría que esto quedara entre nosotros. Creo que mi orgullo masculino ya ha sufrido bastante como para que encima lo vayas contando por todo el campamento.

—Como tú quieras. —Cogió la aguja y la enherbró otra vez—. ¿Necesitas algo antes de que empiece? —le preguntó con dulzura—. Un trago de whisky, tal vez... o algo para morder.

—Sí, una cosa.

—Dime.

La cogió, la puso encima de él y la besó.

Camelia gritó y forcejeó, pero Simon la sostuvo con fuerza y la besó apasionadamente mientras le acariciaba la espalda con posesividad, y sus piernas se entrelazaban.

Sólo quería calmar su orgullo herido y marcarse un tanto; quizá fuese infantil, pero a él le parecía de lo más lógico. Sin embargo, era embriagador tener a Camelia entre sus brazos, desatando la extraordinaria pasión que había procurado ocultar tras las interminables noches en vela y las horas de duro trabajo. La atrajo hacia sí y la besó con ternura, explorando con la lengua la dulce y oscura humedad de su boca, persuadiéndola, suplicante, intentando hacerle entender lo que, al parecer, no sabía expresar con palabras.

Camelia permaneció unos instantes inmóvil, notando cómo se evaporaban los últimos vestigios de autocontrol.

Y a continuación gimió y presionó su cuerpo contra el de Simon, su esbelta suavidad se fundió con las duras superficies y curvas de él, que tan maravillosamente familiares y excitantes le resultaban. Entrelazó los dedos en su enmarañado cabello aclarado por el sol, sintiéndose repentinamente ansiosa por notar su tacto, sus besos, su deseo. Si el fuego que había entre ellos era erróneo, entonces su vida entera era un error. Era lo único en lo que podía pensar mientras abría la boca y le regalaba besos por su elegante y marcada mandíbula al tiempo que con los dedos le desabrochaba frenéticamente los botones de su arrugada camisa de hilo.

Lo deseaba con una desesperación abrumadora, más de lo que había deseado nada en toda su vida. De modo que se concentró únicamente en la sensación que le producía su imponente cuerpo, que se removía debajo de ella, en su masculino aroma, que le embriagaba los sentidos, en el sabor a la vez salado y dulce de su preciosa piel bronceada, que tentaba su lengua mientras Camelia descendía por la tensa columna de su cuello, mordisqueándolo, lamiéndolo y besándolo.

«Te deseo», confesó en silencio, aunque tampoco era necesario que lo dijese en voz alta. Le sacó la camisa y besó los marcados músculos que esculpían su pecho.

«Te necesito», añadió, abrumada por la intensidad de su propio deseo. Siguió descendiendo por la dura superficie de su barriga. Simon dejó de abrazarla con tanta fuerza; sus caricias eran cada vez más castas y tiernas.

No sabía qué fuerza era ésta que los unía, pero era más potente que cuanto había conocido jamás. Más poderosa que sus ansias de independencia, más misteriosa que los secretos de la Tumba de los Reyes y más amedrentadora que el viento oscuro que, desde la muerte de su padre, había proyectado sus sombras sobre ella. Era una fuerza contra la que no podía luchar. Una fuerza contra la que, hasta cierto punto, tampoco quería luchar.

Jadeó y apoyó su mejilla contra el musculoso vientre de Simon, buscando alguna forma de explicarle cómo se sentía.

De pronto un fuerte ronquido inundó la tienda.

Camelia levantó la mirada, confusa. La expresión de Simon era casi aniñada, ahí tumbado con la cabeza felizmente apoyada en su almohada, completamente ajeno tanto al torbellino emocional que ella sentía como a sus apasionados besos. Debía de estar verdaderamente agotado, pensó. No le había mentido al decirle que había estado trabajando día y noche para conseguir que la bomba funcionase.

Moviéndose despacio para no despertarlo, Camelia bajó de la cama y, con cuidado, tapó a Simon con una manta antes de coserle rápidamente la herida y vendársela.

Y después se sentó frente a su mesa y, con los ojos empañados, se quedó mirando fijamente el diario de su padre, preguntándose de dónde sacaría las fuerzas para soportar el dolor cuando, al fin, Simon la abandonara.

Capítulo 15

—Despierta, chico —ordenó Oliver.

Simon gruñó y hundió la cabeza en la almohada.

—No quiero gusanos, Oliver. Ni estiércol. Lárgate.

—Tenemos que hablar con usted —insistió Zareb.

—Hágalo cuando me haya despertado. —Simon se tapó la cabeza tirando con fuerza de la manta y se puso de lado.

—Sé que estás cansado, muchacho —comentó Oliver con tranquilidad—, pero estoy seguro de que querrás oír lo que tenemos que decirte.

—Por el modo en que hablas, intuyo que no me gustará —dijo arrastrando las palabras—. ¿Qué problema hay? ¿Se ha acabado el estiércol?

—Me temo que es más grave que eso.

—¡Genial! ¿De qué se trata?

—Por desgracia, la bomba ha sufrido un pequeño percance.

Simon se destapó y lo miró con incredulidad.

—¿Qué quiere decir que ha sufrido «un percance»?

—Se ha caído —explicó Zareb—. Y se han producido algunos daños.

Simon se levantó de un salto de la cama de Camelia y, corriendo, salió de la tienda a la luz matutina sin prestar atención a lo que le contaba Zareb.

Los trabajadores, con expresión grave, estaban arremolinados alrededor de los enfangados terraplenes de la excavación. Al acercarse, Simon supo que estaban observando a Camelia, a Badrani, a Senwe, a Lloyd y a Elliott, que se movían por el agua fangosa, al parecer, en busca de algo. Entonces desvió la vista.

Y vio en el suelo los restos destrozados de su bomba de vapor.

Miró atónito la máquina hecha añicos. No era posible. Anduvo hasta la bomba lentamente. Tenía que estar soñando. Alargó un brazo y la tocó vacilante. El acero estaba caliente al tacto de su mano.

O sea, que no era un sueño. Era real.

Una furia total y absoluta se apoderó de él, tan intensa que le dejó momentáneamente sin habla.

—¿Podrás arreglarla?

Se volvió y vio a Camelia. Su cabello era una maraña dorada que colgaba sobre sus hombros, su vestido estaba empapado de agua y barro, y tenía las mejillas y la frente llenas de suciedad.

—Ten. —Abrió las manos mojadas y le enseñó un variado surtido de tornillos, tuercas, clavijas y demás piezas pequeñas y rotas de la máquina—. Las he encontrado en el agua. El resto también ha encontrado unas cuantas piezas. —Su voz era tensa—. Seguiremos buscando mientras empiezas a repararla.

Simon la miró con impotencia. Debajo de las manchas de suciedad su bello rostro estaba pálido y su elegante frente estaba arrugada por la preocupación. Sin embargo, sus ojos del color de la salvia lo miraban abiertos y esperanzados, iluminados por la magnitud de su propia determinación y quizás incluso la increíble confianza que, al parecer, tenía en él. Y al contemplar las profundidades de esos ojos extraordinarios, de pronto se sintió abrumado, tanto por lo maravilloso que era que ella creyese que él podía arreglar aquel desastre como por la absoluta certeza de que eso era imposible.

—Camelia —empezó a decir en voz baja y ronca—, no puedo arreglar esto.

—Te prometo encontrar todas las piezas —repuso fervientemente—. Buscaremos día y noche, si es necesario. En cuanto las tengas todas podrás volver a ensamblar la bomba.

Simon sacudió la cabeza.

—Aunque encontremos todas las piezas, no podré arreglarla. Los mecanismos de la válvula están gravemente dañados; la caldera se ha roto; los dientes de expansión están tremendamente torcidos y el eje se ha partido. No puedo arreglarla.

—Pediremos a Ciudad del Cabo los recambios que necesites. —Cerró el puño y apretó con fuerza el montón de tornillos y clavijas, negándose a aceptar la realidad—. Haz una lista, y Zarbe y yo iremos esta misma mañana a Kimberley para ver si allí conseguimos alguna pieza; el resto lo encargaremos en Ciudad del Cabo.

—No es tan sencillo, Camelia. La mayoría de las piezas las he diseñado yo y un soldador londinense las ha fabricado especialmente para mí. Son únicas.

—En ese caso le escribiremos una carta a tu soldador y le pediremos que nos haga más.

—Eso nos llevará meses, Camelia.

Ella lo miró directamente a los ojos, esforzándose por dar una imagen fuerte y decidida. Pero su labio inferior temblaba mientras se agarraba con fuerza de la falda sucia y arrugada. Estaba tan destrozada como él, pensó Simon. Sus trabajadores la miraban serios y en silencio, esperando para ver cómo reaccionaría a este último desastre. Eso fue lo que la mantuvo entera; era una luchadora, pero en ese momento, también era líder.

No podía permitir que el miedo y la decepción pudieran más que ella; de lo contrario, los pocos trabajadores que quedaban acabarían creyendo que, al fin, había sido derrotada.

Y se irían.

—Lo siento, señor Kent. —Avergonzado, Badrani se acercó despacio a Simon y a Camelia con la cabeza agachada—. La culpa ha sido mía. Anoche estuve yo de guardia. —Se arrodilló arrepentido frente a Camelia—. Castígueme como crea oportuno, mi señora.

—No pienso castigarlo, Badrani —le aseguró Camelia—. Levántese, por favor, y cuénteme qué pasó.

—Han sido los malos espíritus —declaró Badrani mientras se ponía de pie—. Llegaron tarde, cuando todo el campamento dormía, y me hechizaron para que yo también me durmiese. Cuando me desperté, la máquina estaba hecha añicos y habían tirado las piezas al agua.

Oliver lo miró con incredulidad.

—O sea, que se durmió cuando le tocaba hacer guardia.

—Fueron los malos espíritus —insistió Senwe, leal a su amigo—. Lo hechizaron.

—Yo más bien diría que la bebida lo hechizó —replicó Oliver, que frunció las cejas con reprobación—. ¿Qué bebió antes de la guardia?

—Sólo leche con miel —contestó Badrani.

—Vamos, hombre, no pretenderá que me crea que un tipo robusto como usted no bebe más que leche por las noches.

—Todos los khoikhoi bebemos leche desde que nacemos —intervino Zareb—. Hace que estemos fuertes.

—Si no me cree, mire en mi cantimplora; todavía no la he vaciado. —Badrani se sacó el recipiente hecho con cáscara de huevo de avestruz que llevaba colgado al cuello y se lo dio a Oliver—. Ahora ya no estará buena, pero anoche estaba fresca.

Oliver cogió la cantimplora y escudriñó su interior para cerciorarse. Mientras miraba el líquido blanco un sutil aroma le subió por las aletas de la nariz. Sorprendido, se acercó más el recipiente e inhaló de nuevo.

—¿Qué es? —inquirió Simon.

Oliver levantó la vista, serio.

—Láudano.

—¿Estás seguro?

—Sí.

Badrani frunció sus negras cejas confundido.

—¿Qué es el láudano?

—Un producto que da sueño, joven. Alguien puso láudano en su leche para que se durmiera.

—La miel debía de contrarrestar su sabor amargo —añadió Simon—; por eso no lo notó.

—Badrani, ¿se llenó usted mismo la cantimplora? —preguntó Lloyd, que había salido del agua para ir a reunirse con ellos.

Badrani asintió.

—Pero luego la dejé en mi tienda para que estuviese fría hasta que empezara la guardia.

—Así que cualquiera pudo haber entrado en su tienda y echarle unas cuantas gotas de láudano —comentó Camelia.

—Entonces ¿no fueron los malos espíritus?

—No —contestó Camelia—. No han sido los malos espíritus.

El alivio se reflejó en el rostro del guapo guerrero.

—Sea o no culpa de los malos espíritus, tenemos un serio problema —constató Simon con pesar—. La bomba está rota y la excavación sigue inundada.

—Yo diría que el problema es incluso más grave que eso, chico —añadió Oliver—. Hay algún desgraciado que intenta ahuyentarnos de aquí.

—Oliver tiene razón. —Empapado y lleno de barro, Elliott salió del perímetro de la excavación y le dio a Simon otro puñado de tornillos y tuercas de la bomba—. Las bombas anteriores que Camelia alquiló también sufrieron daños, pero nunca hasta este extremo. Quienquiera que haya hecho esto sabía lo que hacía. —Paseó la mirada por los trabajadores que estaban allí—. ¿Vio ayer alguno de ustedes a alguien entrando en la tienda de campaña de Badrani, antes de que iniciara su guardia?

Los nativos se miraron unos a otros nerviosos y a continuación sacudieron vehementemente sus cabezas.

—No creo que fuera ninguno de mis hombres, Elliott —objetó Camelia—. Son buenas personas, trabajan duro y respetaban a mi padre. Dudo que hallan hecho algo así.

—No obstante, no han ocultado el hecho de que consideran que ha caído una maldición sobre la excavación —argumentó Elliott—. Si de verdad creen que la Tumba de los Reyes existe, está claro que no quieren que sea descubierta. Prefieren hacerte perder el tiempo y seguir cobrando mientras, en secreto, sabotean tus esfuerzos.

—Cuando los africanos luchamos, lo hacemos abiertamente, lord Wickham —dijo Zareb con fingida docilidad—.

No es propio de nosotros mentir y engañar como acaba de sugerir.

—Lo lamento, Zareb, pero lo cierto es que no todos los nativos son como usted —replicó Elliott con naturalidad—. Alguien ha hecho esto, y es evidente que no han sido los malditos espíritus, sino alguien que quiere impedir la continuidad de la excavación.

—Lo que creo que es evidente es que esté o no ese canalla entre nosotros, no parará hasta conseguirlo —comentó Oliver.

—Razón por la cual tenemos que cogerlo —insistió Elliott.

—Puedo hacer que más hombres vigilen el campamento por las noches, pero no serán muchos más —sugirió Lloyd—. Todos trabajan de sol a sol y por la noche están demasiado cansados para vigilar el campamento.

—¿Por qué no hacemos que seis hombres duerman en tres turnos diferentes durante el día para que así por la noche puedan estar de guardia también en tres turnos distintos? —propuso Camelia—. Si vigilan el campamento de dos en dos, uno siempre podrá dar la alarma si algo le sucede al otro.

—La idea es buena —dijo Elliott volviéndose a Simon—. ¿Y usted qué opina, Kent? ¿Podrá arreglar la bomba? Porque, si me dice que sí, ahora mismo me meto en el agua y me pongo a buscar más piezas.

Simon miró a Elliott sorprendido. Wickham tendría que estar encantado de que la bomba se hubiese roto. Era un fracaso más de Camelia, un argumento más a su favor para que abandonase la excavación. Pero Elliott miraba a Simon con decisión, aparentemente deseoso de ayudar de alguna forma. Simon pensó que lo que intentaba era demostrarle a Camelia que la apoyaba; al fin y al cabo, tenía muchas más posibilidades de ganarse su estima si al menos fingía defender su sueño. O tal vez Elliott abrigara en secreto la esperanza de que Camelia encontrase al fin la Tumba de los Reyes; pese a que afirmaba que ya no creía en su existencia, cabía la posibilidad de que en su fuero interno sí lo creyese. Fuese por la razón que fuese, en lugar de recomendarle a Camelia que se diese por vencida estaba tratando de ayudarle, justo cuando ella necesitaba más apoyo que nunca.

Sólo por eso, Simon le perdonó por ser un idiota y un engreído.

—Es posible que pueda arreglarla. —No quería darle demasiadas esperanzas a Camelia y que después se llevara una decepción—. No lo sabré hasta que la haya examinado realmente y vea la gravedad de los daños. Pero aunque la arregle, Camelia, quiero que entiendas que tardaré semanas o incluso meses.

Camelia asintió. Semanas. Meses. Tiempo durante el cual debería serguir pagando a sus trabajadores con el poco dinero que le quedaba. Antes de irse de Londres, lord Cadwell aceptó a regañadientes invertir dinero en su excavación. Asimismo había conseguido convencer a sus acreedores londinenses de que le dieran algo más de tiempo, asegurándoles que en breve podría empezar a devolver los enormes préstamos. Pensó que con la ayuda de Simon no tardaría en extraer el agua de la excavación y finalmente encontraría la preciada Tumba de los Reyes.

La destrucción de la bomba había sido un duro revés.

—De acuerdo. —De algún modo logró fingir tranquilidad, pero por dentro tenía ganas de gritar—. Simon, si me haces una lista de lo que crees que necesitarás, Zareb y yo iremos a Kimberley en el carro esta misma mañana y lo pediremos. Hasta entonces seguiremos sacando el agua con cubos, como hemos hecho hasta ahora.

—Muy bien, ¡a trabajar! —exclamó Lloyd—. Traigan junto a este terraplén de aquí todos los cubos y recipientes disponibles en el campamento. Cuando el nivel de agua descienda, buscaremos más piezas de la bomba. ¡Tengan los ojos bien abiertos! ¡Ya hemos perdido media mañana!

—Vete a cambiar, Camelia —sugirió Elliott con suavidad—. Yo seguiré buscando.

—No hace falta que me cambie hasta que me vaya a Kimberley, Elliott —repuso Camelia—. Me quedaré aquí y también seguiré buscando.

Simon la observó mientras bajaba de nuevo a la excavación y empezaba otra vez a buscar a tientas en el agua fangosa. Elliott suspiró e hizo lo propio.

—Esa chica es muy valiente —dijo Oliver al ver cómo hundía los brazos hasta los hombros en el charco oscuro—. Debe de tener antepasados escoceses.

—Tisha tiene espíritu africano —le informó Zareb—. Por eso le puse ese nombre. Significa «voluntarioso». Lo supe nada más verla.

—¿Y qué le pareció a lord Stamford que llamase así a su hija? —inquirió Simon.

—El señor estaba encantado de que yo la considerase una chica fuerte —contestó Zareb—. Cuando Camelia vino a África, su padre no las tenía todas consigo. Era menuda, y estaba pálida y perdida; era como una flor delicada. Le daba miedo que no pudiese soportar vivir tan lejos del mundo en el que había crecido. Por eso decidió llevársela a la tierra que ella conocía, a Inglaterra.

—¿Y por qué no lo hizo? —quiso saber Oliver.

—Porque enseguida se dio cuenta de que África hervía en el corazón de Tisha. África, su padre y la búsqueda de la Tumba de los Reyes. Durante muchos años no ha habido nada más en su vida. Pero el corazón puede cambiar —añadió con seriedad—, y lo que un día le llena no necesariamente le llena al día siguiente.

—Camelia nunca se irá de África, Zareb —declaró Simon con total seguridad—. Ella pertenece aquí, y lo sabe.

—No me refería a Tisha —repuso Zareb mirándolo fijamente.

Simon apartó la vista, repentinamente incómodo.

—Si quieren esa lista, será mejor que empiece ya. —Le lanzó una última mirada a Camelia, que seguía inclinada sobre el charco enfangado buscando más piezas de la bomba—. Con su permiso.

Camelia cogió aire y se sumergió en la agradable y purificadora agua del río, desprendiéndose de las capas de barro, polvo y desesperación de ese día. Cerró los ojos y avanzó por la suave y fresca oscuridad con rápidas brazadas, estirando mucho los brazos mientras con las piernas se impulsaba hacia delante, deslizándose a través de la extensión de ébano salpicada de estrellas. Procuró no pensar en nada más que en la sensación del agua que la rodeaba y la sostenía mientras se movía por ella. Continuó nadando, alejándose del montículo de tierra en el que había dejado la toalla y el camisón, y de la roca en la que Zareb, Harriet, Oscar y Rupert estaban sentados vigilándola con una linterna que le sirviese de guía.

Alejándose de la excavación, de la bomba hecha añicos de Simon y de las temerosas miradas de los nativos, preocupados de acabar también siendo víctimas de la maldición de Pumulani. De la ira de Elliott y la frustración de Simon, perceptible pese a su esfuerzo por ocultarla. De Oliver y de Zareb, que habían intentado animarla y ayudarle a mitigar la aplastante sensación de derrota que había amenazado con apoderarse de ella al ver la bomba en la enfangada excavación de su padre.

Y alejándose del doloroso recuerdo de su querido padre, que murió sin saber si el trabajo de toda una vida culminaría en un brillante descubrimiento o en una locura absurda.

Salió a la superficie y respiró. El sonido que emitió fue más un sollozo que una inhalación de aire. Se apresuró a respirar varias veces más, bien alto y con regularidad, por si Zareb la había oído llorar y se preocupaba de que algo le hubiese pasado.

—¿Estás bien, Tisha? —preguntó Zareb con inquietud.

—Sí, estoy bien. —Estaba de pie en la orilla del río, con Harriet en un hombro y Oscar en el otro, escudriñando la oscuridad—. Me había quedado sin aire, eso es todo.

—No deberías alejarte tanto —protestó—. Acércate un poco.

—Enseguida voy. Quiero nadar un poco más.

—Hace fresco, Tisha. Si coges frío, te pondrás enferma.

—Nunca me pongo enferma.

—Te pusiste enferma en el barco.

—No me marearé por nadar en el río de noche.

—Pero podrías resfriarte y tener fiebre. —Cogió su toalla y la sostuvo en lo alto—. ¡Venga, Tisha! Es tarde.

—Ahora mismo voy.

Se puso boca arriba para flotar, dejando que el agua formara un velo alrededor de su cabeza con su enmarañado y sedoso cabello, y sin poder oír lo que Zareb le decía. No quería desobecerle, pero tampoco quería salir ya del agua. No se oía nada salvo el susurro del agua; era como la llamada de una concha marina que anhela el océano. Suspiró y cerró los ojos.

«Mira hacia arriba.»

Sorprendida, abrió los ojos.

Se extendía sobre ella un manto negro y sedoso, salpicado de un puñado de titilantes estrellas plateadas. La luna se había escondido detrás de unas espumosas nubes, que suavizaban su luz nacarada, por lo que las estrellas brillaban incluso más que antes; eran como diminutas joyas en medio del aterciopelado cielo nocturno africano.

«Las estrellas te guiarán.»

Sobresaltada, miró a su alrededor. Zareb se había vuelto a sentar en la roca y le ofrecía nueces a Oscar.

—¿Has dicho algo, Zareb?

—Decía que deberías acercarte, Tisha. El agua está fría.

—¿No me has dicho nada sobre las estrellas?

—No, pero hoy brillan mucho. Si quieres observarlas, deberías hacerlo desde aquí.

—Dame un minuto más. —Con cautela, flotó boca arriba una vez más.

De nuevo estaba rodeada por el río. Se quedó completamente inmóvil, aguzando los sentidos, tratando de escuchar.

«Las estrellas te guiarán.»

—¿Has oído eso? —preguntó Camelia mirando en dirección a Zareb.

—¿El qué?

—Esa voz.

—Yo no he oído nada, Tisha. —Zareb miró a su alrededor—. Aquí no hay nadie más. Tal vez hayas oído a los hombres, están cantando en el campamento.

—No, no son voces cantando.

—Entonces debe de ser un animal.

—Tampoco.

Zareb estuvo un buen rato en silencio.

—¿Qué te ha dicho esa voz, Tisha? —inquirió con tranquilidad.

De pronto Camelia se sintió insegura y estúpida. Seguramente habría sido fruto de su imaginación; demasiadas horas
de sol.

—Nada.

Esperó a que Zareb le hiciese más preguntas, pero no dijo
nada.

Volvió a tumbarse boca arriba en el agua. Un par de minutos más y saldría para irse directamente a la cama. Era evidente que necesitaba dormir.

«Deja que las estrellas te guíen.»

Esta vez no se movió. Se quedó donde estaba, flotando en
el agua, intentando decidir si estaba enloqueciendo. Aunque
a juzgar por la normalidad de cuanto le rodeaba, no creía que
se estuviese volviendo loca.

«Deja que las estrellas te guíen.»

Zareb siempre había confiado en que las estrellas lo guia-
ban; era una de las razones por las que detestaba Londres. El
implacable velo de humo, hollín y nubes no sólo bloqueaba
los rayos del sol, sino que además le impedía a Zareb ver las
estrellas por la noche. Le daba igual la ordenada estructura de
la ciudad con calles, plazas y carreteras, lámparas de gas y señales de tráfico.

Sin estrellas, Zareb estaba perdido.

Camelia permaneció tumbada un instante más, respirando apenas. El río seguía meciéndola con suavidad. Aguzó el oído, pero no escuchó nada más. Confusa, se volvió y nadó hasta Zareb.

Y entonces oyó el rugido de un león.

—¿Qué pasa, Tisha? —preguntó Zareb con rostro realmente preocupado mientras ella se apresuraba a salir del río con la camisa y la ropa interior empapadas, y cogía la toalla que él le ofreció—. ¿Estás asustada?

—Tengo que ver la roca. —Se envolvió deprisa con la toalla y se puso las botas.

—Es tarde, Tisha —objetó Zareb—. Ya la verás mañana por la mañana, no se moverá de donde está.

—Tengo que verla ahora, Zareb.

—Por lo menos sécate y ponte esta ropa seca. No me iré de aquí hasta que te cambies. —Se puso de espaldas para darle un poco de intimidad mientras se vestía.

Y después sacudió la cabeza estupefacto cuando Oscar y Harriet empezaron a chillar para avisarle de que Camelia se había ido sin él.

Capítulo 16

—¡Simon, despierta!

Simon abrió un ojo con dificultad y frunció el ceño.

—¿Qué le pasa a mi forma de dormir que hace que todo el mundo quiera despertarme?

—Hemos estado excavando en el lugar equivocado —le informó Camelia.

—Maravilloso; cuéntamelo mañana. —Cerró el ojo y hundió la cabeza en la almohada.

—¡Simon! Hemos estado excavando en el sitio equivocado. ¿Acaso no te importa?

—Lo único que me importa ahora mismo es dormir unas cuantas horas más.

—Tienes toda la vida para dormir, Simon. —Le agarró de los hombros y lo sacudió con brusquedad—. ¡Despierta!

Él se puso boca arriba y la miró furioso.

—Si éste va ser siempre tu modo de despertarme, Camelia, te anticipo que nuestras mañanas van a ser bastante difíciles.

—Necesito que me escuches.

—De acuerdo; te escucho.

—¿Estás suficientemente despierto para entender lo que te he dicho?

—Estoy suficientemente despierto para entender que, si no te escucho, no me dejarás en paz. Que creo que ya es bastante.

—Hemos estado excavando en el lugar equivocado, Simon.

—Sí, ya me lo has dicho. Por lo que deduzco que sigues creyendo que hay una tumba.

—¡Pues claro que hay una tumba!

—Sólo quería asegurarme. ¿Tienes idea de dónde está?

—No estoy segura. Esperaba que tú me ayudaras a resolver el puzzle. Se te dan bien esa clase de cosas.

—¿Qué clase de cosas?

—Ya sabes, lo de pensar de una forma extraña.

—¿Pretendes convencerme de que te ayude a base de insultos?

—No te he insultado —contestó Camelia—. Ya te comenté que tú no ves las cosas como la mayoría de la gente. Donde la gente ve un impedimento, tú ves posibilidades. Eso es lo que hace que seas brillante.

—Si fuese brillante, habría construido una bomba capaz de seguir funcionando aunque la arrojasen a un charco gigante de barro —replicó Simon con sequedad—. O al menos habría elaborado un plan secundario razonable por si alguien destrozaba la bomba y la dejaba casi sin posibilidad de arreglo. Eso es lo que habría hecho un estratega brillante, cosa que obviamente yo no soy.

—Es imposible prever cada pequeño detalle que pueda salir mal.

—Yo no diría que hacer añicos un motor de vapor y lanzarlo al barro sea un pequeño detalle.

—¡Olvídate del motor de vapor, Simon! —Exasperada, Camelia se volvió para salir de la tienda—. ¿Vas a venir o no?

—Depende. ¿De verdad crees que soy brillante?

—Sí, increíblemente brillante. ¡Y ahora ven! —Abrió la abertura de la tienda con energía y desapareció en la oscuridad.

Suspirando, Simon bajó de la cama y se puso las botas cansado.

—...y luego si miras este león, también lo puedes interpretar de varias formas —continuó Camelia con seriedad, señalando el dibujo del león que había en la roca mientras Zareb sostenía la linterna—. Puede que el león esté a punto de atacar a uno de los antílopes o a un guerrero, lo que significa que simboliza peligro. Pero también es posible que sea el propio león el que esté en peligro, porque podría ser agredido por los antílopes o recibir un disparo de uno de los guerreros. O quizá en realidad no es un león, sino un chamán que ha adoptado la forma de un león; en cuyo caso no pueden matarlo y tampoco corre ningún peligro, ya que se considera que los chamanes son capaces de trascender las formas animales que en algunas ocasiones adoptan. Pero, si es así, ¿por qué lo dibujaron?

Simon bostezó.

Camelia le lanzó una mirada de irritación.

—¿Me has estado escuchando?

—Por asombroso que te parezca, sí. Y eso a pesar de que me has obligado a levantarme de la cama en plena madrugada después de haber estado dieciséis horas reparando tu motor de vapor. Creo que merezco al menos cierta indulgencia a la hora de bostezar.

—¿Qué crees que significa eso?

—Que necesito dormir más.

—¡Me refiero a las pinturas rupestres!

Simon suspiró.

—La verdad, no lo sé, Camelia. La arqueología es tu especialidad, no la mía. Lo que no comprendo es a qué ha venido ese impulso de hacerme venir aquí de noche para debatir el significado de estos dibujos. ¿No podías esperar hasta mañana?

—No.

—¿Por qué no?

—Porque en estas pinturas hay estrellas. —Señaló las descoloridas estrellas amarillas que había encima de los antílopes y los guerreros—. Me he pasado años estudiándolo y sacando la misma conclusión que mi padre: que las estrellas simbolizaban la parte mítica del dibujo. Pero ahora creo que mi padre se equivocó. No creo que las estrellas simbolicen la espiritualidad de los animales o un chamán. Creo más bien que son una especie de guía; puede que hasta un mapa para indicarnos dónde está la tumba.

—¿Qué clase de mapa?

—No lo sé —reconoció ella—. Por eso quería que le echaras un vistazo. Zareb y yo lo hemos estado estudiando durante más de una hora hasta que al final he ido a despertarte; no hemos podido descifrar el significado de las estrellas.

—Tal vez no signifiquen nada, Camelia.

—Significan algo —insistió ella—. Son una guía. Estoy convencida de ello.

—¿Por qué de repente estás tan segura?

Camelia titubeó. De algún modo pensó que aquél no era el momento adecuado para decirle a Simon que unas voces extrañas le habían susurrado cosas en el río.

—Es un presentimiento; como me sucedió cuando llegamos a la costa africana. Tú mismo me dijiste que a veces la intuición es lo único en lo que podemos confiar.

Simon se volvió a Zareb.

—¿Y usted qué opina, Zareb?

—Creo que esta noche Pumulani le ha hablado a Tisha —contestó con seriedad—. A lo mejor la Tumba de los Reyes ha accedido a ser descubierta.

—Entonces ¿por qué no le da una pista más clara que no sea este misterioso jeroglífico de estrellas, leones y chamanes?

—Pumulani habrá tenido sus motivos para permanecer oculto. Y cuando finalmente decida salir a la luz, también tendrá sus motivos. No podemos entenderlo todo.

Simon suspiró. Como estaba bastante claro que Camelia no iba a dejarle volver a la cama, pensó que por lo menos podría intentar entender de qué demonios hablaban Zareb y ella.

—De acuerdo, pues —empezó diciendo mientras se concentraba en la enorme roca—. Aquí tenemos el león, aquí los antílopes y aquí los guerreros, que, por cierto, están un poco escuálidos. Entonces, aquí arriba hay varias estrellas. Veamos, hay... cuatro, cinco, seis estrellas.

—Cinco —le corrigió Camelia.

—Yo veo seis.

—Pues sólo hay cinco —insistió Camelia—. Mira, ¿lo ves? Mi padre dibujó cinco en su diario —explicó mientras abría el cuaderno de notas de su padre para enseñárselo.

—Puede que tu padre dibujara sólo cinco, pero yo sigo viendo seis —repuso Simon—. Zareb, ¿le importaría acercar un poco más la linterna, por favor?

Zareb se acercó y un haz de luz dorada iluminó la gastada superficie de la antigua roca.

—¿Ves como hay seis estrellas? —concluyó Simon señalando cada una de ellas.

—Lo último que has señalado no es una estrella —objetó Camelia—. Es la roca, que está un poco gastada. A lo mejor fue cincelada con algo.

—La cinceló la persona que esculpió una estrella —insistió Simon—. Cuatro ojos ven mejor que dos. Mira, pasa el dedo por encima y te convencerás de que es una estrella .

—Es posible —admitió Camelia mientras acariciaba la áspera superficie—. Pero aun así, ¿qué significan?

—No sé lo que significan. Yo solo digo que veo seis estrellas, no cinco.

—Está bien. Hay seis estrellas. ¿Qué más ves?

Simon frunció las cejas y contempló la sencilla escena dibujada.

—No creo que las estrellas concuerden con ninguna de las constelaciones aceptadas como tales, de modo que es difícil saber si el artista intentaba dibujar algo concreto en el cielo.

—Quienquiera que dibujase esto era imposible que estuviese al tanto de las constelaciones existentes —intervino Zareb—. Por aquel entonces no tenían telescopios para ver más allá de lo que veían sus ojos.

—En ese caso podría tratarse de una distribución aleatoria de las estrellas, que simplemente nos indica que la escena de caza tiene lugar de noche.

—Pero los cazadores no cazan de noche —argumentó Camelia—. Cazan durante el día, cuando los animales pastan y la luz es buena. Así que el hecho de que el artista dibujase estas estrellas es relevante. Algo tienen que significar. He intentado visualizar líneas imaginarias entre ellas para ver si constituían alguna especie de patrón, pero no he sacado nada en claro.

—¿No te parece que tienen la forma de una cometa? —dijo Simon—. Aunque dudo que aquellas tribus tuviesen cometas.

—¿Dónde ves una cometa? —inquirió Camelia—. Porque si ordenas las estrellas, lo que forman es un triángulo.

—Ahora incluye la sexta estrella que pensabas que era una simple muesca en la roca. Si dibujas una línea de una estrella a otra, ésta última de aquí forma el vértice superior de una cometa. —Simon trazó una línea imaginaria entre las estrellas para enseñárselo—. ¿Lo ves? Es una cometa.

Camelia abrió los ojos desmesuradamente.

—Es un escudo —constató con un susurro.

Simon se encogió de hombros.

—Llámalo como quieras. Personalmente, creo que se parece más a una cometa que a un escudo.

A Camelia se le iluminó la cara de alegría.

—¡Claro! ¡Cómo no me he dado cuenta hasta ahora! Es un escudo suspendido en el cielo entre los antílopes y el león.

—¡Genial! ¿Y eso qué significa?

—El escudo representa la protección; intenta proteger algo o a alguien —explicó Camelia exaltada—. Y está dirigido hacia el león, o sea, que a quien protege es al león.

—¿Desde cuándo un león necesita protección?

—Es un león simbólico —le informó Zareb—. Representa a un espíritu poderoso.

—Y está colocado totalmente de cara a los guerreros y los antílopes —prosiguió Camelia—, y no tiene ninguna intención de salir corriendo, porque está custodiando algo... ¡La Tumba de los Reyes!

Intrigado, Simon enarcó las cejas.

—¿Y dónde está la Tumba?

Camelia se mordió el labio, indecisa. Alargó el brazo con cautela y acarició con el dedo el trazo que dibujaban las estrellas de la roca. Al llegar a la última estrella, la que estaba en el vértice superior del escudo, sintió calor en el dedo. Vaciló, insegura.

Y entonces el dedo empezó a descender lentamente por sí solo y se detuvo en el león.

—Está detrás del león —anunció Camelia en voz baja.

Simon echó un vistazo a la infinita oscuridad que los rodeaba.

—¿Y dónde es eso? Por desgracia, el dibujo no nos da ninguna pista y de haberla habido, ya se ha borrado.

«Deja que las estrellas te guíen.»

Camelia levantó la cabeza para mirar al cielo.

—Mira —susurró.

Simon también miró hacia el cielo. Había seis estrellas formando un escudo, que titilaban en contraste con el mar negro.

—¡Qué raro! —exclamó asombrado—. No recuerdo haber visto antes las estrellas así dispuestas.

Zareb contempló las estrellas y sonrió.

—Las cosas se revelan en el momento oportuno.

—Si desde la estrella de la punta superior dibujamos una línea imaginaria hacia abajo como la que has hecho antes en la roca, Camelia, el león queda más o menos aquí. —Simon señaló un oscuro grupo de arbustos y rocas que había junto al pie de la montaña.

—¡Vamos! —instó ella echando a correr hacia los arbustos.

—¿No podríamos hacer esto por la mañana? —suplicó Simon—. Si tenemos que empezar a remover tierra, preferiría que hubiese un poco más de luz y haber dormido un buen rato.

—Hay que hacerlo *ahora* —insistió Camelia, que se apresuró a examinar los arbustos y las rocas que había a su alrededor—. Las estrellas nos están indicando la dirección adecuada.

—Precisamente porque ya sabemos cuál es el sitio, podríamos dejar aquí una especie de marca —comentó Simon al reunirse con ella—. Sería mucho más fácil hacer esto de día.

—Tal vez Pumulani no esté destinado a ser descubierto a la luz del día. —Zareb se aproximó con Oscar y Harriet sentados majestuosamente sobre sus hombros—. Debemos respetar las señales que nos han sido dadas esta noche.

—Si no buscamos ahora la entrada a la tumba, es posible que perdamos la oportunidad de hacerlo. —Camelia empezó a remover los arbustos en busca de alguna pista que le indicase cuál era el siguiente paso—. Mirad por esta zona y moved cuanto veáis; pero tened cuidado, sería una pena estropear las reliquias que pudiéramos encontrar.

—Oscar, ya que estás aquí, ¿qué tal si buscas tú también? —Simon bajó al mono del hombro de Zareb y lo puso en el suelo—. Si encuentras algo, a lo mejor te daré una torta de avena. —Complaciente, Oscar corrió hasta una enorme roca y empezó a gesticular con exageración fingiendo empujarla con las patas.

—¡Qué extraño! —Camelia arqueó las cejas al ver un espeso montón de matorrales frente a la roca—. Estos matorrales son más espesos que los demás.

Se acercó hasta ellos y comenzó a rebuscar, intentando averiguar si ocultaban algo debajo.

Satisfecho de su trabajo, Oscar trepó a la roza que había tratado de empujar y extendió una pata reclamando su premio.

—¡Tampoco te ha costado tanto esfuerzo! —exclamó Simon.

Oscar puso cara de bueno y extendió la pata un poco más.

—Está bien, supongo que mereces algo al menos por haberlo intentado. —Simon se apoyó en la roca, metió la mano en el bolsillo y extrajo de él una torta de avena, que partió por la mitad—. Media para ti —dijo dándole la mitad a Oscar— y media para Harriet, que todavía no ha podido irse a dormir. —Se alejó de la roca y le dio a Harriet su trozo de torta.

—El león —susurró Camelia.

Confuso, Simon miró de nuevo hacia la roca.

Ahí estaba, borroso pero inconfundible, el tosco contorno de la cabeza de un león. Había permanecido oculto debajo de un sinfín de capas de suciedad, parcialmente removidas cuando Simon se había apoyado en la roca.

Camelia corrió hasta ella y se apresuró a sacudir el resto de polvo con las manos.

—¡Mira, está aquí! El león... ¡exactamente igual que en la otra roca!

—Lo más probable es que los guerreros tapasen el dibujo con barro y después plantasen esos arbustos delante para asegurarse que quedaba oculto —reflexionó Zareb.

—¡Hay que mover esta roca! —ordenó Camelia mientras la abrazaba y empezaba a empujar—. ¡Vamos, empujad fuerte!

—Camelia, espera, así no podrás moverla. —Simon examinó la pesada roca unos instantes, pensativo—. Necesitamos algo para levantarla, algo como una barra.

—Aquí no hay ninguna barra.

—No, pero podemos usar unas cuantas piedras pequeñas —decidió Simon mirando a su alrededor—. Nos servirán para sacar una poco de tierra de la base de la roca para que pierda estabilidad. Y luego entre los tres trataremos de volcarla.

Zareb asintió en señal de aprobación.

—A veces las herramientas más sencillas son las mejores.

Los tres se pusieron de rodillas y con las piedras empezaron rápidamente a remover la suave y fragmentada tierra que había debajo de la roca. Al cabo de un rato Simon consideró que habían sacado suficiente tierra.

—De acuerdo, y ahora agarrad la roca con fuerza —ordenó— y cuando cuente hasta tres apoyaremos todo nuestro peso en ella y empujaremos hasta que ceda. ¿Preparados?

Zareb y Camelia asintieron.

—Muy bien, pues, vamos allá. Uno... dos... ¡tres!

La roca se inclinó ligeramente.

—¡A empujar! —gritó Simon—. ¡Venga, más fuerte!

La áspera superficie de la piedra rechinó dolorosamente debajo de las manos de Camelia, cuyo cuerpo empezó a temblar contra el tremendo peso de la roca. Entornó los ojos y apretó la mandíbula con fuerza.

«Empuja —se repetía Camelia monótona y silenciosamente mientras apoyaba todo su peso y su fuerza contra la pesada roca—. Empuja, empuja, empuja...»

La roca se inclinó un poco más.

Y de pronto se le escapó de las manos y volcó con gran estrépito.

Camelia se quedó mirando la estrecha abertura que había en la base de la montaña, oculta hasta ahora por la roca. Del interior emergió un riachuelo negro de enormes y agitadas arañas, que corrían por el suelo como un pequeño ejército enemigo.

Oscar soltó un chillido y se subió al hombro de Simon.

—Supongo que preferirás esperar a mañana para entrar con unas linternas decentes —dijo Simon con una mueca de dolor, porque Oscar le tiraba del pelo.

Camelia sacudió la cabeza.

—Tengo que entrar ahora, Simon. Pero no creo que haya ningún peligro. Los espíritus no me habrían indicado el camino, si no quisieran que entrara.

—No son los espíritus lo que me da miedo; más bien me preocupan los bichos asquerosos que hay ahí dentro y que se deslizan, se arrastran, reptan, muerden y apestan.

—Muy bien, pues espérame aquí. —Camelia cogió la linterna y desapareció por la abertura.

Simon suspiró.

—Sabía que me diría esto. Está bien... Oscar, ¿vienes?

Oscar se abrazó con fuerza al cuello de Simon y enterró la cara en su pelo.

—Lo consideraré un sí. ¿Y usted, Zareb? ¿Le apetece arrastrarse por un diminuto pasadizo oscuro lleno de arañas y Dios sabe qué más en plena madrugada?

—Yo voy donde vaya Tisha —contestó Zareb con solemnidad—. Es mi destino.

—Estupendo, porque creo que será mucho más divertido si estamos los tres juntos.

Simon se arrodilló y se introdujo con esfuerzo en el oscuro agujero, siguiendo el tenue resplandor de la linterna de Camelia.

—¡Mirad esto! —exclamó Camelia emocionada mientras señalaba las pinturas rupestres que había en el angosto pasadizo que recorrían.

Un leve crujido hizo que Simon alzara la vista.

—¿Qué es eso tan asqueroso que cuelga del techo? —inquirió con cautela.

—Murciélagos —contestó Camelia distraída—. Mira estos dibujos, Simon, son guerreros llevando cadáveres, y los hombres que van detrás sostienen obsequios y objetos valiosos.

Sin perder de vista a los murciélagos, Simon arrugó la nariz al percibir el olor a humedad del aire.

—Esperemos que trajeran algo más que unos cuantos animales sacrificados, porque esta cueva huele a piel y huesos descompuestos.

—Incluso las pieles y los huesos son significativas para ayudarnos a entender a nuestros antepasados —le aseguró Camelia.

—Los guerreros que recorrieron este pasadizo debían de ser muy delgados —se quejó Zareb, soltando un gruñido mientras trataba de entrar—. Harriet y Rupert no están acostumbrados a sitios tan estrechos.

Abrió la bolsa de cuero que llevaba colgada del brazo y extrajo a Harriet, que voló sobre su hombro batiendo nervioso sus alas grises. Rupert asomó la cabeza, sacó la lengua cauteloso a la fría oscuridad de la cueva y luego dejó que Zareb lo pusiese en el suelo para poder estirarse y explorar.

—¡Maldita sea! —renegó Simon, que estuvo a punto de tropezar con un esqueleto que había tumbado en el suelo con una lanza al lado—. ¿Éste es uno de los reyes?

Camelia se acercó para verlo de cerca.

—No, seguramente era un guardián. Debió de quedarse aquí para proteger la tumba.

—No creo que le hiciera mucha gracia que pusieran esa roca delante de la abertura —comentó Simon—. Si ésta es la tumba, ¿dónde están los cadáveres y las riquezas?

—Esto es solamente un pasadizo, tenemos que seguir avanzando. —Alumbrando con la linterna, Camelia empezó a adentrarse en la cueva.

—Deja de mover la cola, Oscar, me hace cosquillas en la espalda —protestó Simon siguiendo a Camelia dificultosamente.

Oscar miró hacia abajo, chilló asustado, y luego trepó a la cabeza de Simon, tapándole los ojos con las patas.

—¡Venga, Oscar, para ya de hacer el tonto!

—¡No se mueva! —le ordenó Zareb mientras le sacudía la espalda con las manos.

Simon apartó las patas de Oscar de sus ojos justo a tiempo para ver una cascada de escarabajos, que caían de su espalda y corrían por sus pies.

—¿Por qué no vendría una mujer tranquila y normalita a mi laboratorio? —preguntó con ironía mientras procuraba no pisar los horribles insectos que caían de sus botas—. ¿Una mujer para la que una salida agradable consistiese en dar un paseo por el parque en carruaje una tarde soleada?

—Porque no era su destino —repuso Zareb.

—¿Y cree que lo es arrastrarme por esta oscura y apestosa cueva con un mono aterrorizado y agarrado a mi cabeza, y estar rodeado de bichos diminutos y asquerosos que apenas puedo ver?

—No hacía falta que entrara. La decisión fue suya.

—No quería perderme tanta diversión —musitó Simon mientras apartaba una pegajosa telaraña.

—¡Simon! ¡Zareb! ¡*Venid, deprisa*!

Simon corrió por el pasadizo, intentando ignorar a los murciélagos que colgaban encima de su cabeza y los insectos que chafaba con las botas.

Dobló una esquina y se encontró a Camelia de pie en el centro de una gran cámara, únicamente iluminada por la suave luz de su linterna.

—¡Dios mío! —exclamó asombrado.

Había ocho esqueletos formando un círculo alrededor de la cámara, envueltos en pieles medio podridas de leopardo, cebra y león. Tenían los brazos cargados de pulseras de marfil y oro, y sobre los restos de sus troncos colgaban collares de cuentas hechos con piedras agujereadas y trozos de cáscaras. Perfectamente ordenados alrededor de cada cuerpo, había magníficos cascos, lanzas, puñales y máscaras. Las paredes de la cámara habían sido minuciosamente pintadas con numerosas escenas de la vida tribal, incluyendo batallas entre guerreros, mujeres preparando la comida y cuidando de los niños y animales corriendo por las llanuras africanas.

Simon posó los ojos en la vasija de barro que había junto a cada uno de los reyes difuntos.

—¿Qué hay en esas vasijas?

—Seguramente habrán sólo fragmentos de cuarzo y otras piedras que a las tribus les pareciesen bonitas —dedujo Camelia, echando una mirada al montón de piedras desiguales—. ¡Fíjate en esas pinturas, Simon, son extraordinarias!

Simon cogió una piedra de color claro y la examinó a la luz de la linterna, que Camelia había dejado en el suelo. Intrigado, la rascó en el cristal de la linterna.

Un profundo arañazo estropeó el cristal ahumado.

Simon contempló el arañazo con incredulidad.

—Esto es un diamante.

Escéptico, Zareb enarcó las cejas.

—¿Está seguro?

—No del todo. —Simon buscó a su alrededor y encontró un fragmento de roca en el suelo. Lo cogió y lo frotó contra la piedra para intentar rayarla. Entonces levantó la cabeza lentamente—. Ahora sí lo estoy.

Camelia desvió su atención de las pinturas rupestres.

—¿Cómo puedes estar tan seguro? —preguntó también escéptica.

—Porque un diamante puede rascar cualquier otro mineral, pero no puede ser rascado por otros minerales —explicó Simon—. Y con lo mucho que se parecen esta piedra y las de las vasijas, juraría que están llenas de diamantes sin pulir. —Miró a Camelia con reservada excitación—. ¿Sabes lo que eso significa?

—Significa que por fin viviré bien —dijo Bert silabeando mientras entraba en la cámara llevando una pistola.

Simon se colocó inmediatamente delante de Camelia para protegerla con su cuerpo.

—Hola, Bert —saludó con amabilidad, cerrando el puño alrededor del diamante—. ¿No te parece que estás bastante lejos de Londres?

—Ponga las manos donde pueda verlas, despacito y con cuidado —ordenó Bert—. No jueguen con nosotros, porque ni Stanley ni yo tendremos ningún problema en dispararles.

Zareb levantó las cejas.

—¿Quién es Stanley?

Bert miró cautelosamente por encima de su hombro y luego frunció el ceño.

—¡Stanley! ¡Trae hasta aquí tu enorme culo! Cabeza de chorlito, ¿no ves que estamos trabajando?

—Perdona, Bert. —Stanley entró lentamente en la cámara con una patata a medio comer en una mano y rascándose tímidamente la cabeza con la otra—. Esta cueva es tremendamente pequeña, Bert; no paro de darme golpes en el coco contra el techo.

—Ya te he dicho que no te pusieras de pie, zoquete —le espetó Bert.

—Pero tengo que estar de pie, Bert; ¿cómo voy a caminar si no?

—¡Dios! Pues andas agachado como ese mono que está encima del hombro del inventor, ¿acaso no puedes hacer eso?

—Por supuesto que sí, Bert —contestó Stanley tratando de ser complaciente—. Lo intentaré.

—Muy bien —dijo Bert arrugando la frente—. ¿Por dónde iba?

—Creo que comentabas lo bien que vivirías con estos diamantes —le recordó Simon sin soltar el diamante que llevaba en la mano. Estaba convencido de que si lo lanzaba contra la cabeza de Bert, acabaría con ese gordo cobarde.

Aunque, por desgracia, aún tendría que lidiar con Stanley.

—Exacto —repuso Bert, asintiendo—. Creo que aquí habrá suficiente para comprarnos una bonita casa...

—En Cheapside, ¿verdad, Bert? —le interrumpió Stanley nervioso.

—Cheapside ya no nos conviene, Stanley —se burló Bert—. Con todos estos diamantes podremos vivir donde queramos, incluso en St. James Square, si queremos.

—Yo quiero vivir en Cheapside —insistió Stanley—. Ahí hay una pastelería buenísima.

—Ya no comeremos pasteles grasientos, Stanley; ¡comeremos cordero estofado, ternera hervida y pollo con salsa de crema tres veces al día!

Stanley bajó los hombros, decepcionado.

—A mí me gustan los pasteles.

Bert puso los ojos en blanco.

—De acuerdo, te dejaré seguir tomando pasteles. Y ahora coge la cuerda y ata a esos tres de ahí —ordenó señalando a Camelia, Simon y Zareb—. No quiero que nos creen ningún problema mientras nos llevamos los diamantes.

Stanley se acercó a Camelia.

—Lo lamento, señora —se disculpó—. Procuraré no atarla demasiado fuerte.

—Eres muy considerado, Stanley. —Camelia le sonrió con dulzura al tiempo que alcanzaba el puñal que escondía enfundado en la bota. «Lo tendré en cuenta cuando te clave el puñal.»

De pronto Stanley se detuvo, preocupado.

—Y cuando nos hayamos llevado los diamantes, los desataremos, ¿verdad, Bert?

—¡Pues claro que no los desataremos, gordo estúpido! ¿No querrás que nos sigan?

—Pero si no los desatamos, ¿cómo saldrán? Si van atados, no podrán salir por esa pequeña abertura.

—Eso es, no podrán —concedió Bert, tratando de ser paciente—. Ése es el plan, Stanley. Cogemos los diamantes, volvemos a Londres, y esta señora se queda aquí para siempre con sus esqueletos y esos viejos cachivaches... —Sus labios dibujaron una malévola y amarillenta sonrisa—. Y todos contentos.

Stanley sacudió la cabeza con seriedad.

—Eso no está bien, Bert. El viejo chocho que nos contrató en Londres nunca dijo nada sobre dejarla a ella y a sus amigos atados en una cueva. Lo único que dijo fue que la siguiéramos hasta África y le creáramos problemas hasta que acabase queriendo regresar a Londres.

—Tampoco dijo nada acerca de que no la dejáramos atada en una cueva —señaló Bert razonablemente.

—Pero si los dejamos a todos en la cueva, ¿qué comerán y beberán, Bert? Pasarán hambre.

—¡Por el amor de...! ¡Pues claro que pasarán hambre, pedazo de *simkin*! De eso se trata ¿no? Si se quedan aquí, no podrán hacernos nada, porque se morirán.

Stanley abrió los ojos desmesuradamente.

—¡No podemos hacer eso, Bert! ¡No está bien! Además, ¿qué diría el viejo chocho?

—No se enterará. De todas formas, ese maldito cabrón jamás podría pagarnos lo que hay aquí en diamantes. En mi opinión, hemos venido hasta África porque esta señora no ha tenido la sensatez de quedarse en Londres como tenía que haber hecho —dijo mirando indignado a Camelia—. He estado a punto de palmarla en el viaje y odio este maldito Poo Moo Lanee desde el primer día que llegué. Ahora que he encontrado los diamantes, no pienso irme sin ellos.

—De hecho, creo que fue lady Camelia la que los encontró —objetó Simon amablemente.

Bert se rió con desdén.

—Bueno, pues aquí dentro ya no los necesitará.

—En eso tienes razón. —Camelia intentó aparentar resignación mientras cambiaba ligeramente de posición.

De algún modo, no le parecía justo clavarle el puñal a Stanley. Además, pensó que la verdadera amenaza era Bert, porque era el único que iba armado. En cuanto Stanley se apartara un poco sacaría el puñal y lo tiraría contra Bert.

Pero primero quería averiguar quién los había contratado.

—¿Quién es este viejo chocho del que habláis, Stanley? —preguntó con naturalidad, intentando distraerlo mientras se colocaba mejor para poder darle a Bert con el puñal.

—Es el pez gordo que nos contrató para que la siguiéramos a usted —explicó Stanley—. Quería controlar todos sus pasos.

—¿Es lord Bagley, el arqueólogo? —Habló con voz suave y persuasiva, y añadió—: Ahora ya no pasa nada por decirlo.

—Nunca nos dijo cómo se llamaba. Nos vio una noche a Bert y a mí en Spotted Dick, y nos comentó que había una mujer a la que quería que vigiláramos. Y cada vez que le pasábamos un informe de lo que habíamos visto, nos encargaba otra tarea, como amedrentarla en la callejuela o incendiar la casa del inventor.

—Eso son actos de hombres sin honor —observó Zareb con desdén—. Los espíritus os juzgarán como unos cobardes.

—Un momento, de cobardes nada —replicó Bert ofendido—. Somos sólo un par de estafadores que intentan ganarse la vida, igual que todo el mundo.

—Yo más bien diría que sois un par de bribones despreciables —se oyó a alguien decir en voz baja y débil—; ¡y tú recibirás un disparo en tu asqueroso culo como no sueltes la pistola ahora mismo!

—¡Oliver! —exclamó Camelia sonriente—. ¿Cómo has conseguido encontrarnos?

—Bueno, jovencita, puede que sea viejo, pero huelo los problemas a kilómetros de distancia —le aseguró Oliver sin modestia alguna mientras entraba en la cámara de enterramiento tenuemente iluminada—. Es el resultado de haber criado a este joven de aquí y a todos sus hermanos y hermanas. —Empezó a reír—. Recuerdo aquella ocasión en que decidieron robar una pequeña tienda...

—Estoy seguro de que a Camelia le encantará escuchar la historia en otro momento —le interrumpió Simon, quitándole hábilmente la pistola a Bert—. Mientras tanto, Stanley, espero que no te importe que use tu cuerda para ataros a Bert y a ti juntos.

—No me importa —replicó Stanley alegremente mientras le entregaba la cuerda a Simon—. Pero intente no atar a Bert demasiado fuerte; le entra un poco de claustrofobia cuando no se puede mover.

—¡No puede permitir que la palmemos en esta cueva! —protestó Bert al tiempo que Simon le maniataba—. ¡Eso es un asesinato!

—No tengo ninguna intención de dejaros aquí —los tranquilizó Camelia.

Bert la miró sorprendido.

—¿Ah, no?

—Por supuesto que no. Esta tumba es un hallazgo sumamente importante y tardaré años en analizarla, y extraer las reliquias para estudiarlas y conservarlas. No puedo permitir que estéis los dos aquí, quejándoos e interfiriendo en mi trabajo.

—Yo no me quejaría, señora —prometió Stanley—. Si quiere, podría ayudarle —añadió con timidez—. Se me da bien cargar peso. Yo mismo volqué la bomba de vapor; pesaba muchísimo.

—Gracias, Stanley, eres muy amable.

—¿Y qué piensa hacer con nosotros? —inquirió Bert.

—Deberían ser juzgados por el jefe de los Khoikhoi —gruñó Zareb enfadado—. Os enviaría al desierto sin agua ni comida, ¡y os prohibiría volver hasta que hubierais encontrado la sabiduría!

—Eso me parece un castigo un poco duro, Zareb —repuso Camelia—. Me conformaré con entregarlos a la policía de Ciudad del Cabo.

—¡Camelia! —De repente, Elliott entró corriendo en la cámara con la cara sonrojada y jadeando—. ¿Qué demonios ocurre aquí?

—¡Hemos encontrado la Tumba de los Reyes, Elliott!

Abrumada por la ola de emociones, Camelia corrió a abrazarlo. Después de toda una vida buscando, finalmente había logrado hacer realidad el sueño de su padre. Se alegraba de que Elliott estuviese ahí para compartir la emoción y la alegría del momento, aunque al mismo tiempo sintió una dolorosa punzada en el corazón. Su padre debería haber estado allí con ellos. Apoyó la cabeza en el reconfortante y cálido pecho de Elliott y cerró los ojos, suspirando. En algún lugar, más allá de las seis estrellas que titilaban en el cielo nocturno, sobre la cueva, estaba segura de que su padre los estaba mirando con una sonrisa.

—¿A que es magnífico? —musitó, hablándole a su padre y también a Elliott—. ¡Es exactamente como nos imaginábamos!

—¡Dios mío, Camelia! Claro que es maravilloso, pero tú eres lo único que me importa. —La abrazó con fuerza—. ¿Estás bien?

—Estoy bien. —Se enjugó las lágrimas que asomaban a sus ojos y esbozó una temblorosa sonrisa mientras levantaba la vista y lo miraba—. Estos son Stanley y Bert —continuó señalando a la pareja, ahora firmemente atada. Pensando que tal vez Elliott necesitase algún tipo de explicación que aclarase lo ocurrido, añadió—: Los que han estado entorpeciendo mi camino tanto aquí como en Londres. Al parecer, nos siguieron hasta aquí y han intentado echar por tierra todo nuestro trabajo rompiendo la bomba.

Elliott miró indignado a los dos hombres.

—¿Así que ésta es la escoria que destrozó tu casa y clavó con un puñal esa horrible nota en tu almohada?

Camelia se sintió confusa. Se separó de Elliott poco a poco y lo miró con inseguridad.

—¿Qué has dicho?

—La nota de la que me hablaste; me dijiste que la habían clavado en tu almohada con el puñal favorito de tu padre. ¿Lo hicieron estos dos?

Camelia lo miró fijamente con el corazón encogido. «No», pensó. «No puede ser.» Repitiéndose a sí misma que tenía que haber alguna explicación lógica para el comentario de Elliott, le dijo en voz baja:

—Yo no te dije que la nota había sido clavada en mi almohada con un puñal, Elliott.

—¡Claro que sí! —insistió él—. Me contaste todo lo que ocurrió.

—No, no lo hice. No quise que supieras que habían usado el puñal de mi padre, porque me daba miedo tu reacción. Estabas al tanto de sus supuestos poderes y sabías cuánto cariño le tenía mi padre. Pensé que si te contaba que lo habían utilizado para amenazarme, habrías hecho todo lo posible para evitar que volviese a Pumulani.

—Bueno, pues debió de decírmelo alguien más —repuso Elliott con desdén—. A lo mejor fue Kent.

Simon sacudió la cabeza.

—Lo siento, Wickham, pero nunca he hablado con usted de lo que sucedió esa noche.

—Entonces me debí de enterar por Zareb.

—Yo no hablo de lo que le pasa a Tisha con nadie —declaró Zareb con severidad—. Ni siquiera con usted, lord Wickham.

Elliott los miró impaciente, como si le pareciese absolutamente ridículo darle tanta importancia a una tontería.

—Bueno, pues debió de ser Oliver.

—Yo estoy seguro de no haberle dicho nunca nada, muchacho. —Oliver frunció sus cejas blancas—. Sé por experiencia que es mejor morderse la lengua cuando no sabes de dónde vienen los problemas.

Lentamente, Elliott posó su mirada en Camelia.

Ella también lo miró; sus suaves ojos verdes estaban muy abiertos y brillaban débilmente esperanzados. Notó que estaba luchando por mantener la clama, por creer que había alguna explicación plausible y lógica para el hecho de que supiese lo del puñal. Entonces él se sintió abrumado, tanto por el feroz deseo de Camelia de seguir teniendo fe en él, fe que había ardido en una llama discreta pero constante desde que ella era una niña, como porque acababa de darse cuenta, lleno de dolor, de que le había fallado completamente. No había sido su intención, pero eso apenas importaba. Lo que había empezado como un deseo sincero de protegerla y crearle una vida con él, de algún modo se había convertido en este terrible y desgradable momento. La vergüenza se apoderó de él, mezclada con una ira irremediable, que le hicieron sentir disgustado y frustrado.

¿Qué había sido de esa bella joven que solía mirarlo con admiración y devoción?, se preguntó con pesar. ¿Cuándo había empezado Camelia a alejarse de él hasta estar fuera de su alcance, hasta que, finalmente, cuanto él dijese, hiciese o pensase no despertara en ella nada más que impaciencia o unas leves ganas de desafiarlo? Durante algún tiempo, justo después de la muerte del padre de Camelia, ésta había recurrido a él en busca de consuelo. Entonces Elliott había sentido que ella lo quería y pensó que había entendido lo que él sentía por ella; que, sin duda, había entendido cuánto la quería después de aquel beso en el jardín de lord Bagley.

Pero no había sido suficiente para Camelia, pensó, sintiendo que algo empezaba a romperse en su interior. Le había ofrecido cuanto tenía, incluyendo su apellido, su hogar y su corazón.

Y aun así no había sido suficiente.

—Lo lamento, Camelia —se disculpó con voz apagada y áspera debido al arrepentimiento—. Nunca quise hacerte daño. —Por lo menos eso era cierto. Pero al mirarla a los ojos y ver cómo los últimos vestigios de su confianza se desintegraban lentamente, cayó en la cuenta de que eso no importaba. Extrajo la pistola de la cinturilla de los pantalones y la apuntó con ella, procurando mantener la mano firme—. Me temo que tendrás que darme el puñal que llevas en la bota.

Elliott la observó mientras se agachaba aturdida y sacaba el puñal para tirarlo al suelo, frente a los pies de él.

Se aclaró la garganta y dijo:

—Kent, si no le importa, me gustaría que Oliver y usted dejaran sus pistolas aquí, en el suelo, y que después desataran a mis amigos Stanley y Bert.

—Yo no soy su amigo —protestó Stanley, confundido—. Ni siquiera lo conozco.

—Cierra el pico, Stanley. ¿No ves que este señor intenta ayudarnos? —le espetó Bert.

—Y ¿por qué nos ayuda si no nos conoce? —inquirió Stanley.

—Sí que os conozco, estúpidos, idiotas cobardes —los insultó Elliott—. Soy el viejo chocho del que hablabais, aunque supongo que sin mi habitual disfraz, encorvado como un viejo borracho en alguna esquina apestosa de Spotted Dick, no me parezco mucho al anciano que os contrató.

Bert lo miró atónito.

—¿Usted es el viejo chocho?

—Sí, y debo decir, Bert, que me decepciona mucho que pretendierais robarme estos diamantes; sobre todo porque estáis aquí gracias a mí.

—Sólo bromeaba, señor —se apresuró a asegurarle Bert mientras Simon lo desataba—. ¡Espero que no piense que hablaba en serio!

—Pues yo sí lo he pensado —comentó Stanley.

—¡Cierra la maldita boca, Stanley, y dale un día de vacaciones a tu lengua!

—¡Ah..., ya lo he entendido! Estaba siendo sarcástico. Eso es cuando Bert dice algo en broma, pero finge que es en serio —le explicó Stanley a Oliver, que lo desataba despacio. Frunció las cejas y añadió—: Sí, ya sé que es un poco lioso.

—¿Por qué, Elliott? —Camelia tragó saliva, esfozándose por impedir que las lágrimas que inundaban sus ojos resbalasen por sus mejillas—. Tantos años trabajando junto a mi padre. Te quería como a un hijo, Elliott. Te enseñó todo lo que sabía. ¿Cómo has podido traicionarle de esta manera?

—No era mi intención que acabase así, Camelia —afirmó Elliott—. Tienes que creerme. Durante muchos años creí con la misma pasión que tu padre que la Tumba de los Reyes existía. Pero después de quince años no habíamos encontrado nada. Los trabajadores se marchaban; el dinero se terminaba, y luego murió mi padre, dejando una gran cantidad de deudas. Me encontré de pronto con una madre y tres hermanas solteras que alimentar, varias casas que mantener, criados y facturas que pagar... y los ingresos no eran suficientes para cubrir todo eso.

—No está mal —intervino Oliver en tono burlón.

—Elliott, tu padre murió un año antes que el mío —señaló Camelia—. Podrías haberte marchado justo entonces a

Inglaterra para montar tu empresa, no hacía falta que te quedaras aquí.

—Lo sé. Y ésa era mi intención. Pero la noche en que fui a decirle a tu padre que me iba, lo vi en su tienda de campaña examinando unos diamantes que había encontrado.

Ella lo miró con incredulidad.

—Te equivocas; mi padre no encontró ni un solo diamante en Pumulani.

—Sí lo hizo, Camelia. Pero no quería que nadie lo supiese, ni siquiera tú. Le daba miedo que la noticia se propagase y la excavación se inundase de buscadores de minas, que se peleasen por comprarle o robarle una porción. Y él era consciente de que, si se extraían minerales de Pumulani, se echaría a perder todo lo que tuviese valor arqueológico.

Ella cabeceó, se negaba a aceptar lo que Elliott acababa de decirle.

—Si lo que dices es verdad, ¿dónde están los diamantes que viste en su tienda? No los vi entre sus cosas cuando falleció.

—Me los llevé, para guardarlos.

Oliver soltó una risotada desdeñosa.

—¿Es así como lo llama? En mi época se llamaba robar.

—Necesitaba más tiempo, Camelia —insistió Elliott, tratando de hacerle entender—. Sabía que por derecho los diamantes eran tuyos, pero también sabía que harías lo mismo que tu padre. Necesitaba tiempo para ayudarte a comprender que lo mejor era extraer minerales en lugar de remover eternamente cada centímetro de tierra con escobillas y palas para no encontrar nada de valor.

—Jamás habría consentido que extrajeran minerales, Elliott. Siempre he creído que la Tumba de los Reyes existía. No habría hecho nada que pudiese ponerla en peligro.

—Eso ya lo sabe, Camelia. —Simon miró a Elliott fijamente, debatiéndose entre arrojarle el diamante que sostenía en la mano o esperar hasta estar seguro de que Zareb y Oliver estaban en posición de despojar a Stanley y a Bert de sus pistolas—. Por eso nunca te quiso enseñar los diamantes. No quería convencerte de que vendieras el terreno a la De Beers Company debido al valor potencial que tenía como zona diamantífera. Sabía que te parecías demasiado a tu padre para consentir algo así. Lo que quería era ahuyentarte mientras te convencía de que la tierra no tenía absolutamente valor alguno.

—Pero ¿por qué? —Camelia miró a Elliott suplicante—. Aunque al final me hubiese rendido y hubiese vendido el terreno, ¿en qué te habría beneficiado?

—Mi intención inicial no era ahuyentarte. —Hablaba con voz suave—. Sabes que te aprecio, Camelia. Tenía la esperanza de que te casaras conmigo y después de eso pretendía contarte lo de los diamantes. Pensé que podría hacerte entender que lo mejor para ambos era vender el terreno y establecernos en Inglaterra. —Sus ojos se ensombrecieron—. Pero al no dejar que te conquistase, me di cuenta de que debería adoptar medidas más severas para que te marcharas de Pumulani y volvieras conmigo. Pero por muchos accidentes que provocase o por mucho que pagase a estos idiotas para amedrentarte, no abandonaste el sueño de tu padre.

—¿Eh? ¿A quién ha llamado idiota? —inquirió Bert.

—Esta chica es muy valiente —observó Oliver, mirando a Camelia con cariño—. No se encoge, se sacude el agua.

—Tisha es africana. —Zareb la miró orgulloso—. Es una guerrera.

—Debió de ser muy frustrante para usted, Wickham —intervino Simon—. Supongo que a esas alturas ya habría hablado con la De Beers Company acerca de los diamantes.

—Les hice un par de ofertas —admitió Elliott—. Y, naturalmente, cuando vieron los diamantes estuvieron muy interesados en adquirir el terreno. Les prometí convencer a Camelia de que se lo vendiera a ellos a un precio más que aceptable, si a cambio me pagaban una buena suma de dinero por mis servicios.

—Me sorprende que no negociara quedarse también con un porcentaje de los beneficios de la extracción de diamantes.

—Me lo ofrecieron, pero por muy poco dinero. Y como tampoco estaba seguro de que el terreno tuviera más diamantes enterrados, aparte de los que lord Stamford había encontrado, preferí cobrar el dinero de inmediato.

—¡Qué pragmático! Veo que no le gusta arriesgarse mucho.

—He corrido riesgos durante casi toda mi vida, Kent —le informó Elliott nervioso—. Mi padre juró que me desheredaría cuando le dije que quería ser arqueólogo. Me llamó idiota y prometió que jamás recibiría un penique suyo. Antes de irme a África me echó de casa y me dejó de dar mi asignación mensual convencido de que sin su apoyo económico jamás tendría valor para ir a África.

Sorprendida, Camelia abrió los ojos desmesuradamente.

—Nunca me lo habías contado, Elliott.

—Nunca se lo he contado a nadie, salvo a tu padre. Tuve que decírselo. Lord Stamford había accedido a ser mi profesor, pero de pronto me encontré sin dinero para comprarme el billete a África. Entonces se lo pedí prestado a tu padre, pero él me regaló el billete y se ofreció a pagarme un sueldo modesto. Me permitió hacer frente a mi padre y seguir mi propio sueño. Por eso siempre estuve en deuda con él.

—Y ahora lo traiciona dañando su excavación e hiriendo a su hija. —La voz de Zareb estaba cargada de rabia—. A los espíritus no les gustará nada.

—Pagué mi deuda estando a su lado durante muchos años y creyéndole cada vez que me decía que estábamos a punto de hacer un increíble descubrimiento —se justificó Elliott—. Y acabé con un montón de deudas y el desdén socarrón de la Sociedad Arqueológica Británica. Me consideraban un idiota por haber desperdiciado tanto tiempo excavando en África con lord Stamford. —Su boca formó una tensa línea llena de amargura mientras miraba a Simon—. Pero no fue hasta que Kent viajó hasta aquí que me di cuenta de lo estúpido que había sido.

El significado de sus palabras estaba claro.

—Tenga cuidado con lo que dice, Wickham —le advirtió Simon apretando los puños.

—¿De verdad cree que no estoy al tanto de los jueguecitos que se traen los dos entre manos en su tienda por las noches?

—¡Basta ya! —exclamó Oliver malhumorado—. ¡Ya está bien de tonterías!

—Cierre el pico, lord Wickham —añadió Zareb, que apenas podía contener su rabia—, o me veré obligado a cerrárselo yo.

—¡Cómo no! El siempre leal kaffir que sale en defensa de lady Camelia, aunque haya dos pistolas apuntándole —comentó Elliott mordaz—. Usted tiene parte de culpa de que ella sea como es.

—He dedicado mi vida a protegerla de las fuerzas oscuras. —Zareb lo miró con forzada calma—. Y de usted.

—¡No era necesario que la protegiese de mí, viejo estúpido! ¡Yo habría cuidado de ella!

—Para eso tendría que haber sido suya, señor, y nunca lo fue —replicó Zareb—. No merece semejante privilegio.

Elliott desvió la vista y miró a Camelia.

—Hubo un tiempo, Camelia, en que realmente creí que estábamos hechos el uno para el otro. —Alargó el brazo y le acarició con los dedos su sucia mejilla—. Pero ahora que he visto la vulgar y apestosa escoria por la que te sientes atraída, me considero afortunado de que rechazaras casarte conmigo.

—¿Acaba de decir que la señora se siente atraída por mí? —inquirió Stanley, perplejo.

—De hecho, Stanley, me parece que se refería a mí —le contestó Simon.

—Pero si usted no es vulgar. Sus inventos son más que brillantes.

—Gracias.

—¡Cállate, Stanley! —le espetó Bert—. ¿No ves que estamos trabajando?

Stanley lo miró avergonzado.

—Lo siento, Bert. ¿Qué quieres que haga ahora?

Bert miró a Elliott expectante.

—Atadlos ahí —ordenó Elliott— y empezad a sacar fuera de la cueva esas vasijas de diamantes. ¡Deprisa, maldita sea! Quiero esta cueva vacía y cerrada antes de que nadie los encuentre.

—Entonces ¿eso es todo? —Camelia habló con frialdad mientras Stanley y Bert, a regañadientes, obedecían la orden—. ¿Vas a cerrar la cueva y dejarnos aquí dentro?

—Lo lamento, Camelia, pero dadas las circunstancias no tengo otra alternativa. Jamás imaginé que encontrarías realmente la tumba. Y ahora que lo has hecho, reconoce que es bastante lógico que tanto tú como tus amigos os quedéis aquí dentro. Llevas toda la vida intentando descubrir este sitio; ahora podrás pasar aquí la eternidad.

—Pero ya le he dicho a Bert que eso no está bien —protestó Stanley, haciendo una pausa en el proceso de maniatar a Oliver—. No pienso dejar que la palmen en esta cueva, ¡hay arañas!

—Harás lo que te mande, cabeza de chorlito, si no quieres que os deje a los dos también aquí —amenazó Elliott furioso—. ¿Lo has entendido o necesitas que el desgraciado de tu amiguito te lo explique?

Stanley miró a Bert suplicante.

—No es correcto, Bert.

—¡Cierra la maldita boca y haz lo que te mandan, Stanley! —advirtió Bert, que miraba la pistola de Elliott nervioso.

—Buen consejo —añadió Elliott con sequedad.

Camelia permaneció inmóvil con los puños cerrados a los lados de la falda. Sintió a su alrededor un aire helado que le hizo tomar conciencia del martilleo de su corazón, de los escalofríos que sentía en el cuerpo y de la intensidad con la que le latía la sangre en las venas. Había encontrado la Tumba de los Reyes. Y al hacerlo, había descubierto que su queridísimo Elliott, que había sido un hijo para su padre y un hermano mayor para ella, estaba dispuesto dejar a un lado los años de amistad y cariño a cambio de unas cuantas vasijas de diamantes.

Nada era lo que parecía, pensó con pesar.

«Deja que las estrellas te guíen.»

—Es la hora, Tisha —comentó Zareb en voz baja.

Camelia le lanzó una mirada, confusa, y éste se la devolvió con una serenidad extraordinaria; sus ojos oscuros brillaban de amor y severa determinación.

—Los espíritus han hablado, Tisha —susurró—. Es la hora.

—Nunca se rinde, ¿eh, Zareb? —dijo Elliott—. Todas sus tonterías absurdas sobre los espíritus malignos, las fuerzas oscuras y las maldiciones. La verdad, me asombra que Stamford le confiara su hija a un ignorante y viejo kaffir. —Miró indignado a Camelia antes de concluir—: Todo habría sido distinto si tu padre te hubiese dejado en Inglaterra al cuidado de una buena institutriz inglesa.

—Tienes razón, Elliott —concedió Camelia con suavidad—. Las cosas habrían sido muy distintas. Pero hay algo que dudo que una institutriz inglesa hubiese podido enseñarme.

—¿El qué?

—Esto. —Cogió el meñique de la mano izquierda de Elliott y tiró de él hacia atrás con todas sus fuerzas, desencajándoselo.

Elliott aulló de dolor y se tambaleó, disparando accidentalmente la pistola.

Oscar chilló y saltó sobre su cabeza, cegándolo durante unos instantes. Mientras Elliott forcejeaba para liberarse del mono, Harriet voló para asistir a Oscar y se puso a aletear mientras le daba violentos picotazos a Elliott en la cara y la cabeza.

De pronto, una figura naranja y negra, Rupert, se irguió sobre el suelo y hundió sus colmillos en la pierna de Elliott.

—¡Socorro! ¡Sácadmelos de encima! ¡*Socorro*! —gritó Elliott, que tropezó con los esqueletos de los reyes muertos y volcó las vasijas de diamantes—. ¡Socorro!

Súbitamente, los murciélagos que colgaban del techo de la cueva chillaron y alzaron el vuelo, creando un viento helado mientras salían de la cámara.

—Supongo que no les ha gustado el disparo de la pistola —comentó Oliver, rascándose la cabeza.

Un gran estrépito sacudió la cueva y fragmentos de piedra y nubes de polvo empezaron a llover sobre todos ellos.

—¡Se va a derrumbar! —exclamó Simon mientras corría hasta Camelia y le cogía de la mano—. *¡Salgamos de aquí!*

—¡Venga, Stanley, largo! —gritó Bert, precipitándose al pasadizo tan rápido como sus cortas piernas le permitían.

—¡Ahora voy! —repuso Stanley mientras destaba rápidamente a Oliver y Zareb.

—Oscar, Harriet, ¡ya basta! —Camelia cogió a Rupert del suelo, que se había deslizado hasta sus pies, y se lo enrolló alrededor del cuello—. ¡Hay que salir de aquí!

Harriet le dio a Elliott un último y fuerte picotazo antes de volar hasta el hombro de Zareb. Enfadado, Oscar golpeó a Elliott en la cabeza y a continuación se alejó de él y se encaramó a Simon.

—¿Estás bien, Elliott? —preguntó Camelia apremiante—. ¿Podrás salir de aquí?

Elliott la miró confuso mientras el polvo y fragmentos de roca caían a su alrededor.

—¡Mis diamantes! —Se agachó y empezó a buscar por el suelo de la cueva, intentando recuperar las piedras esparcidas para metérselas en los bolsillos.

—¡Por el amor de Dios, Wickham, deje esas piedras! —gritó Simon.

—¡Son mías! —A cuatro patas, Elliott rebuscaba frenético entre el polvo.

—¡Elliott, por favor! —suplicó Camelia—. ¡Tenemos que salir ya!

—¡Un minuto más!

Una nefasta grieta se abrió en una de las paredes, creando una fisura en las pinturas rupestres entre un grupo de guerreros y el león que estaban tratando de cazar.

—Vamos, Tisha —dijo Zareb—. Tienes que salir de este lugar.

—Elliott, te lo suplico, ¡deja los diamantes! —exclamó Camelia con voz de angustia.

—Sólo unos cuantos más —repuso Elliott, que buscaba a tientas por el suelo.

—Es su elección, Camelia. —Simon le agarró del brazo—. ¡Salgamos!

—¡No puedo dejarlo aquí!

—Si te quedas, morirás —le soltó Simon—. Y aunque esa posibilidad pueda parecerte aceptable, te aseguro que para mí no lo es en absoluto.

Y entonces la cogió en brazos y corrió por el pasadizo, que se estaba desmoronando, seguido de cerca por Oliver y Zareb.

—¡Venga, Stanley, empuja! —le ordenó Simon al ver que se había quedado atascado en la entrada de la cueva.

—No puedo. ¡Me he quedado atascado!

—Desde luego esta noche no puede ser mejor —musitó Simon mientras dejaba a Camelia en el suelo—. Bert, ¿estás ahí fuera?

—Sí, estoy aquí —respondió Bert—. Pero está completamente encajonado, ¡no puede moverse!

—De acuerdo, tiraremos de él un poco hacia dentro y luego veremos si conseguimos que se coloque mejor para poder salir. Oliver y Zareb, hay que cogerle de las piernas. Camelia y yo lo cogeremos por el tronco. ¿Preparados? ¡Estirad!

—¡Eso es! —exclamó Bert desde el exterior de la cueva—. ¡Se está moviendo!

—Muy bien, Stanley, quiero que bajes el hombro derecho y subas el izquierdo para que estés más ladeado, ¿entendido?

—Creo que sí —jadeó Stanley—. Me parece que ahora respiro mejor.

—Magnífico. Ahora mete la barriga y encógete todo lo que puedas. Bert, cuando cuente hasta tres, quiero que tires fuerte y nosotros empujaremos, ¿de acuerdo? ¡Un... dos... tres!

Se oyó un coro de gruñidos y gemidos mientras todos se esforzaban por liberar a Stanley de las garras de la roca.

—¡Es como intentar introducir a un elefante por el ojo de una maldita cerradura! —protestó Oliver al que le temblaban sus ancianos brazos debido al esfuerzo.

Llovió sobre ellos más tierra y piedras. Los rodeó un mar de insectos y serpientes mientras procuraban huir de la cueva, a punto de venirse abajo.

—¡Venga, Stanley! —lo animó Simon apretando los dientes—. ¡Encógete!

—¡Se mueve! —exclamó Camelia.

Stanley se movió un par de centímetros y luego otro par.

Y después salió despedido por la abertura como un corcho gigante y aterrizó pesadamente encima de Bert.

—¡Ahora tú! —Le ordenó Simon a Camelia tras sacar por el agujero a Oscar y a Harriet.

—¿Y Zareb y Oliver...?

—Nosotros saldremos después que tú —prometió mientras sin miramientos los empujaba a ella y a Rupert por la abertura—. Muy bien, Oliver, ¡ahora tú!

—No tardes, chico. ¡No tengo intención de sufrir solo el viaje de vuelta a Inglaterra! —El anciano escocés salió con dificultad de la cueva.

—Su turno, Zareb.

Zareb lo miró con seriedad.

—Los espíritus han hablado.

—Sí, acaban de decirnos que salgamos de aquí corriendo... ¡Así que muévase!

Zareb lo miró fijamente y a continuación inclinó la cabeza con solemnidad.

—Ahora ella es suya. Cuídela.

Con los ojos oscuros llenos de lágrimas, se volvió hacia el pasadizo a punto de derrumbarse.

—¡Por el amor de Dios...!

Simon le agarró por los hombros y le obligó a girar.

—¿En serio cree que me iré de aquí sin usted, Zareb?

—Debe hacerlo —insistió el africano—. Tisha lo necesita.

—Me halaga que piense eso, pero también lo necesita a usted.

Zareb sacudió la cabeza.

—Yo ya he terminado de velar por ella, ahora es su turno.

—¿No será esto una especie de alocada creencia africana? Porque Oliver *jamás* pensaría que tiene que dejar de velar por mí. Todavía cuida de mi madre, y está casada y tiene nueve hijos, ¡por Dios! ¡Incluso diría que cada año tiene más trabajo!

Zareb lo miró con los ojos muy abiertos.

—¿De verdad?

—Me encantaría seguir hablando del tema —silabeó Simon mientras se agachaba al ver que un enorme fragmento de roca caía a su lado—, pero, sinceramente, preferiría hacerlo fuera de esta cueva. ¿Viene conmigo?

Zareb miró con sorpresa la mano extendida de Simon.

Y entonces posó su palma sobre la de Simon, absorbiendo su calor mientras los dedos de Simon se cerraban sobre los suyos, ancianos y curtidos.

—Por supuesto que sí —afirmó con una sonrisa—. Tisha nos espera.

—No hay nada como esperar hasta el último segundo —musitó Simon al tiempo que ayudaba a Zareb a pasar por la estrecha abertura.

Mientras una espesa lluvia de rocas y tierra caía en cascada a su alrededor, Simon se lanzó por la abertura cada vez más estrecha y aterrizó con estrépito en el suelo.

Entonces cogió a Camelia y la cubrió con su cuerpo, protegiéndola con su cuerpo mientras la Tumba de los Reyes suspiraba y se derrumbaba, volviendo a enterrar su cámara secreta.

Capítulo 17

—No tengo más comida —le dijo Camelia a Oscar, que estaba dándole codazos.

Estaba sentada en el suelo con las piernas cruzadas y el valioso diario de su padre abierto sobre su regazo, contemplando con solemnidad la pintura rupestre del león y los guerreros.

—Si te has quedado con hambre, vete a ver a Oliver. A lo mejor te da una última torta de avena antes de irse con Simon.

Oscar siguió tirando de su brazo. Suspirando, Camelia lo levantó para librarse de él. Entonces Oscar se arrimó a ella y la miró con cara de preocupación.

—No pasa nada, Oscar. —Le acarició la cabeza con suavidad, procurando reconfortarle—. Todo irá bien.

—Zareb me dijo que te encontraría aquí.

Camelia se volvió rápidamente y vio a Simon de pie detrás de ella. Iba vestido con su atuendo habitual consistente en una camisa de hilo holgada y unos pantalones, ambos copiosamente arrugados pero limpios. Llevaba a Rupert tranquilamente colgado al cuello y a Harriet posada con majestuosidad sobre su hombro.

—Por lo visto Rupert y Harriet le han cogido cariño a mis cosas —anunció Simon mientras sacaba con cuidado a la serpiente de sus hombros y la dejaba en el suelo—. Harriet no para de sacar cosas de mi maleta para esparcirlas por la tienda, mientras que Rupert se desliza entre mi ropa para esconderse; me ha dado un buen susto cuando estaba a punto de cerrar la maleta.

Camelia observó cómo Rupert se enroscaba junto a la bota de Simon y sacaba la lengua con paciencia a la espera de ver adónde se dirigiría Simon. Por su parte, Harriet aleteó en señal de protesta cuando Simon intentó que se fuera de su hombro. En cierto modo, aunque primitivo, daba la impresión de que sabían que Simon se marchaba.

Camelia se mordió el labio y miró de nuevo la pintura rupestre.

—¿Qué harás ahora, Camelia? —Tras darse por vencido en su intento por deshacerse de Harriet, Simon se sentó en el suelo sin tocar a Camelia, pero lo bastante cerca de ella para que fuera plenamente consciente de su presencia.

Ella siguió acariciando con suavidad la cabeza de Oscar.

—No estoy segura.

—Podrías tratar de volver a excavar la Tumba de los Reyes. Llevaría su tiempo, pero al menos ahora ya sabes dónde está exactamente.

Camelia cabeceó.

—No quiero volver a encontrarla.

Simon la miró en silencio. En sus ojos verdes del color de la salvia había un velo de tristeza, y las ojeras que había debajo de ellos le indicaron que apenas había dormido desde el derrumbe de la cueva ocurrido la noche anterior.

—Lo que le pasó a Elliott anoche fue terrible —dijo suavemente—, pero fue decisión suya, Camelia. Podría haber salido de la cueva con todos nosotros, pero decidió quedarse hasta que fue demasiado tarde.

—No creo que su decisión fuese consciente, Simon. En esa tumba había otras fuerzas, fuerzas que ni tú ni yo podemos entender.

—No me digas que ahora crees en los vientos oscuros y las maldiciones de Zareb. No es un enfoque muy científico para una arqueóloga experimentada como tú.

—Hay cosas que desafían los principios de la ciencia —reflexionó Camelia—. Zareb siempre ha dicho que hay cosas que no podemos saber, porque no estamos destinados a saberlas, al menos hasta que llegue el momento adecuado. Ayer noche la Tumba de los Reyes me permitió acceder a ella y al hacerlo también Elliott se reveló a sí mismo. Las dos cosas estaban intrínsecamente ligadas. No creo que los espíritus hubiesen dejado salir a Elliott de la cueva, aunque lo hubiese intentado. Por eso la enterraron.

—Los espíritus no enterraron la cueva, Camelia —objetó Simon—, fue Elliott. Disparó la pistola y la cueva se vino abajo, ya fuese porque agrietó el techo o porque el eco de la detonación causó temblores en la estructura. Para cada acción hay una reacción y en este caso concreto la reacción física fue el desmoronamiento de la cueva.

—Yo le rompí el dedo a Elliott y por eso disparó la pistola —señaló Camelia—. Si todo se reduce a una acción y su reacción, entonces soy la responsable de la destrucción de la tumba.

—Si no le hubieses roto el dedo a Elliott cuando lo hiciste, Zareb, Oliver y yo habríamos hecho todo lo posible para desarmarlo, con lo que la pistola se le habría disparado igualmente. Creo que hasta Stanley y Bert habrían acabado ayudándonos. Stanley lleva toda la mañaña detrás de mí, preguntándome si hay algo que pueda hacer para demostrarme su agradecimiento por ayudarle a salir del agujero de la abertura. Y Bert se ha ofrecido a ayudar a Oliver con las maletas, aunque creo que se refería a que le ordenaría a Stanley que las llevara. Así que no debes atormentarte culpándote por el derrumbe de la cueva y la muerte de Elliott, Camelia. Me alegro de que Zareb te enseñase ese truquillo del dedo, aunque te confieso —concluyó con una sonrisa— que no pensé eso cuando me lo hiciste a mí.

—Elliott jamás habría intentado hacernos daño, de no haber descubierto la cueva y los diamantes; y jamás habríamos encontrado la cueva, si no hubiese oído esa voz que me habló en el río.

Simon arqueó las cejas.

—¿Qué voz?

—Da igual. —Camelia cerró el diario de su padre y lo dejó a un lado, tratando de ordenar su torbellino de emociones—. Lo único que intento decirte es que tal vez haya cosas que sea mejor dejar como están, Simon. Volver a excavar implicaría un montón de años removiendo la tierra, ¿y para qué? ¿Para sacar las reliquias de su verdadero hogar, cruzar todo el océano y colocarlas en un museo de Inglaterra, donde las pondrían en vitrinas para mostrárselas a miles de personas ignorantes que nunca apreciarían su valor?

—No te reconozco, Camelia. Siempre has defendido que hay que compartir la información del pasado con el resto del mundo.

—Los cadáveres y las reliquias de esa cueva no fueron puestos ahí con la intención de que luego los sacaran para enseñárselos al mundo entero. Aquello es una cámara de enterramiento, Simon. Esas reliquias pertenecen a África y a los africanos que descienden de los jefes enterrados en la cueva, e incluso a los espíritus que velan por ellas. No estaría bien que yo me las llevara.

—¿Y qué hay del sueño de tu padre?

—Mi padre soñaba con encontrar la Tumba de los Reyes y la hemos econtrado.

—Pero el mundo arqueológico no te creerá, si no le proporcionas ninguna prueba. Menospreciarán la historia tachándola de ser excesivamente exagerada o de ser pura ficción.

—Lo sé. Y me duele pensar que el trabajo de mi padre nunca será valorado, después de pasarse la vida entera intentando ganarse el respeto de sus colegas. Pero sé que si estuviese aquí, estaría de acuerdo conmigo. Mi padre amaba la arqueología, Simon, pero su amor por África era aún mayor. En última instancia querría hacer lo que fuese mejor para África, no para su legado.

Camelia había cambiado, pensó Simon, conmovido y admirado por el sereno realismo y madurez que emanaban de ella. La búsqueda que había consumido todos sus pensamientos y su aliento desde que la había visto por primera vez sentada en el suelo de su laboratorio con las enaguas empapadas había desaparecido. Y aunque un velo de tristeza cubría su mirada, Simon intuyó que estaba en paz con la decisión que había tomado.

—Siempre puedes extraer minerales del terreno —sugirió—. Lejos del emplazamiento de la tumba, naturalmente.

Camelia sacudió la cabeza.

—No pienso destrozar la tierra para buscar unas cuantas piedras blancas absurdas. Los diamantes no me interesan lo más mínimo, no tienen ningún valor añadido.

—De hecho, siendo como son una de las sustancias más duras de la tierra, creo que sí tienen cierto valor añadido, al menos desde un punto de vista científico —repuso Simon—. Podrían acabar siendo bastante importantes en los campos de la ciencia y la tecnología. Aunque no logre convencerte de eso, hay algo más que deberías considerar. Elliott le llevó los diamantes que tu padre encontró a la De Beers Company, que se ha mantenido en un segundo plano porque tiene la esperanza de comprarte el terreno. Que los rumores sobre los diamantes de Pumulani se extiendan, es sólo cuestión de tiempo. ¿Qué harás entonces para impedir que otros vengan a remover la tierra?

—Pumulani me pertenece; no permitiré que nadie venga a remover mis tierras.

—Y te admiro por ello. Es posible que consigas protegerlo siempre y cuando puedas tener hombres haciendo guardia constantemente, pero ¿de dónde sacarás el dinero para pagar a esos hombres? ¿Y qué pasará con Pumulani cuando tú faltes?

—Me ocuparé de que siga estando protegido —insistió Camelia.

—Supongamos que consigues proteger el terreno durante los próximos cien años; pasado ese tiempo alguien vendrá a intentar excavar —argumentó Simon—. La cuestión es, ¿tratarán la tierra con cuidado? ¿Cómo tratarán a los trabajadores? ¿Y a qué destinarán los beneficios que obtengan?

—No lo sé. Sólo puedo controlar cómo trato yo la tierra y a la gente que trabaja para mí. No puedo controlar lo que hagan los demás.

—Razón por la cual deberías plantearte extraer tú misma los minerales. Piénsalo, Camelia —le recomendó—. En primer lugar, podrías excavar con todo el cuidado que quisieras, asegurándote de no tocar el emplazamiento de la tumba y conservando cualquier reliquia que encontraras a medida que fueras removiendo la tierra. En segundo lugar, además de darles un trabajo que necesitan, te asegurarías de que los nativos reciben un buen trato y están bien remunerados. Y en tercer lugar, podrías destinar parte de los beneficios a mejorar las condiciones de vida de los africanos.

Era un buen argumento, pensó Camelia. Siempre había menospreciado a las compañías mineras, porque destrozaban la tierra y abusaban de los trabajadores nativos únicamente para que los inversores se enriquecieran. Pero si ella extrajera los diamantes por su cuenta, las cosas serían distintas. Podría asegurarse de que la tierra se removía con cuidado, conservando cualquier reliquia que descubriesen; trataría a los trabajadores con respeto e integridad, y todo lo que ganara podría utilizarlo para ayudar a las tribus de la zona cuando la comida escaseara y para prepararlos para el nuevo mundo que se cernía sobre ellos rápida e inevitablemente. Podría crear una escuela. Quizás incluso podría construir un pequeño hospital para cuando los poderes de las hierbas humeantes y los chamanes no fuesen suficientes. Extraer diamantes de Pumulani no era necesariamente una traición a todo cuanto creía, pensó. No, si significaba mejorar las vidas de los africanos, aunque fuese sólo de unos cuantos.

Aun así, era extrañamente reacia a embarcarse en esta nueva aventura.

—No lo sé. —Hablaba con voz apagada y añadió—: No sé si me quedaré aquí.

Simon la miró confuso.

—No es necesario que vivas en Pumulani, si no quieres. Siempre y cuando contrates hombres eficientes en los que confíes y un buen capataz, estoy convencido de que podrás controlarlo todo desde tu casa de Ciudad del Cabo.

—En realidad, estaba pensando en irme un poco más lejos.

Simon arqueó las cejas.

—¿Adónde?

Camelia inspiró profundamente.

—A Londres.

Él la miró con los ojos muy abiertos.

—¿Por qué?

«Porque no puedo soportar quedarme aquí sin ti —pensó vulnerable y temerosa de los sentimientos que la embargaban—. Porque nada de lo que haga, vea, sienta o toque será lo mismo si tú no estás. Porque si tú te vas y yo me quedo aquí, viviré el resto de mi vida con el corazón desgarrado.»

—Porque quiero ir allí. —Se había imaginado que a Simon le encantaría que ella quisiese irse a Londres con él. Sin embargo, estaba completamente atónito—. ¿Tan extraño te parece?

Él se encogió de hombros.

—Si me lo hubiese dicho cualquier otra mujer, probablemente no. Pero viniendo de ti, que detestas Londres y amas África con todo tu corazón, sí.

—Podría aprender a amar Londres.

—Eso lo dudo. Y aunque así fuera, ¿por qué demonios quieres ir allí, si todo lo que te importa está aquí?

—Porque no todo lo que me importa está aquí. En Londres hay algo sumamente importante para mí.

—¿El qué?

Ella se volvió y lo miró. Haciendo acopio de todo su coraje, susurró con solemnidad:

—Tú.

Simon la miró asombrado.

Y entonces, provocando una profunda irritación en Camelia, empezó a reírse tanto que Harriet se fue de su hombro tembloroso agitando malhumorada sus alas grises.

—No pienso irme a Londres, Camelia —dijo al fin.

Ella lo miró perpleja.

—¿Ah, no?

—Bueno, supongo que si tú vas, tendré que ir contigo, pero preferiría que fuera sólo para hacer una breve visita. Sé que mi familia está deseando conocerte, especialmente después de las historias que, sin duda, les habrán contado Doreen, Eunice y Jack. Pero prométeme que Rupert vendrá con nosotros; de lo contrario, Byron, mi hermano pequeño, jamás me lo perdonaría. Está intentando convencer a Genevieve de que las serpientes son unas mascotas excelentes.

—Pero yo sólo quería ir a Londres para estar contigo —objetó Camelia—. Badrani me ha dicho que estabas haciendo las maletas. Que Senwe y él iban a llevaros a Oliver y a ti a Kimberley para coger el tren que sale esta tarde hacia Ciudad del Cabo.

—Exacto, y si seguís aquí sentados de cháchara, anochecerá y perderé el tren —comentó Oliver con firmeza mientras se aproximaba hacia ellos.

—Sería mejor que se marchase mañana —insistió Zareb que caminaba lentamente a su lado—, todavía no le he preparado los gusanos *mopane*.

—Ésta sí que es una buena razón para que te quedes, Oliver —soltó Simon con agudeza, divertido con la cara de asco del anciano escocés. Se levantó y le ofreció la mano a Camelia para ayudarle a ponerse de pie.

Oliver se rascó su barbilla entrecana, fingiendo que pensaba en ello.

—Me temo que he estado fuera demasiado tiempo —dijo al fin con un suspiro—. Por muy tentadores que sean esos gusanos, Zareb, tendrán que esperar a mi siguiente visita. A lo mejor logro convencer a la familia del muchacho para que se las apañe sin mí unos cuantos meses el próximo verano.

Zareb inclinó la cabeza hacia su amigo con solemnidad.

—En ese caso buscaré los mejores gusanos para dárselos cuando venga a visitarnos.

—Oliver se va —le explicó Simon a Camelia—. Por fin se ha convencido de que puedo arreglármelas sin él una temporada. Creo que ayer vivió demasiadas emociones y tiene ganas de volver a Escocia, donde nadie lo meterá en cuevas inundadas de murciélagos ni estará a punto de matarlo.

—No es para tanto —se mofó Oliver—. En peores líos me han metido tus hermanos y he vivido para contarlo.

—Pero Badrani me dijo que los dos estabais haciendo las maletas para iros a Kimberley —repuso Camelia, todavía confusa.

—Estaba ayudando a Oliver y quiero acompañarlo a Kimberley para asegurarme de que no se equivoca de tren —le aclaró Simon—. Luego volveré.

—¿Por qué?

—Porque aunque me considero bastante abierto mentalmente, no soy tan liberal como para consentir que mi mujer viva en un continente y yo en otro. —Ladeó la cabeza y la miró con fingida seriedad mientras concluía—: Me temo que en esto seré bastante inflexible, Camelia.

Ella lo miró atónita.

—¿Me estás pidiendo que me case contigo?

Simon sonrió.

—Por el ritual que tú elijas y en el lugar que quieras.

—Yo mismo oficiaré la ceremonia ahora mismo, delante de esta antigua piedra —se ofreció enseguida Zareb, dando un paso hacia delante—. Los espíritus que os han unido os observan y harán que vuestra unión sea sagrada.

—¡Eh! Un momento, puede que los espíritus se contenten con eso, pero estos chicos necesitan una ceremonia como Dios manda en una iglesia y con un sacerdote —objetó Oliver—. Me niego a decirles a Eunice y a Doreen que los casó usted frente a una roca con un mono, un pájaro y una serpiente como testigos. Eunice es capaz de traerse un sacerdote en el siguiente barco que zarpe a África.

—Pero tu vida está en Londres —insistió Camelia, preguntándose si Simon era realmente consciente de todo a lo que estaba renunciando.

—No, Camelia —repuso Simon con gran ternura—. Mi vida está contigo. Te he visto en Londres, cariño, y eras muy desdichada. Sin duda tu sitio está en África, con esta luz, esta belleza, los espacios abiertos y todas las oportunidades que te brinda para hacer algo que de verdad valga la pena. Además, no hay que pensar sólo en ti, también están Oscar, Harriet y Rupert. —Miró al trío con resignación—. No sé si podría volver a vivir con ellos en Londres, en una casa pequeña.

—¿Y qué pasará con tu trabajo?

—La ventaja de ser inventor es que puedes trabajar en casi todas partes —contestó, encogiéndose de hombros—. Pero prométeme que iremos a ver a mi familia un par de meses al año. Así podrás irlos conociendo y yo me pondré al día de las nuevas tecnologías europeas, y compraré maquinaria nueva para seguir trabajando aquí. Probablemente en mi ausencia mi familia seguirá empeñada en registrar la patente de todo lo que invente; están convencidos de que algún día inventaré algo importante.

—Y así será. —El rostro arrugado de Oliver se iluminó con una orgullosa sonrisa—. El aparato para hacer puré de patatas que hizo para Eunice era realmente genial.

—Es que Simon es brillante —convino Camelia en voz baja mientras le miraba fijamente—. Siempre lo he sabido.

—Tal vez deberíamos cargar el carro nosotros dos, Oliver —sugirió Zareb con tacto al ver cómo se miraban Camelia y Simon.

—Iríamos más rápido, si el chico nos ayudara —declaró Oliver sin darse por aludido.

—Me reuniré contigo en un minuto, Oliver —le aseguró Simon.

—Eso mismo dijiste hace más de media hora...

—Vamos, amigo —le dijo Zareb a Oliver—. Vuélvame a explicar cómo se prepara ese delicioso *haggis*, por si acaso Simon quiere que le crezca *pelo en el pecho* en su ausencia.

—¡Claro, cómo no! —exclamó Oliver, contento de que Zareb se acordara de ese plato—. Lo más importante es hacerse con unas entrañas buenas y carnosas. Se lavan bien, asegurándose de que limpia toda la sangre, y luego las sumerge durante diez horas en agua fría salada...

Simon esperó impaciente a que los dos ancianos se alejasen por la tierra cobriza bañada por el sol con el cielo de color zafiro de fondo. Por fin, él y Camelia estaban solos.

—Hace tiempo que quiero decirte algo. —Simon hizo una pausa, de pronto vacilante.

—Dime.

Alargó el brazo y le apartó de la frente un sedoso rizo de pelo.

—Te quiero, Camelia —confesó con voz ronca—. Creo que te quiero desde que te vi en mi laboratorio sentada en el suelo y con ese ridículo sombrero en la cabeza. Me da igual que vivamos en Londres, en Ciudad del Cabo o incluso aquí, en una pequeña tienda de campaña dentro del perímetro de Pumulani. Lo único que me importa es estar contigo. Aunque —añadió mientras la atraía hacia sí— como pretendas quedarte aquí durante la estación de las lluvias, espero al menos que por cuestiones prácticas me dejes construir una casa y tener leña. No sé si me apetece pasarme el resto de mi vida cocinando con estiércol quemado.

Camelia le rodeó el cuello con los brazos y sonrió.

—Tienes que darle otra oportunidad al estiércol —bromeó—. Tal vez con el tiempo acabe gustándote el sabor único que le imprime a la comida.

—De acuerdo. Yo comeré *biltong* hecho con estiércol humeante si tú pruebas el *haggis* crece-pelo que Zareb pretende cocinarme. —Bajó la cabeza y empezó a acariciarle la mejilla con la nariz.

—En realidad, creo que será mejor que vivamos en Ciudad del Cabo —se apresuró a sugrir Camelia, entrelazando sus dedos en el desenredado cabello cobrizo de Simon—. Tengo una casa con una cocina que funciona con leña, y que yo sepa, Zareb nunca ha intentado quemar estiércol en ella.

—Me parece un buen pacto —susurró Simon mientras le regalaba lentos besos por la cavidad latiente de su garganta—. Cásate conmigo, Camelia —suplicó en voz baja y ronca mientras sus labios se rozaban—. Cásate conmigo y dedicaré mi vida entera a hacerte feliz.

Una gran felicidad inundó a Camelia, y le hizo sentir fuerte, segura y plena.

—Sí —susurró con fervor—, siempre y cuando me prometas una cosa. —Se apoyó en él fundiendo su cuerpo con el de Simon.

—Lo que sea —dijo él mientras trataba de reprimir su deseo de tumbarla sobre el cálido suelo africano y penetrarla. Ascendió la mano hasta un pecho y lo empezó a acariciar, despertando el pezón—. ¿Qué quieres, mi amor?

—Prométeme que nunca dejarás de quererme. —Camelia puso sus labios sobre los de él y le dio un profundo beso, saboreándolo y removiéndose inquieta contra su cuerpo hasta que Simon creyó que el deseo le haría enloquecer completamente.

—Coge tus cosas —logró decir con voz ronca—. Te vienes conmigo a Kimberley.

Ella lo miró confusa.

—¿Por qué?

—Porque allí hay una iglesia —explicó—. Y esperemos que también un sacerdote que sea del agrado de Oliver.

—¿Quieres que nos casemos hoy?

—Quiero que nos casemos *ahora mismo*, pero como Oliver se niega a que Zareb oficie la ceremonia, me temo que no tengo más remedio que aguantarme hasta que lleguemos a Kimberley. —Entonces titubeó—. ¿O prefieres que esperemos y organicemos una boda más formal?

Camelia se echó a reír.

—A mí ya me parecía bien la idea de que Zareb nos casase aquí mismo. —Se agachó para recoger el diario de su padre—. Vamos.

Simon reparó en Oscar, Harriet y Rupert, que los miraban fijamente, y suspiró.

—Está bien, os dejo venir a todos.

Gritando de alegría, Oscar dio un salto y trepó a la cabeza de Simon mientras Harriet volaba hasta el hombro de Camelia, y Rupert se deslizaba hasta su pierna para que ella lo cogiera y lo colgara alrededor de su cuello.

—Una estampa encantadora —declaró Simon, que no pudo evitar plantarle un beso a Camelia en la nariz—. Debo de ser el único novio del mundo cuya novia se casa acompañada de una serpiente y un pájaro.

—Tranquilo, me los quitaré de encima antes de que empiece la ceremonia —prometió Camelia.

—Si el sacerdote no se desmaya, a mí no me importa —aseguró Simon ofreciéndole su brazo—. ¿Nos vamos?

Camelia pestañeó con malicia.

—¿Tampoco te importa lo que lleve puesto esta noche?

—¡Menudo descaro! —la regañó Simon—. Mi única condición es que esta noche no haya animales en la tienda de campaña. No quiero distracciones.

Camelia se rió y tiró de él para darle un largo y apasionado beso, dejando claro que pretendía atraer su atención tanto esa noche como en el futuro.

Sobre la autora

Karyn Monk escribe desde que era una niña. En la universidad descubrió su amor por la historia. Después de trabajar durante varios años en el ajetreado mundo de la publicidad, decidió escribir novelas históricas. Está casada con un hombre tremendamente romántico, Philip, al que considera el modelo de inspiración de todos sus héroes.

Para más información sobre Karyn entrar en *www.karynmonk.com*

Otros títulos de

Karyn Monk

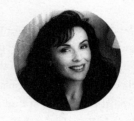

publicados en

books4pocket

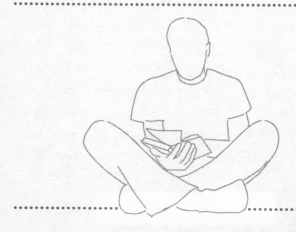

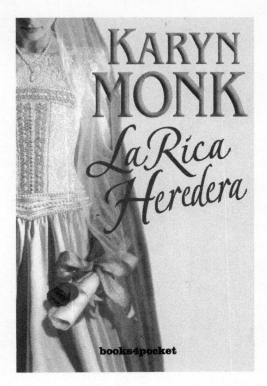

KARYN MONK

La Rica Heredera

books4pocket

Jack Kent no se encuentra a gusto en actos como esa boda, a la que ha acudido por compromiso. Pero todo cambia cuando la novia se descuelga de uno de los balcones y le implora que le permita huir en su carruaje. Aquella joven, que no estaba dispuesta a tolerar un matrimonio impuesto, le atrae desde el principio. Sin embargo, la pasión que nace entre ellos ha de enfrentarse al abismo entre los mundos a los que pertenecen y los propios miedos de Jack, que aún no se reconcilió con su pasado.

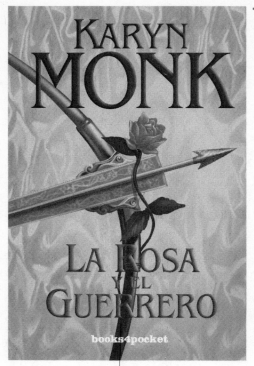

KARYN
MONK

LA ROSA
Y EL
GUERRERO

books4pocket

Escocia, 1216. Cuatro de los más formidables guerreros del
clan MacTier han caído en una trampa, en lo más profundo del
bosque. Iban tras la banda del Halcón, un grupo de forajidos
que asaltaban y humillaban a los miembros de su clan. Estaban
preparados para enfrentarse a hombres aguerridos y bien ar-
mados, y se han dejado vencer por un anciano decrépito y tres
jóvenes que a penas podían con el peso de sus espadas, capi-
taneados por... una mujer.

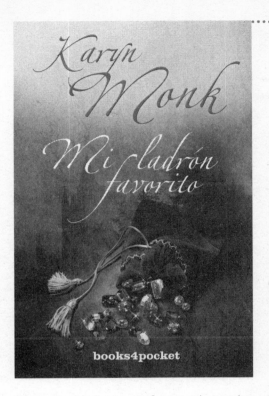

Karyn Monk

Mi ladrón favorito

books4pocket

Harrison Payne es el ladrón más famoso de Londres. Su sorpresa es enorme cuando Charlotte, la joven que le descubre robando las joyas de lady Chadwick, le ayuda a escapar sin asustarse. Pronto sabrá que no se trata de una simple muchacha, sino de una seductora mujer que guarda secretos en su pasado. Su breve encuentro ha servido para despertar en ambos una poderosa atracción, pero se entregarán a un peligroso juego, atrapados entre el deseo y el temor a confiar el uno en el otro...